1 MONTH OF
FREE
READING

at

www.ForgottenBooks.com

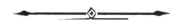

By purchasing this book you are eligible for one month membership to ForgottenBooks.com, giving you unlimited access to our entire collection of over 1,000,000 titles via our web site and mobile apps.

To claim your free month visit:

www.forgottenbooks.com/free1012185

ISBN 978-0-331-08307-1
PIBN 11012185

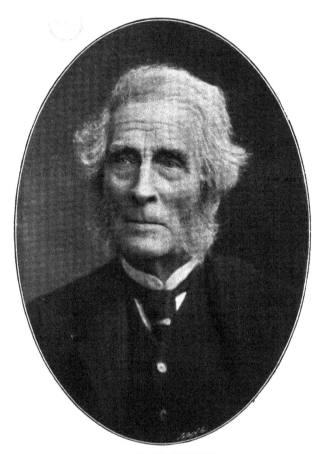

LUTHER HOLDEN

Frontispiece

HOSPITAL

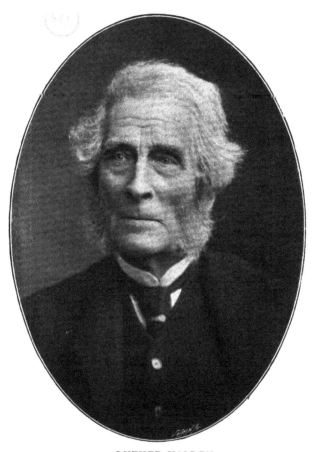

LUTHER HOLDEN

Frontispiece

SAINT
BARTHOLOMEW'S HOSPITAL
REPORTS.

EDITED BY

A. E. GARROD, M.D.

AND

W. M°ADAM ECCLES, M.S., F.R.C.S.

VOL. XLI.

LONDON:

SMITH, ELDER, & CO., 15 WATERLOO PLACE.

1906.

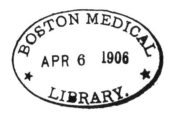
Printed by BALLANTYNE, HANSON & Co.
At the Ballantyne Press

IN EXCHANGE.

The Practitioner, Editor, 149 Strand, W.C.

Royal Medical and Chirurgical Society's Transactions, 20 Hanover Square, W.

Guy's Hospital Reports.

St. Thomas's Hospital Reports.

Westminster Hospital Reports.

King's College Hospital Reports.

Surgeon-General's Office, War Department, U.S.A., per Mr. Wesley, Essex Street, Strand.

Le Progrès Médical.

Annales de Dermatologie et de Syphilographie, Dr. A. Doyon, Uriage les Bains, Isère, France.

Centralblatt für Chirurgie, herausgegeben von F. König, E. Richter, R. Volkmann (Messrs. Breitkopf & Härtel, Leipzig).

The Journal of Nervous and Mental Disease, edited by Charles Henry Brown, M.D., 25 West Forty-Fifth Street, New York.

The Liverpool Medico-Chirurgical Journal, Liverpool Medical Institution, 1 Hope Street, Liverpool.

The Johns Hopkins Hospital Reports, Baltimore, Maryland, U.S.A.

The Bristol Medico-Chirurgical Journal, Dr. P. Watson Williams, Medical School, Bristol.

Transactions of the College of Physicians, Philadelphia, per Smithsonian Institution.

The Journal of the British Medical Association, 429 Strand, W.C.

Transactions of Medical Society of London, 11 Chandos Street, Cavendish Square, W.

West London Medical Journal West London Hospital, per Hon. Librarian.

Archiv f. Verdauungs-Krankheiten, herausgegeben von Dr. J. Boas in Berlin, c/o S. Karger, Charité Strasse 3, Berlin, N.W.

The New York Academy of Medicine, 21 West Forty-Third Street,
per Librarian.

The Archives of Neurology, from the Pathological Laboratory of the
London County Council Asylum, Claybury, Woodford, Essex,
per F. W. Mott, M.D.

The St. Bartholomew's Hospital Journal, per the Editor, St. Bartholomew's Hospital, London, E.C.

The Reports of the Army Medical Department, per the Editor, the
Army Medical School, Netley, Hants.

The Medical Review, per the Editor, 66 Finsbury Pavement, E.C.

The Reports of the Thompson Yates Laboratories, Liverpool, per
Prof. Rubert Boyce, F.R.S.

The Polyclinic, c/o The Librarian of the Medical Graduates' College,
22 Chenies Street, London, W.C.

The Journal of Medical Research, c/o The Editor, 688 Boylston
Street, Boston, Mass., U.S.A.

School of Medicine, Cairo, per Librarian.

CONTENTS.

PAGE

LIST OF SUBSCRIBERS xi

In Memoriam : Luther Holden, F.R.C.S. By John Langton,
F.R.C.S. xxxi

MEDICAL PAPERS.

ART.

I. Clinical Notes on a Tendency to Blood-Clotting during
Life. By Sir Dyce Duckworth, M.D., LL.D. . . 1

II. Alcoholic Neuritis. By Norman Moore, M.D. . . 5

III. A Case of Typhoid Fever followed by Biliary Colic
and the Passage of Gall-stones. By Samuel West,
M.D. 9

IV. Cases of Riedel's Lobe, with Remarks on the Various
Deformities of the Liver. By W. P. Herringham,
M.D. 15

V. Cases of Ascites treated by Deprivation of Salt. By
W. P. Herringham, M.D., and C. F. Hadfield . 25

VI. The Segmental Spinal Sensory Areas Clinically Considered. By H. H. Tooth, M.D. 37

VII. A Case of Aneurysm of the Aorta Communicating
directly with the Superior Vena Cava and with the
left Innominate Vein. By J. H. Drysdale, M.D. . 71

VIII. Albuminous Expectoration following Paracentesis of
the Chest. By P. Horton-Smith Hartley, M.D. . 77

IX. A Case of Complete Transposition of Viscera in an
Adult. By T. J. Horder, M.D. 111

X. On Cardiac Dropsy in Children. By W. Langdon
Brown, M.D. 115

XI. Pulmonary Fibrosis in Childhood. By Clive Riviere,
M.D. 123

ART.   PAGE
XII. A Case of Congenital Occulsion of the Small Intestine.
By C. M. H. Howell, M.B.   135

XIII. A Series of Fatal Cases of Jaundice in the Newborn
occurring in successive Pregnancies.   By G. A.
Auden, M.D.   139

XIV. Cases from the Wards of Sir Dyce Duckworth and
Dr. Champneys.   By H. U. Gould, M.B.   .   . 143

XV. Three Cases of Primary Malignant Disease of the
Liver. By C. S. Hawes, M.R.C.S.   .   .   . 161

SURGICAL PAPERS.

XVI. A Year's Gastro-jejunostomies.   By D'Arcy Power,
F.R.C.S.   169

XVII. Intra - ocular Tuberculosis.   By W. H. Jessop,
F.R.C.S.   183

XVIII. Actinomycosis of the Cæcum, Vermiform Appendix,
and Right Iliac Fossa, including an Account of
Seven Cases. By H. J. Waring, M.S., F.R.C.S. . 197

XIX. Four Cases of Cranio-Cerebral Surgery. By L. B.
Rawling, F.R.C.S.   211

XX. Intra-medullary Teratoma of the Spinal Cord.   By
J. Graham Forbes, M.D.   221

XXI. Two Cases of Diphtheritic Infection of Operation
Wounds. By J. Burfield, M.B., F.R.C.S.   .   . 233

Proceedings of the Abernethian Society for the Session
1904–1905   237
List of Specimens added to the Museum   .   .   . 241
Books added to the Library   289
Summary of Scholarships and Prizes 293
List of Prizemen   294
Hospital Staff 296

INDEX   299

GENERAL INDEX TO VOLUMES XXI. TO XL. (INCLUSIVE) . 305

LIST OF ILLUSTRATIONS.

THE LATE LUTHER HOLDEN, F.R.C.S. . . . *Frontispiece*
From a block kindly lent by the "British Medical Journal."

PLATE I.—DR. DRYSDALE'S CASE OF ANEURYSM OF THE AORTA COMMUNICATING DIRECTLY WITH THE SUPERIOR VENA CAVA AND LEFT INNOMINATE VEIN . . . *To face page* 72

PLATES II. AND III.—SECTION OF LIVER IN MR. HAWES' CASES OF PRIMARY MALIGNANT DISEASE *To face pages* 162 *and* 164

PLATES IV. AND V.—ILLUSTRATING DR. FORBES' PAPER ON A CASE OF INTRA-MEDULLARY TERATOMA OF THE SPINAL CORD . . . . . *To face pages* 224 *and* 228

CHARTS ILLUSTRATING DR. HERRINGHAM AND MR. HADFIELD'S PAPER ON THE TREATMENT OF ASCITES BY DEPRIVATION OF SALT . . . . *To face page* 30

FIGURES IN TEXT—
DIAGRAMS ILLUSTRATING DR. HERRINGHAM'S PAPER ON RIEDEL'S LOBE . . . . . *pages* 16, 17
TWENTY-THREE FIGURES ILLUSTRATING SENSORY SPINAL AREAS (DR. H. H. TOOTH) . . . *pages* 38–70
TRANSPOSITION OF VISCERA (DR. HORDER'S CASE) . *page* 112
CONGENITAL OCCLUSION OF THE SMALL INTESTINE (DR. HOWELL'S CASE) . . . . . . *page* 136
FOUR CASES OF CRANIO-CEREBRAL SURGERY (LOUIS BATHE RAWLING) . . . . *page* 213

LIST OF SUBSCRIBERS.

ACKERY, J., 11 Queen Anne Street, Cavendish Square, W.

ACKLAND, R. C., 54 Brook Street, W.

ADAMS, ALFRED, Looe, Cornwall

ADAMS, Dr. JAMES, 4 Chiswick Place, Eastbourne

ADAMS, JOHN, 180 Aldersgate Street, E.C.

ADAMS, Dr. J. O., Brooke House, Upper Clapton, N.E.

ALCOCK, Dr. R., Shirley House, Hyde

ALEXANDER, J. F., Glendale, Cassio Road, Watford

AMSDEN, W., Lexden House, Seaford

AMY, Dr. G. J., 6 Boulevard Victor Hugo, Nice

ANDERSON, A. R., 5 East Circus Street, Nottingham

ANDREWES, Dr. F. W., Highwood, Hampstead Lane, Highgate, N.

ANDREWS, S., Wote Street, Basingstoke, Hants

ARATHOON, H. C., Surgeon, R.N., The Royal Naval Hospital, Gosport

ARKWRIGHT, Dr. J. A., 13 Welbeck Street, W.

ATKINSON, STANLEY B., Claremont, Cawley Road, N.E.

ATTLEE, Dr. W. H. W., High Street, Eton

AVERILL, Dr. C., Park Green, Macclesfield

BAILEY, Dr. H. V., Pekin, Illinois, United States, America

BAILEY, R. C., 21 Welbeck Street, W.

BAKER, J. C., Ceely House, Aylesbury

BALDWIN, T. P., 51 Stradella Road, Herne Hill, S.E.

BALGARNIE, Dr. W., The Dutch House, Hartley Wintney, Winchfield, Hants

BALL, C. R. H., Hunstanton, Norfolk

BARBER, SYDNEY F., 11 St. Barnabas Road, Highfield, Sheffield

BARKER, TOFT, Corfe Castle, Dorset

BARLING, GILBERT, 37 Cornwall Street, Birmingham

BARRON, W. N., Cranborne Corner, Ascot

BARRS, Dr. ALFRED GEORGE, 25A Park Square, Leeds

BARTON, J. K., *J.P.*, 14 Ashburn Place, Courtfield Road, S.W.

BATEMAN, H. E., 48 Micklegate, York

BATTEN, Dr. R. D., Campden Lodge, Campden Hill Road, W.

BEATH, D. LESLIE, Barnard House, Pulteney Road, Bath

BEAUCHAMP, Dr. SYDNEY, 95 Cromwell Road, South Kensington, S W

BELBEN, Dr. F., Redlands, Kynyeton Road, Bournemouth

BELDING, D. T., East Dereham, Norfolk

BENNION, J. M., Nursted House, Petersfield, Hants

BERRY, JAMES, 21 Wimpole Street, W.

BEVAN, H. C., Blaina, Monmouth, South Wales

BIRD, R., Major I.M.S., *C.I.E.*, c/o Messrs. Grindlay & Co., Agents, Calcutta

BLOXAM, JOHN A., 75 Grosvenor Street, W.

BOKENHAM, T. J., 10 Devonshire Street, Portland Place, W.

Boston Medical Library Association, per Messrs. B. F. Stevens and Brown, 4 Trafalgar Square, W.C.

BOSWELL, Dr. A., Ashbourne, Derbyshire

BOTT, H., Brentford, Middlesex

BOUSFIELD, S., 35 Prince's Square, Bayswater, W.

BOWES, C. K., 2 Marine Crescent, Herne Bay, Kent

BOWES, Dr. T. A., 7 Marine Terrace, Herne Bay, Kent

BOWLBY, A. A., *C.M.G.*, 24 Manchester Square, W.

BOYLE, H. E. G., 50 Welbeck Street, W.

BRANSON, Dr. W. P. S., 59 Gordon Square, W.C.

BREWERTON, E. W., 84 Wimpole Street, W.

BRIGGS, Dr. J. A. O., 37 Noel Street, Nottingham

BRINTON, Dr. R. D., 8 Queen's Gate Terrace, S.W.

BROOK, W. H. B., 8 Eastgate, Lincoln

BROOKS, Dr. J. H., Mile End Infirmary, Bancroft Road, N.E.

BROOKSBANK, Dr. H. L, Thornbarrow, Windermere

BROWN, Dr. W. LANGDON, 37A Finsbury Square, E.C.

BROWNE, Dr. OSWALD A., 7 Upper Wimpole Street, W.

BRUCE CLARKE, W., 51 Harley Street, Cavendish Square, W.

BRUNTON, Sir LAUDER, M.D., *F.R.S.*, 10 Stratford Place, W.

BUCK, A. H., 39 Cambridge Road, Hove

BULL, Dr. G. V., Ashbourne, Derbyshire

BURD, Dr. E. LYCETT, Church Stretton, Salop

BURFIELD, J., St. Bartholomew's Hospital, E.C.

BURN, T. W. B., 79 Mill Road, Cambridge

BURN, Dr. W. B., 189 Balham Road, Upper Tooting, S.W.

BURNETT, Dr. F. M., 34 High Street, Sevenoaks, Kent

BURNIE, W. GILCHRIST, 1 Drewton Street, Bradford, Yorks

BURROUGHES, H. N., 3 Hertford Street, W.

BURROWS, HAROLD, 38 Lyford Road, Wandsworth Common, S.W.

BUTLER, T. M., The Firs, Guildford

BUTLER-SMYTHE, A. C., 76 Brook Street, W.

BUTLIN, H. T., 82 Harley Street, W.

CALVERT, Dr. J., 113 Harley Street, W.

CARTER, Dr. F. H., 117 Upper Richmond Road, Putney, S.W.

CAVE, Dr. E. J., 20 Circus, Bath

CHAMPNEYS, Dr. F. H., 42 Upper Brook Street, W.

CHIPPERFIELD, T. J. B. P., The Green, Hampton Court

CHRISTOPHERSON, CECIL, 28 Eversfield Place, St. Leonards-on-Sea

CHRISTOPHERSON, J. B., Omdurman Hospital, Khartoum, Egypt

CHURCH, Sir WILLIAM SELBY, Bart., *K.C.B.*, 130 Harley Street, W.

CLARK, W. GLADSTONE, Memorial Hospital, Buluwayo, Rhodesia

CLARKE, A. H., 161 Macquarie Street, Hobart, Tasmania

CLARKE, ERNEST, 3 Chandos Street, Cavendish Square, W.

CLARKE, FIELDING (Travelling)

CLOSE, Dr. J. B., 2 Pryme Street, Hull

COLEMAN, F., 129 Harley Street, W.

COLLINGRIDGE, Dr. W., 16 Queen's Road, Richmond, Surrey

COLLYNS, J. B., Dulverton, Somerset

COLT, G. H., St. Bartholomew's Hospital, E.C.

COMBER, C. T. T., c/o Pawling & Co., Victoria Falls, Rhodesia

CONNOR, F. P., Lieut., I.M.S., c/o Messrs. Cook & Sons, Ludgate Circus, E.C.

CONOLLY, CHARLES HAMILTON, Stuart Villa, Crescent Gardens, Wood Green, N.

COOKE, A. S., Badbrook House, Stroud, Gloucestershire

COOKE, Dr. J. G., Fairholme, Walsall

COOMBS, Dr. ROWLAND H., Redburn, Rothesay Place, Bedford

COOPER, Sir ALFRED, 9 Henrietta Street, Cavendish Square, W.

COPE, R., 31 Highdown Road, Hove

CORBIN, J., Adelaide, South Australia

CORNISH, Dr. S., The Old House, Dorking

CORRIE, ALFRED T., Fleet-Surgeon, R.N., Junior United Service Club, S.W.

COURT, E. PERCY, Hill View, Hambledon, Cosham, Hants

COVENTON, A. W. D., St. Bartholomew's Hospital, E.C.

COWLEY, J. S., Upton-on-Severn, Worcestershire

CRACE-CALVERT, Dr. G. A., Llanbedr Hall, near Ruthin, North Wales

CRAWFORD, STEPHEN E., Dunkery, Weston-super-Mare

CRIPPS, W. H., 2 Stratford Place, W.

CRONK, H. G., Repton, near Burton-on-Trent

CROSSE, R. E., East Dereham, Norfolk

CROSSLEY, E. W., Dean House, Triangle, Halifax

CROSSMAN, FRANCIS W., White's Hill, Hambrook, Bristol

CROUCH, C. P., 1 Royal Terrace, Weston-super-Mare

CROWFOOT, Dr. W. M., Beccles, Suffolk

CROWLEY, Dr. RALPH, 116 Manningham Lane, Bradford

CUMBERBATCH, A. E., 11 Park Crescent, Portland Place, W.

CUTHBERT, C. F., 2 Barton Street, Gloucester

CUTHBERT, W. WOOD, Clevedon, Leopold Road, Felixstowe

DALE, C. B., 106 Bristol Road, Birmingham

DARBY, W. S., Station Road, Harrow

DAVIES, Dr. ARTHUR T., 17 Finsbury Circus, E.C.

DAVIS, HALDEN, 7 Hyde Park Square, W.

DAY, DONALD D., 5 Surrey Street, Norwich

DETHLOFF, H. G., Leper Asylum, Bergen, Norway

DINGLE, Dr. W. A., 46 Finsbury Square, E.C.

DIXON, Dr. F. J., 163 Cromwell Road, S.W.

DORAN, ALBAN H. G., 9 Granville Place, Portman Square, W.

DOUGLAS, A. R. J., 500 Lordship Lane, Dulwich, S.E.

DRAGE, Dr. C., Hatfield, Herts

DRURY, Dr. E. G. D., Grahamstown, Cape Colony

DRYSDALE, Dr. J. H., 11 Devonshire Place, W.

DUCKWORTH, Sir DYCE, M.D., 11 Grafton Street, Picca-dilly, W.

ECCLES, Dr. ANNESLEY, 104 Church Road, Upper Nor-wood, S.E.

ECCLES, W. McADAM, 124 Harley Street, Cavendish Square, W.

EDDISON, F. R., Bedale, Yorks

EDELSTEN, Dr. E. A., 370 Brixton Road, S.W.

EDWARDS, F. SWINFORD, 55 Harley Street, W.

EDWARDS, H. NELSON, 31 St. John's Hill, Shrewsbury

ELKINGTON, FRED. V., Fenny Compton, Leamington

ELLIOTT, Dr. J., 24 Nicholas Street, Chester

ELLIS, Dr. W. G., Lunatic Asylum, Singapore

ELMSLIE, R. C., 81 St. Mary's Mansions, W.

EUTING, J., Director, Kais. Universitats- & Landesbibliothek, Strassburg

EVANS, ERNEST R., Hertford

EVANS, E. LAMING, 36 Bryanston Street, W.

EVILL, F. C., The Lodge, High Barnet

EWEN, G. S., Tudor House, Montpelier Road, Twickenham

FAIRLIE-CLARKE, A. J., The General Hospital, Birmingham
FARNCOMBE, E. L., Fairlea, Chudleigh, Devon
FAULDER, T. J., 50 Welbeck Street, W.
FAVELL, R., Brunswick House, Glossop Road, Sheffield
FERGUSON, Dr. G. B., Altidore Villa, Pitville, Cheltenham
FINIGAN, Dr. D. O'C., 5 Windsor Road, Ealing, W.
FIRTH, Dr. C., 196 Parrock Street, Gravesend
FLEMING, J. KENNETH S., Capt. I.M.S., c/o Messrs. Grindlay
  and Co., Bombay
FLETCHER, A C., The Charterhouse, E.C.
FLETCHER, Dr. H. MORLEY, 98 Harley Street, W.
FLINT, Dr. ARTHUR, Westgate Lodge, Westgate-on-Sea
FORBES, Dr. J. G., 1 Duke Street, Manchester Square, W.
FRENCH, GILBERT, Thorn Croft, Chiswick, W.
FROST, CECIL S., Ochil Hills Sanatorium, Milnathort, Kinross-
  shire
FURNER, Dr. WILLOUGHBY, 13 Brunswick Square, Brighton

GABB, C. B., 3 Wellington Square, Hastings
GARDNER, Dr. H. W., 23 St. John's Hill, Shrewsbury
GARRATT, Dr. G. C., Chilworth, Summersdale, Chichester
GARROD, Dr. A. E., 9 Chandos Street, Cavendish Square, W.
GASK, G. E., The Warden's House, St. Bartholomew's Hospital,
  E.C.
GAY, JOHN, 137 Upper Richmond Road, Putney, S.W.
GAYTON, Dr. F. C., Asylum, Brookwood, Woking
GEE, Dr. S., 31 Upper Brook Street, W.
GIBBINS, H. B., The Limes, Ashtead, Surrey
GIFFARD, H. E., Denham House, Egham, Surrey
GILBERTSON, J. H., The Limes, Hitchin
GILES, L. T., 4 Filey Road, Scarborough
GILL, R., 72 Wimpole Street, W.
GILLESPIE, T., Forest Lodge, Shirley, Southampton
GILMOUR, R. WITHERS, St. Luke's Hospital, Old Street, E.C.

GLEDDEN, Dr. A. M., 22 College Street, Sydney, N.S.W.

GLOVER, Dr. L. G., 17 Belsize Park, N.W.

GLYNN, Dr. THOMAS R., 62 Rodney Street, Liverpool

GODSON, Dr. CLEMENT, 82 Brook Street, Grosvenor Square, W

GOODCHILD, N. JOHN, 9 Highgate Road, N.W.

GOODSALL, D. H., 17 Devonshire Place, W.

GOODSALL, Dr. F. W. W., 49 Holborn Viaduct, E.C.

GORDON-SMITH, H., 17 Dartmouth Park Road, Highgate, N.W.

GOULD, H. U., Guildford House, Farnham

GOW, Dr. W. J., 27 Weymouth Street, W.

GRANT, Dr. DUNDAS, 18 Cavendish Square, W.

GREEN, F. K., Cleve Side, Newbridge Hill, Bath

GRELLET, CHARLES J., Bancroft, Hitchin, Herts

GRIFFITH, Dr. W. S. A., 96 Harley Street, W.

GROSVENOR, Dr. W. W., 4 Clarence Street, Gloucester

GÜTERBOCK, Dr. E., Margarethen Strasse, Berlin, W.

HABERSHON, Dr. S. H., 88 Harley Street, W.

HADFIELD, C. F., Moraston, Ross

HAIG, Dr. ALEXANDER, 7 Brook Street, Grosvenor Square, W.

HAGGARD, THOMAS, 10 Hans Crescent, S.W.

HALL, Dr. ARTHUR J., 342 Glossop Road, Sheffield

HALL, Dr. F. DE HAVILLAND, 47 Wimpole Street, W.

HAMER, Dr. W. H., 55 Dartmouth Park Hill, N.W.

HAMILTON, W. G., Capt. I.M.S., c/o W. Watson & Co., Bombay

HANCOCK, Dr. C. J. SORTAIN, 33 Fairlop Road, Leytonstone

HARDING, C. O'B., West House, Chiswick Place, Eastbourne

HARDY, F. W., Major, R.A.M.C.

HARMER, W. D., 45 Weymouth Street, W.

HARRIS, J. D., 45 Southernhay, Exeter

HARRISON, Dr. CHARLES, 30 Newland, Lincoln

HARRISON, H. LEEDS, 104 Marine Parade, Worthing

HARTLEY, Dr. P. HORTON-SMITH, 19 Devonshire Street, W.

HAWES, COLIN S., Hotel Victoria, Davos Platz, Switzerland

HAY, K. R., 20 St. James's Place, S.W.

HAYNES, Dr. F. H., 23 Lansdowne Place, Leamington

HAYNES, G. S., 4 Trinity Street, Cambridge

HEATH, Dr. A., 24 Normanton Road, Derby

HEATH, CHARLES, 3 Cavendish Place, W.

HEATH, Dr. W. L., 90 Cromwell Road, South Kensington, S.W.

HENSLEY, Dr. PHILIP, United Service Club, S.W.

HENSTOCK, Dr. J. L., Viña del Mar, Chile, South America

HEPBURN, Dr. M. L., 66 Wimpole Street, W.

HERRINGHAM, Dr. W. P., 40 Wimpole Street, W.

HEWER, E. S. E., 6 Church Street, Stratford-on-Avon

HIGGINS, ALEX. G., Bury Bar House, Newent, Glos.

HILL, Dr. ALEXANDER, Downing College Lodge, Cambridge

HILL, Dr. A. CROFT, 169 Cromwell Road, S.W.

HILLABY, A., Richmond House, Pontefract

HIND, A. E., Portland House, Midvale Road, Jersey

HIND, HENRY, Blytheholme, Victoria Avenue, Harrogate

HOGARTH, A. H., St. Bartholomew's Hospital, E.C.

HOGG, A. J., Leslie Lodge, Haven Green, Ealing, W.

HOLDEN, Dr. G. H. R., 168 Castle Hill, Reading

HOLLIS, Dr. W. A., 1 Palmeira Avenue, Hove

HORDER, Dr. T. J., 141 Harley Street, W.

HORNE, Dr. W. JOBSON, 27 New Cavendish Street, W.

HOWELL, C. M. H., 53 Queen Anne Street, W.

HUGGINS, S. P., 114 Lower Richmond Road, Putney, S.W.

HUGHES, D. WATKIN, Wymondham, Norfolk

HUGHES, J. B., Roe Street House, Macclesfield, Cheshire

HULBERT, H. L. P., Borough Hospital, Croydon

Hull Medical Society's Library, Church Institute, Albion Street,
 Hull, per Hon. Librarian

HUMPHRY, Dr. L., Lensfield, Cambridge

HURST, WALTER, Atlanta, Georgia, U.S.A.

HUSBAND, W. E., 14 Lansdown Place East, Bath

HUTCHINSON, J., 15 Cavendish Square, W.

HUTTON, E. R., 42 West Green Road, South Tottenham, N.

IREDALE, J., Mablethorpe, R.S.O., Lincolnshire

IZARD, A. W., 215 Lambton Quay, Wellington, New Zealand

JAMES, D. PHILIP, Heullan, Sydney Street, Wellington, New Zealand

JENKINS, Dr. E. J., Australian Club, Sydney, New South Wales

JESSOP, W. H., 73 Harley Street, W.

JEUDWINE, W. W., Lieut. I.M.S., o/o Messrs. Grindlay & Co., 54 Parliament Street, S.W.

JOHN, D., 182 Nepperhan Avenue, Yonkers, New York, U.S.A.

JOHNSON, Dr. MURRAY L., 1209 Broadway, Oakland, California, U.S.A.

JOHNSON, W. H., 725 Commercial Road East, Limehouse, E.

JOLLIFFE, W. J., Yafford House, Shorwell, Isle of Wight

JONES, Dr. E. LLOYD, 59 Trumpington Street, Cambridge

JONES, Dr. H. LEWIS, 143 Harley Street, W.

JONES, MARTIN LL., 2 Victoria Square, Aberdare, Glamorgan

JONES, Dr. ROBERT, London County Asylum, Claybury, near Woodford, Essex

JONES, T. C. LITTLER, 1A Rodney Street, Liverpool

JONES, Dr. W. BLACK, Llangammarch Wells, R.S.O., Breconshire

JOWERS, L. E., 51 Marina, St. Leonards-on-Sea

JOWERS, R. F., 55 Brunswick Square, Brighton

KAY, W., Bentley Cottage, Bentley, near Farnham, Hants

KEATS, W. J. C., The Camberwell Infirmary, S.E.

KEETLEY, C. R. B., 56 Grosvenor Street, Grosvenor Square, W.

KENNEDY, Dr. W. WILLOUGHBY, 8 Russell Street, Calcutta

KIDD, Dr. P., 60 Brook Street, W.

KING, R. H., Twyford, Berkshire

KINGDON, J. R., Nelson Street, King's Lynn

KNIGHT, CHARLES VOUGHTON, 48 London Road, Gloucester

KNIGHT, Dr. H. E., Brooklands, Rotherham, Yorkshire

KOCH, Dr. W. V. M., Hong Kong, China

LANGTON, JOHN, 62 Harley Street, W.

LANKESTER, OWEN, 5 Upper Wimpole Street, W.

LATHAM, Dr. P. W., 17 Trumpington Street, Cambridge

LAUCHLAN, H. D., 136 Lower Richmond Road, Putney, S.W.

LAURIE, CASPAR R., Alma Place, Redruth

LAWRENCE, Dr. H. CRIPPS, "Rahere," Tavistock, Devon

LAWRENCE, L. A., 9 Upper Wimpole Street, W.

LEDWARD, H. D., Norton Way, Letchworth

LEE, Dr. W. E., Santhapuram, Muswell Hill Road, Highgate, N.

Leeds, Medical Faculty of the University of

LEGG, T. PERCY, 141 Harley Street, W.

LEONARD, Dr. N., Laurence House, Westcliff-on-Sea.

LEVY, A., 42 Welbeck Street, W.

LEWIS, H. K., Medical Library, 136 Gower Street, W.C.,
four copies

Library of St. Bartholomew's Hospital, E.C.

LLOYD, G. W., Brough, E. Yorks

LOCKWOOD, C. B., 19 Upper Berkeley Street, W.

LOUGHBOROUGH, W. G., St. Bartholomew's Hospital, E.C.

Low, Dr. C. W., Stowmarket, Suffolk

LOWE, G. J. R., St. Catherine's, Lincoln

LOWE, Dr. WALTER G., 5 Horninglow Street, Burton-on-
Trent

LYSTER, A. E., Great Baddow, Chelmsford

MACDOUGALL, Dr. J. A., "Letterewe," Cannes, France

MACKAY, E. C., Fernside, Hilder's Hill, Hendon

MACLAREN, NORMAN, 23 Portland Square, Carlisle

MACREADY, J. F. C. H., 42 Devonshire Street, W.

MAIDLOW, Dr. W. H., Ilminster, Somerset

MARCH, J. OGDIN, Amesbury House, Amesbury

MARK, Dr. LEONARD P., 49 Oxford Terrace, Hyde Park, W.

MARSH, HOWARD, 14 Hertford Street, Mayfair, W.

MARSH, Dr. N. P., 7 Abercromby Square, Liverpool

MARTIN, E. L., 110 London Road, Chelmsford

MARTYN, REGINALD, St. Bernard's, St. Andrew's Road, Exmouth

MASTERMAN, E. W. G., Jerusalem, Syria. Book post. *Vid* Trieste and Adriatic mail

MATHEWS, Dr. F. E., Welsh Row House, Nantwich, Cheshire

MATTHEY, A., Georgetown, British Guiana

MAUND, J. H., Brackley House, Newmarket.

MAW, Dr. H. T., The Old Home, Westcott, Surrey

MAXWELL, Dr. J. L., c/o E. P. Mission, Tainan, Formosa

MAXWELL, J. P., c/o E. P. Mission, Eng-chhun, Amoy, China

MAY, Dr. E. HOOPER, Tottenham High Cross, Middlesex

MENZIES, J. HERBERT, 47 Earl's Court Square, S.W.

MICKLETHWAIT, G., 1 Driffield Terrace, The Mount, York

MILES, W. E., 17 Devonshire Place, W.

MILLER, JOHN, 14 East Southernhay, Exeter

MILSOM, E. G. D., 50 Welbeck Street, W.

MOBERLY, SYDNEY C. H., Alwyn House, Winslow, Bucks

MOLESWORTH, T. H., St. Margarets-at-Cliffe, nr. Dover

MOORE, J. LANGFORD, Dispensary, St. Bartholomew's Hospital, E.C.

MOORE, Dr. NORMAN, 94 Gloucester Place, Portman Square, W.

MORLAND, E. C., Villa Emilia, Davos Platz, Switzerland

MORRICE, Dr. G. G., *J.P.*, 17 Royal Terrace, Weymouth

MORRIS, Dr. C. A., *C.V.O.*, 28 Chester Square, S.W.

MORRIS, EDWARD, 7 Windsor Place, Plymouth

MORRISON, Dr. J., 11 Brook Street, W.

MORTIMER, J. D. E., 4 Burton Court, Lower Sloane Street, S.W.

MOSELEY, C. K., 14 Northgate Street, Ipswich

MUNDY, H., Florida Road, Durban, Natal

MURIEL, J., Hadleigh, Suffolk

MURPHY, J. KEOGH, 16 Pembridge Crescent, W.

MURRAY, F. E., Graaf Reinet, Cape Colony

MYDDELTON-GAVEY, E. H., 16 Broadwater Down, Tunbridge Wells

NANCE, H. CHESTER, 55 St. Giles' Plain, Norwich

Newberry Library, Chicago, per Messrs. B. T. Stevens & Brown, 4 Trafalgar Square, W.C.

NEWBOLT, G. P., 42 Catherine Street, Liverpool

NEWTON, LANCELOT, Alconbury Hill, Huntingdon

NIXON, J. A., Dr., Royal Infirmary, Bristol

NOKE, F. H., Lieut. R.A.M.C., Roseleigh Cottage, Church Walk, Thames Ditton

NOON, L., Manor Road, Farncombe, Godalming

NORBURY, W., 12 Moreton Gardens, South Kensington, S.W.

ODLING, T. F., per Hickey & Borman, 14 Waterloo Place, S.W.

OGLE, Dr. J. G., South Redlands, Reigate, Surrey

O'KINEALY, F., Major, I.M.S., c/o King, Hamilton & Co., 7 Hare Street, Calcutta, India

OLDFIELD, JOSIAH, 5 Harley Street, W.

ORMEROD, A. L., 99 Holywell, Oxford

ORMEROD, Dr. J. A., 25 Upper Wimpole Street, W.

ORTON, G. H., 7 Campden Hill Road, Kensington, W.

PANK, HAROLD, Hamilton Place, Market Rasen, Lincs

PARDINGTON, Dr. G. L., Glynlee, Tunbridge Wells

PARK, Prof. ROSWELL, 510 Delaware Avenue, Buffalo, New York

PARKER, C. A., 141 Harley Street, W.

PARKER, G. D., 106 Gipsy Hill, Upper Norwood, S.E.

PARKER, G. R., 4 High Street, Lancaster

PARKER, Dr. R. DERWENT, Caledon, Cape Town

PATERSON, H. J., 9 Upper Wimpole Street, W.

PATERSON, W. B., 7A Manchester Square, W.

PAYNE, J. E., Park Grange, Sevenoaks

PEACEY, Dr. W., Rydal Mount, Mead, Eastbourne

PEARSE, R. E. FRANKLYN, Jagersfontein, South Africa

PENNEFATHER, C. M., Deanhurst, Harrow

PETERS, A. E., High Street, Petersfield, Hants

PHILLIPS, Dr. LL. C. P., 11 Sharia Bostane, Cairo, Egypt

PICTON, Dr. LIONEL JAS., Holmes Chapel, nr. Crewe

PIERCE, Dr. BEDFORD, The Retreat, York

PINKER, H. G., 6 Dalby Road, Cliftonville

Plymouth Medical Society, per J. Elliot Square, 22 Portland
    Square, Plymouth

POULTER, A. R., 67 Gordon Mansions, Francis Street, W.C.

POWER, D'ARCY, 10A Chandos Street, Cavendish Square, W.

POWER, HENRY, Bagdale Hall, Whitby, Yorkshire

POYNDER, Dr. F. C., East Grinstead, Sussex

PRATT, Dr. ELDON, Henfield, Sussex

PRICKETT, Dr. MARMADUKE, 27 Oxford Square, Hyde Park, W.

PRIESTLEY, J. G., 3 Buckingham Gate, S.W.

PRITCHARD, Dr. OWEN, 37 Southwick Street, Hyde Park, W.

PRYCE, H. VAUGHAN, 104 Bethune Road, N.

QUARTEY-PAPAFIO, Dr. B. W., Momo's Hall, Accra, Gold Coast,
    West Africa

QUENNELL, JOHN C., Brentwood, Essex

Radford Library, St. Mary's Hospital, Manchester, per
    Librarian

RANKING, Dr. J. E., 18 Mount Ephraim Road, Tunbridge Wells

RAWLING, L. B., 16 Montagu Street, Portman Square, W.

READ, Dr. MABYN, 42 Foregate Street, Worcester

REECE, Dr. R. J., 62 Addison Gardens, W.

REES, FREDERICK J., St. Bertha, Talbot Road, Wembley

REICHWALD, MAX B., Burnbrae, Beckenham

REID, Dr. T. WHITEHEAD, St. George's House, Canterbury

REYNOLDS, H. W., 28 St. Saviour Gate, York

RICE, Dr. EDWARD, Prior's Close, Sutton Courtenay, Abingdon, Berks

RICHARDSON, W. G, 19 Saville Row, Newcastle-on-Tyne

RISK, E. J., Lieut.-Col., R.A.M.C., c/o Messrs. Holt, Laurie and Co., Bankers, 3 Whitehall Place, London

RIVERS, Dr. W. H. R., St. John's College, Cambridge

RIVIERE, Dr. CLIVE, 19 Devonshire Street, W.

ROBERTS, Dr. CHAS. H., 21 Welbeck Street, W.

ROBERTSON, Dr. F. W., Ravenstone, Lingfield Road, Wimbledon, S.W.

ROBINSON, G., *J.P.*, 5 Harpur Place, Bedford

ROBINSON, HAYNES S., 35 St. Giles' Plain, Norwich

ROSE, F. A., 42 Devonshire Street, Portland Place, W.

RUNDLE, H., 13 Clarence Parade, Southsea

RUSHWORTH, NORMAN, Beechfield, Walton-on-Thames

RUST, H. R. G., Wethersfield, Braintree, Essex

RUST, J., 30 St. Mary's Road, Higher Crumpsall, Manchester

St. Bartholomew's Hospital, The Governors of, twelve copies

ST. CYR, J. B. DUMAINE, Aux Cayes, Hayti, West Indies

St. Mary's Hospital, Manchester, per Secretary, Thomas Browning, Esq.

SALE, J. C., Inglewood, Skegness, Lincs

SANDILANDS, Dr. J. E., 9 Sussex Villas, Kensington, W.

SAUNDERS, A. L., 112 Maida Vale, W.

SCHOLBERG, Dr. H. A., University College, Cardiff

SCHOLBERG, P. H., Taltal, Chile, S. America

SCHOLEFIELD, E. H., County Asylum, Lancaster
School of Medicine, Cairo, Egypt
SCOTT, Dr. JOHN, Bromley, Kent
SCOTT, S. R., 44 Welbeck Street, W.
SELBY, Dr. P. G., Teynham, Kent
SEWELL, E. P., Capt. R.A.M.C.
SHADWELL, H. W., 61 Lupus Street, S.W.
SHARPIN, E. C., 19 Bromham Road, Bedford
SHAW, Dr. T. CLAYE, 30 Harley Street, W.
SHEAF, Dr. C. A. ERNEST, Toowoomba, Queensland, Australia
SHELLY, Dr. C. E., Hertford
SHORE, Dr. T. W., 6 Kingswood Road, Upper Norwood, S.E.
SIDEBOTHAM, Dr. E. J., Erlesdene, Bowdon, Cheshire
SIMMONS, H. C., *J.P.*, Standerton, Transvaal
SIMPSON, S. H., Florence Road, Boscombe, Bournemouth
SKELDING, Dr. H., St. Loyes, Bedford
SLOANE, J. S., 82 London Road, Leicester
Small-Pox Hospital, South Mimms, Barnet, per Dr. Claughton
    Douglass, R.M.O.
SMITH, E. A. CLOETE, 1 Westbourne Street, Hyde Park, W.
SMITH, F. A., Captain, I.M.S., c/o Messrs. William Watson
    and Co., Bombay
SMITH, H. L., Buckland House, Buckland Newton, Dorset
SMITH, Sir THOMAS, Bart., *K.C.V.O.*, 5 Stratford Place, W.
SOWRY, G. H., 4 King Street, Newcastle, Staffs
SPICER, HARRY, Staff Surg. R.N., The Admiralty, S.W.
SPICER, W. T. HOLMES, 5 Wimpole Street, W.
SPREAT, F., Whetstone, N.
Stamford Infirmary Medical Book Society, Stamford
STATHAM, H., The Redings, Totteridge, Herts
STAWELL, Dr. R. de S., Castle Gates, Shrewsbury
STEEDMAN, J. F., Arcall, Prentis Road, Streatham, S.W.
STEPHENS, J. W., Tymawr, Cardigan, S. Wales
STEVENS, Dr. A. FELIX, The Hawthorns, Stamford Hill, N.
STEVENS, C. R., Capt., I.M.S , 6 Middleton Street, Calcutta

STIRLING-HAMILTON, J., Woodgates, Southwater, Horsham

STRUGNELL, F. W., Grove End House, Highgate Road, N.W.

STRUGNELL, Dr. W. T., 213 Brixton Hill, S.W.

STUART-LOW, W., 45 Welbeck Street, W.

STUBBS, P. B. TRAVERS, Wynberg, Cape Town, South Africa

STYAN, Dr. T. G., Chapel Place, Ramsgate

SURRIDGE, Dr. E. E. N., Knutsford, Cheshire

SYLVESTER, G. H., Lieut-Col., R.A.M.C., c/o Messrs. Holt & Co.,
   3 Whitehall Place, S.W.

SYLVESTER, K. F., The Court House, Trowbridge, Wilts

SYMONDS, Dr. H., Kimberley, South Africa

SYMPSON, Dr. E. M., Deloraine Court, Lincoln

TAIT, Dr. E. S., 48 Highbury Park, N.

TAYLER, Dr. G. C., Trowbridge, Wilts

TERRY, HENRY G., 2 Gay Street, Bath

THOMPSON, G. H., Buxton, Derbyshire

THURSFIELD, Dr. H., 84 Wimpole Street, W.

TOOTH, Dr. H. H., *C.M.G.*, 34 Harley Street, W.

TRECHMANN, MAX L., 131 St. George's Road, S.W.

TRIST, J. R. RIGDEN, 22 Vernon Terrace, Brighton

TROUTBECK, Dr. H., 151 Ashley Gardens, S.W.

TURNBULL, Dr. G. L., 47 Ladbroke Square, Notting Hill, W.

TURNER, C. H., Lieut. R.A.M.C., c/o Messrs. King & Co.,
   Bombay

UPTON, H. C., 28 Medina Villas, West Brighton

URWICK, Dr. R. H., 11 Dogpole, Shrewsbury

VALÉRIE, JOHN, Gothic House, Devonshire Road, Balham, S.W.

VAN BUREN, Dr. A., Haslemere, Ashford, Middlesex

VAUGHAN-JACKSON, H. F., Potter's Bar, Middlesex

VERDON-ROE, Dr. S., 47 West Hill, Wandsworth, S.W.

VERLING-BROWN, C. R., Carnavon, Cavendish Road, Bournemouth

VERRALL, T. J., 97 Montpelier Road, Brighton

Victoria General Hospital, Halifax, Nova Scotia, per
. Librarian

WALDO, Dr. F. J., 40 Lansdowne Road, W.

WALLER, T. H., Thorneybrook, Chelmsford

WARD, S. E., Rectory Lodge, Brasted, Sevenoaks

WARE, Dr. A. M., 13 Launceston Place, De Vere Gardens, W.

WARING, H. J., 37 Wimpole Street, W.

WATERFIELD, N. E., Khartoum, Sudan, Egypt

WATERHOUSE, Dr. J. H., 19 Avenue Victoria, Scarborough

WATSON, C. GORDON, 44 Welbeck Street, W.

WATTS, H. J. M., Salford House, Tonbridge, Kent

WEAVER, F. K., Blenheim Lodge, Waterden Road, Guildford

WEBER, Dr. F. PARKES, 19 Harley Street, Cavendish Square, W.

WENHAM, H. V., 2 Redington Road, Hampstead, N.W.

WEST, C. E., 132 Harley Street, W.

WEST, Dr. SAMUEL, 15 Wimpole Street, W.

WHITE, Dr. C. PERCIVAL, 22 Cadogan Gardens, S.W.

WHITE, Dr. C. POWELL, The Pathological Laboratory, St Thomas'
Hospital, S.E.

WHITE, Dr. HENRY, 39 Maningham Lane, Bradford, Yorkshire

WHITEHEAD, H. E., 475 Caledonian Road, N.

WHITWELL, A. F., The Castle House, Shrewsbury

WICKMAN, Dr. A., 325 Washington Street, Newark, N.J.

WIGHTMAN, C. F., Royston, Herts

WILBE, Dr. R. H. W., York Lodge, 21 Finchley Road, N.W.

WILKS, Dr. GEORGE, Ashford, Kent

WILKS, Dr. J. H., 43 Montgomery Road, Sheffield

WILLARD, S. D., 48 Hertford Street, Mayfair, W.

WILLETT, A., 36 Wimpole Street, W.

WILLETT, Dr. EDGAR, 22 Queen Anne Street, **W.**

WILLEY, Dr. THOMAS, Graham House, Shorncliffe Road, Folke-
stone

WILLIAMS, J. T., Rossall House, Barrow-in-Furness, Lancashire

WILLIAMSON, Dr. H., 84 Wimpole Street, W.

WINKFIELD, ALFRED, 26 Beaumont Street, Oxford

WOMACK, Dr. F., 115 Alexandra Road, Hampstead, N.W.

WOOD, FREDERICK, 12 Lewes Crescent, Kemp Town, Brighton

WOOD, W. VINCENT, Wrington, Somerset

WORTHINGTON, R. T., 10 Marine Parade, Lowestoft

WREFORD, H., The Firs, Denmark Road, Exeter

WRIGHT, Dr. J. C., Park Road, Halifax

WYER, Dr. OTHO F., Epperston House, The Avenue Road,
Leamington

WYNNE, GRAHAM S., Amersham, Bucks

York Medical Society, 1 Low Ousegate, York, per Hon. Secretary

YOUNG, E. E., North Staffordshire Infirmary, Stoke-on-Trent

NOTICE TO SUBSCRIBERS.

It is particularly requested that Subscriptions be remitted without delay, as an acknowledgment of the receipt of the volume. If not paid for before the Thirty-first day of March 1906, the volume will be charged as a Non-Subscriber's copy.

Cheques and Post-Office Orders to be made payable to Mr. W. M°ADAM ECCLES, 124 Harley Street, London, W.

Price to Subscribers, Six Shillings; to Non-Subscribers, Eight Shillings and Sixpence.

An Index to the first twenty volumes, prepared by Sir William Church, is issued in a separate volume, price 3s. 6d. to Subscribers, 5s. Non-Subscribers.

An Index to the second twenty volumes, prepared by Mr. M°Adam Eccles, is issued with this volume, but may be also had separately, price 3s. 6d. to Subscribers, 5s. to Non-Subscribers.

January 1906.

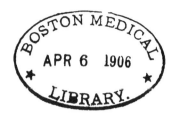
𝔍n 𝔐emoriam
LUTHER HOLDEN, F.R.C.S.

On Friday afternoon, February 10, 1905, all that was mortal of the late Luther Holden was laid to rest in the quiet church-yard at Upminster, a country village in Essex, to which he was much endeared by many happy family associations and ties, and of which his brother, the Rev. P. Melancthon Holden, had been the rector for many years.

Mr. Alban Doran, to whom I am much indebted for many interesting details of Luther Holden's family, tells me that it traces its ancestry to William Holden of Wednesbury, in Staffordshire, who lived at the end of the seventeenth century, and married the daughter of a Monmouthshire gentleman named Hyla. In Bagnall's History of Wednesbury, 1854, the pedigrees of the Holden and Hyla families are carefully narrated. Fourth in descent occurs the name of the Rev. Henry Augustus Holden, the father of Luther, who was born in 1784, and was brought up at Daventry in Northamptonshire. He entered the Indian Army, but after a short service he retired with the rank of lieutenant, and entered Worcester College, Oxford, with the object of entering the Church. Whilst still an undergraduate he married his second cousin, Mary, the daughter of Hyla Holden, of Wednesbury, to whom were born eight children, five being sons; two, the first and the fourth, entered the Church, the third settled in Canada, and the youngest, a midshipman in the Royal Navy, died young.

Luther Holden, the second son, was born on December 19, 1815, in Birmingham, at the house of his grandfather Holden. His father, after graduating M.A. Oxford, took Holy Orders, and was appointed to a curacy at Wolstanton in Shropshire, and in order to increase his stipend took resident pupils for their education. With these Luther Holden received his education, but he seems never to have been at a boarding school, although one of his brothers was at Shrewsbury School.

Luther Holden's father subsequently held a curacy at War-
minster, near Banbury, but never became a beneficed clergyman
of the Church of England.   A small fortune having been
bequeathed to him, he resided for a time at Brighton, and then
came to London, living in Addison Road, Kensington, for many
years, until his death in December 1870.   His house was the
resort of many well-known divines and wits.[1]

Mrs. Luther Holden has kindly communicated to me some
particulars of her husband's early life.   She tells me that she
once asked her husband his reasons for entering the medical
profession, when he said, "Well, when I was a little fellow and
my father a poor curate, I observed that the doctor who attended us drove a nice horse, and I thought if I was a doctor
I should have a horse too."   He was always interested in and
devoted to animals, and he used to say that animals had rights,
and we had duties towards them.   This love for all kinds of
animals clung to him, and was a characteristic feature of his
life.   Holden was, moreover, fond of sport in all its phases,
and he used to tell the story, that one day whilst on the river
Thames rowing with some friends, the boat capsized, and all
were precipitated into the water.   All but one managed to save
themselves, and he was discovered lying in the boat, after it
had righted itself.   To their great relief his friend was rescued,
and proved to be L. L. Worship, who became his life-long
friend, and practised his profession at Riverhead, near Sevenoaks for over forty years.

Luther Holden was well grounded in French, for at the age
of twelve years he was sent to Havre to school, so that he
might in the companionship of French boys learn to speak the
language correctly and fluently.   His progress was so rapid
and thorough that at the age of thirteen he obtained the prize
for composition, which was presented to him by the Mayor of
Havre, and the book, a French dictionary, remained to the last
one of his most treasured possessions.

At the age of seventeen Luther Holden entered the medical
school of St. Bartholomew's Hospital as a pupil of Edward
Stanley, one of the surgeons, to whom he was apprenticed,
and with whom he lived for five years at Lincoln's Inn Fields.
Stanley, who had in 1826 published his "Manual of Practical
Anatomy for the use of Students engaged in Dissections," had
an appreciative regard for Holden's skill as a dissector, and as

---

[1] Mr. Doran has received much information from the Rev. Dr. Holden, the
elder brother of Luther Holden, from his niece, Mrs. Miller, from Mr. A.
Willett, his colleague at St. Bartholomew's Hospital, and from Bagnall's
History of Wednesbury (Wolverhampton, 1854).

an admirable and clear teacher of Anatomy, and did all in his power to advance his professional success. After taking his diploma as a member of the Royal College of Surgeons of England in 1838, Luther Holden studied at Berlin for twelve months, and subsequently for a similar period at Paris. His means at this latter period seem to have been somewhat limited, for he arrived in Paris with only thirty pounds in his pocket, but he was so keen in prosecuting his studies that he determined to make the best use of his meagre financial resources. With this object he shared his room in Paris with a fellow-student, an Italian, and this intimate friendship first aroused his admiration of Italian literature, and awoke a keen desire to critically study Dante in the original, which to the end of his life was one of his favourite pursuits and recreation. He had an intuitive aptitude for the acquisition of modern languages, and was thoroughly at home in French, German, and Italian ; he was also a well-read scholar of Greek and Latin.

Holden, in his Hunterian Oration, strongly advocated the cultivation of Greek and Latin literature—whether the Royal College of Surgeons, or even the Universities, insist on its study or not—"for," he says, "it will ever be held in the highest estimation. The more completely it should happen to be set aside for a time, the greater would be the force of the inevitable reaction which would bring it again into power."[1] Holden was a strenuous upholder of a classical training, for he states that, "if we set aside classical education, we shall be ignoring the value of the best system of training which exists." He further gives his own experience as a teacher of forty years as to the advantage of classics in training the mind of students, for he expresses his strong conviction "that students who have had a public-school training have a fuller development of the logical faculty—a more cultivated memory, a greater grasp and power of combination." In continuation, he says, "I have no hesitation in saying that I can teach such pupils more in two months than others who have had no like education in six."

His twelve months' sojourn in Paris gave him a larger insight into the continental methods of teaching anatomy, far in advance of that in vogue in the English schools, so that on his return to his native country he lost no time in strenuously advocating the continental methods of teaching anatomy. He always inculcated the axiom that anatomy was a science of sight, and not of faith, and throughout his whole career as a

[1] Luther Holden, the Hunterian Oration, 1881, pp. 34–35.

teacher at St. Bartholomew's he determined that his aim should be to demonstrate anatomical structures as described in the manuals, so that all his pupils could see and believe. Transcendental Anatomy, therefore, had few charms for him.

Holden qualified as a member in 1838, and on December 24, 1844, he was elected a Fellow of the College by examination, and at the time of his death he was the Senior Fellow, being the sole survivor of the twenty-four successful candidates who passed with him.

For some time he taught unofficially in the dissecting-rooms, for he was not elected Demonstrator of Practical Anatomy till the year 1846. As an unofficial teacher, he soon attracted a large and appreciative class of pupils, whose fees gained him not only a considerable income, but, what he valued far more, many life-long friendships. In the year 1843 Holden took rooms in Old Jewry, and three years afterwards he removed to 39 Ely Place, where he remained till 1852. His first surgical appointment was that of Surgeon to the Metropolitan Dispensary, Fore Street, which office he held for some years.

It was as a Demonstrator of Anatomy that Holden displayed his undoubted power as a teacher, and was seen at his best. His genuine love of Anatomy, his natural aptitude for neat dissection, his untiring industry, his habitual courtesy and patience, his clearness of description without any circumlocution, and his power to bring to view the details of complicated dissections, whilst his constant sympathy with the members of his class in their difficulties in their elementary stage of professional life, made him an ideal teacher of Anatomy, and secured for him the devoted attachment of his pupils.

It was in the year 1857 that I first entered as a student the Anatomy Class in the rooms of which Mr. Holden and Mr. Savory were then the Demonstrators, and I was thus early much impressed with the different standpoints from which they viewed the best methods of teaching Anatomy.

Luther Holden was ever ready to help all, and even in many instances to dissect a not inconsiderable part for those who did not care to do it themselves, and he would thus endeavour to secure the interest of the student in his work by his contagious persuasiveness, and he was usually successful in his endeavours. Savory, on the other hand, when asked to examine "a man on his part," would answer, "Have you read it up for yourself?" if not, he would tell him that after he had done all in his power to arrive at a knowledge of the part he had dissected he would gladly do so. Mr. Holden's method was to help all; Mr. Savory's was to make all help themselves. The combination of the two methods made a perfect whole in the teaching of practical Anatomy: for the aim of one was to assist, encourage, and interest the weaker members of his class; the aim of the other was to strengthen and to make self-reliant its stronger element.

The gentle and refined personality of Luther Holden secured for him at once the affection of every member—especially the younger—of his class, and all his pupils felt they had in him a sympathetic teacher and a friend willing and able to help them in their anatomical problems and difficulties.

Whilst holding the office of Demonstrator Holden wrote in 1850 his "Manual of the Dissection of the Human Body," published by S. Highley, of Fleet Street, in four separate parts, which were not illustrated. It was subsequently issued as a single volume, fairly copiously illustrated, and passed through five editions.

Subsequently, in the year 1855, another work appeared from Holden's pen, entitled "Human Osteology," which from the first marked a distinct advance in the study of the bones. The illustrations on stone, etched by the late Mr. Thomas Godart, the Librarian of the Medical School, have never been excelled as engravings of the highest order. To Holden is due the conception of marking out on the bones the origins and the insertions of the muscles, the former in red and the latter in blue outlines, and his idea has undoubtedly proved of untold value to the student.

Luther Holden's next promotion was in June 1859, when he was elected joint-lecturer with Mr. Skey on Descriptive and Surgical Anatomy. In the lecture theatre his attractive and breezy, but not quite eloquent, style secured for him the wrapt attention of his audience, for it felt that Luther Holden was lecturing on a subject he knew and loved to teach. Holden told the writer of this memoir that he was never so much at his ease in the lecture theatre as he was in the dissecting-rooms, for he felt strongly that anatomy could only be learnt by personal dissection and examination of the dissected subject, and not by means of lectures, which constituted a considerable part of the methods of imparting knowledge in mediæval times when books were scarce and costly and the desire for knowledge was great.

In July 1860 Luther Holden was elected Assistant-Surgeon to the Hospital when he was forty-five years of age, but owing to the retirement of Stanley, Lloyd, and others, the changes in the staff were many and promotions were rapid, so he was, after five years' service as Assistant-Surgeon, elected full Surgeon in August 1865.

Holden was, in the year 1868, elected on the Council of the
Royal College of Surgeons, and was subsequently re-elected for
another term of eight years.   After holding the post of Junior
and Senior Vice-President he was elected in 1879 President of
the College, which he held for one year.   He had previously
been appointed a Member of the Court of Examiners in 1873,
and held this appointment for ten years, retiring at the end
of his second term of five years in 1883.   In 1881 he delivered the Hunterian Oration on the life and work of John
Hunter, and towards the latter part of the lecture he stated,
"I have no hesitation in calling Antiseptic Surgery Hunterian."
Holden had for many years held the appointment of Consulting
Surgeon to the Foundling Hospital in Guildford Street, and
this office he held till his death.   He always took a deep interest
in its welfare so long as he resided in London ; but on his
retirement into the country he confided the surgical care of
the Foundling children to Mr. Alfred Willett, his former
colleague.

He was presented by his old pupils and friends with his
portrait by Sir J. E. Millais, on his retirement from the
active staff of the Hospital, and he forthwith transferred it
to the Governors of the Hospital.   It is painted as a side
view, three-quarter length portrait, and is pronounced by all
as an admirable likeness.   The painter has been happy in
catching Holden's pose and expression of his face and hands.
To some the painting seems rather thin, lacking the body
and richness of colour so marked in his portrait of Sir James
Paget which hangs on its immediate left in the great hall
of the Hospital.   A small etching of the portrait was subsequently presented to each subscriber of the testimonial, but
this possesses no artistic merit.

After Luther Holden retired from the office of Surgeon to
the Hospital, he was elected one of the Consulting Staff.   He
forthwith lived at his country residence, Pinetoft, in Rushmere,
near Ipswich, where he possessed a small estate.   He not
infrequently made visits to London and so renewed his old
friendship with his former colleagues at the Hospital and the
College of Surgeons, but of late years he rarely came to London,
and then chiefly to visit some life-long friends at Putney.

Holden usually spent the winter months abroad, visiting
with his wife one year the Nile as far up as Wady Halfa ;
another year exploring India and Ceylon, and as late as
1896 he went to the Cape and the Transvaal, and much
enjoyed his new experience in South Africa.

Luther Holden married, as his first wife, Miss Sterry, about the time he was appointed Assistant-Surgeon to the Hospital, and secondly, in 1868, to a lady of the same family, who still survives him. There was no family by either marriage.

He died at Putney, at the house of his valued friends, with whom he was staying at the time, on Monday, February 6, 1905, in his ninetieth year.

Holden in his will gave abundant proof of his good will and interest towards his *alma mater;* for he bequeathed £3000 to the Medical School for a scholarship in surgery and £500 towards the building fund of the Hospital; in addition he gave £1000 to the Foundling Hospital, of which he had been the Consulting Surgeon for many years. He further directs, on the demise of his widow, that his freehold residence at Rushmere with the furniture are to be sold and the proceeds, together with £10,000, divided between St. Bartholomew's Hospital and the Foundling Hospital in equal shares.

Luther Holden was not a frequent contributor to surgical literature, and his papers on clinical subjects are chiefly found in the Medical Gazette, the Medical Times and Gazette, and in the St. Bartholomew's Hospital Reports.

They chiefly had reference to individual cases of interest, one of which referred to a patient suffering from "extra-ordinary anomalous affection of the nervous system in a boy," in vol. iii. p. 299, and the sequel of the case after operation in vol. viii. p. 228. It was in the Hospital Reports that his original papers on "Medical and Surgical Landmarks" first appeared in vol. ii. p. 195 *et seq.,* and in vol. vi. p. 70 *et seq.,* and in 1876 were published as a separate volume. This treatise was another example of Luther Holden's aptitude—nay, almost genius—for bringing anatomical knowledge to bear on the operative practice of surgery.

As an examiner, Holden was always considerate to the candidate and at the same time just to his office on the Court of Examiners. By some he was accounted a too lenient examiner, but he appeared to me that he was endeavouring always to lead the candidate up to his real worth, and trying to elicit the candidate's knowledge of his profession and not to demonstrate his ignorance. He endeavoured to give as high marks as he deemed just to the candidate and to the Court, but his sympathies were with the examinee whenever he thought that it was nervousness and not ignorance which prevented him bringing out his best knowledge. Holden's questions were short, concise, simple, so that the candidate was never at a loss to grasp the meaning of any question, and he never forgot the courtesy and consideration due to the student. He always recognised the double part which an examiner ought to take in the course of an examination; the first, the art of examining so as to bring out the knowledge of the candidate; the second, the gift of rightly assessing the marking value of the candidate's answers. He had the courage of his opinions, and his decisions were rarely wrong.

Holden was promoted to the Surgical Staff somewhat late in his career, so that he always let his anatomical knowledge get the upper hand of his surgical practice; and he never entered into the full spirit of an important and complicated operation.

He was rightly popular with his class, for he was in his element when teaching at the bedside, and the care and patience with which he marshalled his facts, and his review of the signs and the symptoms of his patient's disease, showed that he did his best to lead his class through the quicksands of error to a correct diagnosis. At the bedside, Holden was never in a hurry, and he always recognised that more mistakes occurred from want of care and method than from want of knowledge.

Holden was not a rigid disciple of aseptic surgery in the strict sense, but he strongly inculcated and practised one of the most important principles of the Listerian system, which is that of perfect cleanliness in every detail, and on which Sir W. Savory laid so much stress in his address on Surgery at the Cork meeting of the British Medical Association.

Holden had in great measure retired from active public and professional life for many years, so that his sphere of action had long passed to the sphere of memory; yet the memory he has left to us of his life and his work tells us that he raised the character of the school with which he was connected for over thirty years; that he was a fine and suggestive scholar; that he was a popular and an appreciated teacher, and that he was prized by his intimate friends.

[J. L.]

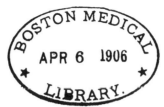
SAINT BARTHOLOMEW'S HOSPITAL REPORTS.

CLINICAL NOTES RESPECTING A TENDENCY TO BLOOD-CLOTTING DURING LIFE.

BY

SIR DYCE DUCKWORTH, M.D., LL.D.

The conceptions as to the formation and purpose of fibrin in the blood have varied with the progress of knowledge in animal chemistry and physiology. As physicians, we are more particularly concerned with the several conditions of the blood in which we find a marked tendency to form clots, one sometimes described under the term "hyperinosis." Physiologists have not yet completed their observations, on this matter. The study of the whole subject of thrombosis, or clotting, has in recent years enlarged our views regarding several morbid conditions involving many organs of the body.

It is obvious that there must be some cause or causes for clotting of the blood within the circulatory system since that fluid tends normally to preserve its fluidity, and we now know that the fault may lie either in the quality of the blood itself, or in its containing vessel, or that, perchance, both blood and vessel may be concerned in the occurrence. In its grossest form we meet with the formation of clot in the sacs of aneurysms, where the process is generally regarded as a *vis medicatrix*, and one that we strive to promote, and so in this case, as in others, we have clear evidence that such deposition occurs during life, and is not solely a property of the blood when withdrawn from its containing vessels. Sir John Simon, in his masterly lectures on General Pathology, delivered over fifty years ago, remarked that the coagulation of fibrin was its *rigor mortis*.

VOL. XLI.

Till lately we have not had much clinical knowledge respecting the presence of, or a tendency to, hyperinosis in our patients. Physiologists tell us that the effect of undue viscosity in the blood is too small to produce any important influence on the quality of the pulse. I should have been inclined to expect that the tension would have been heightened to some appreciable degree in such cases, although the occurrence of clotting is met with in the opposite conditions of plethora and marasmus. Dilution of the blood, induced by injection of normal saline solution, is affirmed to accelerate the velocity of the blood-stream. A rise of temperature is alleged to diminish its viscosity, thus relieving peripheral resistance, and loosening the labour of the heart. The effect of carbonic acid, æther, and chloral hydrate is to be regarded as increasing the viscosity of the blood.

The researches of Dr. Wright have recently led to an increase of our knowledge respecting the tendency to coagulation of the blood. His method, fully described in the *Lancet* of October 14, 1905, affords a ready way of determining this quality, and his suggestions for counteracting it constitute a valuable contribution to clinical practice. He has shown that by dosage with lime salts, the chloride, or preferably the lactate, of calcium, the coagulation of the blood may be accelerated promptly, and thus a tendency to hæmorrhage, or the control of it when in progress, may be averted or secured. The same results were obtained with magnesium carbonate. Dr. Wright and Mr. Paramore have further shown that milk, which is rich in lime salts, has a considerable influence upon blood-coagulation, and that its use in large quantities requires to be fully considered in the case of disorders associated with a tendency to superfibrination. I will consider this matter later.

We are probably not mistaken in believing that superfibrination is a consequence of disordered function or the effect of some variety of disease. It has long been held that this condition prevails in all inflammatory states, hence the significance formerly attached to the "buffed and cupped" characters of the blood when removed by venæsection if they happened to occur. This result of retarded coagulation is, however, not peculiar to the blood met with in the course of inflammatory conditions.

The determinants of thrombosis which are now commonly recognised are found to be associated with (a) a feeble state of the circulation, due to weakness of the heart, leading to local stagnation ; (β) injury to, or alteration of, the *intima* of vessels

(Cruveilhier's doctrine), or (γ) direct interruption of their lumen by the intrusion of foreign matters. There are, however, other predisposing conditions to be considered. The occurrence of thrombosis as a sequel of severe fevers of infective origin is almost certainly associated with the local toxic effect of micro-organisms. These have been found in the case of enteric fever, the general lowered vitality of the patient predisposing to such an occurrence.

The variety of marantic thrombosis following long illnesses due to cachexia and failing powers, especially in cases of cancer and chronic tuberculosis, is probably independent of microbic invasion.

The association of thrombosis with cancer may own a local origin from direct intrusion of new growth into the lumen of a vessel, but an explanation is far to seek at present for the occurrence of clotting in a femoral vein as much as six months before the recognised onset of cancer of the stomach. Such cases were noted by Trousseau, and, strangely enough, he was the victim of such an occurrence himself, and foretold the sequel of it.

There remain, too, other conditions predisposing to super-fibrination of the blood. The disorder first recognised by Paget as gouty phlebitis is one which appears to depend on the state of the blood, whatever that may be, which commonly prevails at the onset of regular or classical gout. The peccant matter appears to alight on the *intima* of one or more veins, and to spread more or less to larger ones, the joints escaping (abarticular gout). In some of these cases there is certainly a traumatic factor which determines the point of selection, the phlebitis leading to local thrombosis, but in others no special exciting cause can be ascertained. The proclivity or habits of the patient in these cases are commonly such as lead up to ordinary articular attacks of gout.

It may be regarded as fairly certain that a diet rich in proteids tends to promote undue superfibrination of the blood and an excess of purin bodies, and thus a so-called gouty proclivity is engendered. The experience of Salvenmoser in the late Professor Ludwig's laboratory at Leipzig, related to me by Sir Lauder Brunton, proved that the blood of rabbits fed on bran and cereals tended to coagulate rapidly, while a diet of green vegetable food promptly overcame this condition, and so enabled experiments upon blood-pressure to be carried on which otherwise were found impossible owing to rapid clotting taking place.

It is not improbable that the use of potable waters rich in lime salts may also induce hyperinosis, and a diet consisting largely of milk is known to have this effect, ordinary milk containing more lime than the *Liquor Calcis* of the *Pharmacopœia* (according to Drs. Wright and R. Hutchison) (*i.e.* gr.ss ad f$\mathfrak{z}$i.). This fact has a clinical importance in relation to the common dietary employed in cases of enteric fever where there is sometimes a tendency to venous thrombosis, and suggests the use of milk diluted with water, to which sodium citrate may be added, or, in many cases, of whey and cream.   Dr. Wright, indeed, regards the free use of milk as particularly undesirable if thrombosis has already occurred, as tending to solidify the clot, and so render it either a more dangerous missile, or more likely to seal up the involved vein permanently.

The condition of the blood in the pregnant woman is probably one tending to viscosity, and its quality after parturition may fairly be described as loaded, and prone to favour clotting.   The altered circulation, the uterine scar, and the rapid involution of the womb may be regarded, as was pointed out some forty years ago by Dr. Robert Barnes, as important factors in the process.   Hence the occasional tendency to phlegmasia alba, or the ghastly occurrence of a travelling thrombus with fatal pulmonary arterial embolism, even in cases conducted with all aseptic methods.   A due consideration of the tendency to hyperinosis should lead us to recognise the importance of a rational dietary in such cases.

It is probably a less difficult task to induce a hyperinotic state than to promote subfibrination of the mass of the blood. Dr. Wright is, however, confident in the use of citric acid in full doses as an agent to promote the latter condition, thus producing what he terms decalcification of the blood, and he employs half drachm doses, well diluted, several times a day, with speedy effect.   By diminishing the intake of rich animal food, by increase of simple diluents and of well-prepared green vegetable food, we may hope to control a tendency to superfibrination and thrombosis.   This should be borne in mind in the case of the pregnant woman who, certainly in the upper ranks of life, is often overnourished, and is too apt to indulge in sedentary habits.

In cases where there is a tendency to languid circulation, together with hyperinosis, the use of alcohol in some form is indicated, both to promote a more vigorous circulation, and to act, as it appears to do in some measure, in lessening superfibrination.

Inasmuch as æther is alleged to promote the viscosity of the blood, it remains for anæsthetists to consider the advisability of employing it in cases where this tendency is suspected.

ALCOHOLIC NEURITIS.

BY

NORMAN MOORE, M.D.

Three cases of neuritis due to chronic alcoholism which have been admitted to Hope ward during the past year seem worthy of record.

The most severe was that of a married woman, aged 36, who was admitted on January 13, 1905, and left the hospital for the Convalescent Home at Swanley on May 3.

The history of the case was that the patient had been drinking every day for several years; that she generally drank whisky, but was never absolutely drunk, and that she had become very untruthful. At the beginning of November 1904 she complained of a tingling, "pins and needles," in her hands and legs. The tingling was succeeded in her legs by pain and loss of power, and on Christmas day 1904 she was unable to walk. On January 10, 1905, she became what her friends described as "delirious," not noisy, but seeing strange figures and things passing across the room. Nevertheless she continued to eat well and to sleep well.

Her appearance on admission suggested chronic habits of intemperance. Her cheeks, nose, and chin were very red with some acne; her expression was one of excitement. Her tongue was covered with white fur, and was tremulous when protruded. Her utterance was broken; her words were indistinct, and her answers hesitating. Her hands were tremulous. She was very thin. She stated that she took beer at supper and whisky very seldom; that her appetite was good, and that she slept well.

On examination nothing abnormal was discovered in her chest or abdomen, and there were no signs of renal disease. Her pulse was regular and soft.

There was some hyperæsthesia of the forearms, but no paralysis of any muscle of the arms. Sensation to touch was natural. The legs showed some paresis, which was most marked in the extensors, but there was no paralysis. Foot-drop was present, but not to an extreme degree.

She complained of great pain when the calf muscles were pressed, as well as of "pins and needles" and "burning." Ordinary sensation was normal. Neither knee-jerks nor plantar reflex were obtained.

There was nothing abnormal about the movements of the eyes.

During the following week she slept after small doses of chloral, and ate fairly well; but had delusions and tremors, and at times complete loss of control of bladder.

Sometimes her pulse became very feeble. Diarrhœa was present for two days.

She generally lay in a muttering, half conscious state from which she could be roused to answer questions, but answered feebly and irregularly. She took her food very slowly. She was so thin that it was difficult to prevent abrasions over the great trochanters and sacrum. She generally lay with her legs drawn up, sometimes on her back, and sometimes on her side. Massage seemed to improve the condition of her legs. Some days she seemed a little more intelligent than on others.

By February 16 but little improvement had taken place. Her temperature was often slightly raised without obvious cause, and sometimes rose to 101 or 102, and some rise continued throughout her illness. Occasionally she was noisy.

In the last week of February a sore which had formed over the sacrum had made some progress in healing, but this seemed the chief improvement. Her mental condition was unaltered and her tremors as well marked as before. She took food fairly well most days, and slept after chloral, chloralanide, bromide of potassium, sulphonal or trional.

On March 2 she seemed to answer questions better, but a week later her mental condition seemed worse, though her face showed a less demented expression.

In the first week of April her mental condition was decidedly improved. She was allowed to sit up in the evening and began to walk with help. Massage evidently did her legs good. She steadily improved from this forward, and by the end of the month had a natural expression; was able to walk fairly well; had gained a little flesh, and had a good appetite. Her knee-jerks were absent. Her mental condition became rational; she was aware of the cause of her illness, and resolved to avoid it in future. She left for Swanley Convalescent Home on May 3.

This was the most severe case of alcoholic neuritis in which I have seen recovery take place. The treatment, in addition to one of the sedatives at night mentioned above, consisted of bromide of potassium gr. x. three times a day from January 13 to February 16, and after that of cod-liver oil.

From January 15 to January 26 she was given 2 oz. of brandy in the day if her pulse indicated its necessity.

On admission the patient's emaciated and demented condition made her seem as one far advanced in a disease certain to end fatally, and without the admirable nursing and attention in every variation of her symptoms which she received from the sister of the ward, recovery would have been impossible.

Another married woman with less severe alcoholic neuritis was admitted on June 29, 1905. She also recovered and left on October 3. Her age was 41, and on admission she complained of severe pain in her arms and legs, accompanied by some loss of power in them.

The pain began in the middle of May 1905. She said that her legs and body had wasted, but she was not generally emaciated. Her statement about drink was that she took a little whisky and water occasionally. She complains of bad appetite, of sickness in the morning, and imperfect sleep.

On admission no signs of visceral disease were discovered except some bronchial rales. Her tongue was clean but tremulous. Her legs were so weak that she could only just walk, and the left leg was the weaker of the two. Knee-jerks were not obtained. There was some anæsthesia on the inner, anterior, and posterior surfaces to a point some way above the knee of both legs. The hands were very tremulous. The venules of the face were somewhat enlarged.

On June 30 she vomited both before and after breakfast, and complained of much pain in the legs, especially in the left foot and calf. Her temperature was normal, and continued normal on some days, or one degree raised throughout. Her mental condition was unstable, and she was inclined to weep. The general tremor was marked. Ten days later the legs were still very tender and their muscles weak. Her tongue and hands were tremulous, and the grip of both hands feeble. Knee-jerks were absent.

On July 18 the pain was somewhat less, but the tremors still distinct and the leg muscles feeble. Her appetite and sleep were improved. A week later foot-drop was distinct, but the pain along the legs was less. The tremor remained.

On August 8 she had more power in her legs and feet, and had gained more still by August 15. Knee-jerks were absent. On August 19 these were obtained for the first time, and there was more muscular strength, but some pain remained.

On September 1 pain was still severe, but the tremor was

less, and on September 12 the patient could walk, though not with ease. At the end of September she was able to walk well and was free from pain.

She had some bronchial catarrh for about seven weeks, which was treated by expectorants. Antipyrin sometimes relieved the pain in the legs, but phenacetin was less effectual. Bromide of potassium and chloral were given to procure sleep. For the first ten days brandy, at first two ounces a day, and then one ounce seemed necessary. On October 3 she left the hospital in fair health and anxious to avoid excess in stimulants.

The third patient was a widow, aged 32, but looking much older, who was admitted with a large tuberculous cavity in her left lung, and with melœna.

She said that she had drunk much beer, gin, and brandy, and on admission had a rough, uncivilised manner, which altered for the better under the influence of the kindness and sympathy of the sister and nurses.

Her father drank, and died with ascites and jaundice. Her mother became insane.

The patient had had aching of the legs for three weeks.

On admission there was severe pain in the calves when pressed, but no paralysis. The knee-jerks were absent.

On March 6 the tenderness and absence of reflexes were unaltered. Three weeks later the tenderness was still present in a marked degree. The knee-jerks continued to be absent, but the neuritis diminished and ceased to be evident soon after May 9, while the symptoms due to her tuberculous lungs, peritoneum, and intestines, and her enlarged, fatty liver increased till her death on June 8.

She was given chloralanide to procure sleep, and the pain in her legs seemed relieved by wrapping them in thermogene wool.

From March 3 to March 12 she had no alcohol, then 2 oz. of brandy in the twenty-four hours when necessary, and after April 18 Port wine or brandy 3 oz., as her general condition obviously needed stimulant.

The pain in each of these cases was relieved by treatment and by cessation of the cause of the neuritis. In cases where the general debility is as extreme as in the first, some alcohol may be necessary, but in all cases of this kind of neuritis it should be altogether disused as soon as possible. The careful use of bromide of potassium, of chloral, or of some other sedatives to procure sleep at night is certainly advantageous, and the fact that such drugs are likely to be necessary for some time makes it desirable to vary their nature and also to avoid the continuous use of opium or of morphia.

A CASE OF TYPHOID FEVER

FOLLOWED BY

BILIARY COLIC AND THE PASSAGE OF GALL-STONES,

EACH ATTACK BEING ATTENDED BY A RIGOR AND FEVER,
WITH REMARKS UPON THE RELATION BETWEEN
TYPHOID FEVER AND GALL-STONES.

BY

SAMUEL WEST, M.D.

A married woman, aged 42, was admitted into the hospital with a mild attack of typhoid fever. The diagnosis would have been uncertain if it had not been that she had a son in this hospital and a daughter in the London Hospital, both suffering from typhoid. The temperature became normal four days after admission. After fourteen days' convalescence, on January 18 she suddenly became very sick, had a severe rigor, which lasted twenty minutes, and the temperature rose to 103°, and a little later to 104.6°, gradually falling during the next twenty-four hours to normal again. A good deal of pain was felt in the epigastrium and in the back at about the same level for several hours. The cause was not obvious until slight jaundice developed two days later. The stools were then rather light in colour, but no bile appeared in the urine. The gall-bladder could be just detected on palpation. Ten days later, on January 28, an exactly similar attack occurred with another rigor, and the temperature rose to 104°. The pain in this attack was felt higher up along the sternum and behind along the dorsal spines. The temperature was normal the next day, but rose again in the evening to 103°, and then continued raised about 1½° above normal for two days longer. The jaundice on this occasion was deeper and the gall-bladder more easily felt.

An interval of a week followed, and then occurred a third and more severe attack of pain with another severe rigor and a temperature of 103.4°.

The fever continued on this occasion for a week, being markedly intermittent, touching normal every morning, but rising to about 103° each evening for the first three days, then touching 100° only for three days. For the next week it remained unsteady, reaching 100° on alternate evenings and dropping below normal in the morning.

The gall-bladder was now quite distinct and very easily felt through the lax and thin abdominal walls.

The stools were frequently examined for gall-stones, and on February 13 twelve small facetted ones were discovered. They consisted of cholesterin.

From this time the jaundice rapidly subsided, and the patient left the hospital well a month later.

There was no history to be obtained of previous jaundice or of any attack at all resembling gall-stone colic. The abdomen had been examined in the usual way on admission and no enlargement of the gall-bladder observed. It was only after the attack of pain that any enlargement was found ; at first not definite, and only becoming very obvious about the time of the third attack. When the patient left the hospital the gall-bladder was still distinctly felt ; it was hard and contracted, and must have contained several other gall-stones.

An attack of severe abdominal pain with a rigor and vomiting in the second week of convalescence was naturally very alarming. It was clear that it was not due to perforation, to peritonitis, or to constipation, and it was not till the occurrence of jaundice that the cause became obvious. Then the question arose whether there was not pus in the gall-bladder, and whether an operation might not be necessary. The short duration of the fever and the patient's general condition rendered suppuration unlikely. In the third attack, when the fever was more continued, this question, of course, arose again, and with more urgency. However, an operation was again decided against, and the patient made a good recovery.

The formation of gall-stones has always been difficult to explain. Formerly it was referred to some chemical defect in the bile itself, the result of morbid conditions of the blood or humors of the body. This theory, which was a relic of humoral pathology, did not admit of demonstration. A step in advance was made when catarrhal conditions of the gall-bladder or bile-ducts were shown to be very common antecedents. With the development of the germ theory of inflammation the catarrhal conditions would naturally be referred to microbic infection. Thus the microbes would excite catarrhal inflammation, and the catarrh lead to the change in the bile which ended in the separation of the cholesterin and bile salts and the formation of gall-stones. But it is clear that microbes may play a more direct part in the process, and themselves excite directly the decomposition-changes which are necessary, and there is reason to believe that this is the case. In health bile is sterile —*i.e.* contains no microbes, but it frequently does in disease. Various organisms have been found; *e.g.* bacterium coli comune, staphylococcus albus, streptococcus pyogenes, the typhoid bacillus, and others. Many of these are common in the duodenum, from which naturally the infection would be expected to take place. Stagnation, or defective flow of bile, is the condition which most favours infection, the germs then passing readily from the duodenum into the ducts. Such stagnation or diminished flow is the result of high temperature of any kind, but especially when associated with septic fevers. Thus may be explained the slight degrees of jaundice which are so common in almost any fever. If in addition to such stagnation microbic infection occurs, the result would be catarrhal inflammation or even suppuration, according to the nature of the infecting germ, or, under other circumstances, the bile might be decomposed and gall-stones be produced.

Further investigations have shown that the mere presence of micro-organisms is not alone sufficient to lead to the formation of calculi. For this the catarrhal state of the mucous membrane must be added. The three ingredients of biliary calculi are mucus, cholesterin, and a substance called bilirubin calcium. Healthy bile prevents the deposition of this last substance, but if albumen be present this inhibitory action is prevented. Thus a catarrhal condition of the mucous membrane leads to the presence of mucus and albumen and the deposit of bilirubin calcium and cholesterin. Hence if the two conditions are required for the production of calculi—viz. micro-organisms and catarrh—it is possible for micro-organisms to be long present in the gall-bladder without harm in the absence of catarrh; and this we know may be the case.

A great deal of work has been done of recent years on the subject in connection with typhoid fever.

The typhoid bacillus has been found almost constantly in the gall-bladder in typhoid fever (Chiari).

Many instances of inflammation or suppuration in the gall-bladder, in the course of typhoid fever, have been recorded, in which typhoid bacilli have been found, and from which pure cultures have been obtained.

Richardson showed that the typhoid bacilli clumped in the bile of typhoid patients, and suggested that these clumps might form the nuclei of gall-stones. The typhoid bacilli have been actually demonstrated by him and others in the centre of gall-stones. Even experimental proof is not wanting, for gall-stones have been produced by the introduction of typhoid bacilli into the gall-bladder of animals. Lastly, living typhoid bacilli have been found in the gall-bladder months or even years after the attack of typhoid fever.

The direct association, then, of typhoid fever and gall-stones is completely established pathologically. Clinical evidence is now abundant. The present case is a good example of it.

Bernheim, so far back as 1889, referred to two or three instances of hepatic colic in the course of typhoid fever in patients who had had none before, and he asks the question whether typhoid fever does not predispose to biliary calculi.

Dupré records a case in which hepatic colic followed typhoid fever. An operation was performed eight months later. The patient died in a septic condition. Post-mortem, calculi were found in the gall-bladder, which with some of the ducts was in a condition of acute inflammation, and in the pus the typhoid bacilli were demonstrated.

Dufourt gives a series of cases of typhoid fever followed by biliary colic in patients who had never had symptoms of it before.

In this series the first attack of colic occurred
in the 2nd month after the fever in 2 cases
    ,, 3rd   ,,   ,,   3 ,,
       4th   3
    ,, 5th   1
    ,, 6th   ,,   ,,   4 ,,
  after 6 months ,,   ,,   6 ,,
In four of these, in the 10th, 12th, 18th, and 25th months respectively.

One case had indefinite pains during the fever, but distinct colic did not occur till two months after.

A similar case to this is recorded by Gilbert and Girode in a woman of 45 who had a mild attack of typhoid with slight gall-bladder pains during it. Colic became severe and necessitated operation five months later, when calculi as large as a hazel-nut were found and removed. From the contents of the gall-bladder a pure cultivation of typhoid bacilli was obtained.

A similar case to this occurred in a nurse at St. Bartholomew's Hospital, who was in the Hope Ward with a very severe attack of typhoid fever, during which she had several alarming attacks of abdominal pain. These in the end proved to be biliary colic, for she became jaundiced. She had never suffered before from either colic or jaundice. She made a good recovery and left the hospital. About four months later biliary colic recurred; the gall-bladder was opened, and the gall-stones removed.

REFERENCES.

BERNHEIM, Dict. Encycl. de Dechambre, art. Ictére, 1889.
DUFOURT, Rer. de Med., 1893, p. 274.
CURSCHMANN, Typhoid Fever, English transl., 1902.
GILBERT AND GIRODE, C. R. Soc. Biolog., 1893, p. 958.

CASES OF RIEDEL'S LOBE, WITH REMARKS ON THE VARIOUS DEFORMITIES OF THE LIVER.

BY

W. P. HERRINGHAM, M.D.

It will be within the experience of all that unusual cases come in company, and it so happened that I had never to my knowledge seen the condition which the following cases illustrate until last year.

CASE 1.—Alice Hughes, 34, housewife, was admitted, August 26, 1904, to Lawrence, then taking cases for Hope.

Present Attack.—For 4 months she has been getting a little thinner. For 2 months she has felt some pain after food, and

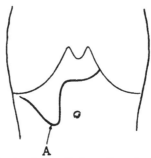

FIG. 1.—Alice H. *A* points to the hepatic projection in each figure.

has had nausea. On August 22 she was in her usual health. The next day she felt a sudden pain below the ribs on her right side, and noticed a lump at that place. On the 24th and 25th the pain grew worse; she vomited several times, and sweated with the pain, and her urine became like very strong tea. On the 26th she came to the hospital, and was in great pain during the journey, the jolting of the tramcar making the pain go through the lump like a knife.

Previous History.—Rheumatic fever and jaundice in 1887; was in bed for a few days. Never any colic.

Catamenia began at 10. Regular. Married at 21; 11 pregnancies, 9 children, of whom 4 died in infancy, and 2 miscarriages.

On Admission.—No jaundice. Well nourished. A little bronchitis.

Heart natural.

In the abdomen a hard lump, moving freely with respiration, below the right ribs, running down to below the level of the navel, having a sharp inner edge continuous with the lower margin of the liver above, and a less distinct outer edge, but a rounded margin below. It can be pushed forward from the loin, and back into the loin, apparently, from behind. This may be partly due to the displacement of the right kidney, which appears to be behind the mass. Percussion is impaired over most of the mass, but there is resonance over its lower end. Its surface is smooth, and it is a little tender. It cannot be separated from, and is apparently a projecting part of, the liver. The upper margin of hepatic dulness is at the sixth rib. The left kidney is somewhat depressed and enlarged.

August 26.—Jaundice began. It lasted until September 9. The pain ceased almost from the day of admission. The rounded swelling at the lower end of the lump diminished, but the hard mass with a sharp inner edge remained as before.

She had a slight rise of temperature (100.8° F.) on the morning of the 28th; but, with that exception, no fever at all. The urine was free from albumin.

She was discharged, feeling perfectly well, on September 16.

The patient was seen again on November 3, 1905, and stated that she had had no symptoms beyond a slight aching. The projecting lobe was not so hard, but easily to be felt, and of the same dimensions as before.

CASE 2.—On September 28, 1904, Mr. G. F., aged 56, was sent to me by Mr. Cooper of Barnstaple.

History.—He had been quite healthy until thirteen years ago, when he went to Central Africa for a year. He lived an exposed life, and acquired attacks of asthma which have lasted ever since. They were brought on by damp and exposure. Damp, chill, or fatigue will bring them on now. He has had such an attack for the last six weeks. He does not, however, cough or spit with them. The feeling is merely one of constriction round the chest.

Three years ago he had an attack of acute pain in the region of the gall-bladder, and has had similar attacks since. He has had slight jaundice with them, and the urine has been as dark as porter. He has never seen any gall-stones. In the last attack his temperature was about 102° F. for a fortnight.

He feels quite well between the attacks except that he is very constipated. He has had no other illnesses.

Present Condition.—His heart and lungs are quite normal.

The abdomen exactly resembles that of Alice H. There is a projection running down from the liver to just below the umbilicus, on the right side, which is tender, and has a sharp inner edge continuous with the lower margin of the liver in the epigastrium. Pressing it gives him the tickling in the throat which he says marks his attacks of asthma. Fig. 1 would accurately represent the tumour.

The urine contained no bile, albumin, or glucose.

I felt sure that this was a case of cholecystitis with a piece of liver dragged down over the adherent gall-bladder. I thought it possible he might even have had suppuration, and at any rate that he was in constant danger of it. But nothing would persuade him to undergo an operation.

Mr. Cooper writes to me (Nov. 1905) that this gentleman has been quite well since I saw him.

CASE 3.—Emma Fieltkan, 36, housewife, was admitted to Elizabeth Ward on May 22, 1905.

History.—Has been healthy until seven months ago. She was then confined ; had a healthy labour and puerperium. Three

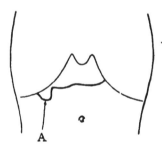

FIG. 2.—Emma F.

days after getting up she was taken with sudden pain in the right hypochondrium. She vomited repeatedly during the six hours that the attack lasted. There was no jaundice.

These attacks have recurred since. The pain is always in the same place, and the attacks seem to have been produced by exertion. She has never had indigestion. The urine has not been altered.

Present Condition.—Well nourished and healthy-looking.
The only abnormalities lay in the abdomen. This moves well,
but is a little tender on deep palpation, especially in the right
hypochondrium and epigastrium. The liver dulness begins at
the sixth rib in the right nipple line, and reaches the costal
margin. But projecting below the ribs a tumour, evidently connected with the liver, can be felt in the region of the gall-
bladder. It extends about 1½ inch below the ribs, is rounded
below, and might well be the gall-bladder except that it is not
movable laterally, and it has a sharp edge on its inner side.

This was taken to be a projection of the liver substance overlying a gall-bladder in which was a stone which by occasionally
blocking the cystic duct gave rise to the attacks of pain.

There was no pyrexia, and no history of rigors or sweats; so
that it did not seem likely that there was any suppuration
going on.

I asked Mr. Power to perform cholecystotomy.

At the operation the reason for the descent of this piece of
the liver was apparent. Some gall-bladders, when distended,
stand free of the liver. But this one adhered so tightly to the
overlying tissue that it had to be carefully dissected away before
it could be exposed and opened. These adhesions had evidently
pulled this piece of the liver down with the gall-bladder as the
latter dilated. A single stone, about 1 inch long, was found
lying close by the opening of the cystic duct. There was no
pus in the gall-bladder.

Partial enlargements of the liver have long been recognised,
but it was not until Riedel's paper appeared that this particular
class was separated from others.

Such partial enlargements fall into three groups.

The first is a mere malformation.

The second is by the majority of pathologists ascribed to
external pressure.

The third, which Riedel was the first to recognise, is due
to disease of the gall-bladder or some neighbouring organ.

I. Deformity due to malformation.

It is so common to see small abnormalities, an increase in
the number of sulci, or an irregularity of the lobules, that
Klebs thinks we are hardly justified in calling any form the
normal type. Such minor changes, however, matter little, as
they are not perceptible during life.

But occasionally (we have had eleven cases in about 3000
necropsies) one lobe, usually the left, exists only in an undeveloped form, and the other enlarges so greatly as to produce
in the abdomen a palpable hepatic tumour. This is a regular
variation the cases closely resembling one another. The

following is the description of such a case taken from the note, by Dr. Garrod, in the P.M. Records.

"The left lobe was reduced to a small leaf-shaped structure, thin, and with indented margin. The right lobe was large, and had its long axis nearly parallel with the long axis of the body. It was broken up into lobules by a number of deep fissures. Structure natural. No indication of gumma."

The left lobe is not always thin: it is sometimes a small globular body. The right lobe may reach down below the crest of the ilium. The gall-bladder usually lies not vertically as in the normal liver, but obliquely or even horizontally. The right lobe is not only large enough to compensate for the absence of the left, but is usually larger than the whole of a normal liver. The following are the weights in ten of our eleven cases. In nine the left lobe, and in one the right, was undeveloped. The right and left lobes were hypertrophied respectively.

MALES.

Case 1. Age 38, Left lobe undeveloped.   Liver weighed 81 ounces.
  ,, 2. ,, 39,   ,,   ,,   ,,   ,,   78   ,,
  ,, 3. ,, 43,   ,,   ,,   ,,   91   ,,
  ,, 4. ,, 49,   ,,   ..   ,,   ,,   68   ,,
  ,, 5. ,, 73, Right lobe   ,,   ,,   ,,   57   ,,

FEMALES.

Case 6. Age 16, Left lobe undeveloped.   Liver weighed 51 ounces.
  ,, 7. ,, 21,   ,,   ,,   ,,   ,,   64   ,,
  ,, 8. ,, 47,   ,,   ,,   ,,   52   ,,
  ,, 9. ,, 65,   ,,   ,,   ,,   40   ,,
  ,, 10. ,, 71,   ,,   ,,   ,,   46   ,,

The tendency is evident for the right lobe not only to replace the tissue of the left, or *vice versâ*, but to be developed beyond that point. It is only in the two old women that the rule is not obeyed.

II. The second class is composed of the cases which we call tight-lace liver, the Germans *Abschnür-* or *Schnür-leber*, and the Italians *fegato cordato* or *strozzato*. The right lobe, which is elongated in the vertical direction, is marked by a shallow transverse indentation over which the capsule is thickened, and often by vertical sulci. The accepted pathology is implied in the names given to it. The transverse depression is ascribed to stays, and the sulci are said to be creases due to lateral pressure.

Sometimes there is more than this. The transverse furrow may be so deep that nothing but a thin bridge of tissue unites the main part of the liver with the part below. The liver seems then to have an accessory lobe hanging from it. This is usually on the right, but sometimes on the left lobe.[1]

The cause of this latter variety is, I think, still uncertain. It is never found, so far as I know, in men,[2] and thus far corresponds to the slighter form. But such a case as the following is difficult to explain by mere pressure.

> A woman of 30 had noticed for eight years a tender tumour in the middle line of her abdomen, which produced various forms of pain and discomfort. Langenbuch thought it most likely to be hydatid, but on opening the abdomen found an accessory lobe with a fibrous isthmus, hanging from the left lobe. He cut it off. It weighed 370 grammes (over 14 ounces). The woman nearly died of bleeding the same night, but eventually recovered.
>
> She had worn stays up to eight years ago, but not since then. She had tied her clothes round her waist instead. Langenbuch thinks that the stays caused the elongation, but protected it, and that the painful symptoms, which appeared after she left off stays, were due to strangulation, by petticoat strings, of the already elongated part.

Such an explanation I find it hard to believe. Moreover, congenital deformities have been recorded in infants which closely resemble this. Chaillons[3] showed the liver of a new-born child which had a supernumerary lobe, shaped like a pear, lying to the left of the gall-bladder at the right of the umbilical vein. It is remarkable that the lobe adhered to an umbilical hernia, and had probably been dragged down by it. It is said that Cruveilhier described a similar case, but I cannot verify the reference.

In one case at least the isthmus or pedicle contained no bile ducts.

> A woman of 36 had for twelve years noticed a lump in the right side of the abdomen. It had lately grown fast, while she had wasted, but it had throughout given rise to attacks of severe pain accompanied by vomiting, though not by jaundice. It was found to be an accessory lobe hanging from the right lobe by a pedicle which contained no bile ducts. It weighed 3¾ lbs. when removed, and was thought to contain an early sarcoma.[4]

[1] Langenbuch, Berl. kl. Wochenschft., 1888, vol. xxv. p. 37.

[2] M'Phedran describes a case of deformity in a man. It was, however, unlike the usual form, and the diagnosis rests merely upon palpation as no operation was performed. In such a case I doubt if I should trust my own fingers, and I do not incline to trust those of another.—Canad. Practit., 1896, vol. xxi. p. 401.

[3] Bull. Soc. Anat., 1898, p. 572.

[4] Martin, Birmingham Med. Rev., 1898, vol. xliii. p. 92.

It is probable, therefore, that this class may have to be divided into malformations and acquired deformities, or that in some of the cases congenital abnormality is increased by external pressure.

III. There is a third class in which, owing to disease in the gall-bladder or in neighbouring organs, a tongue of liver is prolonged downward from the right lobe. This is the class which Riedel first distinguished.[1] In 1888 he described and figured six cases which, with attacks of pain in the right side, presented a tumour in connection with the liver which was not the gall-bladder, or not the gall-bladder alone. Bastianelli[2] thus describes it. "This part of the lower border of the right lobe has the form of a thin tongue, comes down as far as the navel, or even further, reaching a length of 10 or more cm., has its left or internal edge palpable or sharp, the right usually to be made out only at the lowest part, while above it is lost in the margin of the liver. It is movable with the latter. Its extremity, the tip, as it were, of the tongue, is more or less rounded, broad, or conical, and often beneath or internal to it the fundus of the gall-bladder is palpable."

Such a prolongation of the liver as this differs from a tight-lace liver in two respects: it shows no indentation, but is level with the rest of the hepatic surface, and it has a sharply defined inner edge.

But such tongue-like processes are by no means in themselves a proof of cholecystitis. Riedel's statement is that "when the abdomen under the process is painful or tender, when symptoms of cholecystitis or of hepatic colic occur, the presence of the process points to an underlying tumour of the gall-bladder." He referred to cases in which such a lobe was present without disease of the gall-bladder, and indeed produced instances where the tongue was attached to a diseased or displaced kidney as evidence that it could be caused by the dragging of inflammatory adhesions.

Many cases have been recorded in which neither cholecystitis nor any other neighbouring inflammation has existed. Some, indeed, have caused no symptoms and have been found unexpectedly in post-mortem examination.[3] Others have been operated upon for symptoms of various degrees of severity. Two such cases have occurred in the hospital during

---

[1] Riedel, Berl. kl. Wochenschft., 1888, p. 577. See also his Gallenstein-krankheit, 1892.

[2] Policlinico, 1895, vol ii. p. 145.

[3] Rolleston (Dis. of Liver, p. 12) quotes and figures such a case contributed by Fisher, and mentions one of his own.

the ten years 1894–1903, and are described in the Statistical Reports by the Surgical Registrar.

In 1898 (Statistical Tables, p. 131) a woman aged 41 was admitted with a hard movable swelling in the right lumbar region, which was thought to be a movable kidney. The right kidney was found to be fixed; the movable body was a linguiform process of the right lobe of the liver. This was fixed to the abdominal wall by the insertion of three deep sutures.

This patient had been admitted in 1896 for pain which was ascribed to a movable kidney. The right kidney had been stitched to the posterior abdominal wall. The pain returned as soon as she left the hospital, and it was thought that the kidney had broken loose. It was not until the tumour was exposed from the front that it was recognised as a projection from the liver.

An exactly similar case was shown at a society by Langenbuch in 1890.[1]

In 1903 (Statistical Tables, p. 176) an envelope-folder, aged 29, first noticed pain in the right side of her abdomen in July 1901. This increased in severity, and as she was unable to follow her occupation she was admitted in February 1902, and appendicectomy performed. At this operation the presence of an accessory lobe to the liver was observed. Pain still persisted, and in October 1902 she was shown at "Consultations," when opinions were against operative measures. On February 20, 1903, as the pain was still unrelieved, she was readmitted. Laparotomy was performed and the projecting mass of liver substance cut away.[2]

IV. The last cause of true deformity of the liver is syphilis. Gummata sometimes produce massive areas of fibrous tissue, which in contracting form deep fissures, and much distort the lobes. I remember a case in our wards in which a tumour thought to be renal was, after the woman's death, found to be the right lobe of a liver scarred by syphilis. The following case is an instance.

A cachectic woman of 43 was admitted to hospital with ascites and an abdominal tumour. At the operation a large tumour was found hanging from the liver and was removed.

[1] Langenbuch, D. Arch. f. klin. Med., 1890, vol. xvi. p 1241.
[2] Lockwood reports this case and another.—Lancet, 1903, vol. ii. p. 223.
Both these seem to have been tongue-like processes, and in each the gall-bladder was natural.

The woman died next day. The tumour was the right lobe of a syphilitic liver. There was lardaceous disease of the spleen and kidneys.[1]

The diagnosis of these cases is often very difficult. In the first place the tumour may not be noticed at all, as in Lockwood's case, until the abdomen is opened. Next, when noticed, it may be easily mistaken for a renal tumour, or a displaced kidney. I made the mistake myself in my first case. But, while not knowing what else to call it, I was puzzled by two points—the sharpness of the inner and lower edges, and the apparent continuity with the liver. When once these points are recognised I do not think a mistake is likely.

But many accessory lobules, which I have placed in the tight-lace class, do not present these signs. The lobule is rounded, and it is separated from the liver by a sulcus so deep, and an area so resonant, that it is really impossible to tell it from a kidney. Such a case has not actually occurred to me. But knowing that it existed, I have made the reverse mistake. I saw, with Mr. Bailey, a lady who had jaundice, colic, dragging pain, tenderness, wasting, and the whole collection of symptoms of gall-bladder disease. She had a large, rounded tumour, which was so movable in respiration, and pushed back so little in the loin, that I thought it was probably an accessory lobe. When, however, cholecystotomy was performed and the gall-stone duly removed, it was quite plain that the round tumour was the kidney, and not any part of the liver.

If the swelling is recognised as hepatic it has to be distinguished from the gall-bladder. It occurs in circumstances which generally coincide with dilation of the gall-bladder, and this would naturally be the first explanation of the tumour that would come to mind. But whereas a gall-bladder is rounded at the sides and below, and unless adherent is movable from side to side, a Riedel's lobe has a hard sharp edge on its inner side which is continuous with the lower margin of the left lobe, and also in most cases a lower border whose thin sharp margin can be taken between finger and thumb. If the gall-bladder is, as sometimes, prolonged below the liver, this point cannot be made out.

I think there can be no question that if any serious symptoms arise laparotomy ought to be performed, and the gall-bladder explored. If this is not done there is always a danger of

---

[1] Wagner, Verhandl. d. deutsch. Gesellsch. f. Chir. xix. Congress, 1890, p. 29. In the discussion which followed Lauenstein quoted a similar case with like result.

. suppurative cholecystitis, and of many still more serious consequences. But unless there is pain or tenderness, I should leave it alone. In my first case I did not advise operation, because it was the first attack of serious colic or jaundice; and she has been well for a year since then. But I think if the case were to occur again I should feel the risk of such a course too great and should advise operation.

CASES OF ASCITES TREATED BY DEPRIVATION OF SALT.

BY

W. P. HERRINGHAM, M.D.,

AND

C. F. HADFIELD.

During the last few years many experiments and observations have been made upon the part played in metabolism by the chlorides.

It was known long ago that the excretion of chlorine was in some pathological conditions much reduced. Redtenbacher made a series of observations on pneumonia in 1850, and many other febrile conditions were soon afterwards found to show the same phenomenon.[1]

It was early concluded, too, from a comparison of intake and output, that in these cases chlorine must in some way be retained within the body, and it was successively suggested—

1. That it formed some close compound with the albumen of the blood;

2. That the kidneys were so affected by the fever that they could not excrete chlorine;

3. That water was retained in the blood, and that the chlorine was retained with it in order to form normal saline solution.

Of these the first and third are not consistent with the facts of chemical analysis, and the diffusible character of the chlorides makes the second improbable.

4. Lastly, the process of osmosis was invoked. Von Moraczewski stated that the tissues contained more water than in

---

[1] In Garratt's elaborate paper on "Metabolism in the Febrile State in Man" (Med. Chi. Trans., 1904, vol. lxxxvii. pp. 163-324) will be found a full account and a bibliography of the chloride question, so far as it relates to fevers. I am much indebted to it.

health, and that the sodium chloride was a necessary constituent of the tissue fluid.

Hijmans van der Bergh thought that the blood became hypertonic, and that the extra molecules passed out into the tissues until equilibrium was established.

These hypotheses are speculative. We do not to this day know where, or wherefore, chlorine is retained.

Of late the study of cryoscopy, or the determination of the freezing point of a liquid, led by von Koranyi of Budapest, has contributed to turn attention to the inorganic constituents of blood and urine. The freezing point of a liquid varies according to the number of molecules that the liquid contains, regardless of their size or weight. It is depressed as the molecular content rises. Osmotic pressure, which also depends upon the number of molecules, rises with the molecular content. The depression of the freezing point below that of water is therefore an expression of the osmotic pressure of any liquid.

Blood is remarkably stable. Its freezing point in health is almost always − 0·56 or 0·57° C., and when it is altered by the processes of health, such as digestion, or by those of disease, such as hæmorrhage or suppression of urine, it has a remarkable power of recovering its molecular equilibrium. This must be carried out by osmosis, and, as the large organic molecules are very indiffusible, the diffusion will be that of the inorganic bodies. Of these the chlorides are the chief, and the importance which they thus seem to possess in redressing the molecular balance of the blood by passing into or out of it as required, has procured them in France the name of "the small change of the circulation." Cryoscopy has been applied to the urine too, but the cryoscopic changes in the urine are too wide in health to allow of their being useful in disease.

Stimulated by these ideas, chemical analysis was applied to the urinary excretion of chlorine in renal disease. It was soon proved that in many cases there was much irregularity, and that in some there was retention. But, as usually happens, nature was found to be little amenable to theory, and the variations of chloride excretion appeared to be independent of any pathological classification. Chloride retention could not, for example, be assigned to any particular anatomical lesion.

Meanwhile another method of investigation was brought into play. We owe chiefly to the French the experimental process which they call "provoked elimination." In it certain substances are administered to a patient in large known doses, and his excretion of them is compared with the standard of health under similar doses. Thus, sugar is used, though its results seem unreliable, to test the adequacy of the liver. For the kidneys, methylene blue, iodide of potassium, and salicylate of sodium had been employed. In 1902 Claude and Mauté wrote a paper on the excretion of chlorides under forced doses (*chlorurie alimentaire experimentale*), and in 1903 Mauté published a book upon the subject. Patients with nephritis vary greatly in their power to excrete 10-gramme doses of sodium chloride. Mauté felt able to say that the prognosis became worse as this power was impaired, and that in that case the intake of chlorides should be proportionally diminished.

Widal and his pupils, Lemierre and Javal, had likewise been giving forced doses of salt. But they used it to study the question of œdema. Renal œdema is so capricious that a few cases of disappearance under a diet poor in chlorides are not of great weight. But in 1903 Widal had a patient in whom he could really show a connection between the two. Whether the diet was of milk or of meat and bread, the abstraction of all possible salt removed the œdema, and the addition of 10 grammes of salt brought it back. Between March 31 and May 25 they altered the diet seven times, always with this result. Zambelli [1] has repeated this experiment with success.

It is only, however, in a few patients that such attempts are successful.

Turning from artificial conditions to those which naturally arise in disease, Achard and Lœper concluded that a connection, though not a close connection, could be found in nephritis between retention of chlorides and œdema. They compare the effect of retention to that of forced dosing, as accumulating chlorides in the body. They discuss various pathological theories, and are convinced that retention cannot be fully explained by renal impermeability alone.

The long series of experiments, and the longer array of theories which I have thus summarised, are of doubtful value. Throughout them runs a possible source of error in the dissimilarity of terms. The chemical analyses have determined for chlorine alone. The theories all apply to the sodium salt. It has without exception been considered that the chlorine whether in the blood, the lymph, or the urine, was there as sodium chloride. The chlorine has been determined, the weight altered to correspond to the sodium salt, and the amount finally stated in terms of this latter.

Seeing that human life is, as it were, a span long, this

[1] Il Morgagni, 1905, May and June.

procedure is natural, for each determination of sodium takes about a fortnight. But it is not exact. Garratt and myself, who have each independently determined sodium in many cases, have found that sodium does not necessarily correspond with chlorine (see Garratt's paper, p. 203). Garratt is of opinion, and it is one which I share, that the two may have different uses. What chlorine is used for Heaven alone knows (I am paraphrasing Garratt), but sodium may possibly be required to neutralise a pathological acid, as we use it, by injection or by the mouth, in the acid poisoning of diabetes.

One of us, from previous work, had learnt that cases of ascites commonly excreted very little sodium and chlorine. It seemed, therefore, worth while to extend the trial of this method to cases of ascitic effusion. Therefore the following four cases—the first three of ascites, due to hepatic cirrhosis, and the latter a case of renal ascites and anasarca—were treated by deprivation of salt, at intervals, over a considerable period of time. The results are, naturally, not entirely conclusive, but seem to afford sufficient ground for making trial of this treatment in cases of recurring ascites.

We have no proof, and it is not contended, that the treatment has any good effect on the underlying pathological condition, but, if it can prolong the periods between successive tappings, even as much as 20 per cent., the advantage to the patient will be great.

The four cases have not been picked out as convincing examples. They are the only cases that occurred during the period in which the treatment was being tried.

The charts give the best general view of the results, and almost explain themselves. The continuous black curve shows the girth of the abdomen in inches, and the red one the amount of urine passed. In order to avoid complexity in the curve, the urine was taken as averages of each period of three days. The periods during which the patients were taking saltless diet are shown by the thick black lines at the top of the chart, and the exhibition of any drug likely to affect the ascites is also indicated in a similar manner.

In Case IV. the intake and output of chlorine is also charted.

The term saltless diet is used for convenience, and does not indicate a diet absolutely free from sodium chloride. Except for a short period at the commencement of the treatment of Case IV. (when he was on "dieta lactis"), the patients were on the ordinary "dieta dimidia" of the hospital (bread, 400 g.; meat, 120 g.; milk, 1200 cc.; potato, 150 g.; butter, and rice pudding). During the saltless periods they were allowed no added salt; they were supplied with bread and butter free from salt. Also their meat, vegetables, &c., were cooked without any added salt, and in water free from salt.

Our thanks are due to Sir Dyce Duckworth and Mr. Waring for permission to use measurements made while Case II. was under their care.

Case I.

T. F., male, chemist's assistant, æt. 50, was admitted to Colston on October 11, 1905, for swelling of the abdomen.

H.P.C.—For many years he has had morning diarrhœa, and for the last three months morning vomiting. In July 1905 his abdomen began to swell, and on August 20 he was tapped in the London Hospital, and 15 pints of fluid withdrawn.

He has had frequency of micturition (especially at night) for several years, but recently his urine has been scanty. He says he has always been a moderate drinker, and that he has never had syphilis.

C.O.A.—Patient has a sallow complexion, and his conjunctivæ are rather yellow. Chest natural, except for some displacement of viscera by the ascites. The abdomen is distended by fluid; no viscus can be felt. There is some œdema of the back and scrotum, and the legs are much swollen.

Pulse, 108: regular; good volume and pressure. Artery slightly thickened.

Temperature, 98·4°; *respiration,* 24.

Urine.—Scanty; contains albumen, blood, and granular casts. No bile.

The patient was tapped on October 15, and his liver could then be felt an inch below the costal margin. He was then put on saltless diet. By November 9 his girth had not increased, so he was given ordinary diet again, and for a few days he took 90 grains of added salt a day. The effect is seen in the chart and the appended figures. On December 26 the saltless diet was begun again. After a few days he lost his appetite and did not seem well (probably due to the onset of the febrile attack which followed), and the diet was relaxed again. Subsequently, however, he was able to resume it without any inconvenience.

At three different times he had sudden febrile attacks, attended with vomiting, anorexia, and much hæmaturia. Each of these lasted three or four days, after which the urine gradually cleared up.

On April 19, 1905, the patient was discharged at his own request, as his girth was remaining stationary. He was subsequently twice readmitted to be tapped.

On June 21, 1905, he was again admitted. He was now in a semi-comatose condition. He gradually became worse, and died on July 9.

At the *post-mortem* his liver was found to weigh 48 oz., and to be invested by false membrane, which could be stripped off, leaving a smooth, thickened, glissous capsule. The liver substance cut very toughly, and showed much fibrous tissue surrounding the lobules, some of which were bile stained. The spleen weighed 12 oz., and there was perisplenitis.

The kidneys weighed: right, 6 oz.; left, 5 oz. They were both engorged; the capsule split on trying to strip it, and the glands showed under the microscope the lesions of chronic diffuse nephritis.

The effect of the saltless diet in retarding the accumulation of the ascites is sufficiently shown by the chart and the following figures (Table I.). As also in Case II. and Case III., the result of the deprivation seems, as one might expect, to persist for some time after it has been discontinued.

TABLE I.

Period.	Ward.	Diet.	Days.	Ascetic Fluid Resulting.	Average Daily Increase.
1	Colston.	{ Saltless, { Ordinary.	24 } 40 }	26 pints. {	? ? 13 fluid ounces.
2	,,	Ordinary (Saltless 5 days).	16	25 ,,	? 31.25 ,, ,,
3	,,	Ordinary.	21	25 ,,	23.8 ,, ,,
4	,,	Ordinary.	22	26 ,,	23.6 ,, ,,
5	,,	Saltless.	42	27 ,,	13 ,, ,,
6 {	Colston. At home.	Saltless. Ordinary.	20 } 23 }	32½ ,,	?
7	At home.	Ordinary.	20	32½ ,,	32 ,, ,,

CASE II.

Mrs. S. G., machinist, æt. 45, was admitted to Elizabeth on April 25, 1905, for swelling of the abdomen and legs.

H.P.C.—For the last two years she has noticed increasing swelling first of the legs and feet, and later of the abdomen. During the same time she has suffered from frequent morning vomiting. The vomit is frequently streaked with blood, and three months ago she brought up about half a pint of blood. She has also been passing very little urine. Since the birth of her last child, eight years ago, she has suffered from bleeding piles. She has been slightly jaundiced for two years, and recently she

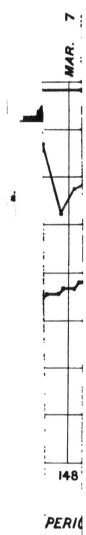

MAR. 7

148

PERIC

13 per

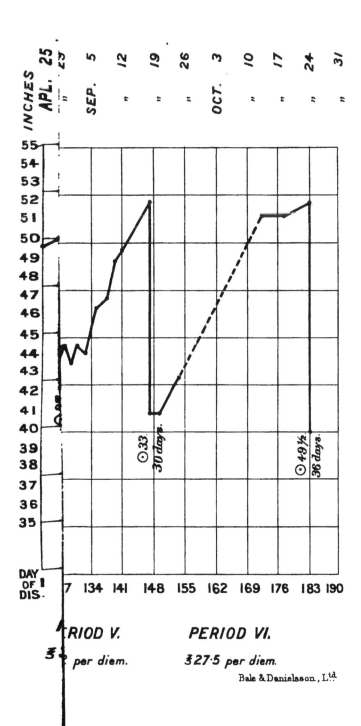

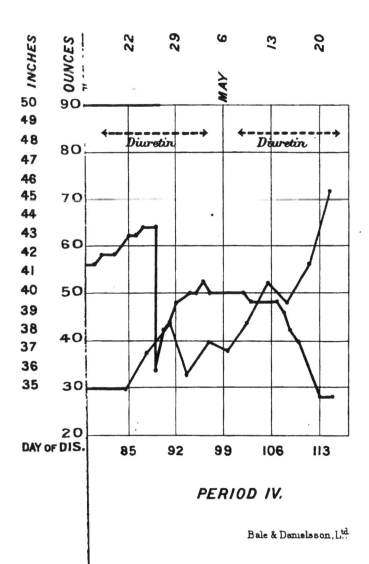

PERIOD IV.

Bale & Danielsson, L.ᵗᵈ

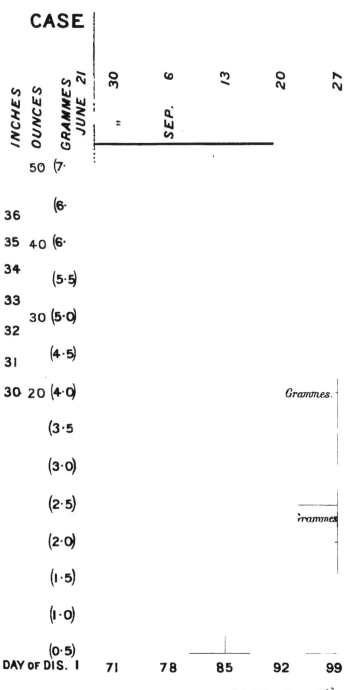

CASE

INCHES OUNCES GRAMMES

JUNE 21
" 30
SEP. 6
13
20
27

50 (7·

(6·
36

35 40 (6·

34
(5·5)

33
30 (5·0)
32

31 (4·5)

30 20 (4·0)   Grammes.

(3·5

(3·0)

(2·5)   ·rammes

(2·0)

(1·5)

(1·0)

(0·5)
DAY of DIS. 1   71   78   85   92   99

Bale & Danielsson, L^{td}

has lost her appetite and thinks she has lost flesh. Always subject to dyspepsia and constipation.

P.H.—No history of syphilis. Takes a pint and a half of ale and a little gin daily.

C.O.A.—Slightly jaundiced, with some dilated venules on cheeks. Tongue furred; abdomen distended by fluid, and some dilated veins are seen on its upper part. The liver could not be felt, but, after tapping, was found to extend 2½ inches below costal margin. There was considerable œdema of the feet and legs.

Pulse, 86: regular; good volume; pressure, 150 mm. mercury. Artery just palpable.

Temperature, 98·6°; *respiration*, 24.

Urine.—Scanty (about 20 oz.). Sp. gr. 1022; acid. No sugar or albumen. Throughout it was quite impossible to measure her urine. It never showed any evidence of kidney disease.

Paracentesis abdominis was performed four times, and then she was discharged at her own request in order to look after her family, and return if necessary.

Later she was admitted to Faith, under Sir Dyce Duckworth (there being no vacant bed in Elizabeth), with her abdomen enormously distended. She was tapped twice. A few weeks later taken into President, under the care of Mr. Waring, with a view to the operation of parieto-portal venous anastomosis. As she was unwilling to have this done, she was transferred to Elizabeth, where she was tapped on the following day, as she had been very greatly distended for many days.

From the chart and Table II. below it will be seen that the ascites accumulated more slowly when the patient was on a saltless diet, and that during the period immediately following the good effect seemed to continue for a time.

She never suffered in any way from the lack of salt, and throughout her general health was exceedingly good.

The period during which she was taking diuretin is charted, but the drug did not make any obvious difference to the amount of urine passed.

Addendum.

Nov. 28, 1905.—The patient was admitted and saltless diet ordered at the time of the last tapping in the table, date Oct. 24. She now requires tapping again, and thus the present interval under saltless diet is only thirty-five days.

TABLE II.

Period.	Ward.	Diet.	Days.	Ascetic Fluid Resulting.	Average Daily Increase.
1	Elizabeth.	Ordinary.	15	28 pints.	37.3 fluid ounces.
2	,,	Saltless.	41	36 ,, [1]	17.5 ,, ,,
3	,,	Ordinary.	31	28 ,,	18 ,, ,,
4	At home.	,,	28	48 ,,	34.3 ,, ,,
5	Faith.	,,	30	33 ,,	22 ,, ,,
6	At home.	,,	37	49½ ,,	26.7 ,, ,,

CASE III.

J. L., male, street musician, æt. 52, was admitted to Colston on January 28, 1905, for swelling of the abdomen.

H.P.C.—Swelling of the abdomen was first noticed two years ago. For one year he has suffered from frequent diarrhœa and morning retching. Slight jaundice has been noticed for six weeks. Recently there has been some frequency of micturition, especially at night.

P.H.—He has been accustomed to take much ale and some spirits. He has had syphilis. At one time he suffered from what appears to have been alcoholic neuritis.

C.O.A.—Skin is bronzed, conjunctions are yellow, and there are dilated venules on the cheeks. Some old-standing ozœna. Tongue furred. Heart and lungs compressed and displaced by ascites. Abdomen contains free fluid, and the liver can just be felt by dipping. Maximum girth, 40½ inches. Some œdema of the legs.

Pulse, 88 : regular ; average volume and pressure. Artery just palpable.

Temperature, 98·4° ; *respiration*, 20.

Urine.—Rather scanty. Sp. gr. 1020. Neutral. Contains some bile but no albumen.

The patient remained in the same condition, with no further increase in ascites until February 15, after which the girth rapidly increased and rendered paracentesis necessary. Following this the reaccumulation was still more rapid, and he was tapped again in 15 days. In the period of saltless diet which followed, paracentesis had not to be performed again for 37 days.

The patient was then again given ordinary diet, and the

---

[1] The drainage obtained at this paracentesis was unusually good. The fluid continued to run for nine hours. At the end there was no sign of ascites, and the girth was less than on any other occasion.

ascites began to return. Soon after, however, the urine increased rapidly in quantity, and the intraperitoneal fluid correspondingly diminished, until on May 20 there was no sign of free fluid in the abdomen. This rapid diuresis may have been helped by the diuretin he was taking, though previously the drug seemed to have little effect.

Apart from the rapid and apparently spontaneous improvement, the effect of the saltless diet may be seen on the chart and in Table III.

TABLE III.

Period.	Diet.	Days.	Ascitic Fluid Resulting.	Average Daily Increase.
1	Ordinary.	? 18 [1]	15 pints.	? 16.6 fluid ounces.
2	,,	15	15½ ,,	20.7 ,, ,,
3	Saltless.	37	15 ,,	8.1 ,, ,,
4	Ordinary.	26	"Hydrops ad Matulam."	

[1] These figures refer only to the time during which the ascites was increasing, and are therefore incorrect, as there was a considerable amount of fluid in the abdomen on admission.

CASE IV.

F. W. J., male, bricklayer, æt. 20, was admitted to Colston on June 21, 1905, for swelling of the face and limbs.

H.P.C.—He caught a "chill" ten months ago, and a month later began to notice swelling of his back and legs. Since then he thinks he has passed less urine than natural, but he has never seen any blood in it. Three months ago his face began to swell. He has twice had to spend some weeks in bed owing to the swelling and stiffness of his legs. He has not suffered from headache, vomiting, twitchings, or diarrhœa.

There is no history of scarlet fever or any other illness.

C.O.A.—Patient has a good deal of swelling of the face, especially round the eyes, and a certain amount of general anasarca. The ophthalmoscope shows nothing unnatural. The tongue is furred. There is some emphysema, and there is hydrothorax at both bases. Heart natural. The abdominal wall is puffy, and there is free fluid in the peritoneal cavity. Considerable œdema of the back and legs.

Pulse, 88: regular; good volume; pressure, 160 mm. mercury. Artery thickened.

Temperature, 99°; *respiration,* 24.

Urine.—25 oz. Sp. gr. 1020; acid. Albumen, 1·2 per cent.; urea, 2 per cent.

After lying in bed six days the anasarca had appreciably diminished, and he was put on saltless diet. On this treatment he improved slowly, and on July 17 there was no free fluid in the abdomen ; the bases of both lungs were more resonant, and the œdema of the back and legs much diminished. The arterial pressure had fallen to 130 mm. mercury. On August 9 he had some venous thrombosis in the right leg, which soon cleared up. On August 22 he was allowed to take a measured amount of salt with his meals, the "saltless diet" being otherwise continued as before. On August 27 there was more fluid in each pleural cavity, and undoubted free fluid in the peritoneum. No increased œdema of the legs. After this the patient got up daily and took a drachm of salt every day. The œdema of the legs and loins distinctly increased, and the general anasarca returned to a certain extent. The shifting dulness in the abdomen is much more marked, and suggests a greater increase in ascites than is shown by the girth measurements.

Careful estimations of the sodium chloride taken, and of the chlorides excreted in the urine were made for a considerable period, and the results are given in the chart and in Table IV., expressed as grammes of chlorine. As in most urinary analyses, the results show such large daily variations that it is difficult to be quite certain that there was retention of chlorine. However, the figures actually obtained certainly indicate a considerable retention, and a retention which was more marked the more salt was taken.

TABLE IV.

The amount of salt contained in the "saltless diet" is an unknown and presumably a constant quantity and is therefore neglected.

Period 1.	Saltless diet . .	Average daily output = 2.69 grammes.
,, 2.	Saltless diet, with 0.8 gramme added salt.	Output should be 2.69 + 0.8 = 3.49 grammes. ,, actually found = 3.1 ,, Chlorine retained = 0.39 gramme.
,, 3.	Saltless diet, with 2.4 grammes added salt.	Output should be 2.69 + 2.4 = 5.09 grammes. ,, actually found = 3.35 ,, Chlorine retained = 17.4 grammes.

The impression left upon us by these cases is that this treatment has, at any rate in some cases, a considerable effect upon the accumulation of dropsical fluid. The deprivation of salt appears to delay the reaccumulation more than any other means at our disposal. It is not so effective as the spontaneous increase of urine. This is always the most favourable event in a case of dropsy. But diuresis is very little under the control of drugs.

The failure of diuretics to produce it in cases of dropsy is indeed so generally the rule that we do not believe the diuresis that cured our third patient was due to our medicines. Short of this a saltless diet seems to have a greater effect than any treatment by derivation.

We did not try forced doses of salt, as we wished rather to test the therapeutic than the pathological question.

THE SEGMENTAL SPINAL SENSORY AREAS CLINICALLY CONSIDERED.[1]

BY

H. H. TOOTH, M.D.

The exact localisation of lesions of the spinal cord is a subject which has made great strides of late years, owing to the researches of many writers, among them Ross, Mackenzie, Head, Thorburn, Allen Starr, and, in the laboratory, Sherrington. By the aid of knowledge gained from many sources lesions may now be located with an exactness which, a few years ago, would have been quite impossible; and compression lesions, such as tumours, are approached and dealt with by the surgeon with the least possible damage to the vertebral column, and with surprisingly favourable results. In the following remarks an attempt is made to illustrate, by means of cases, the upper limit of the altered sensation which follows a lesion of segments of the cord at the levels most useful in practice. Many of these lines of altered sensation are probably correct, and will not in the future be subject to much alteration, but no doubt some will be considerably modified as time goes on. The lesion which gives information of the greatest value is the simple root lesion, but obviously these are comparatively rare, and in most of our cases there is also compression or damage to the spinal cord with resulting paraplegia.

It is of the utmost importance, in this study, for the student to think in term of segments, not peripheral nerves. The roots, both anterior and posterior, which mark the division of the cord into segments, on leaving the vertebral canal, become so intermingled in the plexuses that lesions of the finally rearranged nerve-trunks produce widely different clinical pictures from those of similar lesions of the roots.

[1] This formed part of a paper read before the Abernethian Society, Nov. 1904.

It must also be borne in mind that the area of skin and group of muscles served by a segment are shared more or less by the neighbouring segments, with the resulting overlap which is so marked a feature in the monkey. A practical result of this is that the upper line of anæsthesia, even in complete lesions of the cord, is never sharp, but graduated, as it were, from a slight alteration to some or all forms of sensation, to absolute loss of sensation, often some two or three roots lower. This is not indicated in most of our diagrams; from the point of view of exact localisation by sensation, it is important to take, as the surest guide, the line below which the sensation is *altered*, if ever so slightly, from the normal,

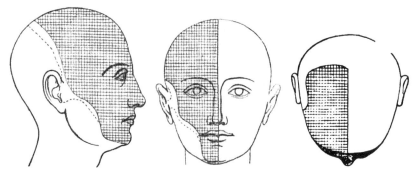

Fig. 1.—Skin field of fifth nerve. The cross-shaded area represents that of complete loss of all forms of sensation. The dotted line indicates the extent of Cushing's area of relative anæsthesia.

whether in degree or kind. Speaking generally, the tendency of the surgeon should be to operate rather above than below the level indicated by the chart of sensation.

I have to thank my colleagues of the National Hospital for their kindness in allowing me to make use of their notes and charts. The cases chosen to illustrate the following remarks are selected from large numbers of cases of lesions at all levels of the cord, and the diagrams are most of them due to the patient labour of some generations of resident medical officers, to whom also I tender my thanks.

The posterior limit on the head and face of the skin field of the fifth nerve gives us the anterior line of the upper cervical roots, and it is important to define this line as accurately as possible. The now common operation of removal of the gasserian ganglion enables us to do this with some certainty, and Fig. 1 may be taken as an example of the distribution of loss of sensation after this operation, making a liberal allowance for individual variation. This subject has been studied with great care by Professor Cushing.[1]

In most cases this observer finds that the posterior line of complete analgesia and anæsthesia does not represent the line or final distribution of the nerve, but that there is another line still farther back, between which and the analgesic line there is a slight alteration of tactile sensation only, represented in Fig. 1 by the dotted line. Possibly this field indicates to some extent the overlap of the fibres of the upper cervicals, including even, perhaps, Cervical 3, as it does in the monkey. It will be seen that besides extending the field of the fifth by an inch more or less beyond the analgesic line, this line defines the sensory distribution of the ear or a part of it. This field then includes the tragus, and just the crus of the helix, but no other part of the pinna; it dips over the tragus to include the anterior half of the external auditory meatus, and that half of the tympanic membrane which lies in front of the dividing line of the malleus.[2]

CERVICAL 1 and 2.—It is probable that the skin field of cervical 1 is very small, if indeed it exists at all. Sherrington,[3] for instance, fails to find it in the monkey. He, however, definitely delimits a skin field for Cervical 2. This has for its anterior border the posterior border of the fifth nerve field. The posterior border was defined by cutting the third and remaining cervical roots, together with those of Dorsal 1 and 2, the sensitive area (the "remaining æsthesia") being that of Cervical 2. This line in the monkey runs from a point 1.5 cm. below the external occipital protuberance outwards 2 cm. below the root of the pinna, just below and behind the angle of the jaw to the lower edge of the cricoid. The skin field therefore includes the external ear. Louis Bolk,[4] in an elaborate and valuable anatomical research, defined in man a skin field for Cervical 2 which corresponds essentially with that of Sherrington; but it is much smaller in extent, as might be supposed, for the scalpel cannot be expected to disclose the ultimate distribution of nerves. According to Bolk, Cervical 2 claims the greater part of the pinna and a narrow strip along lower border of the jaw—that, in fact, left after Krause's operation.

[1] Cushing, The Sensory Distribution of the Fifth Cranial Nerve. Bulletin of the John Hopkins Hospital, vol. xv. 1904, p. 213.

[2] Cushing, *op. cit.*, p. 217.

[3] Sherrington,'On the Peripheral Distribution of the Fibres of the Posterior Roots of Spinal Nerves. Phil. Trans., vol. 190 B., 1898.

[4] Louis Bolk, Die Segmental Differenzirung des Menschlichen Rumpfes, u,s,w, Morpholog, Jahrbuch, Bd. 25, 1898,

The overlap of these skin fields is so extensive, and the area thus assigned on the face to Cervical 2 so narrow, that it is difficult to dissociate this area from that of Cervical 3.

Fig. 2[1] is the sensation chart from a case of torticollis, in which Mr. Ballance divided certain spinal nerves on the left side close to their exit from the vertebral canal. The case lacks, of course, the segmental accuracy of root lesions within the theca, but the distribution of altered sensation on the face and head is so definite that it suggests a root rather than a peripheral distribution, and corresponds with the area defined by Sherrington and Bolk. The loss of sensation to all forms is absolute over the area proper to Cervical 2. Below this there is an area including the whole of the neck on that side to the tip of the shoulder nearly, the sixth cervical spine behind and to somewhat below the clavicle in front, over which there was slight relative hypoalgesia only ; that is, the area proper to Cervical 3 encroaching on that of Cervical 4 somewhat.

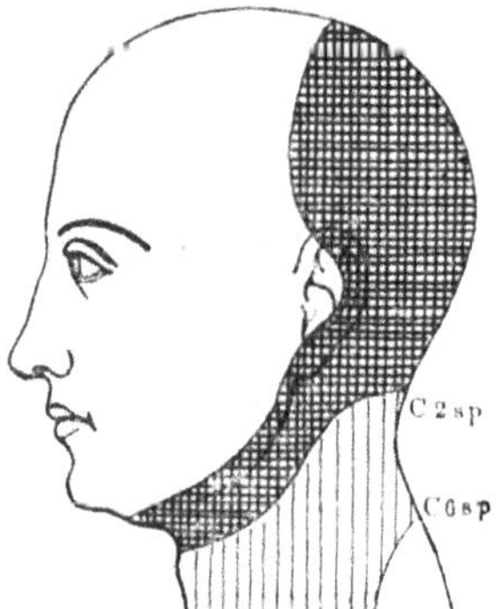

It will be noticed that the upper line of Cervical 2 skin field skirts the concha of the pinna, taking in the lobe, helix, and anthelix, but leaving the concha unaltered. We have traced the posterior line of the fifth to the tragus, so that we have here a little isolated area, including, probably, the posterior wall of the external auditory meatus, for which another nerve supply must be found—the vagus, as suggested by Sherrington.[2]

FIG. 2.—Area of complete loss of sensation (deep cross-shading) following section Cervical 2 root fibres. Slight relative analgesia (vertical shading) over area of Cervical 3.

CERVICAL 3.—The literature on this root area is not large, and is dealt with by Mr. Thorburn[3] in connection with a case

[1] In this and the succeeding diagrams (with the exception of the final three) the parts shaded indicate the extent of altered sensation. The form of sensation affected is shown by the direction of the shading lines : *i.e.* tactile, *horizontal* ; pain, *vertical* ; temperature, *oblique.* Where it is desired to make a comparison between areas in the same chart as regard *degree*, use is made of thick or fine lines.

[2] Sherrington, *op. cit.*, p. 64. This interesting point is discussed also by Cushing, *op. cit.*, p. 229.

[3] Thorburn, A Case of Tumour of the Axis Illustrating the Functions of the Third Cervical Spinal Segment, Brain, vol. xxvi. 1900, p. 120.

of tumour of the body of the second cervical vertebra. The muscles of respiration were absolutely inactive; and respiration was carried on only by the sternomastoid and trapezii. The upper limit of altered sensation (hyperalgesia in this case) was apparently a line running from the spine of the axis horizontally round along the lower jaw margin to the chin, encroaching, therefore, on the area believed to be proper to Cervical 2, as shown in Fig. 2 ; but the line of complete analgesia corresponds closely to that shown in Fig. 2—that is, from the second cervical spine behind to the junction of neck with chin in front. The lower limit is the line of the clavicle in front, but the vertebral point behind is not defined. It is probably the sixth cervical spine.

CERVICAL 4 has for its upper limit about the line of the clavicle in front and the seventh cervical spine behind, its lower line being the second rib in front dipping down at the shoulders to somewhere about the insertion of the deltoids, and rising again behind to about the third dorsal spine. Its shape suggests the milkman's yoke.

CERVICAL 5.—About this area there is little dispute. It is probably not represented on the trunk at all, but on the outer or radial aspect of the arm or forearm from about the middle of the deltoid above to the wrist-joint below, its boundaries on the flexor and extensor aspects of the arm being somewhere short of the median line.

The following instance of injury to the fifth cervical root lacks the certainty conferred on a case by surgical operation, a post-mortem verification, but the area of altered sensation is checked by the very definite muscle symptoms which point to a lesion of the fifth cervical anterior as well as posterior roots. Dr. Ormerod has kindly allowed me to refer to this case.

CASE I.—G. M., a soldier, was thrown from a trap in March 1898. He fell on to his right side. On regaining consciousness he found he could not move his right arm, hand, or fingers, and that he had violent pain in that shoulder.

He was six months in a military hospital, and in April 1899 was operated upon in the Westminster Hospital, but with no benefit. Finally he was admitted to the National Hospital under the care of Dr. Ormerod. Mr. Ballance decided that nothing could be done surgically, and so the patient was discharged.

The muscles wasted and paralysed were as follows : the right supra- and infra-spinati, deltoid, teres major and minor, serratus magnus, pectoralis major (upper or clavicular part, not the

lower or sternal) biceps, brachialis anticus, supinator longus;
in other words, the muscles usually considered as belonging to
the fifth cervical segment. There. was an area of hypoalgesia
as shown in Fig. 3. Bearing in mind the great overlap of
root areas shown experimentally by Professor Sherrington, this
is probably all that can ever be expected in the matter of
degree of analgesia from a single root lesion, and it would be
obviously undemonstrable in an animal.

It is probable that Cervical 5, 6, 7, 8, Dorsal 1, 2, and ? 3 are
not represented as *single root areas* on the trunk at all ; or if so,
only by a band so small as to possess small localising value.

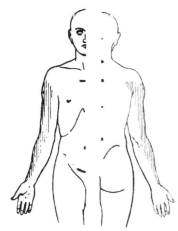

But of course an upper limit
of anæsthesia is definable in
cases of pressure or destruc-
tive lesions of the cord at these
segmental levels, and there is
reason to believe that there is
a zone from, say, the second
rib in front to, say, the fourth
rib which is common to these
root levels; this will be more
fully discussed later.

I am indebted to the kindness of Sir William Gowers
for the following case of compression lesion at the fifth
cervical segment.

FIG. 3.—Hypoalgesic area following
lesion of Cervical 5 posterior
root. Case I.

CASE II.—J. P., a man
æt. 47, was admitted on March
17, 1902. In July 1901 he was
wet through, and his clothes dried on him. Three days after
this he noticed a numbness of the right fingers gradually spread-
ing up the arm. In three weeks the right arm hung paralysed
at his side, and the right side of the body became numbed
during this time. In a month the right leg became weak, and
soon after a tight (girdle) feeling appeared across the abdomen,
and the left leg became paretic. In four months both legs
were paralysed, and the left arm began to show signs of
paralysis. In six months he lost control over his bowels; the
bladder was paralysed.

On admission in March 1902 he was paraplegic, all limbs
rigid, and movements much limited. The highest muscles of
the fifth cervical group were affected—*i.e.* the deltoids and
supra- and infra-spinati were weak, but the pectorales appear
to have been spared.

The upper limit of sensory change is shown in Fig. 4. It runs through the angulus Ludovici in front and about the first or second dorsal spine behind (a little high, perhaps, for this segment). The degree of sensory change was slight, and variable in different parts of the body. The interest in the

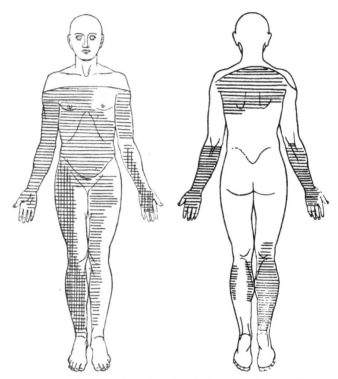

FIG. 4.—Compression lesion, Cervical 5 segment. Case II.

case is, for our present purpose, the upper limit, which gives also the lower limit, probably of Cervical 4.

Sir Victor Horsley operated about six weeks after admission. On removal of the laminæ of the third and fourth cervical vertebræ, the cord was seen to be pressed backwards by an extra-dural growth, the maximum of pressure being at about the fourth vertebra, corresponding, therefore, to about the fifth cervical segment. Above this point the cord pulsated well. The growth was scraped away as far as possible, and in doing so the fourth root, which was much involved, was unavoidably removed with the growth. There was a slight return of pulsation in the cord below the compressed spot after this procedure. It was hardly to be expected that a permanent result could be obtained, but it is recorded that in September, five months after, there was considerable improvement.

The upper limit line assigned to Cervical 5 segment corresponds closely with that of other writers, for instance, Allen Starr.[1]

The next three cervical segments—*i.e.* 6, 7, and 8—are represented as small skin fields on the hand principally. Possibly they may exist also as thin mesial strips, as suggested by Starr,[2] down the back and front of the arms, but this can scarcely be demonstrated in man owing to the overlap. The arrangement probably approximates that made out by Sherrington (*op. cit.*) in the monkey, but it would appear that the overlap in the monkey is much greater than it is in man.

From a clinical point of view it is sufficient to conceive a line drawn down the middle of the ventral, and another down the middle of the dorsal, aspects of the arm and forearm, to about the level of the wrist, and to regard this line as a common upper limit on the arm to the skin fields of Cervical 6, 7, 8, and Dorsal 1 and 2.

CERVICAL 6 skin field includes the thumb and first finger, and probably half the second finger, so that its posterior border may be said to split the second finger.

I have not found a case that satisfactorily illustrates this skin field, but that part of the right hand of Fig. 5 which is unaffected below the wrist-level is that proper to Cervical 6.

CERVICAL 7 area is a small strip on the hand, dorsal and ventral, included between a line drawn down the middle of the second finger and another splitting the ring finger. Its anterior boundary is shown in the diagram below (Fig. 5), on the right side (of the body); on the left side the line more nearly corresponds with the situation of the eighth cervical area.

CASE III.—The patient was a young woman, G. B., æt. 19, under the care of Dr. Bastian, admitted July 24, 1896. The first symptom, as is so often the case, was severe, paroxysmal, local pain, and situated in the region of the right biceps, four years before admission.

This went on without other symptoms until ten months before admission, when weakness of the right leg began to develop, followed in three months by paralysis of the left

---

[1] Starr, Local Anæsthesia as a guide in the Diagnosis, &c. Brain, vol. xvii. 1894, p. 502.
[2] Starr, *op. cit.*, p. 506.

arm, mostly of the extensors, and later by weakness of the left leg, so that she ultimately became quite paraplegic, with occasional incontinence of urine. Three months before admission a hard lump appeared in the right supraclavicular triangle, which gradually increased to the size of an orange.

The line of anæsthesia to touch (Fig. 5, transverse shading) splits the second finger of the right hand, runs up the mid-

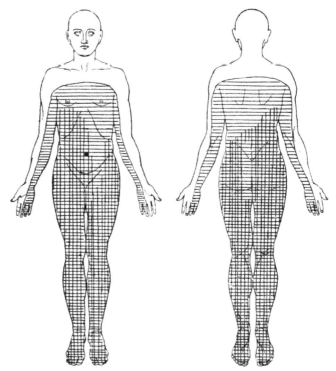

FIG. 5.—Upper limit of Cervical 7 skin field in the right hand, and of Cervical 8 in the left. Case III.

ventral line across the thorax along the second intercostal spaces, and down the left arm much in the same line as on the right, but apparently sparing the second finger. One may infer, then, that the pressure on the cord was more pronounced and extensive on the right side, and this is confirmed by the line of analgesia (vertical shading) shown to reach higher on the right side of the body than on the left, both back and front.

The motor symptoms were more marked in the right hand than the left. There was marked paralysis of the small hand muscles on both sides (Dorsal 1), weakness of the extensors of the forearm on the left side, of the flexors on the left.

Sir Victor Horsley removed the laminæ of the fifth, sixth, and seventh cervical vertebræ, and found that the cord was tightly

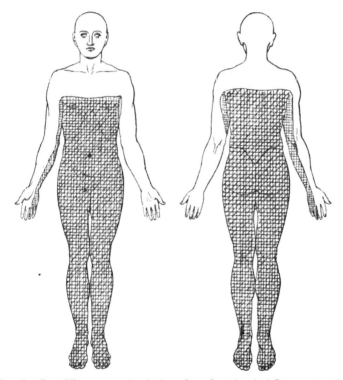

Fig. 6.—Case IV., compression lesion of cord at Cervical 8 segment. On the right arm are shown the sensory area, which includes Cervical 8, Dorsal 1, 2, and 3. On the left Dorsal 3 only.

squeezed by new growth at the level of the seventh cervical segment. There was no improvement, and the patient died five days after operation.

CERVICAL 8 claims the rest of the hand and fingers—that is, the ulnar half of the ring and the little finger, a distribution which coincides closely with that of the ulnar nerve.

It is shown in Fig. 6 on the right side, in so far as the hand is concerned, the area from the wrist to the elbow belongs to

Dorsal 1, and the rest of the anæsthetic area on the arm to Dorsal 2 and 3. On the left arm is indicated the skin field of Dorsal 3 only.

CASE IV.—The patient was a man, T. S., admitted on October 6, 1903, under the care of Dr. Beevor with the following history. Twelve months before admission he felt a "stinging" sensation in the right fourth interosseous space gradually extending up the ulnar side of forearm and back of arm to shoulder. Ten months' painful cramps in the legs, followed four months after by weakness of left leg, later of right, with rigidity of ankle. Three months before admission numbness of legs and feet appeared, and in six weeks there was numbness in the right little finger, since which time he has been quite paralysed and unable to leave his bed. On admission the right arm muscles were generally flabbier and weaker than those of the left; he was completely paralysed below, the breathing being chiefly diaphragmatic. On October 29 Sir Victor Horsley operated, removing the laminæ of the seventh cervical and first two dorsal vertebræ. There was found considerable pachymeningitis and a small cyst on the posterior aspect of the theca. On the right side, at the level of Cervical 8 and Dorsal 1 posterior roots, was a small tumour which compressed the cord. The patient went downhill steadily, and died on March 3, 1904.

We now come to more debatable ground—namely, the position on the forelimbs of the skin fields of the upper dorsal segments.

All writers seem to agree that Dorsal 1 occupies the ulnar aspect of the forearm, from the elbow probably to the wrist. The question, still undecided, is the extent of the fields of Dorsal 2 and 3 on the arm.

In Fig. 7 the upper limit of altered sensation is that of Dorsal 1, but it also includes, of course, on the arm, the skin fields of the two segments below.

CASE V.—The patient was a young woman, L. A., æt. 29, admitted on May 28, 1902, under the care of Dr. Buzzard, with the history, that three months before, she suddenly began to suffer from severe paroxysmal pain in the left shoulder shooting down the left arm, and very much worse at night. One month later it ceased on the left side, and appeared in the right arm and between the shoulders. This lasted six weeks.

One month before admission the legs became weak, first the right and then the left, and for fourteen days she had been unable to stand. No bladder trouble.

Soon after the pain came on, three months ago, the hands became weak, and, from her description, the fingers must have assumed the position of the claw hand.

On admission, the right arm was wasted down the ulnar side; there was hollowing of the interosseal spaces, and flattening of the hypothenar eminence. The grasp was feeble, and

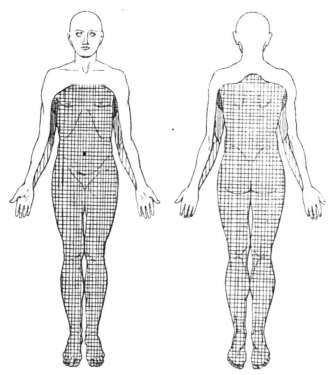

FIG. 7.—Compression lesion of cord at Dorsal 1 segment. The skin fields on the arm of the two first dorsal segments are suggested by degrees of hypoalgesia (vertical shading), the distal being Dorsal 1. Dorsal 3 shows impairment of touch and pain sensation (crossed shading).

accompanied by extension of the wrist. In the left hand the wasting of the small hand muscles was still more marked. This group belongs to the first dorsal segment.

The lower extremities were markedly paretic; that is, all movements could be performed, but feebly, and there was marked spasticity with increased reflexes.

Sensation (Fig. 7).—The upper line of alteration runs from the ulnar side of the wrist up the arm, near the mid-ventral line, across the thorax through the second interspace. Dorsally the line on the arm corresponds in position to that on the ventral aspect, and it runs across the back, cutting the second dorsal spine. In this diagram the area thus marked off on the arm is divided into three divisions by Dr. Singer, who made the clinical note, according to the degree of hypoalgesia. Thus there was a just discernible blunting to pain over the distal division (Dorsal 1), better marked over the middle area (Dorsal 2), and blunting to touch and pain over the small proximal division (Dorsal 3). On the body the anæsthesia to touch and pain becomes more pronounced as we pass down, to be complete below the lumbar region.

On June 4 Sir Victor Horsley operated, removing the laminæ of the seventh cervical and first and second dorsal vertebræ. The bones were found to be softer and more vascular than natural. A circular band of organising granulation tissue about half an inch wide was found constricting the cord between the seventh cervical and first dorsal segments. This was but slightly adherent to the dura, but below it the cord was not pulsating. On removing the band pulsation returned immediately. On the left of the theca also was found a small pocket containing fluid pus; this was thoroughly cleaned out. The operation was entirely successful, and in two days there was a return of sensation in the legs.

The patient was discharged three months after admission, nearly well.

I have not been able to find cases satisfactorily demonstrating the skin fields of Dorsal 2 and 3, but the area of Dorsal 3 is indicated in Fig. 6 on the left side. See also Figs. 7 and 8.

Head places Dorsal 2 on the dorsal half of the upper arm extending nearly to the elbow, and Dorsal 3 on the corresponding ventral half.[1] The arrangement figured by Sherrington in the monkey, however, is probably more nearly that which obtains in man.

The representation on the arm of Dorsal 2 segment, then, is probably a field bounded ventrally and dorsally by the midventral and dorsal lines distally by the elbow and proximally by a curved line corresponding to the junction roughly of the upper with the middle third of the distance between the axilla and the elbow.

The upper third, including the axilla, is probably occupied by the skin field of Dorsal 3. Dorsal 1 and 2, therefore, are detached from the trunk like the cervical areas.

[1] Head, on Disturbances of Sensation, with especial reference to the Pain of Visceral Disease. Brain, vol. xvi. 1903.

In this connection we may refer to an interesting communication by Wallenberg [1] reporting a case of stab wound involving the third dorsal spinal root on the left side. An area of altered sensation was found on the inner aspect of the left arm much as shown in Fig. 8, but smaller in extent. The writer also figures a narrow zone of altered sensation along the third costal cartilage from the sternum to the nipple line, and another posteriorly along the spine of the scapula, so it would appear that this root is represented in the body, and this observation confirms the position of the little pain area, Dorsal 3, on the chest in Head's diagram.

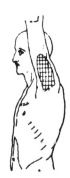

FIG. 8. — Skin field of Dorsal 3 root according to Wallenberg. There is indicated also a small patch of hypoalgesia on the third costal cartilage.

Summary of Distribution of Skin Fields on the Upper Limb.

It will now be seen that the skin fields proper to the segments Cervical 5 to Dorsal 2, and probably also Dorsal 3 inclusive, are situated mainly, if not entirely, on the upper or forelimbs, Cervical 5 occupying the radial aspect of the whole arm to the wrist, and Dorsal 3, 2, and 1 serially from the axilla to the wrist occupying the ulnar aspect. Probably these areas nearly, if not quite, meet in the mesial ventral and dorsal lines, therefore shutting off, as it were, the cervical areas 6, 7, and 8, and conducting them to the hand, as described above. Some writers (Kocher, Allen Starr) figure these little hand areas as long thin strips down the mid-ventral and dorsal aspects of the arm. If this is the arrangement it must be exceedingly difficult to demonstrate, and it is more probable that the areas of the forelimb are disposed in a radial fashion round the mid-ventral and dorsal lines, as shown by Sherrington in monkey, and Louis Bolk in man. The cases quoted in this article are nearly all of them cases of lesion of the spinal cord, not purely of posterior roots. Therefore in every case there is more or less alteration of sensation below a line on the trunk. This line is the continuation of the mid-ventral and dorsal lines of the forelimbs across the body, and probably runs in the second interspace in front (ventrally), and cuts the third dorsal spine behind (dorsally). This line, then, is common to segments Cervical 6, 7, 8, and

[1] Wallenberg, Stichverletzung des dritten linken Dorsal Nerven am Ganglion spinale. Neurolog. Centralblatt, 1901, p. 888.

Dorsal 1, 2, 3, and without the knowledge of the areas on the forelimb exact diagnosis of seat of lesion in the cord would be an impossibility, and an error of five or six roots from the actual lesion would be quite possible.

This common line is indicated in the final diagrams (Figs. 21 and 22) by a thick black line.

Segmental Areas on the Trunk.

The segmental areas on the trunk have been charted with great exactness by Dr. Head, but the method used by him was that of referred pain due to lesions of visceral organs, and the distribution of herpetic eruptions, and therefore the areas assigned by him to the first three dorsal roots on the trunk are of more morphological than diagnostic interest, as regards lesions of the cord at any rate.

From the point of view of localisation we may consider that a lesion of each segment of the cord gives rise to a band of altered sensation round the body, the upper limit of which is fairly constant for each segment. Head's bands are sharply delimited, those due to spinal cord lesions are rarely so, and purely root lesions are the least sharply delimited owing to the extensive overlap between neighbouring root areas.

It will simplify matters if we refer to only the four trunk areas which are associated with well-known landmarks. If these are known the intermediate zones may be placed with quite sufficient accuracy.

DORSAL 5 includes the nipples, but as these landmarks are somewhat inconstant, it would perhaps be better to define the upper limit of Dorsal 5 area as the fourth interspace in front and the fourth or fifth spine behind, but this requires more accurate information than Case VI. affords.

CASE VI.—M. R., a woman æt. 36, was admitted under the care of Sir William Gowers on September 29, 1899, with the history that six months before admission, after a wetting, she had some numbness of the legs for which she laid up for three days, but had no further trouble until six weeks before admission. Then she began to suffer from pain in the left leg, with stiffness and dragging, followed in two or three days by similar symptoms in the right leg. She finally became paraplegic with retention of urine.

The chart (Fig. 9) shows the extent of the altered sensation the day before operation—namely, the fourth rib in front and the sixth spine behind (probably the true dorsal level, for this segment should be at least two spines higher than this diagram shows).

At the operation on November 8, by Mr. Ballance, the cord was found to be not pulsating below the fourth or third dorsal lamina. Unfortunately the note is not more explicit on this point, but under one of these laminæ, probably the fourth— that is, at the fifth segment—there lay on the theca a small

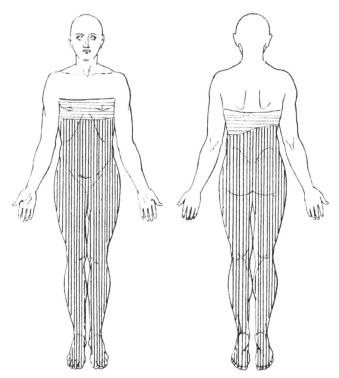

FIG. 9.—Upper limit of altered sensation in compression lesion of cord at level of Dorsal 5 segment.   Case VI.

tumour about ⅜ inch in diameter. It had hollowed out for itself a little cavity in the cord, such as would take the tip of the little finger. Some new growth continuous with this could be traced up on the outer surface of the theca for about 1 inch lying on the right side, and hollowing out in the bone a similar cavity. On removal of the tumour pulsation returned in the cord below.

The patient was able to walk before leaving hospital; that is, seven months after operation.

DORSAL 7.—The upper limit of the skin field of Dorsal 7 is easy to remember, and the landmark is a fairly constant one—namely, the xiphoid cartilage in front, and the sixth dorsal spine behind, as shown in Fig. 10. This case corresponds closely with the one reported by Dr. Hale White,[1] in which an abscess in the vertebral canal was found at this level.

CASE VII.—H. H., a man æt. 47, was admitted on June 17, 1905, to the National Hospital under the care of Sir William Gowers.

Ten years before admission he had noticed a loss of temperature and pain sensation in the left leg, but tactile sensation was not in any degree altered. Five or six years before admission there had been a similar condition of the right leg which eventually became affected more deeply than the left, and the loss of temperature sense, finally extended to the trunk, was high at the lower margin of the costal arch. All this time tactile sensation has been natural.

For eight years also his gait had been affected, owing to a progressive weakness of the right leg, so that dancing became a difficulty to him, though he could still walk several miles. But gradually both legs became weaker.

Two and a half years before admission the dragging of the right leg became more pronounced; but there seems to have been considerable recovery of the left, for on admission there appeared to be little if anything wrong with that leg.

For five or six years also he had suffered from a dull aching pain in the small of the back, and for the same time some difficulty in starting micturition, but no incontinence of urine.

On admission there was nothing abnormal discovered in the upper part of the body, upper limbs, or head.

Trunk.—The respiratory movements were chiefly diaphragmatic. The abdominal muscles were rather rigid, and those on the right side were subject to frequent spasms; but there was no loss of power, for the patient could rise from the lying to the sitting posture without using the hands.

There was slight tenderness of fifth and sixth dorsal spines.

Legs were both rigid; with frequent reflex spasms, most on the right side, and principally extensor. The right leg was almost completely paralysed, but the movements of the left seemed fairly powerful.

[1] Hale White, On the exact sensory defects produced by a Localised Lesion of the Cord. Brain, vol. xvi. 1893, p. 375.

The gait was feeble and spastic, and he dragged both feet in walking, but the right most. Knee-jerks both exaggerated, right most so. Plantar reflex, extensor response.

Sensation.—There was alteration of sensation below a line running through the tip of the xiphoid cartilage in front and the sixth dorsal spine behind. This was the line of analgesia which was complete. Tactile sensation was much less deeply

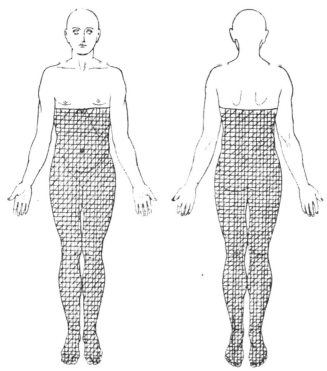

FIG. 10.—·Lesion of cord at Dorsal 7 segment. Case VII. Touch pain and temperature sense impaired. (The upper limit is drawn a little too high in front: it should touch the tip of the xiphoid cartilage.)

affected, and reached to a level $1\frac{1}{2}$ inch below the analgesia line, somewhat more pronounced on the right side than the left.

Thermal anæsthesia to heat was co-extensive with the analgesia, but to cold on the right side reached a level about $\frac{1}{2}$ inch below the analgesia line, and on the left side only to half-way between that line and the umbilicus.

On June 24 Sir Victor Horsley removed the fifth and

sixth dorsal laminæ. The perithecal fat was found to be pushed backwards, especially that under the sixth lamina. When the fat was removed there was found lying on the right side, and outside the dura, and apparently coming from in front, a small elongated cyst ¾ inch long and of the diameter of a lead pencil.

It was thought at the time to be a hydatid cyst. The history, however, of long loss of temperature sense rather suggests some central growth of which this might have been an outlying part.

The patient remained in hospital until September 8; there was some improvement in the power of the legs, but the sensory symptoms remained unaltered.

DORSAL 10.—The umbilicus, according to Head's diagram, lies between the areas Dorsal 9 and 10. There is, in accord with Fig. 11, a chart of the anæsthesia resulting from a tumour situated upon the tenth dorsal root on the left side.

CASE VIII.—G. P., æt. 36, was admitted to the National Hospital under the care of Dr. Buzzard on October 18, 1898. Three months before admission he had suffered from excruciating pain in the back, between the kidneys. Seven weeks before admission the pain had become less, but his legs became weak, first the left and then the right. For three weeks he had been unable to walk, and for the same time there was numbness of the legs to the abdomen. No sphincter trouble.

On admission the lower abdominal muscles were weak; the umbilicus rose 1 inch on attempting to raise the body from supine position.

Legs.—No wasting or rigidity. Left almost completely paralysed. Right, all movements performed, but very feebly. He could just stand when supported. The sensation as charted at this time shows absolute analgesia of right leg and abdomen to level of umbilicus and behind to first lumbar spine. But the left leg from groin downwards shows only relative analgesia and anæsthesia.

November 3.—The paraplegia was complete, with retention of urine.

November 7.—There was noted absolute analgesia and anæsthesia of both legs and abdomen to 1 inch above the umbilicus, as shown in Fig. 11.

November 22.—Sir Victor Horsley operated, removing first the seventh dorsal lamina; finding the cord pulsating, he removed the eighth lamina, and the theca was found to be pressed back against the opening. There was absolutely no pulsation below the ninth dorsal root level. On incision of the theca for about 3 inches a small, smooth - surfaced tumour was found lying to the left of the middle line in the subdural space, and on the tenth posterior root. The cord was much compressed, and a depression was left on removal of the tumour, which was the size of a large hazel-nut.

The day after operation the level of altered sensation was

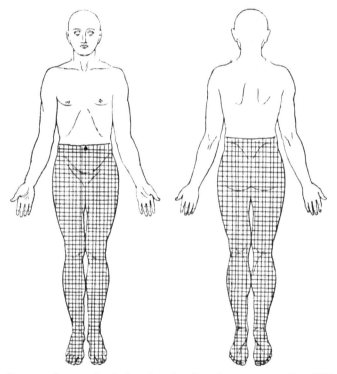

Fig. 11.—Compression lesion of cord at Dorsal 10 segment.   Case VIII.

at least two roots lower, and on November 27, five days after, he could feel as low as the knees and on the soles.

May 6.—He was discharged able to walk.

LUMBAR 1 is placed by Thorburn above the line of Poupart's ligament. In Head's diagram it appears below this line. In all probability Thorburn's conception is the correct one.

Its disposition may be likened to that of an inguinal truss. Its upper limit runs above the pubes, Poupart's ligament, and the anterior superior spine about 1½ inch, and posteriorly about the same distance above the crest of the ilium.

The upper limit of this area is indicated in Fig. 12.

CASE IX.—C. S., a man æt. 48, was admitted to St. Bartholomew's Hospital on August 2, 1904.

On August 1, while moving furniture, he felt weak in his

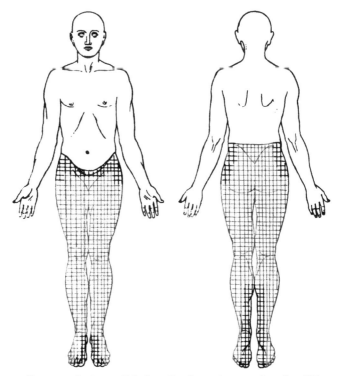

FIG. 12.—Acute myelitis from Lumbar 1 downwards.   Case IX.

legs. On August 2 his legs suddenly completely gave way under him in the street, and he was brought straight from there to the hospital.

There was some slight pain in the loins.

On admission both legs were completely paralysed, flaccid, and devoid of reflexes superficial and deep. At this time there was great alteration of sensation amounting almost to complete anæsthesia and analgesia, below a line through the knees in front in the gluteal region corresponding to Sacral 3;

in other words, the upper limit of anæsthesia indicated a lesion at the level of Lumbar 4. Two days after the upper limit had moved up to the upper third of the thigh (Lumbar 3), and at this time the bladder became completely paralysed with cystitis, and much hæmaturia. Later, the upper limit of anæsthesia, to all forms, settled permanently to a line 2 inches above and parallel to Poupart's ligament in front, and about 1 inch above the crest of the ilium behind (Fig. 12). The sudden onset suggested at first a hæmorrhage into the cord involving the lumbar region, but the patient went steadily downhill, with loss of flesh and persistent cystitis, and died October 4.

Post mortem the cord only was examined and was found to be swollen and softened by acute myelitis through the whole of the lumbar and sacral regions. A careful examination of the cord by serial sections was made in the laboratory of the National Hospital by Colonel Lukis, I.M.S., who found that the highest level of the lesion was Lumbar 1.

LUMBAR 2.—The upper limit of Lumbar 2 is the line of Poupart's ligament, or a little below it, in front and about the crest of the ilium behind.

It is the last of the spinal segments lesion of which gives a *line* of altered sensation encircling the body. It is doubtful whether its root area does surround the body. Reference to the final diagrams (Figs. 21–23) shows that the lower limit of this area is a line more or less horizontal on the ventral aspect of the thigh at about the junction of the upper with the middle third. But the interpolation of Sacral 3, which occupies the genital area, stops the band of Lumbar 2 viewed ventrally; and dorsally it fails to reach a mesial line down the dorsal aspect for the same reason. I have not been able to find an instance of lesion of the cord at this root level. The area therefore must be inferred from the position of the areas above and below.

The remaining spinal segments, Lumbar 3 to Sacral 5 inclusive, are represented on the legs and buttocks only in much the same detached fashion as is seen in the forelimb. The arrangement about mid-ventral and dorsal lines is not obvious, as in the case of the forelimb, but some such plan exists as has been shown in the monkey by Sherrington.[1]

As figured in the final diagrams (Figs. 21 and 22), it will be seen that the skin fields are disposed on the ventral aspect, roughly from above downwards (in the erect position), and on the dorsal aspect from below upwards, the last three sacral

[1] Sherrington, Peripheral Distribution of the fibres of the Posterior Roots of some Spinal Nerves. Phil. Trans., vol. 184, 1893, B. p. 750.

being concentrically arranged around the anus apparently, but more probably around the root of the tail.

Growths in the lower part of the theca are common, and, as they develop, they press upon the roots of the cauda equina. The opportunities of observing pure root lesions are much more frequent, therefore, than in the upper extremities.

LUMBAR 3 occupies about the middle third of the ventral aspect of the thigh, a small part only of the inner aspect owing to the presence of Sacral 2 and 3 (see final diagrams, Figs. 21-23), and about the middle third of the outer aspect of the thigh.

The diagram below was made from a man æt. 38, a patient of Dr. Collier's, in whom was found an abcess in the left loin. The skin fields of Lumbar 3 and Lumber 4 are fairly well delimited on the front of the leg, but the posterior distribution of Lumber 3 does not seem to have been made out. The operation threw no light on the real seat of lesion.

CASE X.—G. L., æt. 38, admitted December 16, 1903, under the care of Dr. Collier, with a history of severe pain in the abdomen just below the costal margin on the left side since May, on and off, for which he had been taking morphia for months. Nothing could be found in the spinal column by examination or skiagraphy except some prominence of the lower dorsal vertebral spines. In February 1904 Sir Victor Horsley excised the eighth left costochondral joint as a probable seat of pain, and the patient was discharged on February 12 apparently much better.

On October 15, 1904, he was readmitted. He said that for some time after the operation he was free from pain, then he began to have a feeling of stiffness about the wound and some pain in the back, and since June 1904 the pain in the back had been continuous almost. Since this date also there had been a feeling as numbness in the front of the left thigh, and there had also been some swelling along the left side of the spine, which was obvious on admission, at about the level of the lowest ribs. The swelling was soft, diffuse, and fluctuating.

Sensation.—On the anterior aspect of the thigh was an area occupying the middle third, as shown in Fig. 13, over which the prick of a pin was so blunted as to be almost unrecognisable as such, and touch also was blunted. This is the area of Lumbar 3, but it should lap round the outer aspect of the thigh to show on the outer third of the posterior as shown in the final diagrams, Figs. 22 and 23. The area below this over which there was only slight blunting to pain and touch corresponds to that of Lumbar 4.

There was no paralysis, but flexion of the left hip was not so strong as that of the right.

The operation on November 24, 1904, by Sir Victor Horsley, is inconclusive as regards localisation. On cutting through

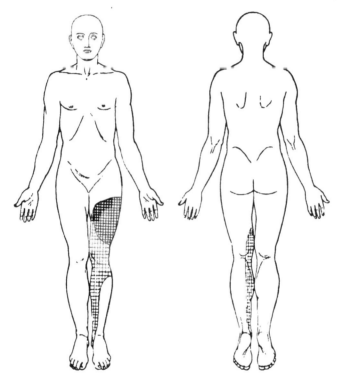

Fig. 13.—Areas of Lumbar 3 and 4 segments. Deep anæsthesia and analgesia indicates Lumbar 3 (in front only); slight, Lumbar 4.

the spinal muscles on the left side, a loculated abscess cavity was found, from which a quantity of pus escaped. It extended a considerable vertical distance and formed a large sac behind the left pleura. Some of the vertebral bodies were found diseased. But it is evident that the affection of the cord or roots was only slight.

LUMBAR 4.—The upper line of the skin field of Lumbar 4 is probably a little above the knee, curved so that the area claims more on the outer and inner aspect of the thigh than on the front. . Owing to the large overlap this outer and inner aspect may be very extensive, and this may explain the large area of the thigh given to Lumbar 4 by Thorburn.[1] The lower or distal limit of this root area is a line which runs on the posterior and outer aspect a little below the knee, obliquely downwards to the line of the shin-bone in front and down that line to a little short of the inner ankle. The inner aspect of the lower third of the thigh, and the whole of the leg to the inner ankle, therefore, is claimed by this segment. It will be seen, however, that the area does not encircle the limb at the knee owing to the strip of Sacral 2, which runs up the back of the leg.

These features are well illustrated by the following case, for the use of which I am indebted to Dr. Beevor, and, for the diagrams, to Dr. Gordon Holmes, then resident medical officer. See also Fig. 13.

CASE XI.—S. Y., a woman æt. 46, was admitted to the National Hospital under Dr. Beevor's care on October 17, 1904. Three years before she had suffered from a tumour of the left breast, which was amputated eighteen months after.

For twelve months she had been losing flesh.

About four months before admission she began to suffer from severe sharp pain in the left leg, along the inner side of the tibia, which would sometimes extend to the knee and above it to the hip on the outer side. Two months after this similar pains appeared in the right leg, but never so severe as in the left. At this time also great pain developed in the small of the back, especially on movement or rotation.

All this time she suffered from progressive weakness of the legs, first in the right, then in the left, so that she had been unable to walk for nearly three months. Seven weeks before admission she had considerable difficulty in passing water, particularly in starting the flow.

On admission the scar of the operation wound of the left breast was firm and healthy-looking, and there was no evidence of recurrence of the growth.

The patient was unable to stand, and the movements of the legs generally were very feeble, those of the left more so than the right.

There was no trace of rigidity. Knee-jerks: right, a trace;

[1] Thorburn, The Sensory Distribution of Spinal Nerves. Brain, vol. xvi. 1893, p. 355.

left, absent. Ankle-jerks absent. Plantar reflex, flexor response.

There was prominence of the third and fourth lumbar spines with considerable tenderness on pressure and great pain on movement, also some diffuse swelling on each side of the prominent spines.

The alteration of sensation is shown in this diagram (Fig. 14), made by Dr. Holmes on the date of admission.

There was decided analgesia and less decided anæsthesia

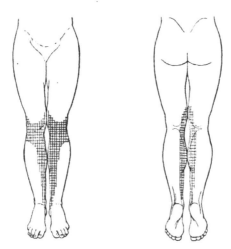

Fig. 14.—Case XI., Oct. 17. Area of Lumbar 4 segment. Touch and pain sensation slightly affected in the right leg ; more deeply in the left.

over the area of Lumbar 4 segment on the left side, and only a slight hypoalgesia of the same area on the right side.

On October 30 another chart (Fig. 15) was made, by which it will be seen that the extent of the area of altered sensation on the left leg had increased so as to include the whole of the anterior aspect of leg and foot below the Lumbar 4 upper line, and posteriorly to reach the upper limit (?) of Sacral 2. The proper root distribution of Lumbar 4 remains on the right side.

On November 6 the chart (Fig. 16) shows involvement of all the roots below Lumbar 4, the upper line of anæsthesia being posteriorly on the buttocks that of Sacral 3.

The patient died on May 16, 1905. Post mortem there was found a malignant growth involving the fourth and fifth Lumbar vertebræ, compressing the roots of the cauda equina.

Microscopical examination showed complete old-standing degeneration of both Lumbar 4 roots, and more recent degeneration of all the roots below this level.

LUMBAR 5.—The skin field of Lumbar 5 appears to admit of little dispute. It occupies the outer aspect of the leg, not including the ankle, which belongs to Sacral 1, and that part of the anterior aspect that is unoccupied by Lumbar 4—namely, all that external to the line of the tibia, and also the dorsum of the foot to the roots of the toes. Posteriorly this area

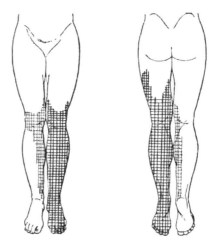

FIG. 15.—Case XI., Oct. 30. Altered sensation indicates involvement of Lumbar 4 roots to Sacral 2 inclusive, on the left side.

occupies only a small part because of the mesially disposed strip of Sacral 1 and 2. I have found no case of isolated lesion of Lumbar 5 segment, but the probable shape of the skin field is indicated in the final diagrams, Figs. 21–23, and also in Fig. 20.

SACRAL 1.—This segmental area is also fairly well defined. It includes the sole of the foot, the toes, and the sides of the foot, including the two ankles; in fact, the part of the foot covered by a golosh, but also extending up the middle line of the posterior aspect of the leg an undetermined distance, probably about half-way to the knee, as a strip about 1 inch to 2 inches wide (Fig. 19).

SACRAL 2.—This area is the least determined, of all the leg areas, both as regards its extent and also its relations with the area next above it—*i.e.* that of Sacral 3. It may be defined roughly as a median strip continuous up the back of the leg with that of Sacral 1. Its configuration as indicated in the final diagram (Fig. 22) must be regarded as provisional only, to be confirmed or altered as cases of isolated lesion arise. At present I know of no such case, and the position of this area must be inferred as lying somewhere between the area of Sacral 3 above and that of Sacral 1 below, as shown in Fig. 19, which is a common one. Some writers, Dr. Head, for instance, figure the skin field of Sacral 2 as surrounding that of Sacral 3, and it is quite possible that that is the true

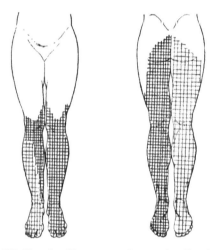

FIG. 16.—Case XI., Nov. 6.   Shows area of sensation, Lumbar 4 to Sacral 3 inclusive.   The upper limit of Lumbar 5 is indicated on the right leg.

arrangement, as is suggested by a consideration of the successive diagrams in the next case (XII.).

SACRAL 3.—This is segmentally represented by an area occupying most of the buttocks, in fact, it may be described as covering all that part of the skin which is pressed when sitting down; so that it presents a somewhat racquet-shaped outline, with the handle of the racquet continued for a short way down the back of the thigh. But this is not all, for this root supplies also a small part, perhaps about a fifth of the upper and inner aspect of the thigh, and with it the genitals, the labia, or the scrotum and penis. This area is well shown in Dr. Head's Case 37,[1] and in Fig. 18 below.

[1] Head, *op. cit.*, p. 82.

SACRAL 4 and 5.—Lesion of these roots gives rise to a circular patch of anæsthesia having the anus nearly in its centre; or more probably the coccyx, suggesting strongly the root of the Simian tail.

These last-described areas, *i.e.* Lumbar 5 to Sacral 15, will be best illustrated by the following case of tumour of the cauda equina.

CASE XII.—K. C., a girl æt. 9, was admitted to the National Hospital under the care of Dr. Beevor on August 7, 1902. Eighteen months before admission, while in church, she suddenly began to cry with severe pain in the left buttock, which has continued with intermissions ever since, but always more severe at night. For six months before admission she had been unable to walk, or stand on the left leg. She had lost flesh generally, and for two months had urethral anæsthesia, so that she did not know when she passed water, during which period also she had suffered from pain round the heel (Sacral 1).

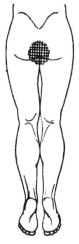

FIG. 17.—Case XII., Aug. 7. Area caused by lesion of Sacral 4 and 5 roots.

On admission the lower spine was rigid, and rotation either way was very limited. There was tenderness on pressure over the second lumbar spine, and some prominence in the sacral region. Both legs more or less paralysed; all movements could be performed, but very feebly.

There was complete incontinence. Knee and ankle jerks absent. Sphincter ani reflex absent. Plantar reflex flexor.

Sensation preserved everywhere except in a small area surrounding the anus, as shown in Fig. 17, from a diagram made by Dr. Grainger Stewart, which was anæsthetic to all forms of stimuli. This is the area of Sacral 4 and 5.

On September 25 the area of loss of sensation to touch and pain had extended on the buttocks, as charted in Fig. 18, it will also be noticed there is a similar loss of sensation on the external genitals. This is the distribution of Sacral 3.

On October 11 the sensory area had still farther extended down the mesial lines of both thighs and legs (Fig. 19), heels, and soles of feet, and in the golosh distribution on the sides and dorsum of feet and toes—the skin fields, in fact, of Sacral 2 and 1. The area of skin affected on the buttocks in this and

the next diagram (Fig. 20) is larger than that shown in Fig.
18, which is a suggestion that Sacral 2 skin field is not merely

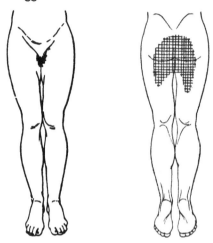

FIG. 18.—Case XII., Sept. 25. Extension of area of altered
sensation proper to Lumbar 3 on buttocks, inner aspect of
upper fourth of thigh and labia.

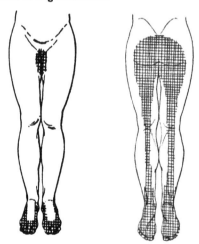

FIG. 19.—Case XII., Oct. 11. Further involvement of roots
Sacral 2 and 1.

a continuation down the leg of the racquet handle of Sacral 3,
but that it has a concentric distribution around Sacral 3.

On November 10 the above observation was confirmed with

the addition that there was found also some alteration of sensation to touch on the outer aspect of the right leg, as shown in Fig. 20, indicating some involvement of Lumbar 5 segment, but the upper line is not typical in its situation.

On November 11 Sir Victor Horsley exposed the sacral and lumbar cord. The theca was large and tense, and on opening it the sacral cord was found to be displaced backwards by a

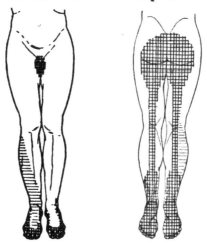

Fig. 20.—Case XII., Nov. 10.   Areas as in the last figure,
but with the addition of a hypœsthetic area in the right leg,
suggesting some affection of Lumbar 5 root.

tumour which lay on its ventral aspect, and further caudal wards along the nerves of the cauda equina.

As much as could be was removed. A month after this there was considerable return of power in the legs, but the distribution of anæsthesia remained unaltered. The patient died on January 1, 1903.

The facts illustrated by the foregoing cases are embodied in the following diagrams, Figs. 21, 22, 23.

The resulting picture is not supposed to be a final one, though many of its details have been defined and accepted by authorities sufficiently often to have therefore stood the test of time. But the diagrams are probably accurate enough to afford a safe guide to the localisation of lesions of the cord and roots for all practical purposes.

Morphologically there is no doubt much room for further accuracy of detail, an end to be attained only in the lapse of time by careful observation.

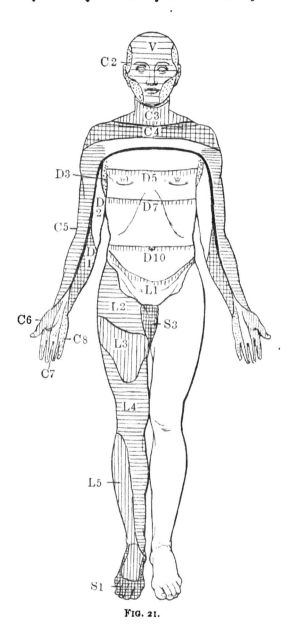

FIG. 21.

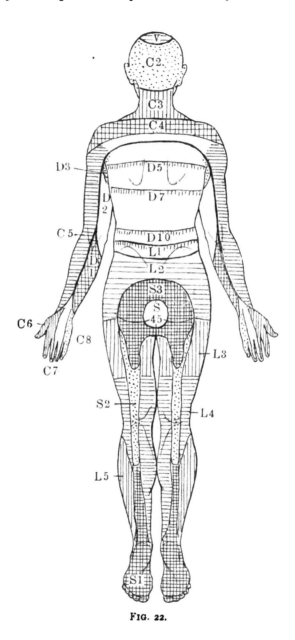

FIG. 22.

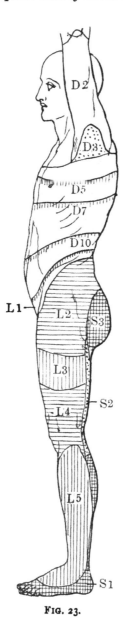

FIG. 23.

A CASE OF ANEURYSM OF THE AORTA

COMMUNICATING DIRECTLY WITH THE SUPERIOR VENA CAVA AND WITH THE LEFT INNOMINATE VEIN.

BY

J. H. DRYSDALE, M.D.

John Thomas D., aged 56, postman, was admitted to Colston Ward on April 29, 1905.

Married. No children; wife no miscarriage.

Previous History. — Syphilis and gonorrhœa thirty years before. Drinks about four pints of beer daily. Winter cough lately.

History of Present Condition.[1]—Patient was quite well, so far as he was aware, till April 1904. On the 27th day of that month, when carrying a heavy packing-case, he suddenly fell and became unconscious. On coming round after two or three minutes he noticed that his face, especially about the ears, was of a blue colour. He was taken to the London Hospital, and remained there under the care of the late Dr. Gilbart Smith two months. Nine months ago he noticed swelling of his face and eyes. (Œdema of the face and head was present a year before—*v.* London Hospital notes.) Three months ago his arms and body began to swell. He has never suffered any pain. Since his illness his voice has been hoarse off and on. No history of dysphagia.

Present Condition.—Patient looks very fat and bloated. The whole face is deeply cyanosed, the lips and ears being almost black. The face and rest of the head are slightly œdematous. The subcutaneous tissue of the neck, especially under the lower jaw, is thickened, and the superficial veins are enlarged. No tracheal tugging.

Eyes. — Conjunctivæ glistening, œdematous, and greatly

---

[1] See also note when in London Hospital, p. 73.

congested.   Pupils equal; they react normally.   Ocular movements natural.

Tongue clean.   Fauces natural.   Vocal cords move naturally.
Pulse, 84; regular; equal on the two sides, so far as could be
determined in face of the œdema.   Hands cold; arms very
œdematous.

Chest.—Barrel-shaped, costal angle wide; moves *en masse*.
The chest-wall is moderately œdematous all over, and covered,
both back and front, with enlarged and varicose veins.   The
cardiac and liver dulnesses are absent.   Owing to the œdema
and fat the percussion note is poor all over the chest.   On
the right side, at the level of the upper border of the second
rib, the note below the inner third of the clavicle and the
sterno-clavicular joint is less resonant than that of the corresponding area on the left side.   The breath sounds are very
feeble everywhere, but no difference can be detected as between
the two sides.   The cardiac impulse is absent, and the heart
sounds are clear but feeble.   All over the front of the chest a
murmur can be heard, the point of maximum intensity being
over the area of impaired resonance at the upper border of the
second rib close to the sternum.   The murmur at this spot is
continuous, occupying the whole period of the cardiac cycle
rising in intensity with each systole and fading gradually away
till it becomes almost inaudible just before the succeeding systolic
re-enforcement.   The diastolic portion is heard over only a small
area, the louder systolic portion alone being perceptible over
the greater part of the front of the chest and over the right side
of the back.   Notwithstanding the thickening and œdema of
the tissues of the neck, a coarse thrill can be felt faintly in the
large veins at each systole.

No abnormal pulsation anywhere over chest-wall.

Abdomen.—The superior epigastric veins are enlarged, but
no enlarged veins nor any œdema is present below the level
of the umbilicus.   Neither liver nor spleen palpable.   No
œdema of legs.

Urine.—Acid: no albumen or sugar.   Temperature subnormal.

Examined with the fluorescent screen, a large aneurysm
could be seen implicating the whole of the ascending portion
of the aorta projecting a considerable distance towards the
right, beyond the edge of the sternum.

May 3.—Patient decidedly more cyanosed.   Complains of
pain in the abdomen; some tenderness over liver.

May 18.—Left arm rather more swollen.   Sleeps a good
deal, but is disturbed by bad dreams.

PLATE I.

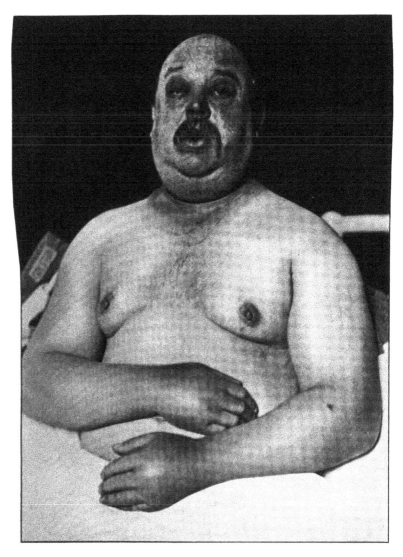

Dr. J. H. DRYSDALE**'s Case of Aneurysm of the Aorta communicating directly
with the superior Vena Cava and left Innominate Vein.

Bale & Danielsson, Ltd.

May 25.—Rather more swelling of both arms. L > R. Wanders very much in his sleep; quite sensible while awake.

June 1.—Œdema increasing everywhere. Says he feels very full in the head.

June 8.—Œdema still increasing; some swelling of the soft palate and pharynx, with slight difficulty of swallowing. Trace of albumen in the urine for the first time since admission.

June 9.—Has had several attacks, during which he falls back and becomes unconscious, respiration ceasing for a few seconds. During some of the attacks slight twitching of the right eyelid and hand were noticed with deviation of the eyes to the right.

June 15.—Patient much worse. He is spitting up some muco-pus. Hands very cold. In the third and fourth intercostal spaces on the right side for three fingers'-breadths outwards from the edge of the sternum, the percussion note is obviously less resonant than before, and the breath sounds are feebler. Signs of fluid at the right base behind. Bronchitic sounds over the left lung.

June 16.—The dyspnœa and the signs of fluid rapidly increased, and the patient died at 3.30 P.M.

By the kindness of Dr. Thompson, the medical registrar of the London Hospital, I am able to append an abstract of the notes taken when the patient was an inmate there.

John T. D. was admitted on April 27, and discharged on June 6, 1904.

He had been ill for two months with pains in the head, shooting up to the side of the neck. He complained of giddiness and staggering. There was dulness over the right upper chest in the first and second spaces in front; there was a very marked systolic thrill over the aortic area, and a systolic murmur over the greater part of the chest; there was œdema of the head and face and cyanosis on exertion; there was a continuous hum heard over the greater part of the right chest and a large portion of the left. The apex beat was displaced downwards and outwards; the pulses were equal; the pupils were equal; the vocal cords moved well, and there was no tracheal tugging. The X-rays showed definite enlargement of the aortic arch. There were signs of diminished air entry into the right upper lobe.

On May 12 he spat up a quantity of blood-stained sputum.

A diagnosis was made of aneurysm of the aorta pressing upon the innominate veins and the upper lobe of the right lung.

Post-mortem Examination.—Marked œdema of the face, neck, arms, and upper part of the trunk, but none of the legs or of the trunk below the level of the umbilicus.

Brain, 48 ozs. "No œdema." Perhaps some slight excess of fluid in the ventricles.

The soft palate and the walls of the pharynx showed a high degree of œdema. The veins of the upper two-thirds of the œsophagus were somewhat dilated, and its walls were swollen and œdematous. The lower third appeared natural.

Larynx, œdematous, but otherwise natural.

Both lungs were congested and œdematous, and each pleural cavity contained about 3 pints of serous fluid.

The heart valves were natural, and there was an obvious hypertrophy.

Apart from the aneurysm, the aorta showed a few scattered patches of atheroma.

Peritoneum.—A few scattered adhesions, otherwise natural.

Stomach, natural. Intestine, somewhat congested.

Liver, 44 ozs.; slightly "nutmeg."

Spleen, 6 ozs.; firm. A few patches of perisplenitis. The other abdominal organs natural.

On opening the chest the whole of the ascending portion of the arch of the aorta was found converted into a globular aneurysm about the size of a cricket-ball. The inner surface of the sac was rough and irregular from atheromatous change, and presented several distinct calcareous plaques. Here and there a few fine filaments of fibrin adhered to the walls, but otherwise there was no sign of any attempt at coagulation. The superior vena cava and both innominate veins at their points of origin were closely adherent to the walls of the aneurysmal sac forming its posterior and lateral walls. In the upper part of the superior vena cava, close to its division, an oval opening, about $\frac{1}{4} \times \frac{5}{16}$ inch, was found communicating directly with the cavity of the sac. About a third of an inch below this was a second small opening, the size of a pin's head, also communicating directly. Half an inch or so to the left of the larger opening in the aneurysmal sac there was a third which admitted a small probe and led directly into the left innominate vein. The superior vena cava and the larger veins of the neck were dilated, and the walls of the jugular and innominate veins were distinctly thickened. The inferior vena cava was natural.

A small portion of lung still covered with pleura formed part of the right posterior wall of the aneurysm, but no leaking or rupture had taken place here or elsewhere excepting always the rupture into the veins.

Considering the comparative frequency with which aneurysm of this part of the aorta occurs, communications between the sac of such an aneurysm and the superior vena cava are exceedingly rare. This is partly due, no doubt, to the fact that the superior vena cava may be pressed upon and displaced to some extent without adhesions being formed between the two vessels, but also and to a greater extent to the well-recognised tendency of aneurysms in this situation to make their way forwards and to the right.

On the first inspection of the patient it was evident that pressure was being exerted on his superior vena cava. The physical signs pointed to some "tumour" in the mediastinum, and when the patient was placed before the screen the sac of the aneurysm could be seen plainly pulsating in the situation of the tumour. The presence of a continuous murmur reinforced at each cardiac systole made the diagnosis sufficiently certain.

The chief point of interest of this case lies in the length of time —more than thirteen months—over which the patient survived the establishment of the communication. The great majority of cases die within a few weeks, or even days, and the longest period of survival I can find record of is seven months (quoted by Pepper and Griffith).[1] The absence of all symptoms before the sudden onset was most probably due to the small size of the aneurysm at that time; the consequent minor degree of external pressure, the signs of which but slowly increased afterwards, must have favoured his long survival. In connection with the communication between the sac and the left innominate vein it will be seen from the notes that the œdema became at a certain date better marked in the left arm. Another point which may be noticed in comparing the notes during his stay in the two hospitals is the great effect that the œdema of the chest-wall had in obscuring all physical signs, and especially in limiting the area over which the continuous murmur could be heard. In the absence of this continuous murmur cases of this kind are difficult or impossible to diagnose, but in this instance the history of the very sudden onset with loss of consciousness followed immediately by cyanosis and œdema was sufficiently striking to suggest the condition even before the physical examination had got beyond the stage of inspection. The condition of the patient contrasts well with another who is attending as an out-patient

[1] Amer. Jour. of Med. Sc., 1890.

at the present time. The physical signs of obstruction of the superior vena cava and of thoracic "tumour" in the same situation as in the first patient are practically identical, but the continuous murmur is absent, and before the fluorescent screen no sign of an aneurysm can be seen. The onset also, it may be noted, was gradual, and the diagnosis is new growth of the mediastinum.

ALBUMINOUS EXPECTORATION FOLLOWING PARACENTESIS OF THE CHEST.

BY

P. HORTON-SMITH HARTLEY, M.D.

PART I.

I am indebted to Sir Dyce Duckworth for permission to publish the following case of albuminous expectoration, which occurred in his wards during the present year. To Dr. Gee also I am indebted for the notes of his unpublished case which is described in Table II. To both I desire to express my cordial thanks.

A Case of Albuminous Expectoration following Paracentesis of the Chest in a Patient suffering from Pernicious Anæmia.

John Abraham Brown, aged 56, butcher, was admitted into Matthew Ward under the care of Sir Dyce Duckworth on April 6, 1905, complaining that during the last twelve months he had gradually been getting paler and weaker. During this time he had also lost 3 stone in weight and had been somewhat constipated.

Past History.—Patient was born at Braintree, in Essex, but since the age of 18 had lived in London. He had always enjoyed good health, was a teetotaller and a non-smoker. His circumstances had always been good. He married thirty-two years ago; had eight children living, while three others died in infancy.

Family History.—His father died of cancer, but otherwise there was nothing abnormal to note.

Condition on Admission.—On admission patient was found to be a man looking somewhat old for his age. He was well nourished, and there was still a good deal of subcutaneous fat, but he was markedly anæmic, and the skin had a slightly yellow tinge. The temperature was 97°. His tongue was pale, moist, and clean. His teeth and appetite were good.

On examining the chest, the apex beat of the heart was found in the fifth space within the nipple line. The cardiac dulness extended .to the third rib above, and to the left border of the sternum. On auscultation a soft systolic murmur was heard at the apex, but apart from this the sounds were natural. His pulse was 74 per minute, small, soft and regular. The vessel wall was somewhat thickened.

The lungs were natural; the respirations 22 per minute.

The abdominal organs were natural.

The knee-jerks were present, and neither ankle-clonus nor Babinsky's sign was obtained.

The skin showed no hæmorrhages.

The urine possessed a specific gravity of 1016, was acid, somewhat dark in colour, and did not contain either albumin or sugar.

The stools were formed and normal in appearance.

An examination of the blood revealed the following changes :—

Red corpuscles	.	.	.	941,000 per cubic millimetre.
Hæmoglobin .	.	.	.	30 per cent.
Colour index .	.	.	.	1.6.
White cells .	.	.	.	8,800 per cubic millimetre.

Under the microscope poikilocytosis was observed in a high degree, but nucleated red corpuscles were not seen.

A diagnosis of pernicious anæmia was made.

The patient was treated with arsenic ($\mathbb{M}$iv.–$\mathbb{M}$vii. of the liquor arsenicalis three times a day) and for a time seemed to improve. His appetite became better, and he appeared less pallid.

On May 27 the improvement was confirmed by a blood examination, which showed the red corpuscles to number 1,100,000, per c.m., and the white corpuscles 7,600. The hæmoglobin was 25 per cent. The improvement was, however, transitory, and in the middle of June he became obviously paler, very weak, and dyspnœic on the slightest movement. On the 12th of the month œdema of his legs and back was noticed, probably dependent upon dilatation of the heart, which at this time made itself apparent, the apex beat being situated in the fifth space, 1 inch outside the nipple line, and the right border of the cardiac dulness extending a finger-breadth beyond the right border of the sternum. The systolic apical murmur conducted towards the axilla was still present.

On July 1 the patient was worse. The legs and loins were œdematous, and the scrotum and penis were in a similar condition, and the œdema caused some difficulty in micturition. In addition a double hydrothorax had developed, the dulness extending on the left side up to the angle of the scapula and on the right to the mid-scapular region. Breath sounds and vocal vibrations were absent over the dull area. The liver was enlarged and tender.

The blood examination made on this day gave the following result :—

Red corpuscles	920,000 per cubic millimetre.
Hæmoglobin	28 per cent.
Colour index	1.5.
White corpuscles . . .	7,200 per cubic millimetre.

Differential count of leucocytes—

Polymorphonuclears	60 per cent.
Lymphocytes	36 „
Eosinophils	3 „
Myelocytes	1 „

Poikilocytosis was present, and a certain number of nucleated red corpuscles were observed.

On July 4 the patient's condition had not improved at all. The œdema and hydrothorax still remained, and on the slightest movement his breath became distressingly short. It was decided, therefore, to aspirate the chest in the hope of affording some relief.

Paracentesis was accordingly performed, at 4.0 P.M., on the right side, in the mid-axillary line, in the seventh space, a Garratt's syphon-apparatus being employed.

The patient lay on his left side during the operation, and the liquid from the syphon tube was received into a vessel placed on the floor by the side of the bed about 3 feet below the level of the puncture. The flow was easy and gradual, and in about fifteen minutes 4 pints of ordinary yellowish serous fluid had been evacuated. The flow then ceased, and the cannula was removed from the chest. During the paracentesis the patient was somewhat anxious and was given brandy, but after the completion of the operation he recovered and appeared for a time quite comfortable.

At 4.50 P.M., however, about half-an-hour after the completion of the operation, he began to cough. At first little or no expectoration was brought up, but after five minutes he began to bring up much liquid, so intimately mixed with ai that it appeared as though foam were welling from his mouth. On auscultating the chest abundant crepitations were heard over both lungs. The attack continued for about ten minutes

(4.55–5.5 P.M.), when the severity of the cough and the amount of liquid brought up diminished somewhat and the patient became more quiet.

But the amelioration of the symptoms was only transient. At 5.15 P.M. the cough returned, and with it the expectoration of foam and fluid. So quickly and in such large quantities were these brought up that when he was turned on to his right side they ran from his nose and mouth. Till 5.50 P.M. the patient remained conscious, endeavouring, by coughing, to free his tubes from the liquid which was slowly drowning him. His strength then gradually failed, he became unconscious, and died at 6 P.M.—one hour and three-quarters after the conclusion of the paracentesis. During the attack oxygen and injections of strychnine were freely employed, but apparently with little or no benefit. Owing to the continual flow of liquid from the mouth swallowing was impossible, and brandy was therefore not administered.

The frothy fluid expectorated was collected and soon resolved itself into a yellowish amber-coloured, albuminous and somewhat viscid fluid, with a layer of foam (now much diminished in amount) resting on its surface. Its appearance so closely resembled that of the fluid removed from the chest that the occurrence of a perforation of the lung at once suggested itself to the sister in charge of the case. The further characteristics of the fluid are more fully set forth below. In all, about 2 pints were brought up.

POST-MORTEM EXAMINATION.

On July 5, eighteen hours after death, I performed the post-mortem examination, with the following result.

Nature of Disease.—"Pernicious anæmia. Fatty degeneration and dilatation of heart. Anasarca and hydrothorax. Extreme œdema of right lung. Death following 'albuminous expectoration.' Arrested phthisis."

External Appearance.—Body anæmic but well nourished; œdematous, especially over the legs and scrotum.

Brain.—44 oz.—natural.

Eyes.—Natural. No hæmorrhages into the retinæ.

Mouth.—Teeth in very good condition. No sign of oral sepsis.

Œsophagus.
Cervical Glands. } Natural.
Larynx.

Trachea and Bronchi.—In the right bronchus and in the lower portion of the trachea was a clot of a light greenish-yellow colour, which lay loose in the air-passages and occupied about ⅛th of their lumen.

Lungs.—The right lung weighed 34 oz. It was in a condition of marked and general œdema, the liquid pouring out when a section was made. A portion cut off floated in water, but only with difficulty. The surface showed no sign of any wound or puncture, the pleura covering it being quite natural. There was no pneumo-thorax. Apart from the œdema the organ showed no morbid change, either to the naked eye or when examined microscopically. There were no clots in any of the pulmonary vessels.

The left lung weighed 16 oz. It showed no œdema, and, except for the presence of a small patch of arrested tubercle at the apex, was natural.

The left pleural cavity contained 4 pints of serous fluid; the right about ¾ pint. Both were otherwise natural.

Heart.—Weight, 9 oz. The right side was much dilated—the tricuspid orifice admitting four and a half fingers. The left side was less enlarged—the mitral admitting two and a half fingers. The muscle was exceedingly flabby, and definite streaks of fatty degeneration were seen in the papillary muscles of the left ventricle. The valves were natural.

The aorta showed a few small patches of atheroma not far from the cusps, but was otherwise natural.

The pulmonary artery and veins were natural. They showed no clot themselves, nor was any clot found in any of their branches.

Peritoneum.—Contained ¾ pint of serous fluid, but was otherwise natural.

Stomach.—Walls thin and atrophied.

Intestines.—Natural.

Liver.—Weight, 60 oz. It gave the iron reaction, but otherwise appeared natural.

Spleen.—Weight, 6 oz.; was soft, but otherwise natural. It did not give the iron reaction.

Pancreas.
Abdomial Lymphatics. } Natural.
Suprarenals.

Kidneys.—Each weighed 4½ oz. Both showed a fair iron reaction, and the right contained on its surface a cyst the size of a small marble. Otherwise natural.

Ureter and Bladder. } Natural.
Organs of Generation.

Bones.—A longitudinal section of the left tibia showed the fatty marrow to be replaced by red marrow throughout the whole bone.

Microscopical Examination.—A portion of the right lung, hardened in formalin and stained by Dr. Riviere, showed practically all the alveoli distended with a finely granular material staining faintly with eosin, and presenting the usual characters of pulmonary œdema. Apart from this the microscopical appearance of the lung seemed natural. The vessels in the walls of the alveoli showed no evidence of passive congestion, there were no desquamated epithelial cells, or escaped red corpuscles in the alveolar spaces, in these respects the specimen contrasting strongly with the appearances seen in œdema of the lung, the result of cardiac failure.

CHEMICAL EXAMINATION OF (A) THE FLUID EXPECTORATED.

Carried out in the Laboratory for Chemical Pathology, St. Bartholomew's Hospital.

When first brought up the expectorated material was so intimately mixed with air that it resembled foam. After some hours the air-bubbles gradually disappeared and a transparent liquid showing the following characteristics was left. In colour it was amber, deeper than that of any ordinary pleural or peritoneal exudation, and deeper than that of the fluid actually withdrawn from the patient's pleura, which, as we shall see, was more straw-coloured in appearance. It showed a slight but definite viscidity, when moved from side to side of the vessel in which it was contained, possessed a specific gravity of 1024, and was faintly alkaline in reaction. Except for some strings of mucus floating in it, and probably coming from the buccal cavity, it was transparent and clear. When filtered from the threads of mucus and tested with glacial acetic acid, no precipitate of mucin was obtained. It contained no sugar; but on boiling became quite solid with precipitated proteid. When tested in the manner described below, the proteids present in it were found to consist of both "albumin" and "globulin," each in large quantities. Albumose and peptone were absent.

Tests.—

On half saturating a portion of the fluid with ammonium sulphate a dense precipitate of "globulin" was obtained, and on filtering this off and boiling the filtrate a further heavy precipitate of "albumin." The filtrate from the latter gave only the faintest xanthoproteic reaction, and no definite re-action with the biuret-test, thus proving the absence of albumose and peptone.

QUANTITATIVE DETERMINATIONS.

With the help of Dr. Hurtley, Demonstrator of Pathological Chemistry in the Medical School—to whose cordial assistance I desire to express my great indebtedness, and who is alone responsible for several of the quantitative estimations made—the following results were obtained:—

1. *Total Proteid.*

> *Method of Procedure.*—100 cc. of the fluid, filtered to clear away the strings of mucus floating therein, were slightly acidu-lated with acetic acid, and then gradually raised to the boiling point. The precipitated proteid was filtered off, washed with boiling water until the filtrate gave no further precipitate with silver nitrate solution, then dried at 110° C., and cooled in a desiccator until a constant weight was obtained.

Estimated in this way 100 cc. of the expectoration were found to contain 4.8054 *grms.* of proteid.

2. *Total Ash.*—Estimated by Dr. Hurtley as follows :—

> 50 cc. of the fluid were evaporated to dryness in a platinum basin, at first over a water bath, later at 110° C. The residue was then gradually burnt over the flame, but never above a dull red heat, until ash only remained. It was then cooled in a desiccator and weighed.

50 cc. of the expectoration were found in this way to contain 0.4992 *grm.* of *total ash*, giving a percentage of 0.9984 *grm.*

3. *Chlorides.*—Estimated by Dr. Hurtley as follows :—

> The total ash obtained in estimation No. 2 was dissolved in water to which a little dilute nitric acid had been added, and the chlorides then precipitated by a known quantity of deci-normal silver nitrate solution. The excess of silver nitrate added was then determined by Volhard's method.

Estimated in this way, 50 cc. of the expectoration were found to contain 0.2164 grm. chlorine, or 0.3566 grm. sodium chloride, if the whole of the chlorine were present in this combination—*giving thus a percentage of 0.4328 grm. chlorine, and 0.7132 grm. sodium chloride.*

4. *The Freezing Point.*—A cryoscopic determination, made at the suggestion of Dr. A. E. Garrod, to whom I am also indebted for many further hints, yielded the following result.

The freezing point of water was found to be 0.08, while that of the expectoration was 0.73. The freezing point was thus lowered 0.65°.

5. *The Pigment.*—As already stated, the expectoration was of an amber colour when viewed by the naked eye. Examined directly by the spectroscope without any treatment, a marked cutting off of the blue end of the spectrum was observed, but no definite bands.

Treated with alcohol and ether, the pigment went readily into solution; but here, again, no bands could be seen in the liquid, but merely a cutting off of the blue end of the spectrum.

(B) THE FLUID REMOVED BY PARACENTESIS FROM THE RIGHT PLEURAL CAVITY.

Let us now contrast the nature of the expectoration just described with that of the serous fluid removed from the right pleural cavity shortly before death. The comparison is of interest since it has been sometimes thought that the albuminous expectoration is nothing more than the pleural fluid coughed up through a wound in the lung.

The fluid removed by paracentesis was of the light yellow colour usually possessed by such effusions, and differed, therefore, in shade from the amber hue of the expectoration. Its specific gravity was 1014; it was not viscid. It was faintly alkaline in reaction. The addition of glacial acetic acid produced no precipitate showing the absence of mucin. On boiling, after faintly acidifying with acetic acid, a heavy precipitate of coagulated proteid was obtained, but the liquid did not become "solid with albumin," as did the expectoration. As with the latter, the proteids were found to consist of albumin and globulin, each in large quantities. Albumose and peptone were absent. The fluid contained no sugar.

QUANTITATIVE DETERMINATIONS.

The methods of procedure employed were the same as those used in the case of the expectoration, and need not therefore be again described in detail. Tested thus, the following results were obtained.   .

1. *Proteid :*—

> 100 cc. were found to contain 1.5357 *grm.* of proteid.

2. *Total Ash :*—

> 50 cc. were proved to contain 0.3919 grm. of total ash, giving a percentage of 0.7838 *grm.*

3. *Chlorine and Chlorides :—*

50 cc. of the liquid were found to contain 0.1839 grm. chlorine, or 0.303 grm. of sodium chloride, if all the chlorine were present in this combination. Expressed as percentages the following figures were obtained :—

Chlorine	. . . .	0.3678 grm. per cent.
Sodium chloride	. . .	0.606 „ „

4. *The Freezing Point.*—A cryoscopic determination showed that the freezing point was lowered 0.53°.

5. *The Pigment.*—When the fresh liquid was examined with the spectroscope, the blue end of the spectrum was found to be much cut off, but, as in the case of the expectoration, no bands could be observed. On further testing it was found that the yellow pigment did not go into solution in ether, or in alcohol-ether, as did the pigment of the expectoration, suggesting that some change had taken place in the original colouring matter, or possibly the difference may have been due to some subtle variation in the reaction of the two liquids.

The following table shows at a glance the points of similarity and of difference exhibited by the two fluids, and proves that in many respects they differ materially from each other.

TABLE I.—*Showing the Chemical Composition of the Expectoration, and of the Fluid Removed by Paracentesis from the Pleural Cavity.*

No.	Expectoration.	Effusion.
1	Faintly alkaline	Faintly alkaline.
2	Somewhat viscid	Not viscid.
3	Amber coloured	Light yellow in colour.
4	Specific gravity, 1024	Specific gravity, 1014.
5	Contained no mucin in solution . .	Contained no mucin.
6	On boiling became solid with precipitated proteid.	On boiling showed a dense precipitate of proteid, but did not become solid.
7	Contained 4.8054 grms. per cent. of proteid.	Contained 1.5357 grm. per cent. of proteid.
8	Total ash, 0.9984 grm. per cent. . .	Total ash, 0.7838 grm. per cent.
9	Chlorine, 0.4328 grm. per cent. . .	Chlorine, 0.3678 grm. per cent.
10	Chlorine expressed as NaCl, 0.7132 grm. per cent.	Chlorine expressed as NaCl, 0.606 grm. per cent.
11	Lowering of freezing point, 0.65°. .	Lowering of freezing point, 0.53°.
12	Contained no sugar . . . : . .	Contained no sugar.
13	*Pigment.*—The liquid showed no absorption bands. The pigment was soluble in alcohol and ether.	*Pigment.*—The liquid showed no absorption bands. The pigment was not soluble in alcohol and ether.

PART II.

Instances of albuminous or serous expectoration following paracentesis are very uncommon, and it may be of interest now to analyse the chief features of those cases which have been recorded. They are not numerous. Records of 40 cases have been found in literature by the writer, and though Riesman [1] in his recent paper, with its excellent bibliography, gives certain further references (to which, unfortunately, access has not been found possible), it is probable that even including these, and also the two new cases described in this paper, the total number of instances recorded does not total 50. Nevertheless, the condition, though rare, is not quite so uncommon as these figures would suggest, since inquiry has proved to the writer that not every case has been recorded.

In the year 1873 a careful analysis of the cases up till then recorded was made by Terrillon [2] in his memorable thesis. Since then other cases have been published, and it seemed to the writer that an investigation of the salient features of the total number might prove of value. The result is set forth in the following table (see opposite page).

Let us now analyse a little more closely certain of the data given in this table.

Sex.—From a study of the table it will be seen that of 42 cases, in 30 the patients were males, in 12 females. This predominance of the male sex is seen both in the fatal cases and those ending in recovery. Of the former, 5 out of the 7 were males; of the latter, 25 out of the 35. This increased liability amongst males, though marked, is not easy to account for.

Age.—Of 34 patients in whom the age is recorded, one (No. 32, published by Dr. Gee in 1886) was in his twenty-first year, but this is the earliest age at which the condition is actually described. An unrecorded case is, however, known to the writer in which the complication occurred after paracentesis in a girl aged 9½, so that tender years are no bar to the affection, though it is undoubtedly very rare in early life.

[1] David Riesman, M.D., Albuminous Expectoration following Thoracocentèse. Amer. Journal of the Medical Sciences, vol. cxxiii. 1902.
[2] Terrillon, De l'expectoration albumineux après la Thoracentèse. Paris, 1873.

TABLE II.—*Showing Certain Points of Interest in Forty-two Cases of Albuminous Expectoration following Paracentesis of the Chest (Arranged in order of Date).*

A. *Cases Ending in Recovery.*

No.	Reference.	Sex.	Age.	Side.	Nature of Disease.	Amount of Fluid withdrawn from Pleural Cavity.	Moment of Commencement of the Attack.	Duration of Attack.	Amount of Expectoration.	Appearance of the Albuminous Expectoration.	Remarks.
1	*Pinault*, Thèse de Paris, 1853. Obs. 2, p. 11. Quoted also by:— *Terrillon*, De l'expectoration albumineuse après la Thoracentèse. Paris. 1873. Obs. 19.	M.	47	R.	Acute Pleurisy with effusion.	2500 cc.	A little time after the paracentesis.	24 hours.	A good quantity, but exact data not given.	"A viscid, greenish liquid, exactly resembling the fluid withdrawn from the pleura."	
2	*Pinault*, loc. cit. Obs. 3, p. 14. *Terrillon*, loc. cit. Obs. 20.	M.	34	L.	Subacute Pleurisy with effusion.	3000 cc.		36 hours.	2 cups full (500 cc.) and more.	"Resembling the liquid withdrawn from the pleura."	
3	M. Beenler's case. *Faussillon*, Thèse de Paris, 1864. Obs. 3. *Marrotte*, Bull. de l'Acad. de Med., 1872, p. 447. *Terrillon*, loc. cit. Obs. 7 and 18 (the case being quoted twice with slight variations by this writer.)	M.	36	L.	Acute Pleurisy with effusion.	3000 cc.	Apparently began during the operation.	6 hours.	2–3 glasses (probably about 350 cc.).	A clear, yellow, serous, and viscid fluid, covered with froth, resembling the liquid withdrawn from the pleura.	

TABLE II.—A. *Cases Ending in Recovery (continued).*

o.	Reference.	Sex.	Age.	Side.	Nature of Disease.	Amount of Fluid withdrawn from Pleural Cavity.	Moment of Commencement of the Attack.	Duration of Attack.	Amount of Expectoration.	Appearance of the Albuminous Expectoration.	Remarks.
4	*Béhier*, Bull. de l'Acad. de Med., 1872, vol. i. pp. 696, 722. *Terrillon*, loc. cit. Obs. 4.	M.	62	1. R. 2. L. 3. L.	Double Hydrothorax, secondary to Morbus Cordis.	1. 800 cc. 2. 1400 cc. 3. 800 cc.	1. 1 hour after paracentesis. 2. 1 hour. 3. ½ hour.	1. 4 hours. … …	1. 800 cc. 2. 1100 cc. 3. 700 cc.	'A frothy serous fluid, rather deeper yellow, but almost absolutely similar to that withdrawn from the chest.'	*Three aspirations each followed by albuminous expectoration.*
5	*Berruyer*, Thèse de Paris, 1872, p. 36. *Terrillon*, loc. cit. Obs. 3.	M.	56	R.	Hydrothorax, secondary to Morbus Cordis.	2500 cc.	½ hour after paracentesis.	½ hour.	"A cupful" (probably about 250 cc.).	"Quite analogous to that withdrawn from the pleura, but rather more viscid and covered with a blood-stained foam."	9 subsequent aspirations (460 cc.–3200 cc. withdrawn) not followed by albuminous expectoration. Death 2 months after the attack. *P.M.*—Aortic stenosis, with pleural effusion limited by adhesions between the base of the lung and the diaphragm.
6	*Marrotte*, Bull. de l'Acad. de Med., 1872. Tome i. p. 446. *Terrillon*, loc. cit. Obs. 8.	M.	24	L.	Acute Pleurisy with effusion.	2000 cc.	Interval doubtful, but at least 1 hour after the paracentesis.		⅓ of a spitpot (about 100 cc.).	A viscid, transparent, citron-coloured liquid, covered with foam.	

							Duration doubtful, but some hours.			
7	Marrotte, Bull. de l'Acad. de Med., 1872, p. 447. Terrillon, loc.cit. Obs. 6.	M.		R.	Acute Pleurisy with effusion.	5000 cc.	"Some hours after the paracentesis."	Duration doubtful, but some hours.	"More than a cup full" (probably about 300 cc.).	"A serous fluid, resembling that withdrawn from the pleura."	One subsequent aspiration (3000 cc.) not followed by albuminous expectoration.
8	Potel, Thèse de Paris, 1872. Terrillon, loc. cit. Obs. 17.	M.	40	R.	Subacute Pleurisy with effusion.	3500 cc.	1 hour after paracentesis.	11 hours.	"Six spit-pots" (about 1500 cc.).	"A viscid, citron-coloured liquid, covered with froth; analogous to that withdrawn from the chest, though of greater density."	
9	Woillez, Traité des maladies signés des organes respiratoires, 1872. Obs. 57, p. 468. Marrotte, Bull. de l'Acad. de Med., 1872. Terrillon, loc. cit. Obs. 5.	M.	22	L.	Acute Pleurisy with effusion.	5500 cc.	"Towards the end of the operation."	Probably only a few minutes.	"A few mouthfuls."	Transparent and yellow.	
10	Bernier, L'Union Médicale, 1873, vol. xvi. p. 51.	M.		...	Acute Pleurisy with effusion.	2600 cc.		Several days.	50-60 cc.	Citron-coloured; covered with foam.	
11	Dujardin - Beaumetz, L'Union Médicale, 1873, vol. xv. pp. 941. 959.	F.	22	R.	Hydro-pneumo-thorax.	360 cc.	½ hour after paracentesis.	Several days.	Probably 50-100 cc. a day.	A viscid liquid, covered with yellowish foam, and showing beneath it on standing a layer of mucopurulent material (see Table VII.).	

TABLE II.—A. *Cases Ending in Recovery* (continued).

No.	Reference.	Sex.	Age.	Side.	Nature of Disease.	Amount of Fluid withdrawn from Pleural Cavity.	Moment of Commencement of the Attack.	Duration of Attack.	Amount of Expectoration.	Appearance of the Albuminous Expectoration.	Remarks.
12	Lande, Mémoires de la Société de Médicine et de Chirurgie de Bordeaux, 1873, p. 371.	M.	...	L.	Phthisis, with recent Empyema.	1. 2000 cc. creamy pus. 2. 1000 cc. pus.	...	1. 2 days. 2. 1 day.	1. 250-300 cc. a day. 2. 300 cc.	Viscid, very frothy, white in colour, with some nummular sputa floating in it.	Two aspirations, each followed by albuminous expectoration.
13	Lande, loc. cit., p. 262.	M.	21	L.	Acute Pleurisy with effusion.	3000 cc.	½ hour after paracentesis.	12 hours.	"Very abundant."	Light yellow in colour, very frothy, resembling in appearance the liquid withdrawn from the chest.	...
14	Lande, loc. cit., p. 264.	F.	25	R.	Acute Pleurisy with effusion.	1800 cc.	1 hour after paracentesis.	10 hours.	More than 1000 cc.	Citron-coloured, slightly viscid, resembling closely the liquid withdrawn by paracentesis.	
15	Rasmussen, Irish Hospital Gazette, Dec. 1873, vol. i. p. 369.	F.	37	L.	Acute Pleurisy with effusion.	5¾ pints.	15 minutes after paracentesis.	Duration doubtful, but some hours.	¾ pint.	Greenish yellow, and similar in appearance to that drawn off by aspiration (see Table VII.).	
16	M. Moutard-Martin's case. Terrillon, loc. cit. Obs. 9.	M.	68	R.	Acute Pleurisy with effusion.	3000 cc.	2 hours after paracentesis.	30 hours.	2 litres.	"Resembling the fluid withdrawn by paracentesis."	

No.	Reference	Sex	Age	Side	Disease	Quantity removed	Interval after paracentesis	Duration	Quantity of expectoration	Character of expectoration	Remarks
17	M. Hérard's case. *Terrillon*, loc. cit. Obs. 11.	F.	27	...	Acute Pleurisy with effusion.	2000 cc.	Interval after paracentesis doubtful.	20–24 hours.	500 cc.	Yellow, and very frothy.	
18	M. Hérard's case. *Terrillon*, loc. cit. Obs. 12.	F.	27	...	Acute Pleurisy with effusion.	2000 cc.	Interval for paracentesis doubtful.	20–24 hours.	500 cc.	Yellow, and very frothy.	
19	*Terrillon*, loc. cit. Obs. 13.	M.	42	R.	Hydro-thorax, secondary to Morbus Cordis.	2000 cc.	At least 1 hr after ...	A day and a night.	2 spitoons (about 500 cc.).	A frothy, transparent, viscid liquid (see Table VII.).	
20	M. Demos' case. *Terrillon*, loc. cit. Obs. 14.	F.	35	L.	Acute Pleurisy with effusion.	2000 cc.	"Some time after paracentesis."	2 days and a night.	5 spit-oups (about 1250 cc.).	"A frothy, lightly coloured liquid, evidently mixed with sputa."	A previous aspiration (200 cc. removed) was not followed by albuminous expectoration.
21	*Terrillon*, loc. cit. Obs. 15.	F.	30	L.	Acute Pleurisy with effusion.	2000 cc.	½ hour after paracentesis.	2 hours.	"Very abundant."	"A frothy, slightly stringy liquid."	
22	M. Vulpian's case. *Terrillon*, loc. cit. Obs. 16.	M.	37	L.	Acute Pleurisy with effusion.	1500 cc.		6 hours.	250 cc.	"A stringy, somewhat frothy expectoration."	...

TABLE II.—A. *Cases Ending in Recovery (continued).*

o.	Reference.	Sex.	Age.	Side.	Nature of Disease.	Amount of Fluid withdrawn from Pleural Cavity.	Moment of Commencement of the Attack.	Duration of Attack.	Amount of Expectoration.	Appearance of the Albuminous Expectoration.	Remarks.
23	*Terrillon*, loc. cit. Obs. 21.	M.	49	L.	Hydrothorax, secondary to Morbus Cordis.	1200 cc.	1 hour after paracentesis.	At least 6 hours.	...	Very frothy, at first blood-stained.	Died two days later. *P.M.*—Double aortic disease with mitral and tricuspid regurgitation. Some effusion in both pleurae. Lobar Pneumonia (red hepatisation) R. lower lobe.
24	*Drivon*, Lyon Médical, 1874, vol. xv. p. 536.	M.	56	...	Chronic Pleurisy with effusion.	1. 1600 cc. 2. 2450 cc.	1. Immediately after paracentesis. 2. "A short time" after paracentesis.	1. ... 2. 24 hours.	1. 2 spit-cups (about 1000 cc.). 2. 750 cc.	Covered with foam, greyish in colour, very viscid (see Table VII.).	Two aspirations, both followed by albuminous expectoration.
25	*Labouldene*, Gazette Hebdomadaire de Med. et de Chirurgie, 1874, vol. xi. p. 654.	M.	21	L.	Acute Pleurisy with effusion.	2655 cc.	Began 24 hours *before* the paracentesis (during which time 120 cc. were brought up) and continued for 7 days *after.*	8 days.	100-150 cc. a day.	Covered with foam, colourless, viscid (see Table VII.).	

No.	Reference	Sex	Age	Side	Disease	Quantity	Time	Duration	Quantity	Character of fluid	Remarks
26	*Laboulbène*, loc. cit., p. 656.	F.	23	L.	Acute Pleurisy with effusion.	3000 oc.		Some hours.	Abundant.	With f em, aly resembling the liquid with-win from the pha.	
27	*Pepper*, Philadelphia Medical Times, Aug. 1874, vol. iv. p. 718.	M.	...	...	Chronic Pleurisy with effusion.	3¾ pints.	18 hours after paracentesis.	24 hours.	"3 gills."	"It laid so closely the fluid win off from the ht as to tact the mice of the fay."	
28	*Prévost*, Gazette Mé i-cale de Paris, 1875, p. 236.	M.	44	R.	Sarcoma of Lung and Pleura, with secondary effusion.	3200 cc. of a reddish-brown hæmorrhagic fluid.	"A few moments after the paracentesis."	Apparently some hours.	500 oc.	A yellow, serous fluid (not hæmorrhagic), covered with a layer of foam.	It aspirated many ies, bt on he hr en did this po-toration low, go l ing taken to aspirate slowly, and completely empty-ing the pha. P.M. (4 months later).—Sarcoma of R. lung and R. pl wn.
29	*Fraser, Donald*, British Medical Journal, 1876, vol. ii. p. 110.	F.	"young married lady."	L.	Recent Empyema of large size.	1 oz. of pus.	"A few hours after para-centesis."	2 days.	"A large quantity."	A clear, trans-lucent fluid.	The clear albu-minous sputum was mixed with the mucopurulent material usually brought up by the patient.

TABLE II.—A. *Cases Ending in Recovery (continued)*.

No.	Reference.	Sex.	Age.	Side.	Nature of Disease.	Amount of Fluid withdrawn from Pleural Cavity.	Moment of Commencement of the Attack.	Duration of Attack.	Amount of Expectoration.	Appearance of the Albuminous Expectoration.	Remarks.
30	Dieulafoy, De la thoracentèse par aspiration dans la pleurésie aiguë. Paris, 1878, p. 30.	M.	…	…	acute Pleurisy with effus dn.	1450 cc.	½ hour after paracentesis.	…	100 cc.	…	Two earlier aspirations (each 1000 cc.) *not* followed by albuminous expectoration.
31	Leichtenstern, Deutches Archiv. f. Klin. Med., 1880, vol. xxv. p. 365.	M.	…	…	"A large Empyema."	…	…	Several hours.	¼ litre.	'Serous. Slightly dd-stained."	…
32	Gee, S. J., St. Bartholomew's Hospital Reports, 1886, vol. xxii. p. 99.	M.	20	L.	Hydrothorax, …ary to malfor-… …tin of he ….	1. 2 pints 13 oz. 2. 1 pint 9 oz. 3. 3 pints 8 oz.	3. "Almost immediately" after paracentesis.	1. Some hours. 2. … 3. 2 hours.	2. "Abundant po…tortation." 2. Some, (but not amb) al b-…is ex-…tion. 3. 2 …	"Viscid, frothy, cl ar (ht with brownish- ed ediment), yellowish-green in ol a. It seemed to om-sit of … mixed with small i…s of mucus …d pa". (see … VII.).	*Three aspirations, all follow ed by albuminous expectoration,* though on he third occasion Dr. Ge remarks, "… W, we …d the … … …n off very slowly." P.M. (2 weeks …)—Malfor-…tin of the R. …de, …de hydrothorax, …d …l dropsy.

33	*West, S.,* Transactions of the Clinical Society, 1896, vol. xxix. p. 169.	M.	40	R.	Ae Pleurisy with effusion.	2 pints.	10 minutes after paracentesis.	3 hours.	1 pint.	" A frothy fluid."	...
34	*Gee, S. J.* The case occurred in St. Bartholomew's Hospital in 1897, and is now first published with Dr. Gee's consent.	M.	52	L	Hydrothorax, secondary to chronic nephritis with bronchitis ad m-physema.	3 pints.	" Immediately after" paracentesis.	2 hours.	1 pint.	"Orange-coloured albuminous sputa."	A second aspiration (3½ pints) was not followed by any albuminous expectoration.
35	*Riesman, D.,* Amer. Journal of the Medical Sciences. Jan.–June 1902, vol. cxxiii. p. 620 (with Bibliography).	F.	48	R.	Sarcoma of media-... ith ... pleural fin, of al or nt, ad lly some tin.	3 pints.	" Toward the end of the tapping.	5–6 hours.	160 cc.	Turbid, amber-coloured fluid, covered with thick froth, and containing a few streaks of blood.	Wo 1 tar pin- tis of 2 nt 3 pits eh we nt fol led by this min. *P.M.* (5 las later).—Sarcoma of the itr ld.

TABLE II. (*continued*).—B. *Fatal Cases.*

o.	Reference.	Sex.	Age.	Side.	Nature of Disease.	Amount of Fluid withdrawn from Pleural Cavity.	Moment of Commencement of the Attack.	Duration of Attack.	Amount of Expectoration.	Appearance of the Albuminous Expectoration.	Remarks.
36	Case of M. Girard. Gaz. des Hôp., 1864. No. 55, p. 218. *Terrillon*, loc. cit. Ob. 2. *Foucart*, Thèse de Paris, 1875. Obs. 7.	F.	25	L.	Acute Pleurisy with effusion.	1000 cc.	"10 minutes after the operation."	Fatal in a minute or so.	"Abundant white foam."	"Abundant white foam."	P.M.—Both pleuræ contained 500 cc. serous fluid. Both lungs somewhat ...ticken, and lower third of R. lung ...ingly ...unh engorged, sinking when placed in ...ter.
37	*Terrillon,* loc. cit. Obs. 1.	M.	32	R.	Acute Pleurisy with effusion.	1200 cc.	25 minutes after the paracentesis.	Fatal in 15 minutes.	350 cc.	A frothy liquid.	P.M.—R. pleura still contained 300 cc. fluid. R. lung ... no injury, but it was œdematous, especially in its ...ter and middle ...bes. The upper lobe of R. Lung and whole of L. Lung ...nd old tuberculous ...stie, with much fibrosis.

No.	Reference	Sex	Age	Side	Diagnosis	Amount removed	Time	Result	Amount brought up	Character of fluid	P.M.
38	Legendre, E., Gaz. des Hôpitaux, Jan. 30, 1875. p. 90.	M.		L.	Acute Pleurisy with effusion.	3000 cc. or more.	"A few moments" after the conclusion of the operation.	Fatal in 5 minutes.	"thick foam" (amount not specified).	"Thick foam" alone brought up.	No P.M.
39	Scriba, E., Deutsches Archiv. für Klin. Med., Band xxxvi. 1885, p. 328. Kredel, Berlin. Klin. Woch., 1882, p. 673.	F.	25	L.	Subacute Pleurisy with effusion.	1600 cc.	*Immediately* after the trocar had been removed and the operation finished.	Fatal in 6 hours.	1000 cc.	Light yellow in colour, covered with foam. "In colour, specific gravity, and albuminous contents just like the pleural effusion."	*P.M.*—Pregnant woman. Old tuberculosis L. lung. Tuberculosis of L. pleura, peritoneum, and spleen. *Extreme œdema of L. lung, less so of R.* Completely filling L. main bronchus, and extending into the finer bronchi of second and third order was a fibrinous clot containing numerous air-bubbles. No sign of puncture of lung.
40	Gee, S. J., St. Bartholomew's Hospital Reports, vol. xxii. 1886, p. 100.	M.	40	L.	Hydrothorax, secondary to lymphadenoma.	3 pints.	3–4 mins. after the paracentesis.	Fatal in 25 minutes.	Apparently a good quantity. "It came out in gushes from his mouth and nose."	Clear, yellow, frothy liquid (see Table VII.).	*P.M.*—Great mass of lymphadenoma in upper part of anterior mediastinum. Small amount of serum in both pleuræ. *Lungs œdematous* and showing no sign of injury.

TABLE II.—B. *Fatal Cases* (*continued*).

	Reference.	Sex.	Age.	Side.	Nature of Disease.	Amount of Fluid withdrawn from Pleural Cavity.	Moment of Commencement of the Attack.	Duration of Attack.	Amount of Expectoration.	Appearance of the Albuminous Expectoration.	Remarks.
41	Hayem and Tissier, Revue de Médicine, vol. ix., 1889, p. 27.	M.	44	R.	Acute Pleurisy with [...].	2500 cc.	20 mins. after paracentesis.	Fatal in a few minutes.	500 cc.	"The expectoration was [...]hy, yellowish-red in colour, and resembled [...] the liquid withdrawn from the [...], [...] kept in being more viscid."	P.M.—Arrested [...] in R. apex. [...] on the surface of both lungs; some [...] in both pleurae. Tuberculous pericarditis.
42	Sir Dyce Duckworth's case (recorded in this paper).	M.	56	R.	Hydrothorax, secondary to pernicious anaemia and dilated heart.	4 pints.	½ hour after paracentesis.	Fatal in 1¼ hour.	2 pints.	Amber-coloured, transparent, viscid liquid, covered with a layer of foam.	P.M.—Pernicious [...]. [...]ion and [...]ion of heart. [...] œdema of R. lung (34 oz.). L. lung natural (16 oz.). No sign of injury to lung.

The following table shows the various ages at which the condition has been noted.

TABLE III.—*Showing the Age-incidence of the Affection in Thirty-four Cases.*

Age	20–30		30–40		40–50		50–60		Over 60	
Sex	M.	F.	M.	F.	M.	F.	M.	F.	M.	F.
Cases ending in recovery	5	5	3	3	6	1	3	...	2	...
Fatal cases	...	2	1	...	2	...	1	...	...	...
Total	12		7		9		4		2	

The table shows that the condition is very rare before the age of 20 and occurs most often between the ages of 20 and 30, while between the three decades of 20 to 50, 82 per cent. of all the cases are included. This age-incidence is doubtless connected in some degree with the fact that acute pleurisy with effusion, to which the complication is most often a sequel, is certainly less common in childhood than in the adult, and more frequent during the years of early manhood.

Side of Chest Affected.—The complication may follow paracentesis whether of the right side of the chest or of the left, but is somewhat more frequent in the case of left-sided effusions. Thus, out of 37 instances it followed paracentesis of the left side on 22 occasions, of the right side on 15. A somewhat similar result, it may be added, was found by Wilson Fox in the case of simple pleurisy with effusion, the left side being affected rather more frequently than the right.

The Nature of the Effusion.—In more than half of the cases recorded, whether death or recovery has ensued, the primary disease necessitating paracentesis has been an acute pleurisy with sero-fibrinous effusion. In a smaller percentage the effusion has been a hydrothorax the result of failing heart or chronic renal disease, or secondary to malignant growth in the chest. In a few cases the effusion has been purulent.

The following figures show the relative frequency of the various conditions.

TABLE IV.—*Showing in Forty-two Cases the Nature of the Effusion which necessitated Paracentesis.*

Acute pleurisy with effusion	23
Subacute „ „ „	3
Chronic „ „ „	2
Suppurative pleurisy or empyema	3
Hydro-pneumo-thorax	1
Hydrothorax from failing heart	6
Hydrothorax from chronic renal disease	1
Serous effusion secondary to malignant disease of the lung and pleura	2
Serous effusion secondary to lymphadenoma	1
Total cases	42

The Moment of Commencement of the Attack.—The time at which this curious and often very serious complication makes its appearance is subject to marked variations. Thus of 35 cases in which the moment of onset is noted, in 3 it occurred before the conclusion of the paracentesis; in 9 either immediately afterwards or within a few minutes; in 11 there was an interval varying from ten minutes to half-an-hour; in 5 the interval was an hour, while in 6 others the interval was even longer, reaching in one case eighteen hours. The following table shows the time of onset in greater detail.

TABLE V.—*Showing in Thirty-five Cases the Moment of Onset of the Condition.*

During the operation	3		
Immediately after the operation	6		
Within a very few minutes	3	}	9
10 minutes after the operation	2		
15 „ „ „	2		
20 „ „ „	1	}	11
25 „ „ „	1		
½ hour „ „	5		
¾ hour „ „	1		
1 hour „ „	5	}	6
1 hour at least after the operation	2		
2 hours after the operation	1		
"A few hours after"	1	}	6
"Some hours after"	1		
18 hours after	1		
Total cases	35		

Duration of Attack.—Just as the onset of the condition is subject to much variation, so is the duration of the attack. It may be rapidly fatal (and when causing death it usually does so quickly), or, on the other hand, may last for several days, and the patient completely recover. In the majority of cases the attack lasts for some hours and then gradually passes off. As the following table will show, the condition does not often last longer than twenty-four hours, and seldom persists beyond two days.

TABLE VI.—*Showing the Duration of Attack in Thirty-nine Cases (Seven of which Proved Fatal).*

A few minutes (all fatal)	3
Under ½ hour (2 fatal)	3
1–6 hours (2 fatal)	10
" Some hours "	6
6–24 hours	10
1–2 days	5
Longer than 2 days	2
Total cases . . .	39

The Character of the Expectoration.—The character of the expectoration varies somewhat according as it is brought up rapidly and in large quantities or is expectorated more slowly, thereby becoming mixed with the ordinary sputum which the patient is coughing up. In the former case it presents a very characteristic appearance. It wells out of the patient's mouth like foam, and when collected separates into two layers, an upper layer of froth and foam, and a lower *clear, translucent layer of yellowish or yellowish green colour, resembling in appearance the pleural exudate*, to which the patients themselves have often spontaneously compared it. This yellow colour (in the case recorded in this paper it amounted to an amber tint) is very characteristic. It is especially noted in the majority of the recorded cases and differentiates true albuminous expectoration from all other varieties of sputa. Occasionally, however, the colour may be masked by the presence of blood.

Another characteristic often mentioned, and present in the case recorded in this paper, is the *viscosity* of this transparent yellow liquid; but this feature varies, no doubt, with the percentage of albumin and other constituents present which, as we shall see, are by no means uniform.

In the more chronic cases where ordinary mucopurulent sputa become mixed with the characteristic liquid just described, a third layer forms on standing owing to the mucopurulent constituents falling to the bottom. The middle layer, however, still retains the characteristics above described.

TABLE VII.—*Showing the Results of Analyses of the Albuminous Expectoration and of the Fluid removed from the Pleural Cavity.*

		Sp. gr.	Reaction.	Colour.	Albumin.	Mucin.	Remarks.
Terrillon, Obs. 13, 1873 (see Table II., No. 19).	(a) Expect.	...	Alk.	...	1.42 per cent.	Much. Faint precip. with acetic acid.	...
	(b) Pleural exudate.	...	Alk.	...	1.61 per cent.		...
Dujardin - Beaumetz. 1873 (see Table II., No. 11).	(a) Expect.	1010	Neutral.	Yellow.	0.1 per cent.	Some.	(a) Also contained 0.236 per cent. urea, and some cholesterin and fat.
	(b) Pleural exudate.	1020		Brown.	6.688 per cent.	"A notable quantity."	(b) Urea=0.058 per cent.
Rasmussen. 1873 (see Table II., No. 15).	(a) Expect.	1015		Greenish yellow.	"Became solid on boiling."	...	"Was similar in appearance to the fluid drawn off from the chest."
	(b) Pleural exudate.	1020		Greenish yellow.	"Highly albuminous."	...	...
Driron. 1874 (see Table II., No. 24).	(a) Expect.	...		...	"Albuminoid and organic matters."		(a) Total solids=2.31 per cent. Organic matters=1.59 per cent. Salts=0.73 per cent.
	(b) Pleural exudate.	...		...	(a) 1.59 per cent. (b) 4.83 per cent.		(b) Total solids=5.47 per cent. Albuminoid matters=4.83 per cent. Salts=0.64 per cent.

Laboulbène. 1874 (see Table II., No. 25).	(a) Expect.						(a) Dried residue=1.647 per cent. Anhydrous mineral matters =0.5 per cent.
	(b) Pleural exudate.						(b) Dried residue=6.5 per cent. Anhydrous mineral matters =0.75 per cent.
Gee. 1886 (see Table II., No. 32).	(a) Expect.	1022	Slightly alk.	Yellowish green.	Highly albuminous.	Distinct quantity.	...
	(b) Pleural exudate.			...	...	...	...
Gee. 1886 (see Table II., No. 40).	(a) Expect.	1025	Faint alk.	Yellow.	"Loaded with albumin."		
	(b) Pleural exudate.	1020	Faint alk.		"Became solid on boiling."		
Riesman, 1902 (see Table II., No. 35).	(a) Expect.	1018	Neutral.	Amber.	3.5 per cent. (Esbach).	(a) Distinct precip. with acetic acid.	Total solids=5.84 per cent.
	(b) Pleural exudate.	1021	Faint alk.	Amber.	4.5 per cent. (Esbach).	(b) None.	Total solids=6.84 per cent.
Sir Dyce Duckworth's case recorded in this paper. 1905	(a) Expect.	1024	Faint alk.	Amber.	4.8 per cent.	None in solution. None.	For further details see full report.
	(b) Pleural exudate.	1014	Faint alk.	Straw-coloured.	1.5 per cent.		

Chemical Analysis of the Expectoration. — From what has been said it will be readily understood that the chemical constitution of the liquid expectorated is by no means constant. This is well seen in the table on the preceding page (Table VII.), in which the various analyses which have been made of the expectoration and of the pleural exudates are recorded. It should be noticed that though sometimes the two fluids approximate in their chemical constitution, there are always points of difference, while often, as in the case recorded in this paper, the differences are most marked.

The Amount Expectorated.—In amount the albuminous expectoration is subject to great variation. In cases rapidly fatal, where the vital powers are low and the expiratory power of coughing greatly diminished, the amount of foam expectorated may be very small before the patient succumbs. In other cases, as much as 2 litres or nearly 4 pints have been brought up.

The following table will give some idea of the varying quantities expectorated. (For details of individual cases see Table II.)

TABLE VIII.—*Showing the Amount of Albuminous Expectoration brought up in Thirty-four Cases.*

Up to 250 cc.	8
250 to 500 cc.	12
500 to 1000 cc.	9
1000 to 1500 cc.	4
1500 to 2000 cc.	1
Total cases . . .	34

Ætiology.—We may now pass from the consideration of the clinical aspect of the condition to a study of its ætiology. Around this question great controversy has raged and three theories have been advocated. It has been held that the condition is the result of—

(1) Perforation of the lung, either by the trocar (Woillez,[1] Marrotte),[2] or as the sequel of the aspiration (Féréol).[3]

(2) Absorption by the lung of the remainder of the effusion.

(3) Acute œdema of the lung, due to the too rapid withdrawal of the pleural fluid and the consequent flooding with blood of vessels whose walls have been damaged and made more

[1] Woillez, L'Union Médicale, 1873, vol. xvi. pp. 1, 14.
[2] Marotte, Bull. de l'Acad. de Med., 1872, p. 446.
[3] Féréol. L'Union Médicale, 1873, vol. xv. pp. 837, 850.

permeable by long compression (Hérard,[1] Moutard-Martin,[2] Béhier,[3] Terrillon,[4] West,[5] and Riesman [6]). Of these three theories there can be little doubt that the latter is the true one.

Against *perforation* must be urged, amongst other objections, the absence of pneumo-thorax during life; the fact that though death may be very rapid, a perforation has never yet been found post mortem; the difference in chemical composition between the expectoration and the pleural fluid; the fact that very often a considerable interval may elapse between the conclusion of the operation and the commencement of the expectoration; and lastly, the occasional occurrence of the condition in connection with empyema.

Against the *theory of absorption,* which hardly commends itself on general grounds, is the physiological fact that absorption takes place into the lymphatics and not into the bronchial tubes.

We are therefore driven back to the theory of an *acute œdema of the lung.* This theory is supported both by general considerations and by the evidence of morbid anatomy. Thus, in the fatal case recorded in this paper, the lung on the affected side weighed 34 oz. (as opposed to the 16 oz. of the left lung), and was in a condition of marked and striking œdema. So also in the cases of Terrillon (No. 37, Table II. *B*), Scriba (No. 39), and Gee (No. 40) œdema of the lung on the affected side was found, extending in the two latter cases to the opposite lung as well, although in a less degree. In the two remaining cases, that of Girard (No. 36; 1864) and of Hayem and Tissier (No. 41; 1889), œdema of the lungs is not described, though the post-mortem reports do not state specifically that it was absent.

On general grounds the theory may be upheld as being a reasonable view and one in harmony with the teaching of physiology, which has shown (Cohnheim) that the vessels of a lung which has been compressed become more permeable to the passage of plasma than those of a healthy organ.

Moreover, the interval which not uncommonly occurs before the expectoration begins, is easily to be understood on this

[1] Hérard, Bull. de l'Acad. de Med., 1872, tome 1, p. 729; L'Union Médicale, 1873, vol. xvi. p. 117.

[2] Moutard-Martin, L'Union Médicale, 1873, p. 962.

[3] Béhier, L'Union Médicale, 1873, vol. xv. p. 974.

[4] Terrillon, De l'expectoration albumineux après la thoracentèse. Paris, 1873, p. 38.

[5] S. West, Trans. of Clinical Society, vol. xxix. 1896, p. 169.

[6] Riesman, Amer. Journal of the Medical Sciences, Jan.–June 1902, vol. cxxii. p. 627.

view. That this interval may, in rare cases, amount to 2, 3, "a few," and even 18 hours (see Tables II. and V.) may suggest at first sight that in these cases at least some other morbid change may be at work. But a consideration of the two following cases in which acute œdema of the lungs, demonstrated post mortem, supervened after 3 and 12 hours respectively, shows that the complication may be in rare cases very considerably delayed. It should be noticed also that in neither of these cases was there any expectoration whatever, possibly because the patients were unable to effect the necessary expiratory efforts. (See Table IX., p. 107.)

In harmony, too, with this opinion is the fact that not uncommonly the complication has followed the *too rapid* removal of *large quantities* of fluid (see Table II.), both of them conditions which would be likely to favour œdema in vessels already predisposed to it. Of late years, owing to the employment of a finer needle, and the care with which the operation is performed, these sources of danger have been to a great extent obviated, and to this must be attributed the comparative rareness of the complication in recent times, as compared with the little epidemic of cases which occurred at the time of Terrillon's thesis.

On the above grounds, therefore, we may conclude that in the vast majority of cases at least the condition is the result of an acute œdema of the lung, the condition being favoured by a too rapid withdrawal of a large quantity of fluid from the pleura.

Aspiration *per se* would seem to have little effect in its production, and if the fluid be drawn off *slowly* and the operation suspended when the patient begins to cough, and too much fluid be not therefore withdrawn, it matters little whether aspiration or the syphon is the method employed.

Prognosis.—As already stated, in the majority of cases, after some hours the cough and sputum gradually become less and the patient in a short time completely recovers. In certain cases, on the other hand, the amount of exudation is more than the patient can expectorate, and he is asphyxiated sometimes within a few minutes of the onset of the complication (see Table VI.). Thus of the 42 cases recorded in Table II., in 35 recovery followed, while 7 proved fatal; giving a mortality of 16·6 per cent.

There can be no doubt, therefore, as to the statistical gravity of the affection when all cases are considered, but we must add that, provided the patient's strength is well maintained, and he be suffering from no serious pulmonary, cardiac, or other complication, the danger in the individual case is certainly

TABLE IX.—*Showing the Chief Features of two Cases of Fatal Œdema of the Lung following Paracentesis, but after a Considerable Interval.*

No.	Reference.	Sex.	Age.	Side.	Nature of Disease.	Amount of Fluid withdrawn from Pleural Cavity.	Moment of Commencement of the Attack.	Duration of Attack.	Post-mortem Report.
1	Case of M. Béhier. *Liouville and Strauss,* L'Union Médicale, 1873, vol. xv. p. 953.	M.	38	L.	Phthisis: acute Pleurisy with effusion.	2500 cc.	3 hours after paracentesis.	Great dyspnœa for 1 hour. Could bring up nothing. Death from asphyxia.	L. lung in a condition of marked œdema. 1 litre of clear yellow albuminous fluid oozing from it on section. No injury of lung or pleura. R. lung.—Acute scattered broncho-pneumonia, with tuberculous infiltration of the apex. Trachea and great bronchi filled and obstructed with thick white foam.
2	M. Dumont Pallier's case. *Béhier,* L'Union Médicale, 1873, vol. xv. p. 957. *Foucart,* Thèse de Paris, 1875. Obs. 5.	M.	46	R.	Lobar Pn. (l. apex): General Bronchitis. R. pleurisy with effusion.	2500 cc.	12 hours after paracentesis.	Patient died suddenly about 12 hours after paracentesis, having had some oppression before death, but no expectoration.	P.M. — Resolving pneumonia. L. apex. — General Bronchitis. Both lungs distended and in a condition of acute œdema.

less. Thus out of the 24 cases of simple pleurisy with effusion recorded in Table II., in one only (4.2 per cent.) was the complication fatal (case 38). In the other six fatal cases (in whom death occurred after 5, 5, 15, 25, and 75 minutes and 6 hours respectively), the following lesions were found in addition to the effusion—

CASE 36. A second effusion on the opposite side.

„ 37. Tuberculous disease with much fibrosis in the opposite lung, which was thus no longer able to functionate.

„ 39. Old tuberculous disease of the left lung; tuberculosis of the left pleura, peritoneum, omentum, and spleen.

„ 40. Lymphadenoma.

„ 41. Tuberculous pericarditis.

„ 42. Pernicious anæmia with dilated heat.

The conclusion which we may draw from the above facts is, that if in a given case albuminous expectoration sets in after paracentesis, undue anxiety need not be felt, provided the patient's strength is well maintained and the other organs are healthy. But if the patient lack strength to expectorate or the heart or other lung be seriously affected, then the condition is a very grave one.

Treatment.—The line of treatment indicated during the attack consists in stimulating the patient and assisting him to expectorate the fluid, which if allowed to accumulate in the bronchial tubes will certainly asphyxiate him. For this purpose brandy must be freely given, with ether and ammonia, and, if necessary, injections of strychnine.. Inhalation of oxygen is also of value if the patient is becoming cyanosed; if full-blooded, venesection should be performed. To prevent the complication, paracentesis, whether by the aspirator or the syphon, should be performed *slowly*, and only moderate quantities of liquid should be withdrawn.

ALBUMINOUS EXPECTORATION APART FROM PARACENTESIS THORACIS.

Before concluding this paper, it may be well to draw attention to the fact that acute œdema of the lung with true albuminous expectoration, exactly similar in all its characters (colour, viscosity, aëration, albumen-contents, &c.) to that met with as the sequel of paracentesis, may occur apart from this condition.

To this fact Rèvillout[1] drew attention in 1873, and a somewhat similar case of acute recurring œdema of the lung with true albuminous expectoration, in an otherwise healthy woman of 59, was recently published by Dr. F. C. Poynder[2] of East Grinstead. In this case the fluid was very frothy, was neutral in reaction, and possessed a specific gravity of 1019. It was highly albuminous, and became nearly solid on boiling, and yielded on quantitative analysis "9.84 grains of albumin per ounce." Of this nature, too, would seem to be the interesting case of Dr. Beddoes, quoted by Dr. Gee in his Lumleian Lectures (1899),[3] and referred to also by Laennec.[4]

In 1875 an instance of albuminous expectoration was recorded by Foucart[5] in a patient suffering from mitral regurgitation.

Although, therefore, admittedly very uncommon apart from pleural effusion and paracentesis, the occurrence of acute œdema of the lung with typical albuminous expectoration cannot be denied.

RÉSUMÉ.

1. *Albuminous expectoration following paracentesis* is a very rare condition, though probably not quite so rare as is generally supposed. Owing to more perfect methods of performing paracentesis it is seen less often now than formerly.

2. Most of the cases occur between the ages of 20 and 50, but it may occur at any later age. It is only very exceptionally seen in children.

3. It is considerably more common in males than in females.

4. It is connected most often with acute pleurisy with serofibrinous effusion, but may follow paracentesis for hydrothorax, however produced, or for empyema. It is rather more frequently connected with disease of the left side than of the right.

5. In one-third of the cases it has commenced during the operation of paracentesis or immediately after it. In one-third it has supervened between 10 and 30 minutes after the conclusion of the operation, and in a further sixth between half-an-hour and one hour. In other words, in five-sixths of the cases (or 83 per cent.) the complication has occurred within

---

[1] Rèvillout, Gazette des Hôpitaux, 1873, pp. 513 and 561.
[2] Poynder, St. Bartholomew's Hospital Journal, September 1905.
[3] Gee, Medical Lectures and Aphorisms, 1902, p. 152.
[4] Laennec, Auscultation Médiate, vol. i. p. 154, troisième édition,
[5] Foucart, Thèse de Paris, 1875, p. 69.

one hour of the conclusion of the operation. In the remaining
17 per cent. it has been long delayed, in one case as much as
18 hours.

6. During the attack there is as a rule much 'coughing, and
abundant fine crepitations are heard on auscultating the affected
side; and in serious cases these may be heard also over the
opposite lung.

7. The *expectoration* is exceedingly frothy, and when collected
settles into two layers, above a layer of froth, below a layer of
translucent light yellow or straw-coloured (sometimes amber,
sometimes yellowish green) fluid, somewhat viscid and containing much albumen. This appearance, which closely recalls that
of the fluid removed from the pleura, is characteristic. If the
liquid is brought up more slowly, it may be mixed with ordinary
muco-purulent sputa, which form a third layer at the bottom of
the vessel.

Chemical analysis always shows differences, frequently very
marked, between the expectoration and the pleural exudate,
showing that the two are not identical.

8. The quantity of expectoration brought up varies from a
small amount to 2000 cc., but in the majority of cases it
ranges from 250 to 1000 cc. (from $\frac{1}{2}$ to 2 pints).

9. The attack commonly lasts a few hours—but it may be
fatal in a few minutes, or may continue for some days. When
fatal it is generally quickly so.

10. The condition is the result of an acute œdema of the
lung, following not infrequently a too rapid withdrawal of
too large a quantity of fluid.

11. The prognosis is grave if the patient is greatly debilitated
and lacks strength to expectorate, or if the heart or opposite
lung, be seriously diseased. In such cases death often rapidly
supervenes. In the absence of such complications the outlook
is favourable.

12. Lastly, acute œdema of the lung with true albuminous
expectoration, characteristic in every respect, may occur apart
from paracentesis, though well-authenticated cases are few in
number.

A ·CASE OF COMPLETE TRANSPOSITION
OF VISCERA IN AN ADULT.

BY

THOMAS J. HORDER, M.D.

Instances of this strange anatomical condition are so rare that a brief account of one recently met with in the *post-mortem* room of St. Bartholomew's Hospital seems to merit a place in the pages of the Hospital Reports.

On September 23, 1905, the body of a somewhat wasted young man, aged 24, came under examination. The patient had been in Rahere Ward for a couple of days only, and was found during that time to be suffering from pulmonary phthisis. The more advanced part of his disease was discovered in the right lung; the position of the heart to the right of the sternum was therefore considered to be due to displacement by fibrosis connected with the tuberculosis. The fingers were clubbed. The patient was so ill that anything like a detailed examination of the chest was not undertaken, and no examination was made of the abdomen. Despite the free use of oxygen and various stimulants, the man died on the day after his admission: he had but come to the hospital to die. The patient's history showed that he had suffered from phthisis for two years past. One year previously he had been an in-patient at the London Hospital, where his chest was aspirated. Some two months afterwards he was examined by the X-rays at Victoria Park Chest Hospital—a fact which suggests that the abnormal position of his heart at this time aroused interest.

The chief points made out at the autopsy were as follows:—

Lungs.—The right consisted of two lobes, and weighed 18 ounces; the left consisted of three lobes, and weighed 24 ounces; both showed the lesions of long-standing phthisis at the apices, and acute pneumonic phthisis at the bases. The most advanced lesions were at the right apex. The pleura was adherent over both apices; the pleural sac contained no fluid. There were no pleuro-pericardial adhesions.

The *heart* was transposed, lying for the most part to the right of the mesial line. A line drawn through the apex and middle of the base cut the twelfth right rib. The whole of

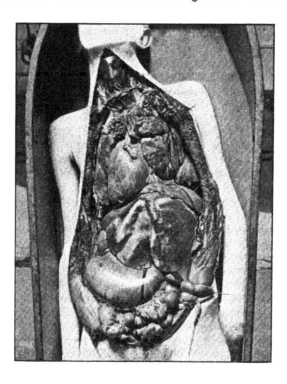

the front part of the organ was formed by the right auricle and right ventricle, except the actual apex, which was formed by the left ventricle. The whole heart was somewhat hypertrophied, and the right auricle was dilated. Nothing abnormal was discovered on opening the viscus—the valves were those appropriate to the respective cavities.·

The *aorta* passed upwards and to the right, the arch curving over the root of the right lung.

The *pulmonary artery* lay in front of the aorta, but passed upwards to the left.

The *superior vena cava* passed directly upwards on the left side and the innominate veins were transposed.

The *vena azygos major* lay along the left side of the posterior mediastinum. The thoracic duct was not identified.

The *vena cava inferior* lay on the left, and the *abdominal aorta* on the right, of the vertebral column.

The *stomach* lay chiefly in the right hypochondrium, its fundus pointing to the right, its pylorus to the left.

The *spleen* lay high up in the right dome of the diaphragm, adjacent to the fundus of the stomach.

The larger lobe of the *liver* was placed on the left of the mesial line; the *gall-bladder* was likewise to the left.

The *sigmoid flexure* occupied the right iliac fossa, the *cæcum* and *appendix vermiformis* occupying the left.

The *kidneys* lay at about the same level on the two sides; perhaps the kidney on the left side lay about half an inch lower than the one on the right.

The *right testis* lay quite one and a half inch lower than the left in the scrotum.

All the organs appeared well formed and free from intrinsic abnormalities. The body was rather above the average height.

A photograph was taken after the anterior thoracic wall had been removed and the abdomen opened. For this purpose the body was placed in the semi-erect position; the viscera are therefore seen at a lower level than natural, having sagged considerably. This is especially the case with regard to the abdominal organs. No such splanchnoptosis was present in reality. The reproduction of the photograph shows the three-lobed left lung, the position of the heart, the large lobe of the liver with the gall-bladder on the left side, the fundus of the stomach and the spleen just above it on right side, and the cæcum with its appendix pinned out on the left.

I am desirous of thanking Dr. Ormerod for his kind permission to record the ·above case, and Mr. Russell Square for taking the photograph.

ON CARDIAC DROPSY IN CHILDREN.

BY

'W. LANGDON BROWN, M.D.

In the following cases I wish to call attention to—

1. The very grave prognosis when œdema of the face comes on rapidly in cardiac affections;

2. Certain risks attending the injection of adrenalin for cardiac failure.

CASE 1.—A little girl, aged 4, was admitted under my care at the Metropolitan Hospital. She was known to have had rheumatic fever ten months previously, and had been attending the hospital with signs of mitral stenosis with regurgitation and some œdema of the legs. Her mother now stated that she had noticed the child's face to be swelling during the last three days; that she was getting very short of breath, and that the urine was scanty, thick, and muddy.

On examination the child was found to be cyanosed and generally œdematous; the pulse was 132, and irregular. The heart's apex was in the sixth interspace, 1½ inch outside the nipple line; the impulse was very diffuse and preceded by a thrill. The cardiac dulness extended upwards to the third rib. At the apex presystolic and systolic murmurs were heard, the latter loud and musical, conducted into the axilla and heard behind at the angle of the scapula. At the pulmonary base the second sound was accentuated. There was some bronchitis, and the liver was palpable. The urine showed a heavy deposit of urates, but only a trace of albumin and no blood or casts.

On the rapid development of the general œdema, involving the face, a very unfavourable prognosis was given. Events fully justified this, for the child died the next day. Unfortunately a necropsy was not permitted, but the condition of the urine made it fairly certain that the kidneys were not the cause of the general dropsy.

In the following case, however, a post-mortem examination was made.

Case II.—A boy, æt. 7, was admitted under my care at the Metropolitan Hospital for shortness of breath with orthopnœa. Ten months previously he had suffered from rheumatic fever, and was ill for four months. On examination his heart's apex was felt in the sixth interspace, ¾ inch outside the left nipple line. The impulse was preceded by a thrill. The cardiac dulness was not increased upwards. A presystolic and a musical systolic murmur were heard at the apex. The pulse was rapid, feeble, and irregular. The urine contained less than 0·05 per cent. of albumin.

Two days later he became cyanosed ; there was a rapid development of anasarca, in which the face shared to a marked degree. This occurred within a few hours. The tongue was very furred, and a urinous smell was noted in the breath. Yet in twenty-four hours the boy passed 40 oz. of urine, acid in reaction, and containing only a trace of albumin. No casts could be found. Though he improved slightly for a time he died rather suddenly a week later. The necropsy revealed double mitral disease, with infarcts in the lungs. The kidneys were merely congested.

Case III.—A girl, aged 3, was admitted to Mary ward under care of Dr. Hensley on March 5, 1903, for cough and shortness of breath. Nine weeks previously she had had diphtheria. For the last two days the feet and legs had swelled, and when she lay down the face had swelled also. On admission she was cyanosed, and the œdema of the face was well marked. The apex of the heart was in the sixth interspace, 1½ inch outside the left nipple line. The area of cardiac dulness extended from the second rib to 1 inch to the right of the sternum and out to the apex beat. On auscultation, a loud systolic murmur was heard at the apex, conducted to the axilla. Many moist sounds were heard in the lungs. The liver was easily palpable, and the abdomen contained no free fluid on admission. The urine was very scanty. Two days later she died, the immediate cause of death being vomiting and hæmoptysis. *Post-mortem*—recent endocarditis of the mitral and tricuspid valves was seen, together with hypertrophy and dilatation of the heart, the myocardium being pale and turbid. There was much ascites. The kidneys were pale, but presented no sign of actual nephritis.

CASE IV.—A girl, aged 6, was admitted to the Metropolitan Hospital under my care on August 25, 1905, for shortness of breath and pain in the chest.

History of Present Illness.—On August 23 she was seized with abdominal pain and some cough. From that time till admission the bowels were not properly opened, only a little mucus being passed. On the morning of admission she became very short of breath and vomited.

Past Illnesses.—Measles and whooping-cough.

Family History.—Nothing important.

Condition on Admission.—The child was dusky, and a little puffy about the face. She lay on her left side, and cried if moved. Respiration, 60; pulse, 140; temperature, 98°. Tongue clean but dry.

Chest—Heart.—A wavy impulse was felt in the fourth and fifth interspace out to the nipple line. The area of cardiac dulness was not increased. There was a distinct cantering rhythm, but no murmur or friction.

Lungs.—At the left apex the breath sounds were harsher than elsewhere. At both bases the percussion note was impaired, and fine hair crepitations were heard.

Abdomen.—A large lump was felt in the right hypochondrium (which proved to be liver) which was not tender on gentle manipulation, but was painful on deep palpation. There was no sign of peritonitis or ascites. Nothing abnormal was felt on rectal examination.

Legs were œdematous.

A specimen of urine passed at the same time as some mucus *per rectum* was filtered off and found to contain a heavy cloud of albumen; apparently more than could be accounted for by the presence of a small amount of intestinal contents. There was no blood in it.

Blood Examination.—40,600 leucocytes. Nothing grew in cultures from the blood.

Two leeches were applied to the chest, and strychnine and digitalis were injected hypodermically, the child's condition appearing extremely grave.

The same evening a natural stool was passed, without blood or mucus.

August 26.—The cardiac dulness was increased up to the second rib, and a finger's breadth to the right of the sternum, the shape of the area being that attributed to pericardial effusion. The rhythm was still cantering, and there was no friction.

The note at the base of the left lung between the angle of

the scapula and the spine was quite dull, and was impaired over the rest of both bases. Fine hair crepitations were heard at both bases with bronchial breathing near the angle of the scapula.

August 27.—At 12.40 P.M. the child became very restless, cyanosed, and almost pulseless, but improved after an injection of strychnine and digitalin. At 3.40 P.M. there was another dyspnœic attack, similarly treated.

August 28.—The child was collapsed, blue, and pulseless at 2.30 A.M. Fifteen minims of adrenalin chloride solution (1-1000) were injected intravenously. She rallied for four hours. At 6.30 A.M. she became collapsed again; she was unconscious and appeared *in extremis.* She was œdematous from head to foot. Ten minims of adrenalin chloride solution were injected intravenously with very little effect. Shortly afterwards the child died.

Post-mortem Report.—General Anasarca.

Chest.—No adhesions; much serous fluid in both pleural cavities. Lungs—broncho-pneumonic areas scattered throughout. Areas of compensatory emphysema were also seen. The upper part of the left lower lobe was collapsed. Pericardium distended with about 2 to 3 ounces of straw-coloured fluid. The veins were much engorged. Heart—extreme dilatation of both sides; no signs of valvular disease.

Abdomen. — Liver — pale, slight fatty change. Kidneys — chronic congestion. Small retroperitoneal hæmorrhage. Stomach and intestines engorged.

Bacteriological Examination. — Cultures from the heart's blood and pericardial fluid were sterile.

This case appeared to be one of broncho-pneumonia associated with rapid dilatation of the heart and pericardial effusion. From the extremely grave constitutional signs throughout and the marked leucocytosis I expected to find evidence of some general infection, but on this point the bacteriological evidence was negative. The appearance of the kidneys and the absence of blood from the urine negatived acute nephritis. For a discussion of the histological changes *vide infra.*

I. *The Significance of General Dropsy in Cardiac Affections.*— Such cases are not very unusual, but in the text-books very little attention is directed to them. Lees and Poynton, in their paper on "Dilatation of the Heart" ("Medico-Chirurgical Transactions," 1898), conclude that there is usually a decided valvular lesion in cases of marked dropsy. Dickinson, in Professor Allbutt's "System of Medicine," vol. v., contrasts the gradual spread of the œdema upwards in cardiac cases with the early œdema of the face in renal cases. These are the principal references to the subject that I have been able to find.

In all the cases here reported the œdema of the face was sudden in onset, and in Case IV. there was no valvular lesion at all, so that they do not fall exactly into these categories.

Recently Bolton [1] has succeeded in producing cardiac œdema experimentally by tying off a portion of the pericardial sac so that the residue of the pericardium was rendered too small for the heart. Free expansion of the heart was thus prevented, and the diastolic filling was interfered with, causing distention of the great veins. If the animal were allowed to live for some days, dropsy of the head, chest wall, and peritoneal cavity occurred, together with dyspnœa, albuminuria, and scanty urine. From observations of the arterial and venous blood pressures it appeared that increased permeability of the capillaries rather than a rise in capillary pressure was the most important factor at work. This altered permeability is brought about by deficient oxygenation of the blood and impaired nutrition of the capillary wall.

The development of œdema in other than dependent parts, then, may be caused by the increased permeability of the vessel wall, either from osmotic changes as in Bright's disease, or by rapid venous engorgement; and it is noteworthy that in all the cases here recorded the œdema was accompanied by cyanosis. This sudden venous engorgement implies a marked failure of compensation due to rapid dilatation. In the last case the pericardial effusion acted like the experimental tying off of a portion of the pericardial sac, and by preventing diastolic filling of the heart greatly increased the venous engorgement. Such rapid dilatation is always of grave prognosis, especially in children, who are notoriously bad at re-establishing compensation. Indeed, this condition has proved fatal within a few days in all the cases I have seen in children.

II. *Certain Risks in the Intravenous Injection of Adrenalin.*—Adrenalin is a most powerful drug, and, like all powerful drugs, is not free from danger. Its use is being widely advocated to-day, and carefully employed it is undoubtedly of service. It is all the more necessary, therefore, that any untoward results which might be attributed to the drug should be placed on record. Elsewhere I have discussed in detail the therapeutic applications of adrenalin (Clinical Journal, Dec. 13, 1905). It has been clearly proved from the researches of Lewandowsky, Langley,

[1] Quoted by Bainbridge, "The Pathology of Dropsy." Practitioner, November 1905, p. 640.

and Elliott that the effect of adrenalin is the same as stimulation of the sympathetic nerves to that part.   As adrenalin is not absorbed as such from the intestine, its use is limited to local application or intravenous injection.   Bearing those points in mind, I ordered intravenous injections in Case IV. if cardiac failure should occur, because of its marked tonic action on the heart.   The first injection caused a decided rally ; to the second the patient did not respond.

Now adrenalin augments the force of the heart's action ; but as by raising the blood pressure it also stimulates the cardio-inhibitory centre in the medulla, reflex slowing may be produced, overpowering any augmentation.   Moreover, by suddenly constricting the peripheral blood-vessels the work of the heart is greatly increased ; failure to meet this increase may result in dilatation of the cavities.   Dilatation combined with vagal inhibition is a danger that would outweigh any advantage derived from the stimulating effect of the adrenalin.   Simultaneous injection of atropin might prevent the vagal inhibition but would not diminish the increased work of the heart.   But nitrite of amyl would flush the peripheral vessels, thus avoiding both extra work and stimulation of the cardio-inhibitory centre.   The effect of both adrenalin and amyl nitrite is about equally sudden and transitory.   My experience with intravenous injections of adrenalin for failing heart leads me to urge the use of amyl nitrite at the same time to avoid untoward effects. The cardiac dilatation in this case could not be referred to the adrenalin as it was very marked before the drug was used.

The mechanical effects of high blood pressure manifest themselves also on the lungs.   Large doses of adrenalin are fatal from asphyxia, the lungs showing intense engorgement and œdema.   The lungs and vessels having no sympathetic vaso-constrictors are unable to protect themselves, and the blood which is being squeezed out of the systemic vessels is forced into them.   Microscopical sections of the lungs in Case IV. showed typical broncho-pneumonic changes in many parts, but in addition they showed areas of intense engorgement, some of the alveoli being stuffed with red corpuscles.   I cannot help thinking that the injections of adrenalin may have been in part responsible for this.

But there is a further risk in the intravenous injection of adrenalin.   Toxic effects have been described in the tissues, especially in the liver and the kidneys, as the result of injections of 20 to 50 mimims into animals.   I therefore examined these organs microscopically.

Liver.—Necrotic areas were scattered throughout, usually

though not invariably situated in the centre of the lobules. The cells here were shrunken, the nucleus apparently occupying the greater part of the cell. Around this came a ring of cells containing large vacuoles, probably of fat; outside this ring the cells seemed healthy. The changes were in fact like those seen in nutmeg liver, but without any signs of central congestion.

Mallory[1] has described a somewhat similar condition of central necrosis chiefly in toxic and infectious conditions, such as diphtheria, acute endocarditis, lobar pneumonia, and acute peritonitis. It would not be worth while, therefore, to lay much stress on the appearances in my case were it not for the close resemblance between them and those described by Drummond[2] and by Drummond and Paton[3] as the result of the experimental injection of adrenalin in animals.

It might be urged that the time elapsing between the injection and death (about five hours) would not allow of such changes occurring; but Paton and Drummond saw early changes in a rabbit's liver in $2\frac{3}{4}$ hours, and distinct changes in $4\frac{1}{4}$ hours.

Kidney.—The glomeruli were natural, but there was extravasation, apparently of blood, into Bowman's capsule. The convoluted tubules showed cloudy swelling; there was desquamation of epithelium in the tubules of the medulla, and the vasa recta were much engorged. Drummond found changes "which varied from congestion of the organ with cloudy swelling of the epithelial cells to a parenchymatous nephritis with desquamation of cells in the tubules." In acute cases he found cloudy swelling of the convoluted tubules.

I am aware that my results are quite inconclusive, all the appearances described in the lungs, liver, and kidney being susceptible of explanation without reference to adrenalin. But their general resemblance to the changes produced by adrenalin is sufficiently close to make it advisable to record them. For it is well to know the worst as well as the best that can be said of a new drug. I am satisfied that an immediate benefit can result from adrenalin injections; the question is, whether this benefit may not be purchased too dearly. In any case, I shall only venture to use much smaller doses for intravenous injections in the future.

---

[1] Mallory, Journ. of Med. Research, vi. p. 264, 1901.
[2] Drummond, Journ. of Physiology, xxxi. p. 81, 1904.
[3] Drummond and Paton, Journ. of Physiology, xxxi. p. 92, 1904.

PULMONARY FIBROSIS IN CHILDHOOD,

BASED ON AN ANALYSIS OF FORTY CASES.

BY

CLIVE RIVIERE, M.D.

Fibrosis of the lung with bronchiectasis takes so prominent a place among the pulmonary diseases of childhood, and the subject is so sparingly dealt with in the text-books devoted to this branch, that I have been tempted to contribute an account of the condition, based on forty cases coming under my own observation. The condition being the outcome of so many pulmonary diseases, as its etiology will show, it might be supposed that the individuals in such a refuse-heap could hardly with advantage be collected together under a single heading, but, clinically, as we shall see, the group exhibits a very distinctive picture of disease. My only difficulty has been with cases, few in number, of bronchiectasis without definite fibrosis, and these, though in their etiology, symptoms, and treatment they are very similar to the cases described, I have elected to omit for the sake of brevity. With regard to the frequency of the condition, some idea of this may be gathered from the fact that nearly two-thirds of the forty cases collected have come under my care within the past two years during my ordinary out-patient work at the Shadwell Children's Hospital and the Victoria Park Chest Hospital, besides a few in the Children's Department at St. Bartholomew's Hospital. For permission to include these last among the cases, I am indebted to the kindness of Dr. Archibald Garrod and Dr. Morley Fletcher.

Etiology.—The etiology of the condition is concisely shown in the following table, based on thirty-three of my cases in which a reliable history could be obtained. It will be seen that the majority originate in broncho-pneumonia and bronchitis, and that especially when these are complications of whooping-

cough and measles.   Another table shows the responsibility of
the infective fevers in the causation of the condition.

Bronchitis . . 13	alone 6		
	with whooping-cough . . 3		
	with diphtheria . . . 2		
	with measles and whooping-cough . . . 2		
Broncho-pneumonia . 14	alone 6		
	with whooping-cough . . 5		
	with measles . . . 3		
Lobar Pneumonia . 4			
Congenital Atelectasis 2			

Total   . 33

INFECTIVE FEVERS.

Whooping-cough . 10	with broncho-pneumonia . 5		
	with bronchitis . . . 3		
	with measles . . . 2		
Measles . . . 5	with broncho-pneumonia . 3		
	with whooping-cough . . 2		
Diphtheria . . 2			

When *broncho-pneumonia* is the starting-point, the attack
drags on to great length, the signs never clear, and, when
health returns, a certain amount of fibroid change is left in the
lung.   Often, after an interval, another attack of pneumonia
ensues, and the lung is further crippled.   These acute attacks
may be repeated at intervals.   In the early stages, could we
inspect the lung, we should doubtless find a dilated bronchial
tree with thickened walls, such as we find after any protracted
broncho-pneumonia, and, as the attacks proceed, inflammation
leading to fibrosis spreads from these tubes into the lung,
the process being probably extended by fibrosing areas of
unresolved consolidation and of collapse.   When the fibrosis
has become considerable, saccular cavitation of the smaller
bronchi ensues, probably through stagnation of secretion in
the tubes of the functionless lung tissue.   In these cases both
lungs may be affected, but seldom with equal intensity.

When *lobar pneumonia* originates the condition, one lung
only is affected, generally part of a lung, and the process may
be limited by quite a sharp line of demarcation.   Lobar
pneumonia is doubtless responsible for most of the apical
cases.

In cases arising in *bronchitis* I have observed that the right middle lobe is very commonly affected, and, seeing the comparative frequency with which collapse occurs in this part of the lung in bronchitis, I am disposed to attribute the fibrosis in most of these cases to such collapse.

Next come two cases arising in early infancy, and probably attributable, in my opinion, to *congenital atelectasis*. In one of these a small area at the base of one lung was involved, in the other the lesion was apical. In the latter no symptoms were observed till six months after birth. Lastly, an untreated *pleurisy* may probably lead to fibrosis, but less commonly, I think, than is generally held. I have seen two cases of pulmonary fibrosis in which the symptoms appeared to be of gradual onset, and in which the possibility of a subacute indurative pneumonia had to be considered. Such cases, I think, may possibly have been of pleural origin.

Pulmonary fibrosis is found at all ages throughout childhood, but its origin can commonly be traced to the early years of life. This we should expect when we consider its common origin in broncho-pneumonia and bronchitis. In the following table the age incidence of my cases appears, and beside it a table of thirty-two of these cases showing the age at which the symptoms were believed to arise. The comparatively large number between the ages of 3 and 5 years is attributable largely to cases of broncho-pneumonia occurring after infancy is past as a complication of the infective fevers.

Age Incidence of Cases.		Age at which Disease Originated.	
Below age of 3 years .	2 cases	From birth to 1 year .	5 cases
3- 5 years .	6 ,,	1- 3 years .	9 ,,
5-10 ,, .	15 ,,	3- 5 ,, .	9 ,,
10-15 ,, .	14 ,,	5-10 ,, .	7 ,,
15-20 ,, .	3 ,,	10-15 ,, .	2 ,,
	40		32

Morbid Anatomy.—This description is based mainly on three of my cases in which I had an opportunity of performing an autopsy. The lung, if affected as a whole, is found lying far back in the chest, the heart and mediastinum are drawn over to fill the vacant space, and with them the opposite lung which is voluminous. When only part of a lung is affected these changes are, of course, much less marked. The lung or its affected part is, as a rule, closely adherent to the chest wall, though the pleura may be little thickened except in rare cases where the process is pleural in origin. When the process is advanced, the lung tissue is firm, tough, and elastic to cut, dark slate-colour or pinkish grey on section, and totally airless.

Through it run the dilated larger tubes; the smaller tubes form saccular cavities throughout its substance, and may contain foul pus. Their walls are red, smooth, and glistening. The fibrotic area may be sharply circumscribed, or the remainder of the lung may show a less advanced change, namely, some increase of fibrous tissue and moderate dilatation of the bronchi, their thickened walls showing as white lines through the section. The lymphatic glands connected with the lung are enlarged, and generally show on section much pigmentation, but little or no fibrosis; they are often quite soft and pulpy.

Histology.—Under the microscope the normal elements of the lung tissue are seen to be replaced by fibrous tissue. In early stages, young fibroblasts are seen infiltrating the alveolar walls and replacing the alveolar exudation. Later these become more elongated, lose their nuclei, and are collected together into bundles of fibrous tissue which run in different directions through the tissue, enclosing numerous blood-spaces in their meshes. The dilated tubes are lined by several layers of cubical epithelial cells, sometimes by a single layer of columnar epithelium, and their walls in some places show a round-celled infiltration.

Position of Lesion.—The following table shows the position of the lesion among my forty cases.

Right Lung.				Left Lung.			
Apex	.	.	. 2	Apex	.	.	. 1
Base	.	.	. 5	Base	.	.	. 6
Whole	.	.	. 5	Whole	.	.	. 16
			12				23

Both Lungs   .   .   .   .   . 5 cases

Symptoms.—The child is generally brought with a history of *cough* dating from some such past illness as the etiology describes. The cough may persist all the year round, or it may be absent in the warm seasons of the year, and only occur with attacks of acute or subacute catarrh in the cold weather. It is accompanied by expectoration, in the summer perhaps only a small quantity brought up on rising in the morning and on going to bed at night, but, during the winter exacerbations, a large quantity is expectorated, perhaps a cupful daily. This may be brought up during a single attack of coughing, or there may be several spasmodic attacks of cough during the day, in many cases followed by vomiting. In a few instances where advanced fibrosis hinders the emptying of the bronchiectatic cavities, the expectoration has a stale odour, or is even putrid.

When this occurs the general health does not appear to me to
suffer to the extent that it does under similar conditions in
adults. The offensive odour may be present for a time only,
and disappear under treatment. Occasionally the cough is dry
and hacking between the acute attacks.

With the sputum *blood* not uncommonly appears either as
streaks, clots, or rarely a brisk hæmoptysis. One of my
patients expectorated a blood cast of a large tube, another
soaked several handkerchiefs at a time with marked relief to
symptoms, and a third, a case of probable fibrosis but not
included in my series, died of a sudden pulmonary hæmorrhage.

General Signs.—The subjects of pulmonary fibrosis are generally small for their age but well nourished. The features are
commonly thick and coarse, the face congested and sometimes cyanosed, and the conjunctivæ somewhat watery. The
paroxysmal cough and some amount of cardiac disability are
doubtless responsible in the main for this facies, and with it
is often associated that characteristic of adenoids and enlarged
tonsils which are very commonly present in these cases. In
some instances where the expectoration is fœtid the skin may
be pale and sallow. *Finger-clubbing* is a marked feature in
cases of pulmonary fibrosis, but it is sometimes absent in well-
marked cases. It was present in 40 per cent. of my series,
and varies from a curving of the nails, with shininess of the
skin at their base, to an enlargement of the whole terminal
phalanx.

Local Signs.—These consist of deficient movement and dulness over the affected region, with distant blowing breath
sounds, and râles which are either dry and rustling, or large,
metallic, and bubbling. In addition, there may be some cavity
signs, amphoric breath sounds, resonant râles, and broncho-
phony. An analysis of my collected cases showed the following
signs to be common.

On *inspection* of the chest, movement is found to be deficient
on one side, generally at the base, and, in marked cases, the
side may be obviously shrunken, the shoulder and nipple
lowered, and the ribs closer together than usual. On measure-
ment, a difference between the two sides of $\frac{1}{2}$ inch to $\frac{3}{4}$ inch in
circumference is common, but this is not often exceeded.
Lateral curvature of the dorsal spine is nearly always present,
the concavity being directed towards the affected side, but in
three of my cases a slight curve was present instead in the
opposite direction, an anomaly for which I can find no explanation. When the left lung is affected, visible cardiac pulsation
may be observed in several spaces owing to uncovering of the

heart's surface, and this may extend out into the axilla from displacement of the heart. When the right lung is fibrosed the cardiac pulsation may extend out to the right nipple line.

On *palpation* the limitation of movement of the affected side is more accurately estimated, and the position of the heart's apex verified. Following the heart and mediastinum, the opposite lung crosses to the affected side, and on *percussion* its resonance may be found ½ inch or 1 inch beyond the sternal margin. The fibroid lung gives a dull, toneless note to percussion, with a noticeable increase of resistance, which often simulates that of fluid. The amount of dulness depends, of course, on the amount of fibrosis, so that many qualities of percussion note may be obtained. In rare cases a tympanitic note may be observed on percussion over large bronchiectatic cavities.

Auscultation.—The character of the breath sounds over the affected area depends on the amount of expansion in the lung, the size and nearness of the bronchiectatic cavities, and also whether these are empty or filled with secretion. The air entry is always feeble, and the breath sounds appear to be distant, or may be practically absent over the most fibrosed part of the lung when this is at the base. Their quality is blowing, sometimes truly cavernous, and some added sounds are generally present. These are either dry or moist according to the nature of the secretion in the cavities. When this is scanty, as at the beginning of an acute catarrh, the sounds may be rhonchus and sibilus, or more commonly and more typically a dry, rustling sound like fine friction. This sound I have often heard described as pleural friction, but its common presence, its alteration with increase of secretion, a peculiar individuality in its character, taken with the almost invariable presence of adherent pleura in these cases, convinces me that it is an intrapulmonary sound. Later on this dry sound may give place to resonant crepitations, or to the large, bubbling, metallic râles which are, when present, so characteristic of multiple bronchiectatic cavities. The signs may be suppressed temporarily through blocking of the tubes with secretion, but a good cough will generally re-establish them.

The *vocal resonance* varies completely with the conditions present. When the base of the lung is affected it is often diminished and somewhat ægophonic, as in pleural effusion; it may be absent. Where the bronchiectatic cavities are large and near the surface, it is bronchophonic, or, rarely, there may be whispering pectoriloquy, especially over the upper parts of the lung. Roughly, it may be said that where the breath sounds are merely bronchial, and especially where distant and bronchial, the vocal resonance is diminished; where the breath sounds are amphoric, the vocal resonance is increased or broncho-phonic.

Over the opposite lung, when this is healthy, the movements are active and the breath sounds harsh. In some cases the unaffected parts of the lungs are emphysematous, and give the signs of this condition. Occasionally the signs of the diseased lung are conducted across the chest to the healthy side, and may puzzle the uninitiated. If this is suspected it is helpful to examine the patient while lying on the diseased side, when the conducted sounds will be found to have largely or entirely disappeared.

For the sake of conciseness I have described the symptoms and signs of fibrosis of the lung as if these were of a stationary character. This is far from being the case, and it is possible that more accuracy might have been obtained if I had divided them into those present during the acute attacks and those present during the quiescent interval.

The *acute attacks* (often subacute) appear to be caused in most cases by a fresh catarrh of the dilated bronchial tubes, in which case a mere exacerbation of the existing condition occurs, and generally an increase in the permanent lung signs. Thus the percussion dulness over the lung may increase, the cavity signs be more clearly brought out, and moist sounds, absent before, will appear. In other cases a definite attack of pneumonia occurs, and the permanent condition may be over-looked till the acute attack has subsided. A third variety of acute attack, occurring in advanced cases, is that caused by cardiac incompetence. The case may present all the symptoms of progressive failure of the right heart, and, if seen for the first time, organic valvular disease may be suspected.

In the *quiescent intervals* the general health may be good, cough slight or absent, and, in cases where bronchiectasis is the main feature, it is truly astonishing how largely the signs in the lung may alter. The evidence of dilated tubes may vanish, and the recollection of former lung signs appear a mere dream till, with the onset of winter, back they all come again exactly as before.

Complications.—When the lower parts of a lung are riddled with cavities, surrounded by tough fibrous tissue adherent to the chest wall, it is obvious that drainage by expectoration or occasional vomiting is bound to be very imperfect. The retained secretion tends to become foul from the growth of

saprophytic organisms, and may contain, besides, more dangerous pathogenic germs.   As a result of the development of the
former, septic absorption may undermine the health, and, as
in a boy of 19 years whom I attended in the last stages, practically lead to death.   As a result of the latter, the patient lives
in constant danger of infection.   Two of my cases developed
empyema over the fibrosed lung, and, of three fatal cases, one,
aged 13 years, died of *broncho-pneumonia* in the healthy lung,
and another, aged 4½ years, of broncho-pneumonia passing on
to *abscess* and *gangrene*.   The third of the three fatal cases,
aged 1 year and 10 months, died with *acute tuberculosis*, though
the fibrosis was not of tubercular origin.   I have not seen a
case of *cerebral abscess* as a complication, though one would
expect it to occur in children as in adults; moreover, none
of my cases appeared to suffer with *lardaceous disease* of the
viscera.

Diagnosis.—This has generally to be made in apical fibrosis
from phthisis, and in basal fibrosis from pleurisy, or from rare
cases of caseous consolidation in young children.

The diagnosis from *phthisis* may be difficult; this disease,
it must be remembered, is very rare in children under 6 years
of age, for in them tuberculosis of the lungs takes a different
form; in children above this age phthisis may occur, but is
not common.   The course of the disease, as described by the
friends, may afford some help; in phthisis it is generally
shorter but progressive; in simple fibrosis it extends over
many years, and dates from an attack of pneumonia, or
bronchitis of the infective fevers.   The difference in the
general appearance of the children is often striking; the
subject of fibrosis is generally well nourished, and presents
a thick-featured, somewhat bloated facies, a contrast to the
wasting and anæmia of tuberculosis.   The signs in the lungs
generally decide the diagnosis.   In fibrosis the sequence of
lobes so regularly followed by phthisis is not observed, namely,
the apex of the upper lobe, the apex of the lower lobe, followed
by the apex of the upper lobe on the opposite side.   Moreover,
in chronic phthisis of children, extensive cavitation generally
occurs, and contrasts strongly with the more moderate dilatations
occurring with apical fibrosis.   Examination of the sputum
may help, but in children a negative result is of no value.
The course of the disease, if the initial diagnosis is doubtful,
will generally give confirmation.   Cases of fibrosis improve
remarkably under treatment, and put on flesh with a rapidity
which the phthisical child can seldom imitate.

Basal fibrosis is easily mistaken for *pleural effusion*.   Especially is it liable to be taken for empyema discharging itself through the lung, since the large quantity of green pus expectorated may closely simulate that of a purulent effusion. On two occasions I have seen a rib resected on the strength of this resemblance. The signs may closely simulate those of fluid—resistant dulness, feeble breath sounds whose bronchial quality is no bar, and perhaps a diminished vocal resonance of ægophonic quality. Add to these finger-clubbing and the likeness is obvious. Points may generally be found, however, to turn the balance, and of these the position of neighbouring viscera comes foremost. The heart is displaced by fluid, drawn over by fibrosed lung, and, though a collapsed lung with chronic pleurisy may ultimately cause retraction of the chest wall and draw over the heart, the diagnosis is then unimportant, since the case is becoming, or will become, one of pulmonary fibrosis. The diagnosis from rare cases of *caseous consolidation* of the lung should not be difficult if it is made a rule not to diagnose fibrosis without evidence of pulmonary contraction. Lastly, it is important to remember, from the point of view of treatment, that the impaction of a *foreign body* in a bronchus, an accident which is likely to occur in childhood, will give rise to bronchiectasis and fibrosis of the corresponding lung.

Prognosis.—This depends on the position and extent of the lesion, and the age and station in life of the patient. Apical cases are probably of more favourable outlook than are those with basal lesions. In the latter, especially when there is considerable fibrosis, drainage of the cavities is bound to be deficient, and the retained secretion is likely to form a focus from which secondary infections may arise. Among three of my cases in which such secondary infections, empyema and broncho-pneumonia, occurred, in all the expectoration was fœtid. It is obvious, then, that the prognosis depends largely on the possibility or otherwise of efficiently draining the dilated tubes. The more advanced the fibrosis, the more marked, as a rule, the bronchiectasis, the more reduced the available lung tissue, and the greater the strain on the pulmonary circulation.

Since the lesion is irremediable, it follows that if it starts in infancy the outlook is worse than if it develops in the later years of childhood. In the poorer classes the exigencies of life greatly increase the risks of those acute attacks which constitute its chief danger; among the well-to-do, change to a warm climate during the winter months would do much to remove the risk of acute catarrhs, and the condition is consequently more likely to remain in abeyance.

Treatment.—The treatment resolves itself into that of the exacerbation and that of the quiescent interval. When the acute attack is due to a definite pneumonia, the expectant line of treatment suitable to that disease will be required, and, at the same time, the heart must be watched, since the fibrosis causes a constant impediment to the work of the right heart, and loss of compensation is much more likely to ensue than during a simple pneumonia. When an acute catarrh of the dilated tubes is present, the treatment is that of bronchitis, the object being to render the secretion liquid and abundant, and then to aid its removal with stimulating expectorants. When the acute attack is cardiac in origin, as it occasionally is, the treatment will be chiefly that employed for loss of compensation in mitral disease.

In the quiescent intervals, or in the less serious exacerbations of slight and apical cases, attention must be directed above all to improving the general health of the child. Such children stand badly the conditions of indoor life customary during the winter of a harsh climate, and, where circumstances permit, they should be removed during the colder months of the year to some spot where abundant sun and still, dry air are obtainable. Failing this, it is probable that a modified outdoor treatment at home would, as in phthisis, benefit the general health, and ward off to a large extent those catarrhs which are both dangerous in themselves and also tend to further the progress of the disease. I have had no experience of such treatment, but cannot but believe that, if judiciously employed, considerable benefit might be derived from it. Cod-liver oil with iron or malt are often useful, especially if creosote be added. Guaiacol may be used instead, and I have had considerable success with thiocol, a creosote derivative which is alike tasteless, soluble, and readily borne by a weak digestion. It may be given in doses beginning at 3–5 grains for children a few years old, and may be largely increased, though the small doses are often quite efficient in improving nutrition and the general well-being. It is best prescribed with syrup of orange or syrup of iron phosphate with or without dilution with water, but these may be omitted if the syrup upsets digestion.

In cases where drainage of the cavities is difficult, the effect of posture may be taken advantage of in clearing the tubes. By stooping, or by hanging the head and chest over the edge of a bed, the cavities empty by gravity into the healthy tubes above, violent cough is excited, and large quantities of phlegm may thereby be got rid of. In addition to this, an occasional emetic may be given, and a course of stimulating expectorants employed. If the sputum becomes foul, it is of the utmost importance that more efficient drainage be secured. Most efficient for this purpose is the method of creosote inhalation introduced by Dr. Arnold Chaplin, and employed with the utmost benefit in cases of bronchiectasis of the adult. I have not seen it tried in the case of children, but see no objection to its use in later childhood when foul expectoration is more commonly seen. The creosote is vaporised in a small room, and the patient endures the vapour for increasing periods daily, from ¼ hour at the beginning up to 1 hour at a sitting. The nostrils are plugged with cotton wool, and the eyes protected with watch glasses framed in adhesive plaster. The irritation of the strong vapour causes effective cough, whereby large quantities of foul sputum are expectorated, and the emptied cavities subjected to the action of the drug.

External drainage of cavities is not applicable to cases of pulmonary fibrosis in children, partly because the dilatations are multiple, and partly because the fibrosed surrounding parts are unable to fall in and close the discharging cavity.

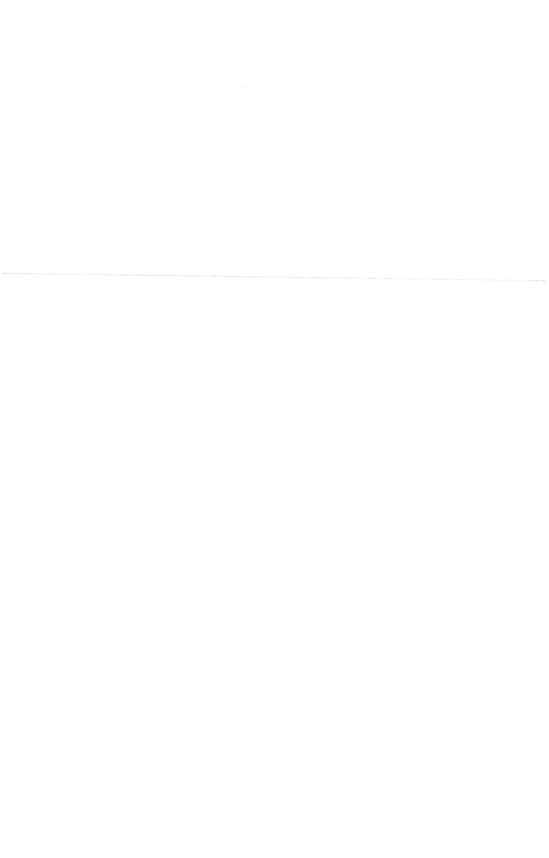

A CASE OF CONGENITAL OCCLUSION OF THE SMALL INTESTINE.

BY

C. M. H. HOWELL, M.B.

E. M. B., aged 4 days, a female child, was admitted to Faith Ward on March 1, with the following history.

She was a full-time child, and the birth had been quite natural. Though small (she weighed only 6 lbs.), she was well formed, and there was no external deformity.

Shortly after birth the child had vomited, and the vomiting had continued up to the date of admission. When first seen in the surgery the vomit contained bile, and there was a history of this bilious vomiting for two days previous to admission. No meconium was vomited. A small amount of meconium had been passed on the day of birth, but from that date till the child died nothing more was passed per rectum.

On examination the heart and lungs were natural; the abdomen was full, but not markedly distended; occasional peristaltic intestinal contractions were visible, and the superficial veins were somewhat full. The cord, which had not yet separated, appeared healthy.

On March 2 the vomiting still continued, but was no longer bilious in character. The child took the small quantities of liquid given to it fairly well, and the food was not immediately rejected.

On March 4, the eighth day after birth, the child died, having become progressively weaker since admission.

The question of operation was raised, and decided in the negative, though the result of the autopsy showed that surgical interference might possibly have proved effective.

The following is an extract from the post-mortem notes of the case :—

"Seven feet from the pylorus the small intestine came to an

abrupt termination, and for a space of 2 inches was wanting. It was then resumed as a patent tube, and extended 2 feet further to the ileocæcal valve. The upper part was considerably distended, and the lower completely collapsed. There was no other abnormality present. The lower portion was intussuscepted into itself for about 2 inches."

The specimen has been added to the museum.

It was noteworthy that meconium was passed soon after birth, and that it was of the ordinary colour, though the bile

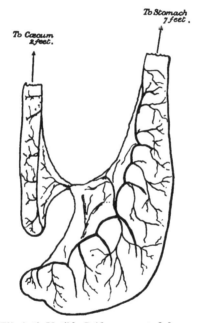

To Stomach
7 feet.

To Cæcum
2 feet.

Elizabeth Matilda Bridgeman, æt. 8 days.

can scarcely have reached the lower portion. In a case recently published by Emanuel in the Lancet, Aug. 12, 1905, in which there were multiple occlusions present, the same fact was noted, and the author quotes observations by Rolleston and Foster stating that in congenital occlusion of the bile-duct on the one hand, and in congenital absence of the liver on the other, apparently normal meconium was passed.

The case is an example of one of the developmental abnormalities resulting in atresia, which may affect the alimentary tract. Such abnormalities are fortunately rare. I can find no similar instance to this case in the post-mortem records for the last ten years at this hospital.

Atresia may occur congenitally in various situations in the alimentary tract. The œsophagus when so deformed is usually obliterated in its lower part—frequently the children so afflicted are born dead, and in many cases other abnormalities occur. The œsophagus is usually divided into two pouches, the lower of which occasionally communicates with the trachea—a condition which can be readily understood from the fact that the trachea and lungs are developed from the ventral part of the foregut.

In the stomach hour-glass contraction and hypertrophic stenosis of the pylorus are met with congenitally. These conditions more commonly occur than œsophageal or intestinal atresia, if we exclude the cases of imperforate rectum or anus.

In the intestine there are three special places where occlusion may occur.

They are :—

1. The duodenum—above Vater's papilla.
2. The duodeno-jejunal juncture.
3. At the spot in the ileum where the omphalo-meseraic duct is given off.

There may also be multiple occlusions, as in the case referred to in the Lancet.

Of the relative frequency with which occlusion occurs at the different localities the statistics differ. Hirschsprung, from analysis of 31 cases, gives 16 in duodenum, 6 in the situation of the omphalo-meseraic duct, and 9 in positions between these two. Gärtner, on the other hand, from 65 cases finds the majority at the omphalo-meseraic duct, fewer in the duodenum, and most of these above Vater's papilla.

An examination of cases of congenital occlusions, more or less complete, of the alimentary tract of which there are records at this hospital, for the period 1896–1905, yielded the following figures :—

Congenital occlusion of œsophagus	o
Hour-glass contraction of stomach	8
Congenital occlusion of intestine	1
(Case referred to above.)	
Imperforate anus or rectum	22
Congenital stricture of rectum	1

I am indebted to Sir Dyce Duckworth for permission to publish this case in the Hospital Reports.

A SERIES OF FATAL CASES OF JAUNDICE IN THE NEWBORN OCCURRING IN SUCCESSIVE PREGNANCIES.

BY

GEORGE A. AUDEN, M.D.

Whether the following series of fatal cases of icterus neonatorum may be referred to one of the pathological divisions of the described forms of jaundice in the newly-born, or whether the cases form a distinct pathological entity, I am not in a position to determine, but as I can only find one parallel series of similar cases described in the literature of jaundice (*vide infra*), the following notes seem worthy of record.

Mrs. G. is a well-developed woman about 38 years of age, whom I have attended in her confinements on several occasions. According to her own account, she has always been a healthy woman, and her labours have been easy. There is no reason to believe that she or her husband have ever suffered from syphilis; and, so far as she has been able to ascertain, there is no similar series of fatalities recorded in the case of any member of her family. She has had twelve pregnancies, the details of which follow.

1st. A full-term boy, born in July 1891. Never jaundiced, but said to have been "very pale," he is now a healthy, well-grown boy.

2nd. A full-term boy, born in May 1893; lived five days; was "born yellow, but became pale and died in its sleep."

3rd. A full-term girl, born in November 1894; lived five days; was "born yellow."

4th. Miscarried at the third month, May 1895.

5th. A full-term girl, born in February 1896; was "yellow when born," and extremely feeble. The yellow colour gradually gave place, in the course of three or four months, to a marked pallor. The child has grown up strong and healthy.

6th. A full-term boy, born in August 1898; was "yellow when born"; lived for six days. A post-mortem examination was made, but nothing was discovered which explained the condition.

7th. A full-term girl, born in September 1900. I saw the child on the third day; it was then deeply jaundiced; the child died of "inanition" on the sixth day.

8th. A full-term girl, born in September 1901. Previously to the birth of this child the mother had taken 15 grains of potassium iodide *per diem* for two months. The child was born at night, and, although carefully examined, no jaundice was visible until daylight, but it was very apparent seven hours later. The colour deepened at first, but by the seventh day had almost entirely disappeared, giving place to a profound anæmia, as if from severe hæmorrhage. During the period of jaundice the urine contained bile pigments in small quantity, and the fæces were yellowish and green. The child took the breast well, and seemed to be doing fairly, but collapsed suddenly on the eighth day. There were no hæmorrhages from the mucous membranes; no ecchymoses, and no vomiting. I have no note of the occurrence or absence of convulsions.

I made a post-mortem examination, but found nothing beyond a marked anæmia of all the viscera, and a soft, friable spleen. The liver and bile-ducts were natural, as also was the heart. An examination of blood-films gave no definite results, but appeared to show a considerable increase in the relative proportion of white blood-cells.

9th. Miscarriage at fifth month, a macerated fœtus; November 1902.

10th. A nearly full-term, still-born child, not jaundiced, August 1903.

11th. A full-term girl, born July 1904. At birth I took especial care to note that there was no jaundice, but the usual red colour of the newborn infant. Jaundice appeared in less than twenty-four hours, and increased for about forty-eight hours. The child became very drowsy; the jaundice then began to disappear, and at the end of the third week had become slight, giving place to a marked pallor. On the twenty-second day convulsions began, succeeding one another almost without intermission for twenty-four hours until death took place. During the period of jaundice bile pigment was present in the urine, but the nature of the stools was always that of a healthy infant, passing from the dark green meconium to the healthy yellow of the second week, although they assumed a dark "chopped parsley" colour shortly before death.

A post-mortem examination was made twenty-four hours after death. The child was well nourished. The spleen was large, soft, and friable. The liver and bile-ducts were normal, as also was the gall-bladder, which was empty, except for a little mucus; the tissues—*e.g.* subcutaneous fat and peritoneum —were bile stained. The heart showed no abnormality.

The cloth in which I removed the organs for histological examination became markedly bile stained. There appeared to be a remarkably small volume of blood in the body.

12*th*. A full-term boy, born August 1905. There was no trace of jaundice at birth. Seven hours later the yellow colour was distinct, and increased rapidly. Forty-eight hours after birth convulsions began, and continued till death occurred on the third day. In order to prevent any possible source of poisoning from the mother, this child was never suckled by her, as the previous infants had been.

The histological examination of the tissues removed from the body of the eleventh child gave no very satisfactory results. The organs appeared to be on the whole normal, and the kidney, the spleen, and the lung showed no changes beyond cloudy swelling of the cells. The umbilical cord also appeared to be quite natural. The liver, on the other hand, was extensively diseased; the cells were the seat of a fine but universal fatty degeneration, and there was a considerable infiltration of small round cells between the liver-cells; bile was present in most of the ducts. There was no cirrhosis, and no localised necrosis. The degeneration was equally developed in all the parts examined. The general aspect of the liver section suggested an acute toxæmia. The blood-films taken from the heart of this child, and from the umbilical cord at birth of the twelfth of the children, gave no definite information, though it appeared that large mono-nuclear leucocytes were present in excess of their normal numbers; the red cells were normal in size and shape, and no abnormal leucocytes were observed. However, in the absence of an estimation of the numbers of red and white corpuscles during life (an examination often pressed, but somewhat naturally always refused), it is obviously impossible to draw any definite conclusions from the examination of the films.

The series of similar cases to which I have referred was recorded by Arkwright in the Edinburgh Medical Journal, vol. xii. p. 156 [1902].

Briefly summarised, the series was one of fifteen pregnancies, the last coming to term when the mother was aged 44. Of these fifteen pregnancies four children survived—the second, the fourth, the fourteenth, and fifteenth. The first child, which lived till 7 months, is not known to have had jaundice, but all the others were affected in varying degrees of severity. Nearly all died in convulsions, but with one possible exception none had any hæmorrhages. The majority died in a few days ; some lived a few months ; none except the four survivors lived beyond 8 months of age.[1]

The interesting points in my own series of cases, with which the other series agrees in the main, appear to me to be :—

I. The appearance in successive children of the same parents.
II. The rapid development within a few hours of birth of a jaundice, which quickly became profound.
III. The occurrence of a generally drowsy condition which usually ended in convulsions, terminating fatally.
IV. The severe anæmia which became more and more marked as the colour of the jaundice waned, and which persisted for a lengthy period in those affected children which survived.
     In none of my series was there any wasting.
V. The "hæmatogenous" characteristics of the jaundice and absence of any form of hæmorrhage.

On the whole, reviewing the clinical history and the post-mortem and histological findings, it appears to me most probable that the disease is an example of an acute toxæmia, due to some profound chemical disturbance, rather than to the products of a bacterial infection.

In the absence of any histological examination of the organs of the still-born children and abortions, it is impossible to determine whether their deaths *in utero* were due to the same cause which produced the jaundice in those born alive, but the inference appears a probable one.

It is a fact worth notice that in both series the pregnancies followed one another in quick succession, and that in both the first child was not affected.

For the histological examination of the organs and the report upon the blood-films I am indebted to Dr. Hugh Thursfield.

---

[1] While the above has been in the press a third series has been reported by Busfield [B. M J. 1906, i. p. 20]. Of the 9 pregnancies of a healthy woman, the 1st never suffered from jaundice, the 2nd suffered but recovered, the 3rd, 4th, 5th, and 6th died of jaundice—the last exhibited the condition on the second day and died comatose on the eighth day. The 7th and 8th were jaundiced, but recovered. The 9th died jaundiced on the fourth day. A post-mortem examination revealed nothing except that the gall-bladder contained bile. There was no distension and no occlusion of the bile-duct. The 10th exhibited jaundice six hours after birth and died on the fourth day. No history of syphilis.

CASES FROM THE WARDS OF

SIR DYCE DUCKWORTH AND DR. CHAMPNEYS.

REPORTED BY

H. U. GOULD, M.B.

In each of the three following cases an acute toxæmic condition obscured the primary cause of disease. The three patients were of about the same age and each exhibited an appearance in which high fever and a semi-comatose condition were the most prominent features and, in the case of each, there was a marked absence of physical signs upon which to base a satisfactory diagnosis.

The first case was one of malignant endocarditis, the probable source of infection being an ulcerated surface on the pharynx. In this instance a prœsystolic murmur was heard on the evening when the patient was brought up to the hospital, but in spite of frequent examinations the murmur was not heard again until five days later, two days before the patient's death. Both these occasions occurred at night and on that account the presence of the murmur could not be verified by other observers.

The appearance of the patient suggested typhus, typhoid fever, meningitis, &c.

The second case was not easy of diagnosis. At first the appearance was very similar to that of the one already mentioned, on the fourth day there appeared somewhat indefinite signs at the right base behind, that pointed either to pneumonia or pleurisy. The illness seems to have followed after a trip to Southend, but whether it was one of those cases of pneumonia with marked toxæmic disturbance and slight local manifestation, or whether it was a case of ptomaine poisoning complicated by pleurisy, is uncertain; the latter appeared the more probable explanation.

It may be mentioned that at the same time there were

under Sir Dyce Duckworth's care two or three other patients
with poisoning from the eating of cockles, one of whom also
had been spending his bank-holiday at Southend.

The third case was one of pneumonia in which death ensued
within eighteen hours of the onset. The chest had been
examined at different times by three or four competent persons
and no sign of pneumonia had been discovered.

CASE I.—H. E. M., aged 13, schoolboy, was admitted to
Matthew ward on April 20, 1904, in a feverish and semi-
comatose condition.

Quite well up to April 12, he went to school on the morning
of that day and while there fainted and was on that account
sent home. In the evening he became feverish, felt unwell
and had a shivering fit. From that time he was kept to bed,
his temperature being 102°-103° daily. On April 18 he complained of pain in his limbs and general tenderness and could
not bear to be touched; he was drowsy all day. There was
no vomiting and no further shivering occurred. There was no
action of the bowels on April 18 or 19.

The boy had always enjoyed good health and had never had
rheumatic fever. There had been no recent illness at home
and there was nothing of importance in the family history.

On being admitted to the hospital and put to bed the patient
lay quietly so long as he was not disturbed, but cried out on
being touched. His complexion was dusky red and his body,
somewhat ill nourished, was covered with what appeared to be
flea bites (? purpuric rash). His temperature was 100.2°; pulse,
100, of low tension; respirations, 28, and shallow. The conjunctivæ were injected, the pupils large and reacted to light.
His mouth was dry, the tongue being glazed but not furred.
In the neck a few small glands were just palpable. There
appeared to be no injury to the head and no affection of ears or
throat was discovered. There was no epiphysitis. The chest
moved equally on both sides, but the expansion was small; the
lungs appeared natural. On examining the heart the apex beat
was found in the fifth space, just outside the nipple line; the area
of cardiac dulness extended to the left margin of the sternum
and upwards to the third costal cartilage. In addition to
natural first and second sounds a proesystolic murmur, somewhat musical in character, was heard at the apex. The
abdomen was full and moved very little in its lower part, but
this was due to the shallow breathing; there was no resistance
or tenderness and the percussion note was natural. The liver
appeared natural, but the spleen was readily palpable. There

were ecchymoses in the region of the left internal malleolus. The urine was acid and had a specific gravity of 1010; there was a trace of albumen, but no blood was present; there was no sugar.

On April 21 the Widal reaction proved negative. A purpuric rash had now developed over the front of the neck and in each axilla. During the day the temperature varied between 101·6° and 104·6°; pulse, 104–136; respirations, 32–40. During the next day the mean temperature was 104° and did not fall below 103°; pulse, 136. The coma increased and the patient no longer cried out when touched. Nasal feeding had to be resorted to at times. The purpuric rash by this time covered the greater part of both trunk and limbs. No cardiac murmur had been heard since the 20th, the heart sounds being natural. The knee-jerks were natural. Urine had been passed involuntarily ever since admission and the bowels had been opened by means of an enema. On April 23 the pupils were unequal, the right being larger than the left; the discs were natural; there was some rigidity of the right leg and, at times, slight retraction of the head and slight arching of the back, but this was not constant. All food had now to be given by nasal tube. During the day there was a blood-stained discharge from the right ear, but this was found to proceed from the external, and not from the middle ear. Lumbar puncture was performed and blood was also taken from the median-basilic vein. (A bacteriological examination detected streptococci in both fluids, the spinal fluid was, however, unfortunately contaminated with blood at the time when it was being drawn off.) The Widal reaction was still negative, whilst a blood-count showed 4,544,000 red corpuscles and 14,000 leucocytes. On auscultating the heart at midnight the proesystolic musical murmur was again heard at the apex, this being only the second occasion on which it was heard. The temperature continued to vary between 103° and 104°, while the pulse-rate was slowly increasing, 140–152, and was of small volume and low tension.

The pulse gradually failed, and the patient died on the afternoon of April 25, no fresh symptoms having appeared.

At the post-mortem examination there were found a few sub-pericranial hæmorrhages. Besides the petechial hæmorrhages in the skin, similar hæmorrhages were found almost everywhere throughout the alimentary and respiratory tracts and also beneath the pericardium and beneath the arachnoid membrane over the convexity of the brain. In the lateral walls of the pharynx, just behind the tonsil on either side, an area, 1 inch in diameter, was covered with a yellow granular membrane. In the pericardial sac were found from 1 to 2 drachms of slightly turbid fluid. The pulmonary, tricuspid and aortic valves were natural, but the mitral valve was completely surrounded as to its free edge with a ridge of recent granulations, soft in consistence and yellow, raised about one-fifth of an inch. There were infarctions of recent date in the spleen and kidneys.

CASE 2.—C. W., aged 14, vanboy, was admitted to Matthew Ward on May 25, 1904, on account of pyrexia and vomiting, being in a semi-comatose condition.

On May 24 the boy, on his return from work, felt sick and vomited several times. He was put to bed and kept on milk and soda. He complained of pain in the abdomen, but slept well all night.

The next day, May 25, at 9.30 A.M., he vomited and was restless; his bowels were opened, the result being a small semi-solid stool. At 11 o'clock he began to wander and a doctor was sent for, who, on his arrival, found the patient unconscious and with a temperature of 104°.

The following further history was obtained: On May 11 the boy had had a fall on his head; on May 21 he had tooth-ache and a swollen face; on May 23 he went to Southend for the day and ate many cockles. It was also said that he had passed no urine for two days.

The patient had always had good health, though he had had coughs from time to time. He had never had fits. The family history threw no light on the case.

On admission, the boy, who was well nourished, lay in a semi-comatose condition; he could be roused a little, but no clear answers could be obtained. He retched occasionally, but was not sick. The legs were drawn up, but there was no other sign of pain or tenderness. The face was flushed, the conjunctivæ slightly injected and the pupils natural; the alæ nasi were not working. The tongue was very dry and glazed and of a red colour. There was some swelling of the right side of the face and there were some carious teeth on that side. The throat, ears and limbs all appeared natural. The chest was well formed and the two sides moved equally, but the expansion was poor; both heart and lungs appeared natural. The abdomen also appeared natural. The urine was acid, its specific gravity being 1020; it contained neither albumen nor sugar.

On the morning of April 26 the bowels were well opened after an enema; the patient was much less drowsy and took food well; his tongue was moist. The temperature was 98·4°, pulse 84 and respirations 26; in the evening the temperature rose to 102·6°, the pulse being 80 and the respirations 26. The following day the temperature was 102° in the morning and 104·2° in the evening, the pulse being 100 and the respirations 32. He was again drowsy and had some cough; on examining the chest some sibili were heard scattered over the right side and friction sounds were heard behind at the right base. On May 28 the sputum was streaked with blood, but the cough was not very troublesome. The bowels had not been opened since the 26th. In the morning the temperature was 103·4°, the pulse 88 and the respirations 32. The temperature fell to 98·2° at noon, but rose again in the evening to 100°, the pulse being 84. On May 29 there was dulness behind at the right base and the breath sounds were weak in that region; the vocal resonance was equal on both sides. The bowels were well opened during the day. The following day the temperature became normal and the general condition was improved. On May 31 there was still a slight cough, the percussion note at the right base was still impaired and the breath sounds in that region were weak. On June 2 the signs at the right base had nearly cleared up, the temperature remained normal and the cough, which had never caused much trouble, had nearly ceased. The patient began to get up on June 7 and was discharged in good health on June 18.

CASE 3.—J. P., aged 12, was admitted to the Surgery Ward on July 18, 1904.

The boy was quite well till the morning of that day, when he awoke, at 2 A.M., feeling ill and vomited. He was brought up to the Surgery at 9 A.M. and admitted.

There was no history of any previous ailment and there was no sickness at home.

On being put to bed he lay quietly in a semi-comatose condition; the breathing was rapid, but the patient appeared to be in no distress. The pulse was rapid, of fair tension and small volume and the temperature was 104°. His face was flushed and his tongue dry. Nothing abnormal was discovered in heart or lungs and the abdomen appeared natural. The urine was highly coloured and contained a trace of albumen.

The coma increased during the day; the chest was examined three or four times, but nothing abnormal was discovered. The temperature rose above 105° in the evening; the pulse gradually failed and the boy died at 10 P.M.

At the post-mortem examination there was found to be consolidation of practically the whole of the right lung.

A Case of Pyrexia and Vomiting, relieved by the Passage of a Round-Worm from the Rectum.

A. T., aged 10, a school-girl, was admitted to Faith Ward on June 11, 1904. She had been quite well until about 11 o'clock that morning, she was then seized with colic and had diarrhœa, the motions being "like blood and flesh." She was said to have had dysentery five years ago.

On admission her temperature was 101·4°, pulse 120 and respirations 28. On examining the chest and abdomen nothing abnormal was discovered. The same evening the temperature rose to 103°, the pulse being 136. Early the next morning a round-worm, 9 inches in length, was passed *per anum*. The temperature immediately fell and became normal within 24 hours. The girl was discharged, shortly afterwards, quite well.

A Case of Rheumatic Fever with Pericarditis, in which there was Rapid Enlargement of the Area of Cardiac Dulness, followed by an almost equally Rapid Return to its former Dimensions.

There was some doubt as to whether this was a case of cardiac dilatation or pericardial effusion. The fact that the endocardial sounds were plainly heard throughout, made the former the more probable; on the other hand, the fact that there was never any cardiac pain or distress, that the pulse was never very irregular and the way in which the pericardial friction disappeared gradually from apex to base, pointed to effusion.

It was a case either of dilatation or effusion; in the latter case the heart must have been rendered adherent to the pericardium anteriorly by old pericarditis.

Lily B., aged 15, a waterproof-maker, was admitted to Faith Ward on June 14, 1904, complaining of rheumatic pains and severe headache.

She had been ailing fourteen days. On June 1 she complained of pains in her right elbow and right knee; she also had a slight cough and had little appetite for food. A week later she began to have severe headache and became worse and, on June 10, had to give up work and take to bed. She complained of pain in her left axillary region when she lay on that side.

Patient has always been delicate and had rheumatic fever

in 1900 and again in 1902; she often gets a "touch" of rheumatism in her hands and other joints.

There was no history of rheumatism among other members of the family.

When admitted to the ward the skin over the right knee, right ankle and tarso-metatarsal joints was red, hot and tender, these joints being painful as well as the right elbow, left knee and left foot. There was some effusion in the right knee and ankle-joints. On examining the chest the heart's apex beat was found in the fifth space, 1 inch outside the left nipple line, and the area of cardiac dulness was somewhat square, extending upwards to the second intercostal space and inwards just beyond the left margin of the sternum. There was pericardial friction all over the area of cardiac dulness; the heart sounds were faint, but otherwise natural, no endocardial murmur being heard. An emplastrum lyttæ was applied over the cardiac region and 10 grains of sodium salicylate were given every four hours. By June 17 nearly all pain had disappeared, though the joints of the right foot were still slightly red and tender. Salicylates were now taken off, as blood had appeared in the urine. No alteration had taken place in the heart's condition. On June 20 there was some return of pain in the joints, so 20 grains of salicin, in cachet, were given six hourly. On June 22 the area of cardiac dulness had increased; it extended 1½ inches beyond the left nipple line in the fifth intercostal space, 1 inch beyond the right margin of the sternum and upwards to the second rib. The apex beat was felt, indistinct and diffuse, in the region of the nipple and the friction sounds at the apex were less clearly heard than formerly, though still plainly audible along the sternum and at the cardiac base.

On June 24 there was again a good deal of pain in the joints. The heart's apex beat was no longer palpable; the area of cardiac dulness was still further increased and extended 3 inches beyond the left nipple line and almost to the right nipple line; upwards it extended to the first intercostal space. The friction sounds were only heard at the cardiac base, whilst in the region of the left nipple a systolic murmur was now plainly heard in addition to the first and second sounds. The veins in the neck were full and pulsated slightly. Four leeches were applied over the cardiac area.

The salicin had been taken off on June 23, as, although the joint pain had been relieved, there was a return of the hæmaturia. The patient was now being given Pot. Cit. gr. xx., Tn. Cinchonæ 3js., Tn. Nuc. Vom. ♏ iv. every six hours.

Towards evening there was a little dyspnœa and slight coughing; the patient, however, was not distressed and slept well during the night. The following day the area of cardiac dulness was slightly diminished, but the apex beat could not be distinguished. A blood-count was made and there was found to be a leucocytosis of 28,000. On July 1 the patient was much better and there was no pain in the joints, but some stiffness; the area of cardiac dulness was less and extended but little beyond the right margin of the sternum; the systolic murmur was still plainly heard near the left nipple and soft friction was heard along the sternum and at the base.

On July 4 the apex beat could be felt 1 inch outside the left nipple line in the fifth space; the area of cardiac dulness extended from the left margin of the sternum to the apex beat; no friction was heard, but there remained the systolic murmur to be heard at the apex and conducted into the axilla. The pulse was regular, of small volume and low tension. There was no pain or swelling of the joints.

From that time forward recovery was uninterrupted; the patient began to get up on July 22 and went to Swanley on August 24, at which time there was very little cardiac enlargement, the apex beat being just outside the nipple line and the area of cardiac dulness not extending beyond the left border of the sternum; there was still a faint systolic murmur to be heard at the apex, but there was no friction. She was quite free from joint pain and felt well.

The temperature from June 14 to 28 varied between 100° and 103°, the pulse being 112–136. After June 28 the temperature gradually fell, it became normal on July 4 and so continued.

There was no hæmaturia or albuminuria after the end of June.

The following case of typhoid fever is of interest on account of the rigor which occurred at about the end of the third or early in the fourth week. The significance of a rigor in typhoid fever is often difficult to estimate at the time of its occurrence; it may indicate some desperate condition, such as perforation of the intestine, or it may, as in this case, pass off without any ill effect, leaving one uncertain as to the cause of the phenomenon. In the following case the whole event took place in a space of less than four hours; up to 11 A.M. the patient appeared to be going on quite well and at 3 P.M. there was no sign that anything untoward had happened.

Emily O'M., aged 12, was admitted to Faith Ward on April 20, 1904, being at that time in the third week of typhoid fever.

She had been drowsy for the last two or three weeks and had not been to school since April 6. During the last seven days she had become more drowsy, had lost flesh and had little appetite for food. The bowels had acted regularly and there had been no diarrhœa.

The family had been short of food lately, but there had been no illness in the house.

· The patient was a fairly well developed child and was some-what drowsy. The mouth was dry and the tongue furred. The heart appeared natural; the lungs gave evidence of a little bronchitis. There was no rash. The abdomen was full and the spleen easily palpable. The urine was acid and had a specific gravity of 1015; it contained no albumen. The Widal reaction was positive.

All went well with the patient up to April 24. During that time the temperature varied between 100° and 104°, the pulse being 116–124. The child was sponged on two occasions when the temperature reached 104°. Nourishment was taken well and the bowels acted naturally once daily, the motions being semi-solid.

On the morning of April 25 the child appeared in her usual condition; at 7 A.M. her temperature was 98° and at 11 A.M. 99·5°, the pulse being 112 and 116. At 11 A.M. patient had a rigor lasting 50 minutes, during which she became cold, somewhat cyanosed and very collapsed, with a running pulse which could not be counted. She complained of no pain and the abdomen moved well. The temperature rose to 105°; the pulse, at first uncountable, was found later to be 140, and later still 152. Brandy and strychnine were administered and, as the temperature rose, the child was first cradled and then sponged.

The state of affairs was alarming, the rigor, extreme collapse and increasing pulse-rate arousing one's fears for the worst. The child, however, speedily recovered and, at 3 P.M., four hours after the onset of the symptoms, she had returned to her previous condition and showed no sign of the recent dis-turbance; the temperature had fallen to 102°; the pulse was 120 and had recovered its volume and tension. Nothing was discovered to account for the rigor.

The patient continued to progress well and the temperature became normal on May 1. Unfortunately a relapse set in on May 6; all went well, however, and the child left the hospital well on July 7.

The two following cases illustrate the difficulty sometimes met with in determining whether the signs found on examining a chest point to consolidation of the lung or the presence of fluid in the pleural cavity.

CASE 1.—May G., aged 17, was admitted to Martha Ward on November 23, 1904, on account of recurring attacks of abdominal pain.

Two years ago she first had an attack of pain in the left iliac fossa; six months later she had another attack similar to the first and ten days ago, on November 13, she had a third attack of pain in the same region.

Menstruation began at the age of 13 and had always been regular; there had been no connection between the periods and the attacks of pain.

The patient had always been delicate and her mother and sisters also were delicate, her mother and one sister having been operated upon for tuberculous glands in the neck.

On examining the abdomen an elastic tumour, the size of a fœtal head, was found moored a little to the left of the navel and not resting on the pelvic brim; the uterus was retroverted.

The chest was well formed; both heart and lungs appeared natural.

On November 30 Mr. Cripps operated and found a left ovarian cyst bound to the abdominal wall by adhesions, the pedicle being partially twisted. The right ovary was four times its normal size and cystic. Double ovariotomy was performed.

The next day the patient vomited several times; the temperature was slightly raised and there was a little coughing.

On December 3 she complained of her throat being sore.

The cough continued and there was a nightly rise of temperature to about 101·5°.

On December 10 the last stitches were removed from the abdominal wound, which appeared quite healthy.

So it went on, the patient being in no distress and, being propped up in bed, she spent the day talking and doing needlework, but the cough got no better and the temperature each evening was raised to 101° or 102°.

On December 23 the chest was again examined and it was found that the right side moved on respiration better than the left. The heart's apex was in the fifth space just inside the nipple line; the area of cardiac dulness and the sounds were natural. At the left base behind and in the left axilla there was dulness on percussion extending nearly to the level of the spine of the scapula; the apex of the lung appeared natural, as did also the right lung. The vocal vibrations were nearly equal on both sides, but slightly increased at the left base behind; on auscultation crepitations were heard over the left base and bronchial breathing was heard over nearly the whole of the left lung and over the inner half of the right back below the level of the spine of the scapula. Vocal resonance was increased over the left base.

The appearance of the chest made the presence of chronic disease, such as fibroid lung, improbable, moreover, there had been nothing very obviously wrong with the chest when the patient was admitted to the hospital. The physical signs pointed to consolidation, while the history, temperature and general condition all indicated the probability of a pleural effusion. There was no expectoration and it had not been possible to collect any sputum.

On December 29 the chest was explored and 33 ounces of clear fluid were drawn off. The lung expanded well as the fluid was removed.

The temperature and cough continued, some muco-purulent sputum was obtained and examined, but no tubercle bacilli were found.

On January 4 the patient was discharged at the request of her parents and was taken home.

CASE 2.—A. M., aged 30, was admitted to Casualty Ward on December 27, 1904, on account of bleeding after miscarriage.

There was a history of 3½ months' amenorrhœa. On December 20 the woman was seized with sudden pain in the hypogastrium and at the same time she noticed a slight "show." On the following day there was bleeding all day, "little and little." On December 22 she awoke flooding and passed a lump of flesh which she thought was the "baby."

She did not lie up and irregular bleedings continued up to the time of admission, clots being passed daily.

The patient has spent some years abroad and has had "malaria" in India and Australia at various times. In June of this year she was in Middlesex Hospital with pleurisy and pneumonia.

On being examined it was found that the uterus was somewhat enlarged and not tender. The cervix was fairly soft and the os was closed, but there was some bleeding into the vagina. The abdomen otherwise appeared natural; the spleen could not be felt; the heart and lungs also appeared normal.

The temperature at the time of admission was 103°, it

became normal later in the evening, but then continued to be irregular for some days.

December 28, morning—temperature, 98.6°; pulse, 86.
	28, evening	,,	103.6°	,,	108.	
	29, morning	,,	100.2°	,,	102.	
	29, evening	,,	105.8°	,,	108.	Rigor.
	30, morning	,,	99.4°	,,	92.	
	30, evening	,,	102°	,,	96.	
	31, morning	,,	98°	,,	96.	
	31, 3 P.M.	,,	104.8°	,,	100.	Rigor.

On December 31 the bleeding still continuing, the temperature being irregular and two rigors having occurred, it was thought advisable to examine the interior of the uterus. Chloroform was administered, the cervix dilated and some pieces of placenta removed by the finger, the uterus being afterwards swabbed out with tincture of iodine.

The patient appeared to be better the next day and the temperature remained normal from January 2 to 6, but then began to rise again. There was no more bleeding.

On January 7 there was a rigor, the temperature being 101°, the pulse 120 and the respirations 24.

From January 9 to 11 the temperature again remained normal.

On January 12 there was a sudden rise of temperature to 104°, but there was no rigor. On January 14 there was another rigor, the temperature reaching 105·8°, the pulse was 116 and the respirations 24.

The patient felt well in the intervals and no explanation was found for the rigors. The heart, lungs and urine all appeared natural, there was no bleeding or discharge from the vagina and the uterus was not tender. Neither spleen nor kidneys were palpable. It was thought possible that the rigors might be malarial in nature, but an examination of the blood gave no evidence of such.

From January 15 to 24 the temperature was normal.

On January 25 there was another rigor, the temperature being 104°, the pulse 124 and the respirations 20.

From January 27 to 29 the temperature varied between 103° and 105°, the pulse being 108–120 and respirations 24–28.

On January 30 the patient complained of pain in her back, loins and lumbar region; the temperature during the day was 101°–104°, pulse 108–136 and respirations 44–60. The sputum was of a prune-juice colour and rather suggested the presence of an infarction in the lung.

On examining the chest, the left base behind was found to

be dull on percussion, in the same region the vocal vibrations and vocal resonance were increased and fine crepitations were heard. There was no bronchial breathing; the heart appeared natural, its apex not being displaced.

The temperature continued above 101°, with an evening rise to about 103° or 104°, the pulse being 140–150 and respirations 50–60. On February 3 patient felt better and the cough was quite loose, the sputum being of a purplish-brown. The left back was dull up to the spine of the scapula and there was distant bronchial breathing just below the angle of the scapula. Vocal resonance was increased over the dull area, but the vocal vibrations were diminished. There were crepitations all over the left base. The heart was as before.

Thus the patient had the signs and symptoms of pneumonia, which appeared from the course of the illness to be of septic origin. The sputum, however, was not that of pneumonia and the woman's appearance, the diminished vocal vibrations, the character of the temperature and the fact that there had been several rigors suggested the possibility of an empyema.

An exploring needle was employed, fluid containing pus was found and 8 ounces of turbid fluid were drawn off.

On February 4, chloroform having been given, a portion of the sixth rib in the posterior axillary line on the left side was removed and several ounces of flaky serum and pus were liberated. Many adhesions could be felt above, below and anterior to the wound.

The temperature gradually fell till February 14 and from that date it continued normal till May 1, when the patient was discharged in good health, the sinus being nearly healed up.

A Case of a Gastric Ulcer Ruptured during Labour.

F. M., aged 24, was admitted to Martha Ward in February 1905, being 38 weeks pregnant and complaining of swelling in the legs. The woman was a primipara.

About January 23, 1905, the patient first noticed swelling of the left ankle, this spread gradually all over that leg and later the right leg became swollen. The voice had recently become husky and weak. The woman had had no headache and no visual symptoms. She had lately passed more urine than usual. There was no previous history of nephritis.

At the time of her admission she was not anæmic, her naso-pharynx was blocked up with adenoids and on that account she breathed heavily and snored at nights.

She had the usual signs of a 38 weeks' pregnancy and the foetal heart was heard beating. There was considerable œdema of the legs, some lumbar œdema, but no œdema of the vulva. The cervix was soft and thinned ; the os admitted two fingers ; a foot presented. The urine contained 0·75 per cent. of albumen.

On February 8, at 3 A.M., the os being fully dilated, the membranes ruptured and a male child was born a few minutes later ; at 5.15 A.M. a female child was delivered by forceps and the placenta came away intact shortly afterwards. Chloroform was given during the birth of both children to save the mother as much as possible. During the birth of the first child, which was a breech case, the vagina was somewhat lacerated in its lower part and had to be sewn up ; the perineum was not injured.

On the following day the temperature was raised and the pulse somewhat rapid. The vulva was œdematous.

On February 11 the temperature was still raised, being about 102°, and the pulse was 120. The vulva was very œdematous and there was some sloughing.

The patient did not complain of pain, she was very drowsy and slept nearly all day and had to be roused for her food, which she took very well.

On February 13 her temperature was 103°-104° and her pulse 120–140. She was still taking her food well and slept in the intervals. She was in no pain and the vulva, which was being syringed with hydrogen peroxide, was cleaning up and becoming less œdematous. The abdomen was rather distended.

On February 15 the abdomen was more distended and there were signs of free fluid in the peritoneal cavity. Blood was taken from a vein for bacteriological examination and streptococci were subsequently grown from it. The patient still took her food well and slept when not disturbed. During the day she asked that she might have some more solid food on the next day. The temperature during the day was 104°-105° and the pulse 130–150.

There was no vomiting throughout.

The woman died on the following day, February 16.

This naturally appeared to be a case of septicæmia following after delivery ; the post-mortem examination, however, showed that the general peritonitis was due to a perforated gastric ulcer. The ulcer was an old chronic one, its base being adherent to the liver by a fibrous band. Evidently during labour the ulcer had been pulled upon by the fibrous band

and ruptured and now the base of the ulcer was attached to the stomach only by a hinge and to the liver by the fibrous band.

The Rupture of a Pelvic Abscess giving the Signs of a Perforated Gastric Ulcer.

A. D., aged 44, was admitted to Elizabeth Ward on March 2, 1905, on account of uterine hæmorrhage.

The woman had been twice married; by her first husband she had had five children, the last of which was born ten years ago; since her second marriage she had had two miscarriages, in July and November 1903. Since the end of 1903 her periods had been regular up to November 1904, then she had six weeks' amenorrhœa and since January 6, 1905 she had been bleeding profusely, on and off, and passing clots.

When admitted she was anæmic; her temperature was normal. Her uterus was retroverted and rather bulky, the sound passing 3¾ inches. There was in the left posterior quarter of the pelvis an elastic body the size of an egg, probably a hydrosalpinx.

On March 4 and 5 tents were introduced into the cervical canal and on March 6 the uterus was curetted, but little mucosa being removed. After the tenting there had been a rise of temperature to 101.4° and in the evening of the 6th the temperature was 102.8° and the pulse 96.

During the next week the temperature remained between 100° and 102°, the pulse being 92. The patient complained of pain in the left iliac fossa and on March 10 examination showed a mass in the situation of Douglas' pouch in front of the rectum, part of it being elastic and part boggy and tender. This mass appeared to be due to perimetritis.

From this time onward the temperature and pulse, though still raised, appeared to be quieting down and the woman no longer complained of pain.

The patient seemed to be going on quite satisfactorily till the evening of March 17, when, at 9.45 P.M., she vomited about 3 ounces of dark brown fluid. After this she was comfortable till 11.45 P.M. and then again vomited, at the same time there was a sudden onset of acute pain localised to an area the size of a five-shilling piece at the costal angle. The pain was not spasmodic but continuous. The patient looked pale and ill and presented the "facies abdominalis." She sweated, but was cold. Her temperature was 100° and her pulse 140, small and irregular. At 1 A.M. on March 18 the condition remained unaltered, the pulse was 140 and at times was felt with difficulty. The abdomen was now fuller than formerly, but not much distended; it moved fairly well and was not more tender than usual, except in the epigastric region. The patient preferred to lie on her right side. There were signs of free fluid in the abdominal cavity and the liver dulness was markedly diminished, the percussion note over it being somewhat tympanitic.

There were, therefore, the signs of free fluid and free gas in the peritoneal cavity and these, together with the brown vomit and acute pain restricted to the epigastric region, called attention to the probability of a perforated gastric ulcer, while, on the other hand, there was the previous pelvic trouble pointing to the likelihood of the general peritonitis being connected with that.

At 4.30 A.M. the temperature was 96.4°, the pulse 140 and the woman very collapsed. Mr. Waring opened the belly and found free gas and a milky fluid in the abdominal cavity. This was sponged out. The appendix was found to be normal. An abscess cavity surrounded by adhesions was found in Douglas' pouch, containing about ½ pint of thick, yellow, stinking pus. This was sponged out and the abdomen closed, drainage tubes being inserted.

The woman did not long survive the operation.

At the post-mortem examination there was found to be pus in both Fallopian tubes and there was evidence of the presence of a large abscess cavity in Douglas' pouch.

There was no perforation of the stomach or intestines.

The two last cases are instances of simple stricture of the rectum following upon pelvic inflammation. Both gave histories that made one a little suspicious of malignant disease and both were in Martha Ward at about the same time.

A. S., aged 42, housewife, was admitted on November 19, 1904, complaining of pain in the right hypogastrium and discharge from the rectum.

There had been a discharge from the rectum ever since the last confinement, two and a half years ago. There had been pain in the right hypogastrium and diarrhœa during the last six months.

The woman was married at the age of 34, eight and a half years ago. She had had 3 children, the last being born two and a half years ago, and one miscarriage six and a half years ago. She had inflammation after the first confinement seven and a half years ago.

On examination, the anus and perinæum were found to be livid, glazy and cracked (due to irritating discharge). The uterus was flexed to the right and fixed; there was a mass, the size of a small egg, situated to the left of the uterus and fixed to it. The cervix was fixed, but felt healthy. Examining by the rectum, about 3 inches from the anus the examining finger passed, through a ring which just admitted the finger; the mucous membrane was healthy. This stricture of the rectum was at the level of the reflection of the pelvic peritoneum and apparently resulted from the old perimetritis which occurred at the woman's first confinement seven and a half years ago.

The bowels were thoroughly cleared out and the symptoms thereby relieved. The patient was discharged on November 25.

B. B., aged 31, housewife, was admitted on November 26, 1904, complaining of abdominal pain and discharge from the rectum.

The woman was in Elizabeth Ward March to April 1903 and was operated upon for left ovarian tumour in the broad ligament. Recovery was uneventful.

On being admitted, the patient was found to have a simple stricture of the rectum similar to, and in the same situation as, the last case. She was treated in the same way and her symptoms relieved.

In conclusion I would express my best thanks to Sir Dyce Duckworth and Dr. Champneys for kindly allowing me to record the cases of the above series.

THREE CASES OF PRIMARY MALIGNANT DISEASE OF THE LIVER.

BY

COLIN S. HAWES, M.R.C.S.

The following three cases may be considered of some interest owing to the comparative rarity of the disease and the relatively great immunity of the native races of South Africa to cancer.

The three patients were Hottentots of the better type, and while one had been born and bred in a town, the other two had lived all their lives in the country. They came under observation in the Albany Hospital, Grahamstown, and I am indebted to Dr. J. B. Greathead and Dr. Bruce-Bays, under whose care they were, for permission to publish these notes.

A complete and thorough post-mortem examination was made in each case (by Mr. Hawes), with the exception that in Case I. the cranium was not opened.

Particularly careful attention was paid to the stomach, intestines, pancreas, gall-bladder, and bile-passages, but in none of the cases was there a trace of any new growth other than that found in the liver. As must always be the case with natives, the histories of the patients were difficult to obtain, and unsatisfactory, but such facts and data as were not rejected are probably worthy of acceptance.

CASE I.—H. J., Hottentot male, giving his age as 17, and not appearing older, was admitted on June 19, 1903, suffering from abdominal distention and dyspnœa. The relatives were positive that the boy betrayed no signs of illness until ten weeks before admission, at which time he began to complain of abdominal pain. Since that date the abdomen had slowly increased in size, and the boy had become gradually weaker.

The patient was much wasted and markedly cachectic.

The abdomen was uniformly distended with fluid so that no abdominal viscus could be felt.

There was some dyspnœa.

A slight icteric tint of the conjunctivæ was present, but no marked jaundice.

On January 20, 18 pints of blood-stained fluid were withdrawn by paracentesis.

The liver could now be felt four fingers'-breadths below the costal margin: the surface was rough and knobbly. A further 14 pints of fluid were withdrawn from the abdomen a few days later. The boy slowly sank, and died on January 27.

Post-mortem examination twelve hours after death.

Head and Neck.—Not examined.

Chest.—Some basal adhesions and slight pleural effusion on both sides.

Abdomen.—Contained 20 pints of blood-stained fluid. *The liver* was very greatly enlarged—the right lobe more so than the left. Weight, after draining, 7 lbs. 8 ozs. On the under surface of the right lobe was a patch of ulceration the size of a crown-piece upon which several small bleeding vessels were visible.

The under surface was covered with irregular knobs, but on the upper surface were only two or three bosses: none of these bosses showed any umbilication.

The new growth affected chiefly the right lobe, in which there was one huge mass, the centre of which had an appearance like recent blood-clot in an aneurysmal sac.

The rest of this focus and other numerous smaller areas of growth were of a yellowish-green hue.

The amount of liver tissue present was roughly about equal to that of new growth.

Microscopically.—The sections showed an advanced condition of biliary cirrhosis with considerable accumulations of newly formed bile-ducts in zones of connective tissue.

The liver cells showed a uniform and advanced degree of fatty degeneration.

There was extreme venous engorgement.

In parts there were groups of cells enclosed in an acinous arrangement of fibrous tissue: these cells had the appearance of being derived from the epithelium of the bile-ducts.

It is perhaps a question whether this case should rather be

PLATE II.

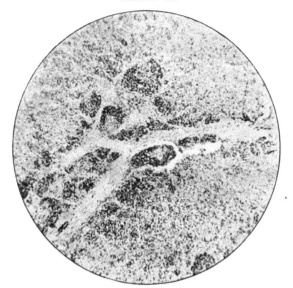

FIG. 1.

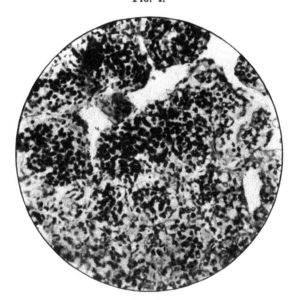

FIG. 2.

Mr. HAWES' Cases of Primary Malignant Disease
of the Liver.   Case II.

To face p. 162

Bale & Danielsson, Ltd.

regarded as one of primary growth of the bile-passages and not of the liver itself: the cancerous cells were, however, by no means confined to the areas of newly formed connective tissue in which there was such marked bile-duct proliferation, but were in many places in close contact with, and displacing, the liver cells.

CASE II.—E. D., female Hottentot, giving her age as 32, was admitted on May 16, 1904, with abdominal distention, vomiting, and dyspnœa.

The patient had been living as servant for some years with an intelligent Englishwoman, who bore out her statement as to approximate age, and corroborated the following details as to her illness.

The patient had been in her ordinary health until five weeks before coming to hospital, at which time she commenced to show symptoms of dyspepsia.

Only three weeks before admission had the woman noticed that her clothes were becoming tight for her, and since then the abdominal swelling had increased rapidly.

There was a doubtful history of some indulgence in alcohol.

The woman was almost moribund on admission. The abdomen was greatly distended with fluid.

There was not jaundice.

An incision was made in the middle line of the abdomen, and over 60 pints of clear fluid let out.

Patient rallied somewhat for a time, and the vomiting ceased, but the heart failed, and death followed forty-eight hours later.

Post-mortem examination eighteen hours after death.

Head and Neck.—Nil.

Chest.—Nothing abnormal of importance.

Abdomen.—The cavity contained about 10 pints of clear fluid.

The stomach was considerably dilated, and the mucous membrane pale and atrophic.

The uterus and appendages were normal.

The liver was greatly and uniformly enlarged, and weighed, after draining for some hours, 8 lbs. 7 ozs.

The surface of the liver was studded with large smooth bosses: there was no ulceration and no umbilication.

On section, the right lobe consisted almost entirely of a single mass of new growth.

There were some twenty other foci of growth in the left and other lobes.

The huge mass in the right lobe had broken down in the centre into a semi-solid substance, but there was no naked-eye hæmorrhage into the growth, which was for the most part of a yellowish-green colour.

Some of the smaller foci were very sharply cut off from the liver substance, and appeared almost encapsuled by bands of fibrous tissue.

  Microscopically.—Liver: Plate II., Figs. 1 and 2.

The two most noticeable features are a marked general cirrhosis and a high degree of venous congestion.

The normal lobular arrangement of the liver is quite destroyed, and in the broader bands of newly formed fibrous tissue may be seen many small bile-ducts cut in various directions.

Numerous distended capillaries are evident.

In the area in which no trace of liver tissue is left the cells of the new growth are arranged in distinct lobules, and at the periphery of these lobules the cells have a definite acinous arrangement, and the nuclei are much swollen, filling about half the cell.

In the centre of the lobule the cells are irregularly arranged in a fine fibrous network, and here also is a marked change in the cells, the nucleus being at one pole, and the protoplasm forming a ring round a large clear vesicle.

CASE III.—H. S., male Hottentot, æt. 16.

The boy was admitted to hospital in May 1904 almost *in extremis*, with enormous abdominal distention and great dyspnœa.

The history was, as usual, difficult to obtain, but his relatives were positive that he had been able to work in the fields "three moons" before coming to hospital, and that his belly had only swelled during the last two or three weeks, and these assertions they firmly maintained.

After admission the abdomen was tapped, and over 30 pints of blood-stained fluid were removed.

The liver could then be felt occupying the greater portion of the abdominal cavity: its upper border was at the lower margin of the third rib, in the right mammary line.

There was some icteric tint of the conjunctivæ, but this was only very slight.

The boy lived three days.

Post-mortem sixteen hours after death.

Head, Neck, and Thorax.—Nothing abnormal discovered.

The abdomen contained several pints of free fluid deeply tinged with blood.

PLATE III.

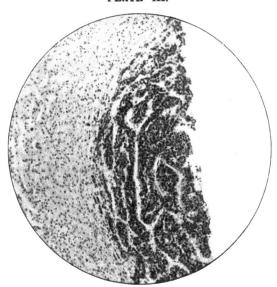

FIG. 1.

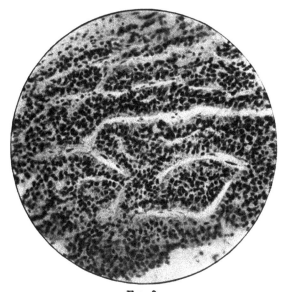

FIG. 2.

Mr. HAWES' Cases of Primary Malignant Disease
of the Liver.   Case III.

To face p. 164.

Bale & Danielsson, Ltd.

The liver was enormously enlarged, and, after draining for twenty-four hours, weighed 9 lbs. 13 ozs.

The growth was nearly uniform in distribution, and the surface was everywhere smooth except where there was some perihepatitis and hæmorrhage from a small ulcerated patch on the right lobe. To the naked eye the whole of the right lobe and the major portion of the left appeared to consist of nothing but new growth.

On section, the growth closely resembled that of Case II., being yellowish-green in colour, and of varying consistency. Some areas were carneous in appearance and friable, showing evidence of recent hæmorrhage in the new growth.

Microscopically.—Liver: Plate III., Figs. 1 and 2.

There were three marked changes.

First. An increase, in size and amount, of the bands of interlobular connective tissue without, however, any marked signs of the formation of new bile-ducts.

Secondly. An intense degree of venous engorgement which has in itself produced a coarse cirrhosis. In parts the liver tissue is reduced by one half and in others almost entirely replaced by a new formation in which can be distinguished a fine stroma indicating the normal liver arrangement, but in which the liver cells are lost, and the spaces almost entirely filled with blood.

Thirdly. The new growth itself is a typical columnar-celled carcinoma, and is not separated by fibrous strands from the liver cells, but is actually in contact with them, the latter being in places flattened, and more or less concentrically arranged round the growth.

There is in parts of the new growth a definitely acinous arrangement.

REMARKS.

In the above notes considerable stress has been laid upon the trustworthiness or otherwise of patients' statements; this is rendered necessary by the extreme ignorance of the South African native with regard to ages, dates, &c.

It is usually admitted that, without the aid of the microscope, the diagnosis of primary carcinoma from sarcoma of the liver is impossible, and that even with the microscope's aid it is by no means always easy.

There would seem to be no doubt that these three cases were all instances of carcinoma, and although they in some points closely resemble that form of primary cancer which is called the "nodular," and in which the organ is exactly like one affected secondarily by cancer, I am strongly of opinion that they were all instances of the form which is called by most authorities "massive cancer" ([1]).   It is true that in none of them was the growth confined to one area or even to one lobe, but it was in each case very obviously of longer standing in the largest focus of disease, and I think there can be little doubt that the main mass of growth in the right lobe was, in all three cases, the original tumour, and that the other foci were metastases from it.

The absence of marked jaundice and of enlarged glands in the portal fissure is said to be the rule in these cases.   These two facts, coupled with the absence of contraction of the fibrous tissue in the growths, fit in with the short duration of the disease which, again, is usual.

Hale White ([2]) found in an analysis of cases "that the remarkable fact comes out that no case lived more than four months after the first symptoms appeared, and that the average duration was only twelve weeks."

The extreme youth of the patients is noteworthy : Hale White's youngest case was aged 23 ([3]) ; Bartholow ([4]) says "it is a malady of advanced life," and Rendu ([5]) says the disease is very rare under 40 and "exceptionally rare under 20."

Although it is acknowledged that cancer is relatively rare among the native races of South Africa, especially among those of Bantu origin ([6]), I have been unable to find any account of the frequency or otherwise of the disease among Hottentots : my own experience, which is very small, would lead me to think that the disease is rare among them also.

Considerable interest attaches to the question of the effect of civilisation upon the cancer incidence among natives.

The Cape Government has recently required from the hospitals receiving Government grants and from the district surgeons a detailed report upon all cases of cancer treated, so that some useful information on the above points should be forthcoming.

For the micro-photographs accompanying these notes, as also for the microscopical sections from which the photographs were taken, and for much help in the description of the specimens, I am deeply indebted to the members of the staff of the Bacteriological Institute, Grahamstown.

REFERENCES.

1. ZIEGLER, Allgemeine Pathologie und Pathologische Anatomie, vol. ii. p. 642. Hektoen and Riesman, Textbook of Pathology, vol. ii. p. 815. Osler, Principles and Practice of Medicine, p. 582.
2. GIBSON'S Textbook of Medicine, p. 784.
3. ALLBUTT'S System of Medicine, vol. iv. p. 205.
4. PEPPER'S System of Medicine, vol. ii. p. 1034.
5. Dictionnaire Encyclopédique des Sciences Médicales (art. Foie).
6. CLEMOW, The Geography of Disease, pp. 67, 68.

A YEAR'S GASTRO-JEJUNOSTOMIES.

BY

D'ARCY POWER, F.R.C.S. ENG.

Last year I placed upon record, in the pages of the St. Bartholomew's Hospital Reports, four cases of gastro-jejunostomy. This year I am able to give an account of sixteen cases in which the same operation was performed, and in only one case with a fatal result. The most interesting of the cases perhaps is No. IV. in this series. I had been somewhat discouraged in operating upon women with chronic dyspepsia apparently due to ulcer of the stomach, because in many cases the improvement seemed to be only temporary. I attributed this to the fact that when the pylorus was functional the gastric contents no longer passed through the anastomosis, which thus became useless. The original symptoms reappeared, therefore, with greater or less severity, and usually within three months. Case IV. was a typical instance of chronic dyspepsia; so after performing the usual gastro-enterostomy I ran a purse-string suture round the pylorus to constrict it without absolutely closing the lumen. Six months after operation the patient had still maintained her initial improvement. For the rest, increased experience has led me to modify the severity of the after-treatment: in the earlier cases I did not allow patients to have anything by the mouth for forty-eight hours after the operation. This period is now shortened to twenty-four hours, and, I think, with advantage to the patient. I still like to select my cases for operation, because it is certain that every case of chronic dyspepsia is not suitable for operation. Many can be cured by less heroic means; but if the surgeon sometimes stays his hand, the physician equally should recognise when he has reached the limit of his resources and not wait until his patient is moribund before he summons his colleague to help him.

CASE I.—*Duodenal Constriction—Post-colic Gastro-Jejunostomy—Cure.*

E. F., a compositor, aged 62, was admitted under my care at the Bolingbroke Hospital on June 23, 1905, saying that for the last two years he had suffered from flatulence and indigestion after food. The attacks had been intermittent, occurring every six months or so, and lasting from three to five weeks at a time. During the attacks the pain occurred some three or four hours after taking food, nausea then supervened, and he had occasionally vomited. He had never brought up any blood nor had he noticed blood in his motions. He had never been jaundiced. The attacks have been getting more severe lately, and in January 1905 he was treated as a medical out-patient at the Bolingbroke Hospital. He improved after his stomach had been washed out systematically and when he was dieted, but he soon relapsed into his former state when he discontinued his visits to the hospital.

The notes state that on admission under my care he was an anæmic-looking man weighing 7 stones 7 lbs. Peristalsis was visible through the abdominal walls, especially in the right iliac fossa, where a swelling was seen to form and disappear. No tumour could be felt, but a succussion splash was heard distinctly nearly down to the pubes. I opened his abdomen on June 24 and found the stomach dilated; the pylorus was bound down to the under surface of the liver, in the region of the gall-bladder, by numerous and dense adhesions. No gall-stones could be felt in the gall-bladder, nor did there appear to be any cancerous growth. I freed the adhesions as far as possible and performed a posterior gastro-jejunostomy by direct suture. The operation was prolonged owing to the great size and distension of the transverse colon.

The patient rallied well from the operation, and for the first thirty-two hours nothing was given by the mouth, but a saline injection was delivered into the rectum every four hours. At the end of thirty-two hours a drachm of peptonised milk or a drachm of albumin water was given alternately every hour. The patient was not sick, and the quantity of nourishment given by the mouth was quickly increased. He was given fish and custard on July 3—the ninth day after the operation—and on July 20 he was discharged from the hospital. His weight had then risen to 7 stones 12 lbs. He was taking his food well without pain or flatulence, and the wound had healed by first intention.

On August 11 the patient came up to the Hospital and reported that his weight was now 8 stones 4 lbs.; that he ate heartily of his ordinary meals, and that he was cured.

CASE II.—*Duodenal Constriction—Post-colic Gastro-Jejunostomy—Cure.*

A. L., housewife, aged 56,[1] was admitted to Paget Ward from Elizabeth, where she had been under the care of my colleague, Dr. Herringham, on January 4, 1905. The patient said that she had been well until two months before admission, when she began to have pain after food. She got worse in spite of all medical treatment, and vomited after taking anything by the mouth. She felt pain under her heart about an hour after each meal, the pain being partly relieved by vomiting. She had twice vomited blood, but had never noticed any melæna: as a rule her bowels are open every other day.

She was given a test meal of tea and toast on New Year's Eve 1904, and her stomach was washed out two hours and a half afterwards. The analysis of the stomach contents showed the absence of free hydrochloric acid and of any organic acid or acid albumin, though the fluid was slightly acid to litmus. There was a little peptone, some starch granules, many squamous and columnar cells, but no blood. The stomach was greatly dilated and reached far below the umbilicus. A blood-count showed the presence of 3,186,000 red corpuscles and of 4000 white corpuscles in a cubic millimetre.

I performed a post-colic gastro-jejunostomy on January 9, 1905: the anæsthetic took seven minutes, the operation twenty-one minutes, and the dressing five minutes, so that the patient was on the table thirty-three minutes. The stomach was found to be greatly dilated, the duodenum being constricted by adhesions which had been formed in connection with the gall-bladder. No new growth was discovered. Examination of the mucous membrane of the stomach removed at the operation showed that it was infiltrated with polymorphonuclear leucocytes, probably the result of inflammation. The glands were of the usual type found at the pyloric end, and did not resemble those situated at the cardiac end of the stomach. They were remarkable, however, in the fact that they contained no oxyntic cells.

The patient was not sick after the operation. She was fed on nutrient enemata for the first thirty-six hours, then upon

[1] Female Surgical Register, vol. v. 1902, No. 2896.

whey and peptonised milk. The wound healed by first intention, and she was discharged cured on February 1, 1905. She reported herself on March 3 as having passed through a severe attack of bronchitis, but that she felt better than before the operation, having neither pain after meals nor vomiting. Her weight was 7 stones 11 lbs., and the scar of the abdominal wound was sound. On August 15 her weight had risen to 11 stones 3 lbs., and had been stationary for many weeks past. She was absolutely free from abdominal pain or discomfort of any kind, and her bowels were open regularly.

Case III.—*Duodenal Constriction—Post-colic Gastro-Jejunostomy—Phlebitis—Cure.*

Mr. E. H., aged 46, had suffered from dyspepsia for many years, and had a sudden hæmatemesis on November 18, 1902. He improved under medical treatment during 1903, but relapsed from time to time. The relapses became more frequent in 1904, until he was quite unable to follow his occupation. He often vomited, the vomiting being worse at night. He had lost a great deal of flesh, and weighed only 8 stones 10 lbs.

I first saw him on April 3, 1905, and found that his stomach was greatly dilated. There was a tender spot on deep pressure just to the right of the umbilicus, but no tumour could be felt, nor was there any perceptible thickening over the pylorus. The liver was of normal size, and there were no gall-stones.

I performed a post-colic gastro-enterostomy upon him on April 8. The stomach was dilated and the pylorus was greatly constricted at a point about 2 inches from the duodenum, and there were numerous adhesions round it. His transverse colon was much distended. The patient made a good recovery from the operation, and the wound healed by first intention. But his convalescence was retarded by a sharp attack of phlebitis in the left leg. He left the nursing home five weeks after the operation, and reported himself on June 19, 1905, as weighing 9 stones 1 lb. He says that he can eat anything again. I found that his stomach was much diminished in size, but it had not quite regained its normal dimensions. On August 15 he came complaining of a little return of dyspepsia, but he seemed well; his weight was 9 stones, and his bowels acted regularly and naturally. His stomach had returned to a natural size.

CASE IV.—*Severe Dyspepsia—Post-colic Gastro-Jejunostomy—Cure.*

E. E. W., housewife, aged 41,[1] was admitted to Paget Ward with a history of indigestion for the last fifteen years. The pain comes on directly after food and is often accompanied by vomiting, which, however, does not relieve her unless it is very copious. She has attended various hospitals for the last eight years, and has been dieted, but has not had her stomach washed out. In July 1904 she brought up about 5 ounces of bright blood after a very severe attack of pain, but she has never passed blood by the bowels so far as she knows. She remained in bed at home for six weeks after this attack of hæmatemesis, vomiting twice a day, and taking only milk and a little fish. She has recently had more severe pain, which begins an hour after taking food. It starts on the left side of the abdomen and travels to the right side in her chest and back. It is relieved by taking fluids. Her weight in 1894 was 8 stones: it is now 5 stones 6 lbs.

On Admission.—The patient was an emaciated and anæmic woman with thin abdominal walls. The abdomen was not distended, but there was visible peristalsis and a point of definite tenderness over the left rectus. No tumour could be detected, nor was the stomach dilated.

I performed a post-colic gastro-enterostomy by direct suture on November 14, and afterwards ran a purse-string suture round the pylorus so as to narrow it considerably. One enlarged gland was found and removed from the gastro-hepatic omentum. The patient made an uneventful recovery, and the wound healed by first intention. She had occasional pain after taking solid food whilst she was in hospital, but she was never sick. She left the hospital on January 18, 1905. I saw her again on June 6, 1905. She was then in excellent condition, looking fat and well, increasing steadily in weight, and able to walk considerable distances without fatigue.

CASE V.—*Dilated Stomach—Post-colic Gastro-Jejunostomy—Recovery.*

A. H., a labourer, aged 34, was admitted under my care at the Bolingbroke Hospital on June 2, 1905. There was nothing noteworthy in his family history except that one brother was said to have died of "cancer of the stomach" at the early age of 32.

---

[1] Female Surgical Register, vol. v. 1905, No. 2493.

The patient said that for the last year he had been suffering from indigestion. The pain usually came on about a quarter of an hour after taking food. He had vomited after food, and thought that he was relieved thereby. His symptoms have been getting worse lately in spite of treatment, and he has been obliged to give up work. He has never vomited blood nor has he had melæna: he has become more constipated of late. His normal weight is about 10 stones 11 lbs., but he only weighs 8 stones 1 lb. at the present time.

On Admission.—He was a healthy-looking and fairly-nourished man whose abdomen moved freely on respiration. No abdominal tumour could be felt, but there was slight tenderness at the epigastrium. A succussion splash was easily obtained in the region of the stomach, and by percussion the stomach was found to reach from the sixth rib above to the mid-axillary line behind and to the middle line in front. The vomit was acid and the urine was normal.

I performed a post-colic gastro-enterostomy by direct suture on June 6, 1905. For the first thirty-six hours after the operation the patient had nothing by the mouth, but half a pint of saline solution was given by the rectum every four hours. At the end of thirty-six hours 2 drachms of hot water and 2 drachms of peptonised milk were given alternately every hour. When liquid was taken by the mouth, it was found that the salines were not retained, so they were given up. Liquid food was taken in increasing quantity, and on the third day the patient had egg and milk and Valentine's meat juice. On June 9 a simple enema was given with good effect. The temperature never rose above 98·6° F. after the operation: the stitches were removed on the tenth day, and the patient left the hospital on June 27, taking solid food and without pain or discomfort.

CASE VI.—*Dilated Stomach—Post-colic Gastro-Jejunostomy—Cure.*

W. L., aged 47, an upholsterer,[1] was admitted into Henry Ward on November 11, 1904, saying that he had suffered from abdominal pain for the last two years. The pain begins high up on the left side of his abdomen and extends downwards. It usually comes on two hours after food, and is accompanied by retching and vomiting. It is relieved if he lies down. He has never been quite free from pain since his first attack, and

---

[1] Male Surgical Register, vol. v. 1905, No. 3226.

he has sometimes been obliged to give up his work for a week at a time on account of the severity of the pain. He has lost 2 stones in weight during the last two years. He has never noticed any blood in his stools, but six weeks ago he vomited a small quantity of clotted blood.

On Admission.—His abdomen moved well and evenly: it was neither distended nor retracted. It was slightly tender at a point an inch and a half above and to the left of the umbilicus. No swelling could be detected, but the stomach resonance was increased downwards, and this dilation was confirmed by distending the stomach with carbon dioxide. A test meal showed the absence of free hydrochloric acid, the total acidity of the gastric contents being very slight.

A post-colic gastro-enterostomy was performed by direct suture on November 24, the operation lasting thirty-two minutes, which included the administration of the anæsthetic and a stop of about four minutes when the patient became collapsed. The stomach was found to be dilated, and there was one enlarged lymphatic gland in the gastro-hepatic omentum. Subsequent examination of the gland did not reveal any evidence of malignant disease. The patient made a good recovery ; his wound healed by first intention, and he left the hospital on December 21, 1904.

He reported himself on January 9, 1905, as being well and cheerful, able to eat everything. He has put on 2 stones in weight, and is going back to work. I saw him again in November 1905, more than a year after the operation, when he said that he had kept well and was free from pain.

CASE VII.—*Dilated Stomach—Post-colic Gastro-Jejunostomy—Recovery—Death a month later.*

E. E., a lady's-maid, aged 55,[1] was admitted to Paget Ward on New Year's Eve 1904, saying that she was well until June 1904, when she began to feel pain in her stomach after taking food. She had been sick after her meals for the last month. She had never brought up blood, but she once passed blood by the bowel. She had been constipated of late. The patient was found to have a dilated stomach which, when distended, reached 3 inches below the umbilicus, extending lower on the left than in any other part. A test meal was given on January 11, the stomach being washed out two hours later. There was no free hydrochloric acid nor any lactic acid.

---

[1] Female Surgical Register, vol. v. 1905, No. 2909.

Another test meal was given on January 13, when no acid at all was found in the gastric contents. A post-colic gastro-enterostomy was performed by direct suture on January 16, the operation taking thirty minutes, exclusive of the anæsthetic. The stomach was found to have a transverse constriction in it near the pylorus, and the anastomosis was made, therefore, on the proximal side of the constriction. The patient vomited twice after her return to the ward. She had nothing by the mouth for thirty-six hours. The wound healed by first intention, and she was discharged on February 17, 1905, with a sound scar, free from pain, and without any sickness. Her weight was 8 stones 7½ lbs.

Microscopical examination of the mucous membrane of the stomach removed at the operation showed it to be of the type found in the intermediate part between the fundus and pylorus. Oxyntic cells were present in fair numbers in the peptic glands. There was no evidence of any inflammation of the mucous membrane.

A month after her return home she died with a swelling in her abdomen, but no post-mortem examination was made.

CASE VIII.—*Chronic Ulcer of the Stomach—Post-colic Gastro-Jejunostomy—Death.*

L. G., aged 27 (unmarried). This girl had suffered for many years from the symptoms of a gastric ulcer situated on the posterior wall of the stomach. She had vomited blood repeatedly, and had been treated in a variety of ways, sometimes deriving benefit but always relapsing again. She had lived entirely on milk and biscuits for many years, and when I saw her she was in an extremely exhausted and emaciated condition. She was habitually constipated, and continually took aperients. I performed a post-colic gastro-enterostomy upon her by direct suture on April 25, 1905. The operation lasted three-quarters of an hour, as there was great difficulty in drawing out the stomach and in localising the gastro-duodenal angle owing to the great size and distension of the transverse colon. I completed the operation by puckering the pylorus with a purse-string suture. The patient proved herself unable to withstand the strain put upon her rallying powers, and she died of exhaustion twenty-four hours after the operation.

CASE IX.—*Cancer of the Bowel—Pre-colic Gastro-Enterostomy—Death.*

E. C., a stationmaster, aged 68, gouty, and the subject of a left inguinal hernia for nineteen years, was seized with a violent attack of sickness at the end of May 1905. During the last three months he had experienced some difficulty in getting his bowels open, and he had felt pain occasionally in the left hypochondrium, the pain extending downwards towards the loin. The attack of sickness lasted two hours and yielded to domestic remedies, but it recurred with greater severity on June 4. During the first attack of sickness his wife discovered accidentally that the patient had a lump in his abdomen. On examination the patient was found to be a healthy-looking man with a good colour. He had a large inguinal hernia on the left side which was partly reducible; on the right side there was an inguinal gland of the size of a walnut. The patient said that he had noticed this gland for five or six years, but did not think that it had increased in size. A large nodular tumour was situated in the left hypochondrium which could be moved downwards towards the pelvis and across the abdomen to the right of the middle line. The tumour was only slightly tender, and I diagnosed it to be a mass of carcinoma involving the transverse colon near its splenic flexure. The examination and handling of the tumour set up symptoms of intestinal obstruction, and as soon as these had subsided I explored his abdomen.

I opened the abdomen on June 9 and found that the tumour was a mass of cancer involving the transverse colon, the small intestine, and the omentum. The constriction of the small intestine was much more severe than that of the colon. I therefore performed a pre-colic gastro-enterostomy by direct suture in such a manner as to throw out of action the affected portion of the small intestine, and I freed, as far as possible, the rest of the intestine from the omental adhesions. The patient rallied well from the operation and seemed comfortable until Wednesday, June 14, when he showed signs of an irreducible inguinal hernia, of which he died on Friday, June 16, without any evidence of peritonitis.

CASE X.—*Pyloric Obstruction—Post-colic Gastro-Jejunostomy—Recovery.*

J. W. H., a gunfitter, aged 40,[1] was admitted with the symptoms of pyloric stenosis. He said that he had been ill

---

[1] Male Surgical Register, vol. v. 1905, No. 2457.

for the last twelve months and was becoming increasingly costive. He was admitted into Charity Ward on September 15, 1905, his weight being then 10 stones. Examination of a test meal showed that his stomach contained free hydrochloric acid and some yeasts, but there was no lactic acid, blood, fragments of a new growth, or sarcinæ, neither were there any Oppler-Boas bacilli.

I performed a posterior gastro-enterostomy upon him on October 4; recovery was uninterrupted, and the patient was discharged on October 28. He was then able to eat the ordinary hospital diet without pain, though it is too soon to say whether he is cured.[1]

CASE XI.—*Chronic Gastritis—Post-colic Gastro-Jejunostomy—Recovery.*

Mrs. S. A. P., aged 50,[1] was admitted into Paget Ward on September 16, 1905, suffering from chronic dyspepsia for the last twelve months. She had been under treatment in the medical wards of the hospital at Stratford-on-Avon. She had been greatly relieved whilst she was there, but always relapsed into her former condition when she returned home. She had suffered much pain and had often vomited blood. For the last three months she had lived on milk puddings and had not tasted meat. On her admission she was an emaciated woman weighing 7 stones, and she had a markedly dilated stomach. A test meal showed the presence of free hydrochloric acid and yeasts in the gastric juice, but there were no sarcinæ or Oppler-Boas bacilli; no blood or fragments of new growth: lactic acid was absent.

I performed a posterior gastro-enterostomy on October 2, and the patient travelled home to Warwickshire on October 28. She had improved greatly, and for several days had eaten fish, mutton, and eggs. She weighed 6 stones 11 lbs. on the day of her discharge from the hospital.

CASE XII.—*Chronic Gastric Ulcer—Hæmatemesis—Post-colic Gastro-Jejunostomy—Recovery.*

B. H., aged 39, a trained nurse,[2] was admitted into Paget Ward on October 17, 1905. She had suffered from painful dyspepsia for several years, and for the last two years the pain has been constant. She had vomited 2 or 3 pints every

---

[1] Female Surgical Register, vol. v. 1905, No. 1971.
[2] *Ibid.*, No. 2222.

two days, and for the last year she had been in the habit of washing out her own stomach. On October 2 she had a sudden hæmatemesis after passing the stomach tube and lost, she estimates, from ½ to 1 pint of blood. On October 5 she had another attack of hæmatemesis which rendered her quite prostrate. She had been unable to eat any meat for the last two years, and from the 2nd to the 5th of October she lived on nutrient suppositories, although she was engaged in nursing a "heavy" case in private. The patient was too ill to allow of any thorough examination. She was kept quietly in bed until October 30, when I performed a post-colic gastro-jejunostomy.

The anterior wall of the stomach, about 1 inch from the pylorus, was scarred transversely by the cicatrix of an ulcer which had involved all the coats and was evidently of long standing. The anastomosis was made on the proximal side of the scar and on the posterior wall of the stomach, which was healthy.

The patient made an uneventful recovery.

She was able to take pounded fish on November 5, and soon afterwards chicken and mutton. She left the hospital on November 23.

CASE XIII.—*Chronic Dyspepsia—Hæmatemesis— Post-colic Gastro-Jejunostomy—Recovery.*

A. G., aged 49, labourer,[1] has been under treatment for dyspepsia since September 15, 1903. On this day he suddenly vomited a large quantity of deeply stained and dark-coloured blood and was afterwards kept in bed for six months. He was under treatment in the medical wards at St. Bartholomew's Hospital in 1905, but later in the year he became worse, and was admitted into Henry Ward under my care on October 24, 1905. He was obstinately constipated, and weighed 9 stones 1 lb. as against his usual weight of 13 stones.

His gastric juice contains free hydrochloric acid, but no blood, lactic acid, new growth, sarcinæ, or Oppler-Boas bacilli. Yeasts are present. The patient suffers greatly from pain, which comes on independently of the kind of food he takes, though it varies with the quantity eaten.

I performed a post-colic gastro-jejunostomy on October 26, and found a dilated stomach partially hidden by an unusually large liver. The patient made an uneventful recovery, but remained constipated though he was free from pain.

[1] Male Surgical Register, vol. v. 1905, No. 2823.

CASE XIV. — *Chronic Dyspepsia — Hæmatemesis — Post-colic Gastro-Jejunostomy — Vomiting — Secondary Gastrotomy — Recovery.*

L. B., a deaf and dumb girl aged 19, laundry-maid, was admitted into the Bolingbroke Hospital on October 1, 1905. She had already been three times in the hospital for the treatment of gastric ulcer, and for the last few months she had been constantly sick after food. Pain comes on directly after taking food, and she had hæmatemesis four days before her admission to the hospital.

We kept the patient under observation for a month, and found that she suffered a great deal of abdominal pain and many attacks of sickness. On October 28 I performed a post-colic gastro-jejunostomy. The walls of the stomach were congested and thickened, and there was so much bleeding from the submucous coat that several ligatures had to be applied.

The stomach was dilated, but no ulcer was seen.

The patient vomited repeatedly on the 28th and 29th October. At 6.30 P.M. on October 29—twenty-eight hours after the operation—she vomited a little blood; an hour later she brought up ½ pint of unaltered blood; at 10 P.M. another ½ pint, and at 11.30 P.M. she vomited ½ pint more blood.

I reopened the abdominal wound at 1 A.M. on October 30 and found that the anastomosis was satisfactory, except that the jejunum was contracted distally and rather kinked. I therefore put in three more sutures to attach the distal portion of the jejunum to the stomach wall in a more direct line.

The stomach was opened by a linear incision carried just above and parallel to the gastro-jejunostomy, so that the inner aspect of the anastomosis could be freely examined. There was no actual hæmorrhage, but at one part of the margin of the anastomosis was a small ulcerated patch of mucous membrane covered with blood clot. I passed a curved needle beneath it and sutured healthy mucous membrane over it, and then applied a ligature to another place which looked as if it were in a similar state. The wound in the stomach was closed with Lembert's sutures, and the abdominal wound was again sutured.

The patient vomited a little altered blood on October 30, and on October 31, as she was still retching, the stomach was washed out and she was then fed by the mouth.

The stomach was washed out again on November 5 for the relief of another attack of sickness, and on the following day it was found that the abdominal wound had suppurated. The suppuration did not prove to be anything serious, and on November 10 the patient was free from pain and taking her food well. She left the hospital on November 27.

CASE XV.—*Pyloric Adhesions—Dilated Stomach—*
Post-colic Gastro-Jejunostomy—Recovery.

G. H., aged 20, a clerk, was admitted into the Bolingbroke Hospital on October 21, 1905, saying that he had been in good health until two years since, when he began to suffer from indigestion. He has a sense of fulness in the chest for hours after a meal, but he has never vomited. He has been increasingly constipated for the last three months, and between June and October his weight has fallen from 8 stones to 6 stones 7 lbs.

I kept the patient under observation until November 3, when I performed a post-colic gastro-jejunostomy. The stomach was dilated ; there were adhesions in the neighbourhood of the pylorus, and the omentum was shrivelled up and very small.

Recovery was quite uneventful; the patient was not sick after the operation, and left the hospital on November 27.

CASE XVI.—*Chronic Gastric Ulcer—Post-colic Gastro-*
Jejunostomy—Phlebitis—Recovery.

F. S., aged 23, a kitchen-maid, was in the Camberwell Infirmary for seven months when she was 19 for a chronic ulcer of the stomach with hæmatemesis: a year later she was in King's College Hospital for four months for the same complaint, and in May 1905 she was admitted to the Wandsworth Infirmary for abdominal pain and sickness.

In September 1905 she became an in-patient at the Bolingbroke Hospital under my colleague, Dr. Campbell Thomson, who transferred her to my care.

I performed a post-colic gastro-jejunostomy on November 3, and found that the stomach was dilated and greatly thickened, especially near the pylorus, the thickening being such as would occur from a chronic ulceration. The patient was not sick after the operation, but the convalescence was retarded by a sharp attack of phlebitis in the left leg which began on November 21.

I am indebted for the notes of the cases at St. Bartholomew's Hospital to my house-surgeons, Mr. G. H. Colt and Mr. A. P. Gibb, and for those at Bolingbroke Hospital to the Resident Medical Officer, Dr. Gerald T. Hughes and to Mr. W. A. Rees.

INTRA-OCULAR TUBERCULOSIS.

BY

WALTER H. JESSOP, F.R.C.S.

When asked to undertake the opening of a Discussion * on Ocular Tuberculosis, I little thought the subject would cover so much ground. I soon found myself obliged to alter the title to Intra-Ocular Tuberculosis, thereby eliminating the extra-ocular diseases, and also those of the protective tissues of the eye (sclerotic and cornea). Even with these excisions my subject is too comprehensive, and I have devoted most attention to tubercular disease of the choroid, especially the chronic form. I must apologise for the way in which some important points have been slurred over, but the short time at my disposal makes it impossible to more than allude to many of them.

TUBERCULOSIS OF THE CHOROID may be conveniently divided into two main sections—(A) miliary tubercle, and (B) the rarer form of solitary or chronic tubercle. Some observers, as von Michel, have described cases of chronic choroiditis of the disseminated type as tuberculous, but this I do not think is yet conclusively proved.

A. *Miliary Tubercles in the Choroid* were first found and described anatomically by Autentrieth in 1808. In 1855 their appearances, as seen by the ophthalmoscope, were recognised by Ed. Jaeger, and in 1858 Manz ([1]) published their microscopical characteristics.

As far as I know, miliary tubercles of the choroid are never primary. They are generally met with in patients the subject of acute miliary tuberculosis, but the proportion of such cases, in which miliary choroidal tubercles have been found, is given very differently by observers.

* Intra-Ocular Tuberculosis Discussion at the Leicester Meeting of the British Medical Association, July 1905.

Till 1867, when Cohnheim [2] stated that tubercles were commonly found in the choroid after death in cases of acute miliary tuberculosis, the association was considered very rare.

Since then the percentage recorded has varied somewhat from Cohnheim's 100 per cent. in 18 cases. Litten [3] in 52 cases of acute miliary tuberculosis, examined after death, found choroidal tubercle in 39 (75 per cent.); Bock's [4] percentage was 82.7; Angel-Money [5] 14 out of 44 cases, or 31.8 per cent.; Stephenson and Carpenter [6] twenty-one times in 42 cases, or 50 per cent., diagnosed by the ophthalmoscope during life. Dr. Thursfield tells me that he found a percentage of about 30 in cases at the Children's Hospital, Great Ormond Street, examined ophthalmoscopically.

I have, with the aid of Mr. Holroyd, looked up the cases of acute general miliary tuberculosis at St. Bartholomew's Hospital for the last ten years, and find that the total number is 244. Of these about 200 were examined by the ophthalmoscope, but not necessarily more than once, and therefore percentages based on such cases would not be very reliable, as it is absolutely necessary that the eye should at all events be examined shortly before death. Of these 244 cases the eyes were examined in 48 cases in the post-mortem room, and tubercle of the choroid was found fifteen times, giving a percentage of 31.25 of cases examined. Of these cases 6 were diagnosed by the ophthalmoscope before death (one twelve days before, and another eleven days before death). Of the 48 cases 47 had tubercular meningitis and the one without meningitis had miliary tubercle of the lungs, peritoneum, spleen, and kidneys.

Relation to Tubercular Meningitis.—For many years it was thought that tubercle of the choroid was rarely found in cases of tubercular meningitis. Dr. Garlick [7] (1869) in 25 cases found the choroidal lesion in only 1 case; Gruening [8] in 50 cases examined after death only in 2 cases; Baxter [9] in twelve years had not a single case; Sharkey only once in three and a half years; Schieck [32] once in 20 cases. In 15 cases of miliary choroidal tubercle at St. Bartholomew's Hospital, no less than 14 had tubercular meningitis.

The percentage is naturally much higher anatomically than ophthalmoscopically as the lesions often occur late in the disease, when it is very difficult to examine the patient. Added to this the lesion being deep in the choroid and covered by the retina it may be easily overlooked by the ophthalmoscope.

The original statement [10] of Gowers, Cohnheim, and Horner, that choroidal tubercle is rarer in tubercular meningitis than in general miliary tuberculosis without meningitis is not according to the latest views. Horner stated that: "It seems as if the pia cerebri takes the place of the pia oculi," and therefore if the pia mater of brain is tubercular, the pial sheath (choroid of eye) is immune.

Gowers[10] observed that choroidal tubercle is more common in cases of tuberculosis without meningitis than those with meningitis. My own opinion is that it is rare to find miliary tubercle of the choroid without tubercular meningitis; just as tubercular meningitis is seldom met with without general tuberculosis. Osler says that tubercular meningitis is always secondary.

Miliary Tubercles of the Choroid occur, as a rule, as small discrete grey round or oval nodules, varying in size from a mere speck, 0.2 mm. to 1 mm., rarely larger unless some nodules become confluent, when the size may be 2 to 3 mm.; the nodules are very slightly if at all raised, the retinal vessels passing uninterruptedly over them. They are generally two, three, or four in number, but as many as sixty-two have been found in the same eye. By the *ophthalmoscope* they are seen as small white, grey, yellowish, or rose-pink discrete spots; they are very slightly if at all raised; the edges are soft and have a moth-eaten appearance; the retina over them is clear, and the contour of the retinal vessels is uninterrupted; in some cases there is a grey stippled appearance due to numerous minute white or grey specks (tubercular dust). The nodule, as seen by the ophthalmoscope, is really much smaller than the real lesion, as owing to its depth in the choroid only the most prominent part from atrophy of overlying tissues becomes visible. It is probably this fact that accounts for the sudden and apparently rapid appearance of the tubercles.

There is no tendency to marked pigmentation, though at times the edges are slightly tinged with greyish black pigment; retinal hæmorrhages are rarely to be found; the vitreous is clear, no opacities being present. Optic neuritis may be present; in 15 cases of miliary choroidal tubercle at St. Bartholomew's Hospital, optic neuritis was said to be present 9 times. The neuritis in these cases was probably due to the accompanying meningeal or cerebral lesion, and quite distinct from the choroidal lesion.

The *position* of the nodules is generally near the optic disk or yellow spot region, and therefore within the equator; but they may, if multiple, extend towards the periphery; a favourite situation is near the retinal veins.

The *acuity of vision* is probably little affected by choroidal tubercles, and this accounts for the fact that their presence gives rise, as a rule, to no definite symptoms.

Microscopical.—The changes are deep—generally in chorio-capillaris layer and from adventitia of the larger vessels. Duckler says that the giant cells are rich in pigment; but Margulies, on the contrary, states that giant cells have no pigment, and are derived from endothelial and connective tissue elements; there is always to be found the tubercular reticulum, numerous endothelial cells, and, quite early in the disease, caseation.

Tubercle bacilli are often to be met with. Haab, who first described the bacilli in tuberculous choroiditis, found them in nearly every case; Lawford [10] in only 2 out of 6 cases, though in all 6 cases tubercle bacilli were found in the meninges.

Ocular Lesions.—The sclera is affected rather than the re-tina; the lesions are often difficult to see post mortem, unless the retina be stripped off.

Diagnosis.—The absence of black pigmentation and of the ringed spots distinguishes choroidal tubercle from disseminated choroiditis. It is sometimes difficult to diagnose from spots of choroidal exudation, but in tubercle the nodules are rounder, the colour greyer or more yellow, the edges not so soft and with the peculiar moth-eaten appearance; in the exudation due to syphilis vitreous opacities are present.

If the nodules are found early in the disease they are an important aid to diagnosis; I have by these means been able to diagnose cases of tubercular meningitis from typhoid fever ten days or so before death.

Prognosis.—As far as I know, patients never recover when the choroid is affected by miliary tubercles, as is also the case in acute miliary tuberculosis.

In the St. Bartholomew's Hospital statistics in 1896 some cases of diagnosed acute miliary tuberculosis did not die, but since that time all such cases have succumbed.

Treatment is confined to relieving the general symptoms of the patient, and no local treatment is of use. I have no knowledge of the effect of tuberculin in such cases.

B. *Chronic, Solitary, Aggregated, or Conglomerate Tubercle of the Choroid* presents clinically quite a different picture to that associated with miliary tubercle of the choroid. In a few cases, however, the later result has been a secondary miliary tuberculosis of the meninges from absorption of tubercle virus from the first focus.

The condition was first diagnosed by Horner [11] in 1878 in the case of a boy 8½ years old (Case 2), and Haab [12] has

				abecess tub. bacilli	of phth.	Cilia
19	F.	6	L.	Nil	...	Choroi ...
20	F.	16	L.	...	...	Conj‌lar meningi pupil i‌p nodules ; ‌‌‌‌‌‌ tubercle ; peritonitis

(1) WEISS. *Arch. f. Oph.*, 1877, Bd. 23, 4, p. 11 15) MACKE‌
(2) HAAB. *Arch. f. Oph.*, 1879, Bd. 25, 4, p. 22 16) BARLO‌
(3) MANZ. *Klin. Monatsblät. f. Augenheilk.*, 188 17) JESSOP‌
(4) HIRSCHBERG. *Neurolog. Centralbl.*, 1882, Ba 18) JESSOP‌
(5) MAREN. Augen-Tuberkulose. Thesis. St‌ 19) McHA‌
(6) SCHÄFER. *Klin. Monatsbl. f. Augenheilk.*, 18 20) St. Bar‌
(7) HAAB. *Klin. Monatsbl. für Augenheilk.*, 188‌

published the drawing—originally in black and white, but lately in colours—very much resembling the drawings taken of my case (No. 17). Von Graefe ([14]) first described the condition microscopically in a large conglomerate choroidal tubercle in a pig's eye. Chelius ([15]) and Arlt ([16]), in the pre-ophthalmoscopic days, spoke of a choroiditis scrophulosa and tuberculosa. (*See* Table.)

Though a rare condition, I have been able to collect and arrange notes of 20 cases; I have carefully excluded from my list all doubtful ones. A table of these cases is appended in order to bring out and compare the chief points of interest.

Sex.—The proportion is nearly equal: nine females and eleven males.

Age.—Eleven cases were under 10 years of age, showing that chronic tubercle is generally a disease of early life. Of these eleven cases one was under 1 year, two between 1 and 2 years, eight between 2 and 10; of the other nine cases one was over 60 years, four between 20 and 40, and four between 10 and 20 years of age.

Eyes.—The left eye only was affected in 10 cases, the right in 6; both eyes in only 1 case; there are 3 cases in which the side was not mentioned. This shows that it is very rare to find both eyes affected.

Family History.—Although tubercular strain found in only 7 cases (35 per cent.), yet in only one was the direct negative mentioned. In the notes of the other cases no mention is made of the subject.

Other Clinical Tubercular signs were found in no less than 16 cases (80 per cent.) at time of visit or soon afterwards; in 1 case (10) signs of phthisis were noted ten years afterwards. Of the remaining 3 cases (6, 8, 9) no mention is made of other signs.

The evidence of these cases is very much against the choroidal tumour being the primary focus of the tuberculosis. Of the other foci of tubercle in these cases tumour of the brain was the most frequently met with—viz. in no less than six patients (Nos. 2, 3, 4, 11, 15, 16), or 30 per cent.; and if the 8 fatal cases are only taken, in every case but two (75 per cent.); tubercular meningitis was found in three cases (1, 15, 20), active pulmonary phthisis in 3 cases.

Signs of local chronic tubercle in other parts—sometimes called surgical tuberculosis—were found in 12 cases, or 60 per cent. This is a very important point as far as diagnosis and prognosis are concerned, as such cases are generally very chronic, and do not by any means necessarily assume the acute state. Looking over the 8 cases without notes of surgical tuberculosis, I think that, with the exception of the two (1 and 2), in which a post-mortem examination was made, they probably also might have been included with the 12. The list below gives the local lesions in the 12 cases.

3. Bronchial glands, caseous and chronic tubercle of most other organs.
5. Maxillary, auricular, clavicular, subclavicular glands affected.
7. Osteitis of thumb metacarpus.
11. Bronchial glands, lupus, submaxillary gland, rickets.
12. Brachial fistula.
13. Cervical glands, abscess of thoracic wall.
15. Gonitis.
16. Bronchial glands.
17. Cervical and episternal glands, many sinuses in arms and legs.
18. Mammary abscess.
19. Submaxillary, axillary, and groin glánds.
20. Lumbar and cervical abscesses.

Death ensued in 8 cases, and in 7 of these notes of the post-mortem examinations are given. Of these 7 cases 3 had tubercular meningitis and 5 coarse tubercle of the brain.

The Examination of the Eye is recorded in 15 cases out of the 20. There was generally one large tubercular mass in the choroid, but occasionally two tumours. In almost every case the tumour was nodular in part; the colour was grey (from a yellow to greenish tinge), white, or white with pink tinge. The position was, as a rule, near the optic disk, and the growth tended to overshadow the disk.

The retina at first passed unaltered over the tumour, and was only implicated later in the disease. In some cases detachment took place owing to tension due to the size of the tumour, as happens in malignant disease. In one case (17) retinal changes occurred as the tumours subsided, and in three cases retinal hæmorrhages were present.

The *vitreous* was stated to be clear in 4 cases, disturbed in 4, and with numerous cells in 1 case. Of the 5 cases in which the vitreous was abnormal, 3 had signs of iritis, and the 1 with marked opacities had hypopyon. With the exception of this last case the expressions "turbid" or "slightly turbid" are too vague to indicate necessarily pathological changes in the vitreous. My own opinion is that as long as the tumour does not involve the ciliary body or anterior portion of choroid vitreous opacities are not found.

Let me enumerate the appearance of a solitary tubercle as seen by the ophthalmoscope in the early uncomplicated stages of the disease.

The tumour, of a greyish or white colour, is generally found as a spherical more or less nodular subretinal swelling. It is situated, as a rule, near the optic disk, which it tends to over-shadow. The retina passes with the retinal vessel clearly over it, but may be detached at the periphery of the tumour. Signs of degeneration — as yellowish spots — may be seen, and occasionally retinal hæmorrhages. Vitreous opacities are rarely if ever present, unless the ciliary body is implicated.

The *sclera* was thickened, infiltrated in 13 cases, and in 2 cases perforated; in 2 cases there was definite scleral swelling.

Microscopical.—The chief signs are giant cells, proliferation of the endothelium and adventitia of the blood-vessels, and areas of caseation; these were found in every case out of 15 examined. Bacilli were only noted in 4 cases, and in one of these cases the specimen had been nine years in spirit. (At St. Bartholomew's Hospital tubercle bacilli were found in a specimen which had been seventy years in spirit.)

Operations.—In nine cases the eye was removed, and one of these only was followed by death from meningitis. In 7 of these cases the operation was excision only; in one (9) excision followed by exenteration for an orbital extension of disease; and in one case (13) exenteration was done at once.

After History.—Of 7 non-fatal cases unfortunately I can find no records; of 4, 1 was alive and well five years after, 2 four years after, and 1 two years after.

Diagnosis.—These cases may be mistaken for glioma, sarcoma, or gumma.

From the intra-ocular stage of malignant disease they may, as a rule, be recognised by there being signs of inflammation or conjunctival congestion, keratitis, iritis, scleritis; the tension, too, is generally rather reduced as against increased or normal tension in malignant disease. In both conditions vitreous opacities are rarely if ever met with, unless the ciliary body is affected or perforation into the vitreous has taken place. Signs of tubercle in other parts of the body aids the diagnosis, as does also injection of tuberculin T. R.

From a syphilitic gummatous mass tubercle of the choroid differs in not being accompanied by vitreous opacities, marked black pigment changes in the choroid and retina, and in not being improved by mercurial treatment.

By the microscope the diagnosis is made from the presence of giant cells, epithelioid stroma, caseation, and sometimes tubercle bacilli.

In all cases of doubt, when the material can be obtained,

the surest way is the inoculation of an animal with a portion of the growth.

Prognosis (1) *As to Life.*—This depends mostly on the other foci of tubercle, which are generally of the chronic variety. In the eight cases of death no less than six had tumours of the brain.

(2) *As to Vision.*—Of the twenty cases the affected eye was removed in sixteen, thus leaving only four for consideration (5, 12, 17, 18). Of 5 and 12 there is no note of vision; in case 17 after four years the vision was $\frac{6}{12}$, and in case 18 after five years the vision was $\frac{2}{3}$.

(3) *As to Ophthalmoscopic Signs.*—Of this I have only my two cases (17 and 18) as proof. Fortunately there are drawings during the whole time (four years) the cases have been under observation. Notwithstanding the gross initial lesions in case 17, the fundus has gradually cleared, leaving very little change except at the periphery below. Throughout vitreous opacities have been absent, black or grey pigmentation of the choroid is absent except slightly now at the extreme periphery, and there is scarcely any change to be seen in the retina where the changes were so marked.

In case 18 the choroidal signs quite cleared up without pigment change; vitreous opacities were absent throughout.

Treatment.—I have had no experience of the effect of tuberculin T.R. in such cases, but I should certainly give it a trial when another case comes under my care.

Of my two cases of recovery, No. 17 has been treated as far as possible by living in the open air and frequent visits to Margate. She has also had cod-liver oil, syrup of iodide of iron, and, locally, atropine and tinted glasses. The usual treatment recommended in such cases has been excision of the eyeball, mainly as a preventive of general dissemination. The after history of cases 17 and 18 certainly negatives this procedure, as does also the extreme doubt of the primary focus being ever intra-ocular.

IRIS.—*Tubercle of the Iris* was first described by Gradenigo ([17]) in 1869; but till lately such cases were known as granulomata of the iris and were scarcely ever really diagnosed. In a perforating staphyloma Köster ([18]) first described bacilli.

Tubercular disease of the iris may be divided into three typical classes: (1) miliary tubercle; (2) solitary or chronic tubercle; (3) tubercular iritis, generally associated with cyclitis.

(1) Miliary tubercle, in which the nodules are found on the surface of the iris, mostly discrete and near the ciliary border

or the margin of the pupil. The tubercles are generally small grey or yellowish points varying in number from five to twenty-five, sometimes with vessels on their surface; the condition may be acute or chronic, and is accompanied by marked ciliary congestion; as a rule the younger the patient the more acute the process. There is usually a tendency for the nodules to coalesce and fill the anterior chamber; the cornea becomes hazy (keratitis profunda) with a deposit of lymph on its posterior surface; the ciliary body soon is affected.

Occasionally the tubercles disappear, but as a rule the eye becomes disorganised and lost for vision, the choroid, sclera, and cornea becoming involved and the eye giving way at the sclero-corneal junction or through the cornea, a staphyloma being first formed.

In some cases general infection may occur, but sometimes the nodules grow slowly and become absorbed. (Leber's "attenuated tubercle.")

(2) The solitary tubercle like that of the choroid is generally a definite tumour, yellow-grey in colour, and nodular (aggregated) in form; it grows steadily and slowly, but is not necessarily accompanied by severe iritis; the position is generally from the lower part of the iris (Haab), or from the ciliary region and intermediate zone of the iris.

Microscopically.—It is seldom circumscribed; there are giant cells, leucocytes, epithelioid cells. Some of the giant cells may be pigmented; caseation soon ensues. Out of ten cases, in seven the ciliary body was also invaded.

In most cases the cornea is soon affected; lymph is present in the anterior chamber and on the posterior surface of the cornea; cyclitis, choroiditis, and scleritis may occur.

The growth is generally forwards and may fill the anterior chamber, but, according to Lagrange, rarely involves the ciliary muscle. When perforation takes place it is at the limbus or near the iridic angle.

(3) Tubercular iritis is of chronic nature and generally occurs with great thickening of the iris and punctate condition of the cornea.

Tubercular iritis has been described as primary by several observers. Denig ([19]) in 80 cases found 67 with no other signs of tubercle; of these 67, 40 were sound in every way, whilst 27 were suspect from hereditary taint, but in 39 of these cases later notes show 19 had tuberculosis of other organs; but 5 had no symptoms for some years.

As far as I know, in every case of tubercular iritis in

which a post-mortem examination has been made, another tubercular focus has been found, and I am inclined to believe with Vossius([21]) and Wagenmann([20]) that primary iritis has not been proved in human eyes.

Diagnosis.—From sarcoma, it is very difficult to be sure in the later stages, but in the early stages the tubercular mass is generally accompanied by marked superficial congestion. From gumma it is almost impossible to diagnose, but the position of the syphilitic lesion is generally nearer the pupillary border. The only perfect method of diagnosis is by injection into the anterior chamber of an animal of some of the material. Tuberculin T.R. may aid diagnosis, as also may mercury.

Treatment.—According to some authorities the eye should always be excised when the case is severe, but I am sure there is great danger of dissemination and tubercular meningitis, as the sclerotic is generally affected. Iridectomy for the solitary form has been practised; iodoform in the anterior chamber (Haab), hetol (Pflüger), air (Köster) have been tried, but tuberculin (T.R.) is probably the best treatment.

RETINA.—Of tubercular disease of the retina, except secondary to that of the choroid, I have had no experience. Arnold Knapp([22]) has described a case of localised tuberculosis at the head of the optic nerve, and Sattler has described a somewhat similar case, but in neither was the change only in the retina, though the choroid was less affected.

CONCLUSION.—In order to direct and limit the discussion on intra-ocular tuberculosis, I have drawn up seven headings, comprising points on which opinions are specially needed and invited. I have, as introduction, briefly considered these points myself.

I. *What is the Relative Frequency of Primary Intra-ocular Tuberculosis?*—Cases of primary intra-ocular tuberculosis have been described, but I have not yet seen a case, and am exceedingly doubtful as to their existence. In most cases it is impossible to be certain, unless an examination after death has been performed. Many such cases were originally described, and I think the chief reason for such statements was the fact that the injection of tuberculous material into the anterior chamber of a rabbit was soon followed by general tuberculosis.

Among the supporters of primary tuberculosis are Köster([18]), v. Michel, Deutschmann, Schmidt-Rimpler, Bach([25]), Denig([19]), Lagrange ([26]), Parinaud ([27]), Greef ([28]), &c.; the extreme opponents are Leber ([29]), Fuchs, whilst Wagenmann([20]),

Vossius ([21]), &c., are uncertain, though more inclined to oppose than to support the theory.

II. *How often is Choroidal Tubercle met with in Acute Miliary Tuberculosis?*—The percentage varies greatly, according to different observers, as high as 82 being recorded; the probability, I think, is that choroidal tubercle is found in about 50 per cent. of the cases post mortem, and in less than that by the ophthalmoscope before death—from 30 to 35 per cent.

III. *What is the Value of Tuberculin* (a) *as an Aid to Diagnosis,* (b) *as Treatment?*—On these points I have had little experience, but certainly agree with most observers now that the old tuberculin is not only unreliable, but sometimes a very dangerous remedy. With the new tuberculin T.R. I have never seen bad results. Von Hippel ([30]) is quite enthusiastic as to its use, and says that even in the most severe cases it effects a cure. His cases have remained cured even for as long as nine years. He uses tuberculin T.R. in hypodermic injections of $\frac{1}{500}$ m.g. of the dry substance, at first every three days if there is no increase of temperature. It is very important to take the temperature day and night. If there is a marked rise of temperature it is expedient to have longer intervals, and not to increase the strength of the dose. If no rise of temperature occurs, then the dose should be raised by the same amount, $\frac{1}{500}$ m.g. till it becomes $\frac{1}{10}$ m.g. After this the immediate increase should be less, and the greatest amount given at one time should not exceed 1 m.g. In very severe cases the treatment may last six months. Schieck ([32]) collected thirteen cases which were all cured by this treatment. Looking at these facts I should certainly treat every case with tuberculin, especially as in Rogman's statistics ([31]) after excision the mortality from tubercular meningitis is so high. Uhthoff, Hess, and Jacoby have all given me proofs of the value of this drug in ocular tuberculosis.

IV. *What is the Danger of General Dissemination as a Result of Excision of the Eye in Intra-ocular Tuberculosis?*—The operation of excision which has been suggested as a general treatment in cases of intra-ocular tuberculosis must fall or stand by the results. Does it lessen or increase the risk of tubercular meningitis or general tuberculosis? Is the disease stayed by it? Is there a tendency in some cases to recovery of vision? The operation of excision of the eye is a mutilation which should only be resorted to in most cases if there is danger of sympathetic inflammation, or if the health is affected to a serious extent by the changes in the eye.

In tubercle in the early stage excision could only be justifiable on the ground that the eye was the only focus of infection, and certainly not if it was only one of many foci. In later stages much pain, great growth of the tubercular changes with complete blindness, may suggest excision. Rogman[31] has collected eleven cases in which death ensued soon after the eye had been excised for tubercle. Of these eleven cases one was over 20 years of age, five between 10 and 20, four between 6 and 10, and one under 2 years.

The time after the excision that death occurred was within one month, three cases; between one and two months, four; between two and three months, one ; and in one year and over, two cases. These last two cases died of pulmonary phthisis, and the six months case of general miliary tuberculosis. The eight who died within three months all died of meningitis, and this seems more than suggestive of dissemination, and indicates the risk of excising a tuberculous eye. The sclerotic was affected in all these cases, and this fact doubtless increases the danger.

In my opinion from these facts I should hesitate very much before excising a tuberculous eye—in the earlier stages because in some cases the manifestations clear up ; in the later stages owing to the risk of general dissemination, especially of tubercular meningitis; in all stages because tuberculin has produced such good results ; and, lastly, because the ocular is probably never the primary lesion. A very great contrast to Rogman's[31] eleven cases of excision, with no less than eight deaths from meningitis within three months, is afforded by Schieck's[32] thirteen cases treated with tuberculin without a fatal result and with cure of the symptoms.

V. *In Tuberculous Affection Limited to the Choroid is there Little Tendency to Pigmentation or Scarring of the Retina or Choroid, and are Vitreous Opacities Seldom Present ?*—In acute miliary tubercular choroiditis I have never found vitreous opacities, and in my two cases of chronic tubercle (17 and 18) they were not present.

As in malignant disease limited to the retina or choroid, so I think in chronic tubercle of the choroid a very important aid to diagnosis is the absence of vitreous opacities.

As to pigmentation and scarring I have been surprised how little remains after severe tubercular disease. As shown in the drawings of case 17 there is scarcely any pigmentation now. Stephenson and Carpenter[6] have described cases with marked pigmentation, especially in the macular region, but cases like their drawings I have generally associated with hereditary syphilis and congenital changes.

VI. *How often in Chronic Phthisis, especially Pulmonary, are there Choroidal Lesions?*

In 466 cases at St. Bartholomew's Hospital of chronic pulmonary phthisis I could find no note of chronic choroidal change. Carpenter and Stephenson[6] found in 119 cases of chronic tuberculosis in children choroidal changes in 11, that is, 9.24 per cent.

VII. *In Chronic Choroidal Tubercle, what are the Signs of " Obsolescent" Tubercle?*

As to this point my own two cases are the only ones I can use, as in them the tubercle bacilli or tubercular inoculation experiments made the diagnosis of tubercle sure, and the lapse of years—four and five—has enabled the so-called " obsolescent" changes to be watched from the commencement. In these, as the drawings show, the changes were not in the macular region, but started near the disk, as was the condition in most of the twenty cases described above. The absence of much scarring and of marked pigmentation seems to distinguish these cases from the syphilitic type.

BIBLIOGRAPHY.

1. MANZ, Archiv. f. Ophth., iv. 2, p. 120.
2. COHNHEIM, Virchow's Archiv., xxxix. p. 49.
3. LITTEN, Volkmann's Klin. Vorträge.
4. BOCK, Virchow's Archiv., xci. p. 434.
5. ANGEL-MONEY, Lancet, 1883, 2, 813.
6. STEPHENSON and CARPENTER, Soc. of Dis. in Children, vol. i. p. 170.
7. GARLICK, Trans. Med. Chir. Soc., lxii. p. 441.
8. GRUENING, Mount Sinai Hosp. Rep., vol. ii. p. 476.
9. BAXTER, Trans. Ophth. Soc., iii. p. 132.
10. GOWERS, Medical Ophthalmoscopy, p. 139.
11. HORNER, Arch. f. Ophth., 1879, Bd. 25, 4, p. 224.
12. HAAB, Arch. f. Ophth., xxv. 4, p. 224.
13. LAWFORD, Trans. Ophth. Soc., vi. p. 348.
14. VON GRAEFE, Archiv. f. Ophth., ii. 1, p. 218.
15. CHELIUS, Lehrbuch der Augenheilk., 1843, vol. i. p. 242.
16. ARLT, Die Krankheiten des Auges, vol. ii. p. 212.
17. GRADENIGO, Annales d'Oculistique, vol. 64, p. 174.
18. KÖSTER, Centralbl. f. d. Med. Wissensch., 1873.
19. DENIG, Arch. f. Augenheilk., xxxi. s. 359.
20. WAGENMANN, Arch. f. Ophth., xxxiv. 4, 145.
21. VOSSIUS, Lehrbuch d'Augenheilk., 3rd Aug., s. 445.
22. ARNOLD KNAPP, Archives of Ophthalmology, xxxii. p. 22.
23. SATTLER, Archiv. f. Ophth., xxiv. 3, p. 227.
24. DEUTSCHMANN, Archiv. f. Ophth., xxvii. 1, 317.
25. BACH, Arch. f. Augheilk., xxviii. s. 36.
26. LAGRANGE, Soc. Franç. d'Opht., 1898, p. 89.

27. PARINAUD, Soc. Franç. d'Opht., 1890, p. 98.
28. GREEF, Lehrbuch d., Path. Anat. d. Aug., s. 228.
29. LEBER, Ophth. Gesellsch. Heidelberg, 1892.
30. VON HIPPEL, Archiv. f. Ophth., lix. 1, p. 1.
31. ROGMAN, Annales d'Oculistique, cxxx. 2, p. 65.
32. SCHIECK, Tuberculin auf die Iris Tuberkulose Habilitations Schrift, 1900, and Archiv. f. Ophth., li. p. 247.

ACTINOMYCOSIS OF THE CÆCUM, VERMIFORM APPENDIX, AND RIGHT ILIAC FOSSA,

INCLUDING AN ACCOUNT OF SEVEN CASES.

BY

H. J. WARING, M.S., F.R.C.S.

Actinomycosis of the abdomen appears invariably to commence in a specific lesion of some portion of the abdominal section of the alimentary canal, except in those rare instances in which actinomycosis of the lung or pleura, by direct extension through the diaphragm, involves one or other of the adjacent abdominal viscera. When the abdomen is the seat of this disease, the pathological process commences most commonly in the cæcum or the vermiform appendix. Which of these two anatomical structures is the more common seat of the actual commencement of the affection is difficult to determine, owing to the fact that in most cases both these portions of the alimentary canal become involved, before the seat of disease is either exposed at an operation by the surgeon, or by the pathologist at a post-mortem examination. According to most observers who have investigated this subject, the vermiform appendix is either the primary seat of invasion of the parasite, or it is so definitely embedded in the " actinomycotic mass " as to justify the assumption that this must have been the case. With this assertion I am not prepared to entirely agree, as a study of the seven cases detailed at the end of this paper warrants the assertion that the cæcum is quite as commonly the seat of the primary focus of disease. If this be true, actinomycosis of the cæcum and vermiform appendix resembles tuberculosis of the same organs, since here the cæcum is the more frequently the seat of the original affection. Some observers have found in the interior of the vermiform appendix, when this structure is affected with actinomycosis, a grain of wheat or barley in which the fungus has been found. I have not noticed this condition in any of the cases which have come under my personal observation, although in two instances the patients affected with the disease have stated that they have been in the habit of eating ears of corn or chewing grain.

Amongst the patients from which the present series has been collected there were two other cases of abdominal actinomycosis, one of which commenced in the stomach and the other in the rectum.   This appears to be about the usual ratio as regards the locality of abdominal actinomycosis.

FREQUENCY.—The seven cases of actinomycosis of the cæcum, vermiform appendix, and right iliac fossa, which are the subject of this paper, occurred in a series of approximately 25,000 consecutive surgical in-patients, and of 650 patients suffering from disease of the cæcum, vermiform appendix, and right iliac fossa.

SYMPTOMS.—The clinical course of actinomycosis of the cæcum, vermiform appendix, and right iliac fossa is essentially chronic in character, and resembles that of the disease when it affects other portions of the body, but it is to be remembered that it is more likely to present acute exacerbations due to mixed infections giving rise to the formation of septic abscesses.   This is dependent upon contamination with micro-organisms from the contents of the adjacent or involved portions of the alimentary canal.

The clinical course of the disease may be divided into the following five stages, viz.—

(*a*) The stage of infection and development;

(*b*) The stage of formation of a tumour;

(*c*) The stage of suppuration, formation of abscesses, and resultant fistulæ;

(*d*) The stage of formation of secondary abscesses, either through the veins or by direct extension to distant parts, as into the subphrenic space;

(*e*) The stage of repair.

The early symptoms of the disease are usually indefinite, and cannot be distinguished from those manifested in an attack of ordinary appendicitis.   When a tumour is formed it is in the region of the right iliac fossa.   It is often characterised by its slow rate of growth, and by its hardness.   This latter characteristic is especially to be noted when the superjacent portions of the anterior abdominal wall have been infiltrated.   Definite abscesses usually form quickly when the diseased areas have become infected with the micro-organisms of ordinary suppu-

ration. When an abscess has formed and its contents are
evacuated, the typical yellow granules of actinomyces can be
distinguished. Naked-eye appearances, however, should not be
relied upon, and a definite diagnosis can only be made when
their indications are confirmed by microscopical examination.
The purulent contents of an actinomycotic abscess are usually
thick and mucoid in character, and have a distinctive odour
which is suggestive of sulphuretted hydrogen. An easy method
of detecting the presence of actinomycosis-like granules, is
to take a sterilised test-tube and collect in it a small quantity
of the pus from a possibly actinomycosic abscess. If this be
allowed to run down the sides of the interior of the tube, the
granules when present adhere to the inner surface of the tube
and can be readily seen with the naked eye, and can also be
collected for examination with the microscope. On several
occasions I have been able to demonstrate the very probable
presence of actinomycosis granules at the time of opening an
abscess. Usually the "granules" have a typical light yellow
colour, but in one case which I examined they were black and
had the appearance of grains of black gunpowder.

DIAGNOSIS.—The diagnosis of actinomycosis of the cæcum,
vermiform appendix, or right iliac fossa, may be suggested from
the slow development of the swelling, and the characteristic
hardness of the tumour when it has extended to the overlying
portion of the anterior abdominal wall, but it can only be
absolutely decided by the demonstration of the actinomyces
fungus in the tissues or in the contents of an abscess cavity
which has either been opened or has burst through the skin.
When an abscess of this nature has burst and has discharged
for some time, it is often very difficult or even impossible to
find the parasite in the discharge from the sinus. This was the
case in one of the patients whose clinical histories are given
below. This is explained by the anærobic character of the
micro-organism.

TREATMENT. — Owing to the tendency of the disease to
infiltrate the surrounding and adjacent tissues, it is not usually
possible to attempt complete removal of the disease by a surgical
operation. The limits of surgery appear to be, incision, evacuation, scraping, and drainage of abscesses immediately they can
be diagnosed, and afterwards repeated irrigation with an antiseptic solution, with iodine, or, better, with a solution of peroxide
of hydrogen. The latter chemical substance appears to be the
most effective agent in arresting the local growth of the parasite.
In addition to these local measures it is necessary to give
potassium iodide internally, the best method being to commence

with 10 grains three times daily, and to gradually increase this until each dose consists of 100 grains or even more. As regards the duration of treatment, this varies considerably. In some cases it is necessary to go on for a year or more.

PROGNOSIS.—The prognosis of actinomycosis of the cæcum, vermiform appendix, and right iliac fossa is usually stated to be bad. I think, however, that it is not so bad as has been stated by many observers. If careful attention be paid to incision and evacuation of abscesses whenever they form, and to prolonged administration of large doses of potassium iodide, I think most cases will recover. If, however, the disease gives rise to pyæmic abscesses of the liver, or to a subphrenic abscess, the affection will usually be fatal.

Out of my series of seven cases four patients recovered and three died.

CASE I.—*Actinomycosis of Vermiform Appendix, Cæcum, and Right Iliac Fossa—Operation—Recovery.*

A man aged 40, a shoemaker by occupation, came under observation on account of pain in the right iliac fossa which he stated followed the reception of a blow in that region. As regards the sequence of events, the patient received a blow in the right iliac fossa eight weeks previous to coming under observation ; six weeks later (two weeks before admission) he had an attack of diarrhœa, vomiting, and pain of a sharp shooting character in the deeper parts of the right iliac fossa. This condition persisted for a week, and then a swelling began to form in the right iliac fossa, and consequent upon this the pains in that region diminished very much in severity. The patient stated that for some considerable period before coming under observation he had suffered from periodical attacks of diarrhœa, but that he never had had attacks of pain localised in the right iliac fossa.

When examined, the patient appeared to be a well-nourished man. The tongue was slightly furred, the temperature 100.4°, and the pulse 88, regular, and of good volume. The bowels were open after the administration of an enema. The urine was normal, and nothing abnormal was noticed in the stools. On examination of the abdomen, it appeared to move fairly with respiration, and to be somewhat full, especially in the region of the right iliac fossa. On palpation a hard mass irregular in outline, slightly tender on manipulation, was found to occupy the right iliac fossa and to extend towards the umbilicus, and also over the brim of the pelvis so as to be readily palpable *per rectum.* The area of greatest tenderness was at a point half-way between the anterior superior spine of the ilium and the umbilicus.

The disease from which the patient was suffering was diagnosed as either tuberculous disease of the cæcum and appendix, or carcinoma of the same region. A point of clinical interest in connection with the physical examination was the extreme hardness of the growth. On account of the uncertain nature of the disease and the possibility of its being inflammatory in character, I decided to explore the mass so as to determine its exact character. An incision was therefore made through the abdominal wall in the right iliac fossa, and over the most prominent portion of the swelling. The hard mass was seen to occupy the right iliac fossa, and to surround the cæcum and vermiform appendix, both of which were involved in what appeared to be a form of new growth, the vermiform appendix being very much enlarged and about three times its usual size. A portion of the indurated tissue was excised for the purposes of histological and bacteriological examination, and when this had been done a small amount of semipurulent matter escaped, in which could be seen small rounded yellow granules of actinomyces. Examination of the portion removed confirmed the "naked-eye" diagnosis. The wound was packed with a strip of gauze, and the patient treated by the administration of potassium iodide, commencing with 20-grain doses three times daily. The wound was daily irrigated with a solution of iodine, and afterwards with peroxide of hydrogen, and the dose of potassium iodide was gradually increased until 100 grains were given in each dose. This method of treatment was continued, and gradually the area of induration diminished until at the expiration of twelve weeks the patient was discharged convalescent. The patient was again seen some months afterwards, when he was found to have completely recovered.

CASE II.—*Actinomycosis of the Vermiform Appendix, Cæcum, and Right Iliac Fossa—Operation—Recovery.*

A woman aged 25, a machinist by occupation, came under observation on account of pain and swelling in the right iliac fossa. She stated that one month previously she suffered from general abdominal pain associated with attacks of vomiting and diarrhœa. The medical man who saw her at this time said she had "inflammation of the bowels." She was treated by rest in bed for a week and given medicine. The abdominal pain, in the second week, became localised in the region of the right iliac fossa, and at this time the patient also noticed a swelling in the same region. For three weeks the swelling in the iliac fossa apparently remained of the same size, the pain became less marked, and constipation occurred, which condition was alleviated by the administration of aperients. The patient then applied for treatment at the hospital, and was admitted. The patient was a somewhat anæmic female, who stated that she had suffered from "anæmia and dyspepsia" for some time, but that she had never had an illness with symptoms similar to those of the present attack. On examination, the abdomen was seen to be not distended, and moved freely with respiration, although in the right iliac region a marked fulness could be readily distinguished. On palpation the right iliac fossa was felt to be filled by a hard solid mass which was somewhat tender on manipulation, but no definite evidence of fluctuation could be detected. The subcutaneous tissues over the swelling were slightly œdematous, and on examination per rectum the swelling in the iliac region could be felt to extend some short distance over the brim of the pelvis. The temperature was 101°, the pulse 96, and the respiration 22. Examination of the urine and fæces revealed nothing abnormal. The diagnosis of appendicitis was made, and an operation recommended. An oblique incision was made through the abdominal wall above the outer half of Poupart's ligament and over the most prominent portion of the swelling. A hard, indurated mass was met with infiltrating the deeper strata of the abdominal wall, and the structures in the right iliac fossa, especially the cæcum and vermiform appendix. The main portion of the mass was found to contain a quantity of shreddy caseous material, and a small quantity of thick pus. This was evacuated, and when examined was found to have a curious sulphurous odour, suggesting the presence of sulphuretted hydrogen, and to contain a number of yellow granules which microscopically had the structure of actinomyces. The caseous matter was removed by scraping, the cavity irrigated with a solution of peroxide of hydrogen, and then packed with strips of gauze. The wound was treated by daily irrigation and packing, and potassium iodide given in doses of 10 grains three times daily. The dose of this drug was gradually increased until it amounted to 75 grains. This method of treatment was continued for four weeks, and during this time the aperture of the incision closed until a small sinus-like opening remained, and at this period two small sinuses developed in the region of the original incision. Four and a half weeks after the operation a swelling was detected in the lumbar region of the right side. This on examination was found to fluctuate ; an incision was made into it, and a small cavity containing caseous shreddy material with granules of actinomyces evacuated. This was also treated by daily irrigation with a solution of peroxide of hydrogen and packed. At intervals during the succeeding six weeks three other similar swellings appeared in adjacent portions of the abdominal wall. These were treated in a similar manner. After this time the sinuses commenced to close up, and seventeen weeks after admission, and twenty weeks after the apparent commencement of the disease, the patient was sent to a convalescent home, whence she returned three weeks later, apparently quite recovered. The patient was heard of later, and was reported to be well.

CASE III.—*Actinomycosis of Cæcum and Right Iliac Fossa —Operation—Recovery.*

A printer, aged 18, experienced, a fortnight before admission, a sudden attack of pain in the region of the right iliac fossa, the cause of which was not apparent. This continued at intervals, until he sought admission to the hospital two weeks later. When examined, a definite swelling could be felt in the right iliac fossa. This was tender on manipulation, but no evidence of deep-seated fluctuation could be definitely detected. Examination per rectum did not yield any further evidence of the nature of the affection. The patient was constipated, but the bowels were freely opened after the administration of an enema. The temperature was 101.2°. There was no evidence of any general peritonitis. The diagnosis was made that the patient was suffering from suppurative appendicitis. An exploratory operation was decided upon. An incision was made over the prominent portion of the swelling in the iliac fossa, and the region of the cæcum and vermiform appendix investigated. The cæcum was found to be the seat of considerable thickening, and to be adherent to the surrounding tissues by moderately firm adhesions. The vermiform appendix itself did not appear to be diseased. No collection of purulent matter was found. The wound was partially closed, and a drainage tube inserted. Three days later an abscess cavity in the region of the cæcum suddenly burst, and a small quantity of thick pus was discharged through the external wound. Pus continued to discharge from the wound, and on investigation of this, typical granules of actinomyces were discovered.

The wound was freely drained, and irrigated at intervals with antiseptics. Potassium iodide was administered internally, 10 grains being given three times daily at first, and this was gradually increased until 40 grains were given three times daily. This method of treatment was continued for four and a half months. The local condition was improved, but there was still a sinus when the patient was discharged. From this sinus a small quantity of purulent matter was discharged, in which occasional granules of actinomycosis could be found. The number of granules diminished very considerably whilst potassium was administered.

On inquiry later, the patient was found to have completely recovered from the affection.

CASE IV.—*Actinomycosis of Vermiform Appendix, Cæcum, and Right Iliac Fossa—Operation—Recovery*

A laundress, aged 29, who had previously been treated for what was supposed to be an attack of appendicitis, came to the hospital three months later, when she was found to have a swelling in the right iliac fossa, which had all the characters of a chronic inflammatory mass, and gave evidence of fluctuation in its deeper part. The diagnosis of suppurative appendicitis was made, and an immediate operation recommended. An incision was made through the abdominal wall over the prominent portion of the swelling, and a short distance above Poupart's ligament. About 1 ounce of pus was evacuated, No search was made for the vermiform appendix. A drainage tube was inserted, and the abscess cavity drained. Induration of the abdominal wall on the right side could be felt to extend upwards as far as the level of the umbilicus. After the operation, a considerable amount of induration of the abdominal wall and the structures in the right iliac fossa remained. There was only a slight amount of purulent matter discharged from the wound. Three weeks after admission a second abscess in the abdominal wall was incised, and about 1 ounce of pus evacuated. A third abscess was incised six weeks later. A bacteriological examination of the matter evacuated showed that it contained granules and mycelia of actinomycosis. When this discovery had been made, potassium iodide in gradually increasing doses was administered. For a time no improvement was noticed, but after the expiration of about two months the induration in the right iliac fossa and in the abdominal wall commenced to diminish. The dose of potassium iodide was increased to 120 grains per day.

This method of treatment was continued at intervals for a year.

At the time of discharge from hospital the patient had only two small superficial sinuses in the abdominal wall from which a small quantity of purulent matter exuded. No granules of actinomyces had been present in the pus for some time.

Some time afterwards the patient was reported to be quite recovered.

CASE V.—*Actinomycosis of Cæcum, Vermiform Appendix, and Right Iliac Fossa—Operation—Death.*

A boy, aged 14, who had suffered at frequent intervals from slight attacks of pain in the right iliac fossa, two days before admission experienced a sudden sharp pain similar to the previous ones, only much more severe. When seen two days later in a medical ward he was found to have tenderness and swelling in the right iliac fossa. Fluctuation could be detected in the central portion of the swelling. The patient was in great pain, and lay curled up in bed; he vomited at intervals; his temperature was 101°, and his pulse 108. The patient improved somewhat after admission, but seven days later, as the swelling still remained in the iliac fossa, surgical treatment was sought. On examination, the right iliac fossa was found to be the seat of a swelling which appeared to contain fluid in its deeper portion. The diagnosis of suppurative appendicitis was made, and an operation advised. This was at once carried out. An incision was made through the abdominal wall over the prominent portion of the iliac swelling, and a short distance above Poupart's ligament. An abscess cavity containing several ounces of very fœtid pus was evacuated. This appeared to be in the lower portion of the right iliac fossa, and in the region of the cæcum and vermiform appendix, although this latter structure was not recognised.

The interior of the abscess cavity was thoroughly irrigated and a drainage tube inserted. Irrigation and drainage were continued, and the local condition improved. The opening closed, but later broke down again, and then closed. The patient was discharged from the hospital, wearing a truss at the seat of the operation wound two months after admission. The presence of granules of actinomyces was not noticed during the period whilst the patient was in the hospital.

He went to the convalescent home, and whilst there three weeks after leaving the hospital he experienced pain in the right lumbar region, and also noticed the formation of a swelling there. He then went home, and gradually got worse, the swelling in the lumbar region increasing in size, and the pain becoming more severe. He again sought admission to the hospital one month after his discharge. When seen, he was found to

have a fluctuating swelling in the right lumbar region, which
extended downwards towards the iliac fossa. An incision was
made into the swelling in the right lumbar region, and a quantity of pus evacuated. The old incision was opened up, and a
drainage tube inserted from one wound to the other. Irrigation
with antiseptics and free drainage were adopted. The patient
did not improve ; copious purulent discharge continued, and the
temperature remained raised, often being 101° in the evening.
One or two small abscesses in the abdominal wall were opened
at intervals. Four months later the general condition of the
patient had become gradually worse, and a swelling was noticed
in the region of the liver. The heart at this time was noticed
to have become enlarged. The patient then had severe
diarrhœa, and at times suffered from cough and dyspnœa.
Six months after readmission the patient died.

Post mortem the vermiform appendix was found to be the
seat of numerous adhesions, no concretion or perforation was
found. On the posterior aspect of the cæcum an ulcer about
two-thirds of an inch in length and half an inch in breadth was
found to involve almost the entire thickness of the wall of the
gut. The margins of this ulcer were soft, irregular, and
slightly undermined. The tissues surrounding the ulcer and
the base were slightly harder than usual. Nothing further
abnormal was found in the other parts of the alimentary canal.
A large extraperitoneal subphrenic abscess, multiple abscesses
of the liver, and abscess of the right kidney, and purulent
pericarditis were found. The subphrenic abscess was apparently due to tracking upwards of the pus behind the colon
and in front of the right kidney, and the purulent pericarditis
to perforation of the diaphragm by the subphrenic abscess.
The abscesses of the liver and kidney were pyæmic in origin.

The subphrenic abscess, the abscesses in the liver and kidney
and the pus from the interior of the pericardium contained
innumerable granules of actinomyces.

Histological examination of the ulcer in the cæcum and the
thickened appendix failed to show the presence of mycelial
threads of actinomycosis.

CASE VI.—*Actinomycosis of Cæcum, Vermiform Appendix,
and Right Iliac Fossa—Operation—Death.*

A clergyman, aged 25, in April 1897 first had an attack
of acute pain in the right iliac fossa which lasted for thirty-six
hours and then subsided. At the beginning of August of
the same year he suffered from a similar attack of abdominal

pain which was limited to the right iliac fossa and was associated with the occurrence of vomiting. On this occasion the pain lasted for four days. The patient then recovered and felt quite well until October 3, when a third attack commenced. On this occasion the symptoms were similar, but lasted longer and necessitated the patient staying in bed for rather more than a week. He again recovered, and remained well until December 2, when a fourth attack commenced. The affection was of slow onset, and was accompanied by the occurrence of severe abdominal pain, mainly located in the right iliac fossa, but there was no vomiting. A swelling or hardness was now noticed for the first time in the right iliac fossa. The patient's condition remained practically unchanged for three weeks, and then he was admitted to the hospital. At the end of July 1897 the patient ate several ears of corn when passing through a cornfield.

When seen, the patient appeared to be in moderate health, and he was not in any sense collapsed. The face was not pallid or anxious in appearance. The temperature on admission was 101.2°, and the pulse 84, and of good volume and tension. On examination of the abdomen, a swelling of considerable size but indefinite in outline was noticed in the right iliac region. The skin over the swelling was œdematous and slightly red, whilst the main mass itself extended into the iliac fossa. The presence of fluctuation could not be detected with certainty.

DIAGNOSIS.—The patient was considered to be suffering from suppurative appendicitis, localised mainly in the right iliac fossa. Immediate operation was advised.

OPERATION.—An incision was made in the right iliac region, parallel with, and a short distance above, the outer portion of Poupart's ligament and the adjacent portion of the iliac crest. When the superficial layers of the abdominal wall had been divided, it was found that the deeper layers were the seat of considerable fibrous thickening, apparently due to long-standing inflammatory processes. After a short search a localised abscess cavity containing a few drachms of purulent matter was found in the right iliac fossa. This was shut off from the general peritoneal cavity by old adhesions and was surrounded by a considerable amount of inflammatory thickening. A microscopical or bacteriological examination of the pus was not made at this operation, owing to the fact that most of it escaped. The wound was plugged with strips of gauze. Subsequently it was dressed daily; the amount of discharge at first was small, and consisted of purulent

matter mixed with a quantity of blood.   After the operation
the induration of the abdominal wall and the tissues in the
iliac fossa increased and extended downwards into the right
side of the pelvis, so that an induration could be felt attached
to the right side of the brim of the pelvis.   This was continuous with the mass felt in the right iliac fossa and in the
adjacent portions of the abdominal wall.   The size of the
swelling somewhat diminished, owing to a continuous discharge
of purulent matter.   A few days after the operation the patient
suffered from temporary difficulties in micturition and defæcation.   These, however, were soon remedied.   Twelve days
after the operation some of the discharge was collected and
examined.   It was found to contain a number of small yellow
granules, each of which had the typical structure of actinomyces.

The administration of potassium iodide was now commenced,
15 grains being given three times a day.   The wound was
also treated locally by irrigation with a solution of iodine.   The
dose of potassium iodide was gradually increased until 70
grains were taken three times a day.   At first the induration
and swelling did not diminish, and numerous actinomycotic
granules could still be found in the discharge.   The affection
also extended in the pelvis, so that the walls of the rectum
became involved.   When the iodide of potassium had been
given for about nine weeks, the swelling and induration in
the right iliac fossa and in the adjacent portions of the
abdominal wall diminished.   The typical granules also almost
disappeared from the discharge.   The patient then left the
hospital.   There was then a sinus in the right inguinal region
from which a small quantity of purulent matter exuded.   The
pelvic induration was less.

Three months after leaving the hospital the patient died.
It was stated that after his discharge he gradually got worse,
and succumbed, owing to the gradual advance of the disease.

No evidence of the performance of a post-mortem examination was obtainable.

CASE VII.—*Actinomycosis of Cœcum, Right Iliac Fossa, and
    Abdominal Walls—Perinephric and Subphrenic Abscesses
    —Abscess of Liver—Death.*

A youth, aged 17, sustained a blow in the right side of the
abdomen, which, he stated, was followed by attacks of pain in
the lower portion of the abdomen and in the region of the right

iliac fossa, at intervals during the succeeding fourteen days. He then recovered, and remained well for about six months. Then he began to get thinner and to have attacks of abdominal pain similar to those which were said to have followed the reception of the injury, only that they were more severe. When examined, this patient was seen to be wasted in appearance, and weighed only 68 lbs. The abdomen was flaccid and moved well, but in the lower part, extending from the right pubic crest and inner portion of Poupart's ligament upwards, almost as far as the umbilicus, and outwards into the right iliac fossa could be detected a hard swelling which appeared to involve the strata of the abdominal wall, and to extend into the iliac fossa and the adjacent portion of the right side of the upper part of the pelvis. The nature of this tumour was indefinite, and it was decided to make an exploratory incision in order to remove a portion of the growth for examination. This was done, and the portion removed was found to consist of caseous material, in which neither signs of tuberculosis, actinomycosis, or malignant disease could be discovered. A few days later, however, a discharge of purulent matter occurred through the operation wound, and on examination this pus was found to contain numerous granules of actinomyces. The wound was then explored, laid freely open, and made to communicate with an abscess cavity which extended into the right iliac fossa in the position of the cæcum and vermiform appendix. The abscess cavity was treated by irrigation and plugging, and, internally, iodide of potassium was given in large and gradually increasing doses. Two days later, intestinal contents with a fæcal odour escaped into the abscess cavity, and thence to the external opening. The patient gradually sank, and died fifteen days later. Post mortem the abdominal walls on the right side and lower part of the abdomen were found to be infiltrated with purulent matter and indurated tissue which contained numerous granules of actinomyces. An abscess cavity was also found in the right iliac fossa, extending upwards behind the cæcum and colon to the perinephric and subphrenic regions. The liver contained a number of pyæmic abscesses, each containing granules of actinomyces, whilst the cæcum was the seat of an ulcer on its postero-internal aspect close to the attachment of the vermiform appendix. This ulcer perforated the wall of the cæcum and allowed an escape of intestinal contents into the abscess cavity already mentioned. Microscopically the margin of the ulcer showed evidence of chronic inflammation, but no evidence of infection with actinomyces was demonstrated. The parts, however, were in a very rotten and decomposing condition at the time of the *post mortem* examination, so that a satisfactory histological investigation was rendered difficult.

For permission to use the notes of some of the above cases, I am indebted to my surgical colleagues at St. Bartholomew's Hospital, and to them I offer my thanks.

FOUR CASES OF CRANIO-CEREBRAL SURGERY.

BY

LOUIS BATHE RAWLING, F.R.C.S.

The four cases, which are here recorded, deserve special mention, as each presented features of special interest.

CASE 1.—*Cerebral Abscess, Secondary to Orbital Periostitis—Operation—Recovery.*

J. S., 39 years of age, was admitted, on May 26, 1905, into Colston Ward under the care of Dr. Herringham. He complained of severe frontal headache, most marked and persistent on the right side. Mr. D'Arcy Power was asked to see the case, and as the upper lid was œdematous, a diagnosis of "orbital periostitis with pus formation" was made, and a local exploration advised. At this time the patient presented no symptoms which suggested any intracranial complication beyond the fact that the headache was persistent and uninfluenced by drugs. The intellect was fairly clear, the pulse 80, the temperature 98°, and a blood-count showed 9000 leucocytes per cubic millimetre. There was no optic neuritis.

On May 28 the upper lid was incised, about 3ij of pus being evacuated, and on digital examination the orbital plate of the frontal bone was found bare of periosteum.

On May 31 the patient was more drowsy. Pulse, 72; temperature, 100·3°. No vomiting, and no optic neuritis.

June 4.—Vomited twice. No optic neuritis.

June 7.—More drowsy. Pulse, 60; temperature, subnormal. Pupils equal and reacted to light. Leucocytosis of 16,500.

June 8.—I was asked to see the case in Mr. Power's absence as a sudden change for the worse had taken place. The man was quite unconscious, the left side of the face paralysed, and the left arm and leg limp and powerless. The temperature was subnormal, the pulse 60, and early optic neuritis present in both eyes, most evident at the upper and inner aspect of the disc. The neuritis was equally marked on the two sides.

Everything now pointed to the presence of a cerebral abscess, and I decided to operate without delay. The question then arose as to the exact site of the trouble, and a difficulty at once presented itself, for experience tells us that a cerebral abscess which is secondary to a bony lesion is almost invariably situated in close proximity to the diseased bone. In this particular case, however, an orbital periostitis, with resultant cerebral abscess formation, was associated with symptoms pointing to implications of the corresponding motor area.

After careful consideration, I came to the conclusion that the abscess involved the anterior, inferior, and external aspect of the right frontal pole, and that the paralytic symptoms resulted from a backward pressure on the corona radiata passing from the Rolandic area. The late onset of the paralysis much strengthened this view, and the symptoms could be very well explained by the secondary œdema of that region and by the possible thrombosis of some of the cerebral veins.

After turning down a suitable flap of the scalp, the pericranium was stripped from an area of bone, about 2 inches in diameter, immediately above the external angular frontal process. A disc of bone was then removed with a 1½-inch trephine. The exposed dura mater bulged outwards and did not pulsate. A fine aspirating needle was introduced for about 2 inches towards the middle line, but no pus withdrawn. The removal of the needle was, however, followed by the escape of two or three drops of pus. The dura was consequently freely incised, and a pair of dressing forceps introduced in such a way that a large ragged cavity, containing about ℥vj of pus, was evacuated. The abscess occupied the greater part of the centre of the frontal pole, and lay, therefore, wholly anterior to the motor area. It was necessary to enlarge the hole in the skull for a short distance in a backward direction in order to ensure efficient drainage. A gentle stream of sterilised water aided in the washing away of pus and brain débris. A large-mouthed drainage-tube was fastened through a hole in the scalp-flap in such a way as to receive all discharge, and a strip of gauze laid alongside and packed loosely into the cavity in the brain substance. During the operation a careful comparison was made between the pulse rate and the arterial pressure, as taken from the left radial artery.

Four hours after the operation the dressings were removed, and fomentations applied.

On June 9 the patient was decidedly better.

On June 11 he could move the left arm, and two or three days later the left leg. Cultures of the pus, taken at the time of operation in a sterilised test-tube, showed plentiful staphylococcus pyogenes aureus.

From now onwards steady improvement took place day by day, and the patient left the hospital for Swanley Convalescent Home on July 18. His condition was then as follows: intellect and memory good, left arm and leg practically as strong as ever, sight excellent, and no traces of optic neuritis. The only defects remaining as a result of the cerebral lesion consisted of some slight facial paresis and a peculiar lisp in

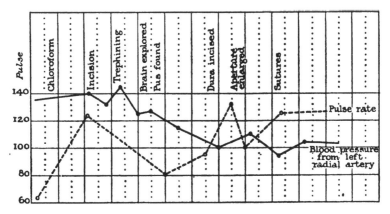

the formation of certain words, especially those beginning with or containing the letter S.

On October 19 the patient was shown at the meeting of the British Medical Association at St. Bartholomew's Hospital, and he then definitely stated that he was well in every way, and perfectly capable of carrying on his duties, which entailed the counting of money, the filing of accounts, and other matters which obviously required a clear intellect.

One of the many interesting features in this case lies in the fact that complete paralysis of leg, arm, and face resulted from an abscess occupying the anterior aspect of the opposite frontal pole. The late onset of paralytic symptoms and their early disappearance after operative measures had been adopted verified my earlier opinion that the motor area was only indirectly affected by backward pressure. The persistence of a slight degree of facial paralysis suggests, however, that the anterior part of the Rolandic area was either directly involved, or else that the vessels supplying or draining that region became thrombosed. It is also remarkable that the general intellectual faculties are absolutely unimpaired after such extensive destruction of cerebral matter.

At the present time the hole in the skull shows no sign of diminution in size, and pulsation is still easily detected over the entire area. I do not anticipate that any appreciable change will take place with regard to these conditions, as experience teaches us that the osteogenetic power of the bones of the vault of the skull is but feeble. The patient is, however, averse to further surgical treatment, though I have advised him to have the hole protected with a silver plate.

CASE 2.—*Old Fracture of Base of Skull—Trephination—*
Cerebral Abscess—Recovery.

A. W., aged 48, was admitted into Charity Ward on March 6, 1905. In November 1903 the patient fell from a trap and struck the left occipital region against the pavement. He was admitted, unconscious, into the Bolingbroke Hospital, and remained in that condition for four to five days. There was profuse discharge of blood and later of cerebro-spinal fluid from the left tympanic cavity.

He was allowed to get up on December 25, and began to walk about in January 1905.

From January till March he suffered from giddiness, unsteadiness of gait, and fits. The fits were not typical in any way, being sudden in onset, preceded by no aura, lasting three or four hours, and with no special movements of arm, leg, or face. They were, however, steadily increasing in frequency and severity.

On admittance, the condition was as follows: He was a healthy though loquacious man; deaf in the left ear; unsteady in gait, and especially so when turning sharply. Knee-jerks normal and no ankle clonus. Eyes normal. An examination of the head revealed no inequality of surface, and though two scars were seen over the occipital region, there was no tenderness on pressure. Both Mr. Cumberbatch and Dr. Drysdale kindly saw the case with me, but nothing very definite could be determined, and at no time did any fits afford a clue as to the exact site of the trouble.

For some time I periodically examined the head carefully, and on April 15 found a tender area immediately above the left auricle.

The whole question was put before the patient, and on

March 1 he was operated on. Special precautions were taken to guard from all possible sources of infection. A large sheet of Keith's rubber dressing was utilised, a hole being cut in the centre, and the rubber passed over the head so as to leave only a limited area exposed. A flap composed of the tissues of the scalp was turned down and the periosteum stripped away from an area of bone, 2 inches wide, above and in front of the external auditory meatus.

The exposed dura bulged and did not pulsate. A dural flap was turned down, and the protruding brain explored with a trocar and cannula. On withdrawing the cannula, cerebro-spinal fluid spurted out to a height of about 2 inches, rising and falling with the cardiac cycle. This ceased in about fifteen seconds, and nothing else was noticed or found beyond the fact that the brain appeared œdematous.

The hole in the skull had been previously enlarged to allow of the turning down of a dural flap, and was covered in with a silver plate.

These plates, as used by me, are made of annealed silver, sufficiently thick to be resistant to any ordinary force, and yet pliable enough to allow of the moulding to the necessary curve. On the night previous to the operation they are hammered out to the required curvature, and always made considerably larger than the estimated size of the hole which is to be covered in.

Previous to the operation the plate is boiled for half-an-hour, and then placed in warm boracic solution till required. At the completion of the operation the plate is clipped with a strong pair of scissors to the necessary size, and the edges pared with an ordinary file. Holes are also bored, three or four in number, in order to allow of the escape of any fluid—blood and cerebro-spinal fluid—which may collect on the deep aspect.

If the brain be explored, cerebro-spinal fluid necessarily escapes for a few days through these holes into the subapo-neurotic tissues of the scalp. This is, however, of but little importance, and the swelling soon subsides.

If, on the other hand, no holes are bored, there is some risk of cerebral compression as the result of the pressure of blood and fluid which may collect beneath the plate. The effused blood would also tend to increase the local formation of fibrous tissue, and by its adherence to dura and cortex predispose to the later supervention of Jacksonian epilepsy.

In this particular case the plate fitted accurately, and the pericranium, which had been previously stripped back from the exposed area of bone, was heaped up round the margin of the plate in order to fix it both temporarily and permanently in position.

The scalp was finally sewn up, and firm pressure applied.

On March 3 the wound was dressed, and all appeared healthy.

The patient's condition was generally good.

On March 4 the man had a fit, which lasted three minutes, and was accompanied by twitchings of the right arm and leg. He was completely unconscious. On coming round, he said he felt quite well, and afterwards slept heavily for many hours. The pulse was 80, the temperature 99°, and there was no headache, vomiting, or optic neuritis.

On March 5 another fit occurred, starting with a cry, lasting seven minutes, and affecting again the right arm and leg. A good night's rest followed.

On March 6 the patient became aphasic, though quite conscious and understanding all that was said. He was at once taken to the theatre, and the scalp flap loosened and turned down. Pus was found on the deep aspect of the plate, and exuding through the holes. Infection had obviously occurred from some source or other. The plate was removed, and the exposed area cleansed and drained.

On March 9 he was much better. No more fits. Temperature, subnormal; pulse, 60–80. No optic neuritis.

Up to March 29 the patient steadily improved. The aphasia diminished, and no symptoms arose which might give rise to anxiety.

On March 30, however, he became suddenly worse. He was apparently unable to understand anything said to him, and the right arm and leg were paralysed. The temperature was subnormal, the pulse 60–70, but there was no vomiting, and the discs were quite clear.

I again explored the wound and found the brain fairly healthy-looking to the naked eye. A trocar and cannula, however, soon exposed a large abscess cavity. This was evacuated, about ℥vj of pus escaping.

On the next day the patient was able to move the right arm, and two or three days later the right leg. From that time onwards he made a steady recovery, and left the hospital at the end of May strong and well, and in a better condition than when admitted.

As instancing his mental condition, it is interesting to note that he conversed fluently in French with a patient in a neighbouring bed, and periodically kept the ward amused by his powers of ventriloquism. The ultimate result was certainly most satisfactory, considering all the troubles he had passed through.

On October 25 a report was received stating that he had suffered from two fits in September, but that the general condition was otherwise fairly good.

Case 3.—*Simple Depressed Fracture of the Vault—*
Trephination—Elevation—Recovery.

T. P., aged 16, was admitted into Harley Ward on May 12 under the care of Mr. Waring, in whose unavoidable absence I was asked to see the case.

The lad had been struck directly above the right ear by the pole of a cart. There was some bleeding from the ear, and though questions were answered, the patient was heavy and stupid, and now and again lapsed into unconsciousness for a few minutes at a time. The pulse was 91, the temperature 97.4°, and the respiration 32. The pupils were equal and reacted to light, and there was no paralysis.

An examination of the head revealed a linear hæmatoma, starting in the region of the anterior aspect of the mastoid process and extending upwards to near the sagittal suture. This certainly indicated a fissured fracture of the vault, but no definite depression could be felt.

With regard to such cases as this I hold strong views, and maintain that when a force is applied directly to the skull of sufficient violence as to result in a fracture, a depressed fracture is the usual result. In other words, I hold the opinion that simple fissured fractures from direct violence are decidedly rare, except when extending upwards on to the vault from a primary basic fracture.

The fracture does not necessarily involve the external table to such a degree that the depression can be felt through the scalp tissues, but it must always be carefully borne in mind that a slight depression of the external table almost invariably indicates a much more extensive depression of the internal table. Such a depression may not give origin to any immediate symptoms, but the irritation of the dura mater, produced by the depressed area of bone, leads frequently to the formation of adhesions between the dura and the bone, and eventually to inflammatory thickening of the dura mater itself. The inevitable result of such lesions consists in the production of one or more of the numerous sequelæ of head injuries, such as melancholia, chronic fixed headache, epilepsy, insanity, &c. Exploration, therefore, is to be advocated in all such cases.

If the wound be compound in nature, this rule should be all the more stringently followed, whilst the conversion of a simple depressed fracture into a compound is a matter of comparatively trivial importance if the strictest precautions be taken with regard to cleanliness. The risk of local infection is not to be weighed in the balance against the leaving of a depressed fracture in the hope that nothing serious may eventually result.

Acting on these principles I decided to operate at once, and the case afforded an excellent example of the views but briefly expressed.

On turning down a suitable scalp flap a fracture was found which extended upwards towards the middle line in the position of the linear hæmatoma. The anterior parts of the parietal bone and of the squamous portion of the temporal bone were depressed to such a degree as to be overlapped by the posterior segment. A 1-inch trephine was placed at about the centre of the free border of the non-depressed area, and the disc of bone removed. The free edge was then nibbled away with Hoffman's forceps in an upward and downward direction till an elevator, resting on the sound· bone, was enabled to raise the depressed fragment to the normal level.

The wound was then sewn up.

The boy slept well during the night, and subsequently made an uninterrupted recovery. He remained in hospital for four weeks, and then went to Swanley. All head cases need as much rest as is possible under the special circumstances, and, acting on my suggestion, the employers of the boy sent him away to the seaside for one month.

On his return he was put to light work only, and is at the present date perfectly well in every respect.

CASE 4.—*Compound Depressed Fracture of the Frontal Bone— Fracture of the Anterior Fossa—Elevation of Depressed Area—Recovery.*

F. R., aged 6, was admitted into Henry Ward on July 15. He had fallen about 14 feet on to cobble-stone, and, though conscious, was drowsy on admittance. A scalp wound was situated over the left frontal region, but so small that the finger could not be insinuated to examine the surface of the bone. A probe, however, grated against a sharp ridge. The wound was, therefore, enlarged in a lateral direction, and the margins retracted upwards and downwards. A very extensive depressed fracture was then revealed, and a complete examination showed that part of the left half of the frontal bone, about 3 inches broad and 2 inches from above downwards, had been driven inwards and to the right, so as to be markedly overlapped by the free edge of the right frontal bone. A fissured fracture extended downwards through the left supra-orbital ridge and inwards across the anterior fossa in the region of the cribriform plate. The free margin of the right frontal bone was nibbled away in an upward and downward direction till an elevator was enabled to raise the depressed area to the normal level. During this part of the operation the state of the patient gave rise to some anxiety, but as soon as the bone was elevated the conditions at once improved.

The membranes were apparently uninjured, but it was deemed advisable to drain the wound for thirty-six hours.

The day after the operation palpebral and subconjunctival hæmorrhage developed in both eyes, appearing first and becoming most marked on the affected side.

The progress of the case was continuous and recovery perfect.

At the present date, October 25, the boy is in an excellent state of health, and the scar, coinciding with the frontal furrows, barely visible.

INTRA-MEDULLARY TERATOMA OF THE SPINAL CORD.

BY

J. GRAHAM FORBES, M.D.

The following case of a teratomatous tumour, involving the cervical region of the spinal cord is of particular interest on account of its great rarity and peculiar histological characters.

William S., aged 5 years and 6 months, was admitted on December 10, 1903, to the Hospital for Sick Children, Great Ormond Street, suffering from paralysis of both arms and legs, due, as was supposed, to cervical caries.

He was under the care of Mr. Collier, to whom I am indebted for kind permission to publish the notes.

The history of the case was as follows:—

At the age of 16 months the boy fell down a flight of stairs, but at the time no ill effects were noticeable. Although a history of injury is not uncommon in cases of tumour of the spinal cord, the accident in this instance had probably little bearing on subsequent events.

He was said to have been always "tottery on his legs," and to have been troubled with looseness of the bowels, and frequent and copious micturition. At the age of three—*i.e.* about June 1901—his head and shoulders were noticed to "droop." After this he was taken to St. Thomas' Hospital, where he attended the out-patient department for some time.

In September 1903 he was brought to the Hospital for Sick Children, and considered by Mr. Collier to be a case of spinal caries on account of the distribution of pain along the course of the posterior cervical nerves and the marked rigidity of the neck. He was provided with a Phelps' spinal box, and subsequently sent to the Convalescent Home for nine weeks.

Family History.—He was the fourth of six children; the

second child died at the age of one week, the third at six months of diarrhœa and vomiting, and the sixth was still-born.

Both parents healthy.

On admission to hospital on December 10, 1903, he is described as a fairly well nourished, poorly developed boy, lying very quietly in bed.

Face.—No paralysis of facial muscles.

Pupils dilated and react naturally.

Tongue slightly furred. No dysphagia. The head is capable of some nodding and rotatory movements, which are painful.

There is rigidity of the lower cervical vertebræ and slight prominence of the 3rd to 7th cervical spines.

Pain is excited by movement and percussion of the cervical spines. There is slight lateral curvature in the dorsal region.

Limbs. Arms. Left.—Almost complete paralysis. He is unable to grasp objects with the hand. The forearm cannot be flexed, and is only capable of slight extension.

The deltoid muscle is partially paralysed.

Right.—Less affected than the left.

There is some power in the hand, and the forearm is capable of slight flexion and extension. The triceps, biceps, and deltoid muscles are partially paralysed.

Legs. Left.—The power of contraction in the quadriceps extensor is diminished, still more so in the hamstring muscles. There is but little power in the calf and anterior tibial muscles.

Right.—Muscles of thigh and leg are even weaker than on the left side.

All deep reflexes are abolished.

Sensation is unimpaired.

There is incontinence of fæces and retention of urine. A catheter is passed twice daily. There is some priapism.

On December 13, with the object of relieving pressure of tuberculous material on the cord, laminectomy was performed by Mr. Collier. The laminæ of the 2nd to 6th cervical vertebræ were removed and the meninges exposed. There was some congestion of the veins of the dura mater, but even after free removal of the laminæ no pulsation of the cord could be noted. At the time no further operation was performed.

On December 20 the patient was doing well.

Urine is drawn off regularly—no improvement in bladder or rectal reflexes. Priapism less marked; the cystitis which had developed shows slight improvement, and the urine is less offensive.

On January 14, 1904, the wound was reopened and a vertical incision was made through the exposed dura mater. Immediately a growth, about the size of a haricot bean, protruded through the incision, apparently growing from the spinal cord and covered by the pia-arachnoid membranes. The bulging portion of the tumour was removed, together with the adherent meninges, and the wound was then closed; for it was realised that as the growth was of intramedullary origin nothing further could be done.

January 16.—Spontaneous micturition occurs at regular intervals.

January 28.—There is now complete paralysis of both arms and legs; knee-jerks and plantar reflexes absent.

The left side of the thorax moves better than the right. Diaphragmatic movements are unaffected.

No facial paralysis. Sensation normal.

Rectum and bladder are emptied spontaneously at intervals.

Sweating is not quite so marked.

He is getting thinner, but is in no pain.

March 17.—He is massaged daily, and is improving.

Pain has been much relieved since operation.

In April 1904 he was discharged.

On August 15, 1904, he was readmitted to hospital. The note says :—

The patient has wasted a good deal in the last 4 months, but has regained some power in the arms. The movements in both arms are good—weaker on the left side than the right. The legs are kept straight by posterior poroplastic splints, but become flexed when the splints are removed.

Patellar reflexes are well marked.

There is no loss of sensation. The bladder and bowels are imperfectly controlled.

Since his discharge from hospital in April a bed-sore has developed on the back.

The patient was discharged on October 25, 1904, *in statu quo.*

After this date he remained at home without showing any improvement. His condition became gradually worse, and death occurred on August 2, 1905, as the immediate result of a terminal bronchitis.

It is unfortunate that no post-mortem examination was made to reveal the extent of the growth and its effect on the spinal cord.

Pathological Report on the Portion of Tumour Removed on January 14.

Measurements.—Length, ½ inch; breadth, ⅓ inch; thickness, ⅓ inch.

On its posterior aspect the tumour is covered by a layer of dense fibrous tissue, probably thickened and adherent meninges. On the reverse side are seen many small strands of well-defined striated muscle fibre, portions of which are embryonic and appear as long fusiform cells with several nuclei arranged in column towards the tapering end of the cell. These structures form the most striking and characteristic feature of the growth. The strands of muscle fibres and cells are separated by broad bands of wavy fibrous tissue and small collections of fat cells. The centre of the tumour is occupied by poorly staining connective tissue, interspersed with inflammatory cells, and a large number of oval and round cells, with fibrillary network, some of which are possibly neuroglia. In the anterior part of the growth is seen a cluster of large multinucleated giant cells resembling the myeloplaxes or osteoclasts of bone marrow, and apparently indicating the existence of young osseous tissue.

The whole tumour is very richly supplied with well-formed blood-vessels, many of which are grouped together and surrounded by cellular connective tissue. There are also large areas of recent hæmorrhage which were probably caused at the time of operation.

Many of the cells lie apparently free in the connective tissue; they stain poorly, showing an oval nucleus with a hyaline margin of protoplasm and shadowy ill-defined processes, and resemble degenerated nerve cells. In addition a few corpora amylacea can be distinguished.

The presence of fully-developed muscle fibre, together with embryonic muscle cells and osteoclasts, clearly shows that the growth is a teratoma. On account of its extreme vascularity it may be defined as a myo-angioma.

Among the many varieties of tumour of the spinal cord hitherto described I have found mention of only one case in which the growth contained striated muscle fibre, and was therefore to be classified as of congenital origin,

PLATE IV.

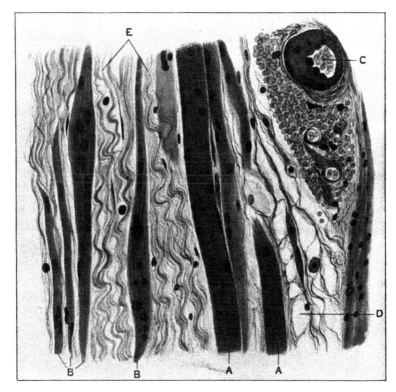

FIG. 1.—Intra-medullary Teratoma of Spinal Cord (× 800 diam.).

    A. Striated muscle fibre.
    B. Embryonic striated muscle fibre.
    C. Blood vessel.
    D. Fat cell spaces.
    E. Wavy fibrous tissue.

All forms of congenital tumour of the spinal cord are remarkably rare. They include myolipoma, and pure lipoma.

Gowers records four cases of lipoma, all of which were derived from the extradural adipose tissue. The age of these cases ranged from 10 months to 4 years.

He has published the only case I have found, in which the tumour contained striated muscle fibre. The patient, an adult, also suffered from locomotor ataxia, not associated with or due to the tumour.

The growth was a myolipoma attached laterally to the conus medullaris. It sprang from the pia mater, enclosing half of the spinal cord from anterior to posterior fissure. Many nerve roots of the cauda equina were embedded in it. The greater portion was composed of round and oval fat cells, in places separated by tracts of fibrous tissue, some of which, together with the capsule of the tumour, were continuous with the fibrous pia matral layer and separated the tumour from the lateral columns of the cord. Within the growth occurred many striated muscle fibres in groups or isolated strands. Their presence suggested the strong probability of congenital origin.

Congenital lipomata are also described in association with spina bifida.

Pick (Prague) describes a case of senile dementia in which *post mortem* there was found marked thickening of the membranes along the dorsal surface of the cord, especially in the lumbar region. On transverse section this thickening was found to be due to hypertrophy of the middle coats of the meningeal arteries, and to the formation of bundles of smooth muscle fibre connected by strands with the hypertrophied muscle of the arterial walls.

The first classified account of tumours of the spinal cord is contained in a paper by Gowers and Horsley read before the Medico-Chirurgical Society in 1888.

Their list includes most of the previously recorded cases, numbering fifty-eight, arranged as follows:—

I. *Extradural*, 20.

Sarcoma (spindle and round celled)	5 cases
Lipoma	4 „
Tuberculous	4 „
Echinococcus	3 „
Myxoma	1 case
Fibro-chondro-lipoma	1 „
Fibro-sarcoma	1 „
Carcinoma	1 „

Enchondroma and teratoma are mentioned, and reference made to angioma and diffuse osteomata.

II. *Intradural*, 38.

Myxoma	12 cases
Sarcoma (spindle and round celled) .	7 „
Fibroma	7 „
Psammoma	4 „
Tuberculous	4 „
Syphilitic	2 „
Parasitic	2 „

Reference is also made to fibro-sarcoma and angio-sarcoma, and to these must be added multiple neuroma, congenital lipoma, and myo-lipoma.

III. *Intramedullary* tumours include, in order of frequency, glioma, glio-sarcoma, and pure sarcoma; also angio-sarcoma, tubercle, and cysticercus.

Further particulars as to age and duration of symptoms are given in tabulated form.

Extradural.

	Average Duration of Case.	Average Age.
1. Lipoma . . .	15 months	10 months–4 years
2. Sarcoma . . .	9 „	18 years
3. Echinococcus . .	6 „	34 „
4. Tubercle . . .	18 „	39 „
5. Carcinoma . . .	18 „	48 „
6. Myxoma . . .	4 years	53

Intradural.

1. Myxoma . .	4 years and 3 months	43 years (19–60)
2. Fibroma . .	3 years and 6 months	44 „
3. Sarcoma . .	2 years	41 „
4. Psammoma .	3 years and 3 months	51 „
5. Tubercle . .	8 months	18 „

The sex is mentioned in fifty-four cases in the proportion of thirty female to twenty male.

Origin of the growths :—

Extradural lipomata spring from the extradural adipose tissue, sarcomata from the periosteum of the spinal column or the outer surface of the dura mater.

Intradural tumours are derived from the inner surface of the dura mater, the ligamentum denticulatum, the arachnoid, or the outer surface of the pia mater.

Intramedullary tumours (gliomata) arise from the neuroglia by proliferation of germinal tissue which has remained in an embryonic state.

The teratomata recorded are due to included portions of mesoblastic and occasionally epiblastic tissue.

With reference to the various causes assigned by patients,

Gowers has pointed out the interesting fact that a history of exposure to cold or injury is common. In sixteen out of twenty-one cases the onset of the first symptoms of tumour was attributed to, or dated from, the influence of one or the other factor, especially in younger patients.

Since the publication of Gowers' and Horsley's list of cases, Lloyd has collected fifty others, including syphilitic and tuber-culous tumours, carcinoma, sarcoma, glioma, and myxoma. Of these 14 per cent. were under the age of 20, four being under 10.

Starr at a later date, 1895, has added to this number, bring-ing up the total of recorded cases to 123.

Herter, in contrasting the age incidence of sarcomatous and tuberculous tumours of the spinal cord, states that in twenty-six cases of sarcoma the majority occurred between the ages of 20 and 50 years, and only two before the age of 20.

And, as a rule, sarcoma of the brain and spinal cord occurs at a later period in life than sarcoma elsewhere.

Fifteen out of twenty-four cases of tuberculous tumour are recorded by Herter between the ages of 15 and 35, and five before the fifth year.

Endotheliomata occur far less commonly in the spinal cord than in the brain. Michell Clarke in 1895, describing a case of endothelioma of the dura mater in the lower cervical region of the cord, alludes to this rarity, and mentions that only five similar cases had been previously published.

Twenty-two cases of parasitic tumours of the spinal cord have been recorded by Maguire, twenty of which were due to echinococcus and two to cysticercus.

According to Starr, malignant tumours of the spinal cord are ten times more common than the benign, and in ratio to tumours of the brain they occur as 1 to 13.

He states that Schlesinger has found 147 cases in 35,000 autopsies, and out of 6540 tumours 151 were situated in the spinal cord and meninges.

His description of the various forms of growth may be briefly summarised in order of frequency.

Sarcoma extends rapidly, invading membranes and posterior surface of cord; more often compressing than destroying it; often multiple; may start from a nerve root, invading both meninges and cord.

Tubercle is found more often within the cord than mem-branes, where it occurs as a solitary tumour; may be found throughout the cord; within the cord as a caseous mass usually beginning in the gray matter.

Echinococcus and cysticercus cysts: rapid growth; cause compression of cord; rarely invade it.

Fibroma usually springs from the inner surface of the dura; grows slowly; lies on and compresses cord; encapsuled and easy to remove.

Gumma occurs in meninges, infiltrating them and cord; growth rapid; diffuse; not encapsuled.

Glioma infiltrates cord, and may involve its whole length; does not involve meninges; growth very rapid and vascular; removal impossible; often associated with sarcoma. Gliosarcoma may involve membranes and cord.

Psammoma occurs in the arachnoid or dura mater lying on the cord; hard; chalky; oval in shape; slow growth; easy to remove.

Myxoma: more often intradural than extradural; never infiltrates cord; single; vascular; may be cystic; slow growth.

Lipoma, often multiple; intradural rather than extradural; soft and encapsuled; slow growth.

Endothelioma: small; often multiple; always meningeal.

Melanosarcoma: may occur secondarily.

Other forms of tumour he describes as pathological curiosities.

Intramedullary tumours occur most commonly in the cervical or lumbar enlargement, extramedullary or meningeal in the dorsal segments, usually on the posterior or lateral surfaces of the cord.

Collins quotes 70 cases, in which, when stated, the sex incidence was 37 male to 25 female; the age limits were 3 years to 65 years, and the average age 40 years. Where the situation was mentioned, 17 occurred in the cervical, 32 in the dorsal, and 8 in the lumbar regions.

His list includes 28 cases of sarcoma, 9 of glioma, 6 of endothelioma, 3 of psammoma, and 3 of fibroma.

Thirty of the 70 cases were operated on, including 12 of sarcoma, 6 of fibroma, 3 of endothelioma, and 1 of myxolipoma. The operation proved successful in 12, partly successful in 8, and failed in 10 cases.

I have verified the references to 26 cases, irrespective of those in Collins' list. The sex incidence was as 15 male to 11 female. 8 occurred in the cervical, 14 in the dorsal, and 4 in the lumbar regions of the cord. They include 8 cases of sarcoma, 3 of glioma, 3 of psammoma, 3 of myxofibroma, 2 of fibroma, 2 of endothelioma, 2 of gumma, 2 of lipoma, and 1 of myolipoma. The ages ranged from 21 to 65 years, and the average was 39 years.

PLATE V.

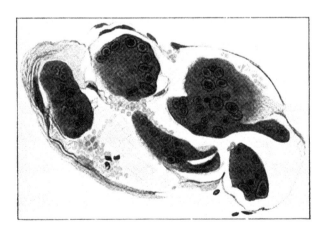

FIG. 2.—Intra-medullary Teratoma of Spinal Cord (× 600 diam.).

A. Corpora amylacea.
B. Blood vessels.
C. Neuroglia cells.
D. Nerve cells.

FIG. 3.—Intra-medullary Teratoma of Spinal Cord, showing multinucleated giant cells resembling osteoclasts of bone marrow
(× 600 diam).

Schlesinger's List of 400 *Cases of Tumour of the Spinal Cord is tabulated as follows, showing order of frequency and situation.*

Variety.	Intradural.			Extradural.				
	Medullary.	Meningeal.	Both.	Meningeal.	Non-Meningeal.	Single.	Multiple.	Total.
Sarcoma	14	56	9	17	11	80	27	107
Tubercle	62	...	...	2	...	55	9	64
Echinococcus	...	5	...	39	...	8	36	44
Fibroma	...	26	2	5	...	15	18	33
Gumma	7	4	15	2	...	19	9	28
Glioma	20	...	...	...	...	20	...	20
Psammoma	...	18	...	...	...	18	...	18
Myxoma	...	7	...	4	...	11	...	11
Lipoma	2	8	...	...	1	8	3	11
Cysticercus	2	5	...	...	1	4	4	8
Glio-sarcoma	...	3	4	...	...	...	7	7
Endothelioma	...	5	...	1	...	4	2	6
Melano-sarcoma . . .	1	...	3	...	...	1	3	4
Neuroma	4	...	...	...	...	3	1	4
Lymphangioma . . .	...	1	...	1	...	1	1	2
Cysts	...	1	...	1	...	1	1	2
Cholesteatoma	1	...	...	...	...	1	...	1
Uncertain	13	12	2	3	...	24	6	30
	126	151	35	75	13	273	127	400

312   88

[BIBLIOGRAPHY OF CASES.

Bibliography of Cases of Tumour of the Spinal Cord.

Sex.	Age.	Duration.	Nature of Growth.	Situation.	Reference.
M.	Adult	...	Myomatous	Throughout the dura mater	Pisk, A., Myomatöse Wucherungen, Prag. Med. Wochenschr., 1895, p. 453.
M. F. 4 cases	Adult 54 10 months to 4 years	12 years 15 months	Myolipoma, intradural Lipoma Lipoma, extradural	Cauda-equina Mid-dorsal	Gowers, Path. Soc. Trans., xxvii. p. 19. Turner, Path. Soc. Trans., xxxix. p. 25. Gowers, Med. Chir. Trans., 1888, p. 377.
1 case	...	...	Fibro-chondro-lipoma, extradural Lipoma	...	Gowers, Med. Chir. Trans., 1888, p. 377.
F.	50	...	Lumbar	Lumbar	Starr, Amer. Journ. Med. Soc., 1895, p. 613.
M.	43	6 months	Myxochondroma	Mid-dorsal extradural	Mader, Ber. d. k. k. Krankenanst; Rudolf, Stiftung in Wien, 1880, p. 301.
12 cases	Average age, 43 ... 45	4¼ years ... 2-3 years	Myxoma, intradural Myxoma Myxolipoma*	Mid-dorsal Mid-dorsal intradural	Gowers, Med. Chir. Trans., ibid. Turner, Clin. Journal, 1904. Oppenheim, Berliner klinische Wochenschrift, 1902, No. 2.
M.	28	...	Myxofibroma	Lower dorsal	Ferrier and Cheyne, Lancet, 1894, i. p. 739.
M.	...	...	Myxofibroma, extradural	Upper dorsal	Gowers and Horsley, Med. Chir. Trans., 1888, p. 377.
F.	38	14 months	Myxofibroma	Lower dorsal	Jackson Clarke, Path. Soc. Trans., xliii. p. 16.
7 cases F.	Average age, 44 40	3½ years 2 years	Fibroma Fibrocystic	Intradural Upper dorsal intradural	Gowers, Med. Chir. Trans., 1888, p. 377. Bennett, Path. Soc. Trans., vii. p. 41.
M.	24	6 years	Fibrosarcoma	Lower dorsal intradural	Ward, Brit. Med. Journ., Oct. 28, 1905, p. 1083.

* Quoted erroneously by Collins (Med. Rec., N. York, p. 882, vol. lxii.), as Myolipoma.

Sex	Age	Duration	Tumour	Position	Reference
F.	19	1 year	Spindle-celled sarcoma	Mid-cervical extradural	Collins, Med. Rec., N. York, vol. xlii. p. 882, 1902.
M., 1 case	25	9 months	Fibrosarcoma	Cervical intradural	Leddiard, Path. Soc. Trans., xxxiii. p.25. *ibid.*
M.	...	...	Fibrosarcoma	Extradural	Gowers, Med. Chir. Trans., *ibid.*
	36	1 year	Spindle-celled sarcoma	Intradural	Collins, Journ. Med. Dis., New York, xxiv. p. 567.
...	...	8 months	Spindle-celled sarcoma	Lumbar	Oladek, New York Med. Journ., 1897, p. 205.
M.	29	16 months	Spindle-celled sarcoma	Lower cervical and upper dorsal intradural	Ross, Med. Record, New York, xliv. p. 193.
M.	28	3 years	Endothelioma	Lower cervical extradural	Mitchell Clarke, Brain, 1895, p. 256.
5 cases	Adults	9 months to 2 years	Endothelioma	Cervical intradural	Mitchell Clarke, Brain, 1895, p. 256.
F.	43	9 months	Fibro-cellular ? endothelioma		Wilks, Path. Soc. Trans., vii. p. 37.
F.	48	2 years	Psammoma	Lower cervical intradural	J. Hutchinson, junr., Path. Soc. Trans., xxxiii. p. 23.
F.	46	12 months	Psammoma	Lower dorsal intradural	Cayley, Path. Soc. Trans., xvi. p. 21.
F.	65	...	Psammoma	Lower dorsal intradural	Bailey, New York Journ. Nerv. and Ment. Dis., xxiii. p. 171.
4 cases	Average age, 51	3 years	Psammoma	Intradural	Gowers, Med. Chir. Trans., *ibid.*
5 cases	Average age, 18	9 months	Sarcoma	Extradural	Gowers, Med. Chir. Trans., *ibid.*
7 cases	Average age, 41	2 years	Sarcoma	Intradural	Ransom and Anderson, B. M. J. T., 1894, p. 395.
F.	50	6 months	Round-celled sarcoma	Lower dorsal extradural	
M.	42	...	Sarcoma	Dorsal	Starr, Am. Journ. Med. Sc., 1895 p. 613.
M.	40	2–3 years	Sarcoma	Mid-dorsal intradural	Collins, Med. Rec., N. York, p. 882, vol. xlii.
F.	23	1 month	Sarcoma	Lower dorsal intradural	*Ibid.*
M.	12 cases, adults		Sarcoma }		Herter, Boston M. and S. Journ., 1893, p. 128.
P.	14 "Young"	Some months	Carcinoma	Cervical extradural	Ogle, Path. Soc. Trans., vii. p. 40.
M.	33	3 months	Glioma	Intramedullary	Fraenkel, Deutsche Zeitung, May 1898.
M.	21	3 years	Neuro-epithelioma	Dorsal intramedullary	Fraenkel, Deutsche Zeitung, May 1898.

Bibliography of Cases of Tumour of the Spinal Cord (continued).

Sex.	Age.	Duration.	Nature of Growth.	Situation.	Reference.
F.	43	15 years	Glioma	Cervical intra-medullary	Hebb, Path. Soc. Trans., xlviii p. 14.
M.	55	1½ year	Gliosarcoma	Lumbar enlargement, intramedullary	Fletcher, Path. Soc. Trans., xlix. p. 6.
F.	29	...	Gumma	Cervical intradural	Bailey, Journ. Nerv. Ment. Dis., New York, Ment. Dis., xxiii. p. 171.
M.	40	...	Gumma	Cervical	Starr, Am. Journ. Med. Sc., 1895, p. 613.
		...	Tubercle	...	Harter, Boston M. and S. Journ., 1893. p. 128.
24 cases	In 15, age 15-35 In 5, age under 5				
4 cases	Average age, 39	1½ year	Tubercle	Extradural	Gowers, Med. Chir. Trans., ibid.
4 cases	Average age, 18	8 months	Tubercle	Intradural	Gowers, Med. Chir. Trans., ibid.
50 cases	{14% under 20} {63% over 20}	...	Gumma, tubercle, Carcinoma, sarcoma, Glioma and myxoma.	...	Loyd, Amer. Text-Book Dis. Child., Philadelphia, 1898, p. 801.
22 cases	...	...	(20) Echinococcus (2) Cysticercus	...	Maguire, Brain, 1888, p. 451.
3 cases	Average age, 34	6 months	Cysticercus Echinococcus	Extradural	Gowers, Med. Chir. Trans., ibid.
...	10	...	Echinococcus	Mid-dorsal	A. Turner, Clin. Journ., 1904, p. 122.
...	...	...	Echinococcus	...	Wood, Inter-Colon. Med. Journ. Australia, Melb., 1896, i. p. 480.

OTHER REFERENCES.

1. Organic Nervous Diseases (M. A. Starr), 1903, p. 390.
2. Beitrage zur Kenntnis der Rückenmarks und Wirbeltumoren. Schlesinger : Jena, 1898.

BIBLIOGRAPHIES.

1. Clifford Allbutt's System of Medicine, vol. vi. p. 920. (Risian Russell.)
2. Zeigler's Special Pathological Anatomy (MacAlister), p. 372.

TWO CASES OF DIPHTHERITIC INFECTION OF OPERATION WOUNDS.

BY

J. BURFIELD, M.B., F.R.C.S.

The following cases were admitted under Mr. Lockwood's care while I was his house-surgeon.

I am indebted to Mr. Lockwood for his permission to publish them.

They are important, I think, because so much depends on the prompt recognition of the nature of such cases.

CASE I.—*Diphtheritic Infection following Cellulitis of the Scalp.*

Alfred H., a well-developed but somewhat anæmic child of 14 months, was brought up to the surgery on Dec. 28, 1904.

When seen in the surgery he was found to be suffering from an inflammatory swelling of the scalp, over the right parietal and temporal bones. As the child's condition was critical (pulse, 160; respiration, 50; temperature, 103°) he was at once admitted to Coborn Ward.

The patient's condition on admission was as follows:—

The child was lying on his left side, with his head somewhat retracted; his breathing was shallow and rapid—60 to the minute. On the right side of his head there was a swelling in the temporal and parietal regions; this was hot and fluctuated, and presented all the signs of acute suppuration. The skin over it was slightly red, but there was no ulceration or open wound, and I suspected the pus to be beneath the aponeurosis of the occipito-frontalis. The tongue was coated with a thick white fur; there was no stomatitis. There was no redness or ulceration of the fauces or soft palate.

Lungs.—The child had bronchitis, moist and dry râles being heard over both lungs back and front.

There was no cardiac lesion discovered.

Past History.—The mother said the child had only been ailing for a week; she had noticed the swelling of the scalp for 3–4 days.

The child's bronchitis and general condition were so bad that incisions into the scalp were made without any general anæsthetic; and pus was found between the aponeurosis and the periosteum. Four incisions were made, and about an ounce of pus let out. The child was very collapsed after the operation. He was given a hot mustard bath; brandy by mouth, and inj. strychninæ hyp. ℳi. These stimulants had a good effect, and the child's condition at once improved.

By January 1 his temperature was 98°, pulse 120, respiration 40; the discharge from his scalp was much less, and the incisions looked clean and were covered with healthy granulations. We all thought that the child had turned the corner, and was on the high-road to recovery.

During the next week the child did not make any progress; the discharge was rather more, and another incision was made just above the pinna, and a small pocket of pus found.

January 8.—The edges of the incisions were becoming ulcerated; in two or three places bare bone can be seen, but nothing like a diphtheritic membrane was ever noticed.

On January 12 Mr. Lockwood saw the child. He ordered a culture to be made from the discharge. The growth was a mixture of diphtheria bacilli and staphylococci.

3000 units of diphtheria antitoxin were at once injected, followed by an equal quantity in 12 hours' time. After the antitoxin the child's condition immediately began to improve again, and the discharge from the scalp was less.

The patient was transferred to Radcliffe.

January 17.—As diphtheria bacilli were still grown from the wound, another injection of antitoxin was given. None were ever found in cultivations taken from the child's throat.

There was now a piece of bare bone as large as half-a-crown near the parietal eminence; the rest of the scalp was healing slowly. There was a slight cloud of albumin in the urine.

February 11.—The child had slight external strabismus of right eye. His general condition had much improved, however; his head was healing, and the exposed bone was nearly covered by granulations. Diphtheria bacilli were still grown from a culture taken from the child's scalp. This was well swabbed with a solution of biniodide of mercury, 1 in 500.

February 22.—Since the last note the child had not been
so well. There was marked ptosis as well as external strabismus
of the right eye. The knee-jerks were absent, and there was
partial paralysis of both lower extremities.

Dr. Ormerod saw the patient and ordered liq. strych. ℳi.
twice daily.

The scalp wound was healing; all the bone was now covered
with granulation tissue. A culture from the scalp still grew
diphtheria bacilli.

March 1.—The child was much better. The paralysis of the
legs had quite disappeared; the external squint was now the only
sign of paralysis.

The further history of the case is unimportant; the paralysis
completely disappeared, although the scalp wound healed very
slowly and grew diphtheria bacilli up to April 18.

The child was discharged on May 23. The scalp wound
was then soundly healed, and the child perfectly well in other
respects.

CASE II.—*Diphtheritic Infection following Cellulitis
of the Abdominal Wall.*

Nellie P., aged 10 months, was brought up to the surgery by
her mother on August 16, 1905.

She then had an inflammatory swelling situated in the
hypogastric region, and extending down to the upper part of
the right labium mageus. There was no ulceration of the skin.
The child's general condition was good. In the surgery a
small incision was made into the swelling, and though the
subcutaneous tissues were very œdematous, no pus was found.

August 19.—The swelling had spread both up on to the
abdominal wall and down towards the perineum. The child was
admitted to Coborn.

On Admission.—The child's temperature was 100.8°;
pulse, 148.

She was perfectly quiet and took no notice of her surround-
ings, giving one the impression that she was suffering from
some kind of toxæmia. There was no inflammation of the
fauces or soft palate, and no dyspnœa.

There was a hard brawny swelling, situated in the hypogastric
region and labia magora; and some superficial ulceration in the
fold of the groin on the right side.

August 20.—Mr. Harmer saw the case and advised several
incisions being made into the indurated area, immediately.

This was done under an anæsthetic, and a small amount of

pus was let out. The vagina was examined, but was not ulcerated, and there was no discharge.

After the operation we thought it just possible that it was diphtheritic infection. A culture was made, and diphtheritic antitoxin was injected, but the child never recovered from the effects of the operation, dying the same night at 1 A.M.

The next day we found that the diphtheria bacillus predominated in the growth from the discharge.

The post-mortem examination showed that the child had no signs of diphtheria in the throat or larynx, and that there was no ulceration of the vagina. The heart's blood was sterile.

I think it is clear that both these cases were in the first instance infected with staphylococcus, which caused the initial cellulitis; and that when this was opened the tissues exposed by the incisions were then infected by the Klebs-Loeffler bacillus.

There is no evidence to prove that the diphtheria bacillus can invade sound skin, and in neither case was there any ulceration or abrasion of the skin over the lesions.

Wound diphtheria is rare, especially when it occurs in a patient free from any other sign of the disease.

I can find no cases of a similar nature in the hospital records during the last ten years.

These two cases are records of failure, the reason being that a correct diagnosis was not made till too late. One of the patients lost her life, and the other child only recovered after a tedious and critical illness, lasting nearly six months. Had a bacteriological examination been made earlier, in all probability both of them would have ended satisfactorily.

Similar mistakes can only be guarded against by a systematic bacteriological examination of every case of "cellulitis," which is not really a disease, but merely a symptom produced by whatever infection there may be present.

PROCEEDINGS

OF

THE ABERNETHIAN SOCIETY

FOR THE SESSION 1904-1905.

OFFICERS.

Presidents . . Mr. R. B. ETHERINGTON SMITH and Mr. T. J. FAULDER.
Vice-Presidents . Mr. J. RIGDEN TRIST and Mr. ERNEST H. SHAW.
Secretaries . . Mr. W. B. GRANDAGE and Mr. W. G. BALL.
Extra Committeemen Mr. L. B. CANE and Mr. J. R. C. TURTON.

October 6, 1904.

The Sessional Address was delivered by Mr. Langton on
Modern Aids to Diagnosis.' Mr. T. J. Faulder was in the
chair.

At the conclusion Mr. Harmer proposed, and Mr. Waterfield
seconded, a vote of thanks to Mr. Langton for his paper, both
expressing regret at Mr. Langton's retirement from the
Hospital staff.

October 13.

An ordinary meeting of the Society was held, Mr. R. B.
Etherington Smith in the chair.

Mr. F. C. Shrubsall read a paper on ' Physical Deterioration'
(illustrated by lantern slides).

October 20.

A clinical evening, Mr. Faulder in the chair.

Mr. Adams showed a case in which the diagnosis lay between
tubercle and leprosy.

Mr. H. H. Clarke showed a case of lympadenoma.

Mr. Shaw showed a case of Charcot's disease of the hip.

The cases aroused a considerable amount of discussion.

October 27.

Dr. C. M. H. Howell read a paper entitled 'Some Notes on Uræmia.'

Mr. R. B. Etherington Smith was in the chair.

November 3.

At the fifth meeting of the Society Dr. W. J. Gow read a paper on 'Labour complicated by Pelvic Tumour.'

Mr. E. H. Shaw (Vice-Pres.) took the chair.

November 10.

Ordinary meeting, Mr. R. B. Etherington Smith in the chair.

A paper was read by Dr. W. P. S. Branson on 'The Clinical Significance of Vomiting in Childhood.'

November 17.

Clinical evening, Mr. T. R. Trist in the chair.

Dr. Ormerod showed five cases illustrative of tabes dorsalis.

Mr. Noon showed three cases, and Mr. Adams two.

November 24.

An ordinary meeting, Mr. Shaw in the chair.

Dr. Tooth delivered an address on 'Exact Localisations of Lesions of the Spinal Cord.'

The address was profusely illustrated by means of diagrams.

December 1.

An ordinary meeting, Mr. T. J. Faulder in the chair.

A paper was read by Dr. J. Valérie on 'Private Practice.'

December 8.

An ordinary meeting, Mr. Faulder in the chair.

Dr. T. J. Horder read a paper on 'The Bacteriology of the Blood—Its Value in Diagnosis and Treatment.'

The paper was illustrated by lantern slides and apparatus used in the study of the blood.

January 13, 1905.

The Mid-sessional Address was delivered by Mr. D'Arcy Power. The subject of the address was 'London in the Early Days of the Hospital.'
Mr. Faulder took the chair.
At the conclusion, a vote of thanks was moved by Dr. Claye Shaw and seconded by Mr. Rawling.

January 19.

Ordinary meeting, Mr. R. B. Etherington Smith in the chair.
Mr. E. M. Niall read a paper entitled 'Some Notes on the Feeding of Infants.'

January 26.

Ordinary meeting, Mr. Faulder in the chair.
Dr. J. A. Willett read a paper on 'The Effects of Heart Disease on Labour.'

February 2.

Ordinary meeting, Mr. R. B. Etherington Smith in the chair.
Dr. J. W. W. Stephens read a paper on 'The Transmission of Parasitic Diseases by Insects.'

February 9.

Clinical evening, Mr. Faulder in the chair.
Mr. Neligan showed cases of enlarged spleen, and of pseudo-hypertrophic muscular paralysis.
Mr. Hadfield showed a case of lymphadenoma.
Mr. Favell showed a case of gout.
A discussion on the cases exhibited afterwards took place.

February 16.

Ordinary meeting, held in the Medical Theatre.
Mr. Faulder took the chair.
Sir William Collins delivered an address on 'Physic and Metaphysic.'
A vote of thanks was proposed by Mr. Faulder and seconded by Mr. H. B. Atkinson.

February 23.

Ordinary meeting, Mr. Etherington Smith in the chair.

Mr. E. Laming Evans read a paper on 'Prevention and Correction of Deformities resulting from Paralyses.'

March 2.

Clinical evening, Mr. Faulder in the chair.

Mr. Elmslie showed a case of achondroplasia.

Dr. C. M. H. Howell showed three cases.

Mr. Shaw showed a case of old infantile paralysis.

Mr. Noon exhibited a case of secondary cataract.

The evening closed with a discussion.

March 9.

Ordinary meeting, Mr. Trist in the chair.

Mr. Faulder read a paper entitled 'Notes on some Diseases of the Rectum.'

March 16.

The Annual General Meeting was held, Mr. Faulder in the .chair.

The Annual Report of the Society was read by the Secretary, and the results of the election of officers for the coming session were declared.

DESCRIPTIVE LIST

OF

SPECIMENS REVISED AND ADDED
TO THE MUSEUM

DURING THE YEAR 1905.

SPECIMENS ADDED TO THE MUSEUM

During the Year ending September 30, 1905

DESCRIBED BY

F. W. ANDREWES, M.D.; W. P. S. BRANSON, M.D,

AND THE LATE EUSTACE TALBOT, M.B.

INTRODUCTORY REMARKS.

THE Museum has sustained a great loss by the untimely death of Dr. Eustace Talbot in the first year of his Junior Curatorship. Partly from this cause, and other changes in the *personnel* of the Museum Staff, the number of specimens added this year is somewhat smaller than it has usually been.

The series to which the most numerous additions have been made is that of Diseases and Injuries of the Eye, which receives 22 new specimens. These have been skilfully prepared and mounted by Mr. E. W. Brewerton, to whom the Curator owes many thanks for assistance in their description. Dr. Williamson has also been active in the preparation of the gynæcological specimens, of which 13 have been added during the year. The remaining specimens include many rare and interesting examples of pathological conditions, but also many good formalin preparations of common conditions, such as tuberculosis of the lung in its various forms. Mention may also be made of the series of bones—marked to show the muscular attachments—presented by Mr. Cornelius Hanbury, and of historical interest, as probably the earliest bones in which this method of marking was ever employed.

The following is a list of the Donors whose names appear in this year's Catalogue:—

Mr. James Berry.	Mr. T. M. Hine.
Mr. Frank Broadbent.	Mr. Norman MacLaren.
Mr. Alban Doran.	Dr. James L. Maxwell.
Sir Dyce Duckworth.	Dr. C. Hubert Roberts.
Mr. H. Duncan.	Mr. H. J. Waring.
Dr. H. Morley Fletcher.	Mr. C. Gordon Watson.
Dr. W. S. A. Griffith.	Dr. F. Parkes Weber.
Mr. Cornelius Hanbury.	

The following is a complete list of the specimens added and remounted, and of the drawings, photographs, and microscopic specimens added during the year:—

New specimens mounted	.	.	.	.	.	93
Photographs added	.	.	.	.	.	1
Drawings added	.	.	.	.	.	1
Microscopic specimens added	.	.	.	.	.	81

The work of revising the old Catalogue has made very little progress during the present year for various reasons, chief amongst which were the inability of Mr. E. H. Shaw to take much part in the work, and the changes in the Museum Staff, which have prevented the Curator's devoting the necessary time to the matter. It is intended to take up this work again in the autumn, and carry it on as quickly as possible.

In the meantime—the condition of the old Catalogues being such as to render reference to the descriptions a matter of much confusion and difficulty—an important departure has been made in the provision of new "scrap-book" copies of the old Catalogues, in which the descriptions of all the existing specimens have been pasted in their proper order. Three such complete Catalogues have already been prepared, each bound in eleven sectional volumes, for use in the Museum. It is proposed to provide two more. The change has proved a very welcome convenience to students and others using the Museum.

ADDENDA.

SERIES I.

DISEASES OF BONES.

CRETINISM.

286b₁. The skull of a female child, twelve years of age, who was the subject of sporadic cretinism. The proportions of the skull do not differ in any marked degree from the normal. The brain-case is well developed, and, if anything, is rather large in proportion to the face. Those bones which arise in membrane are, as a whole, much more completely developed than those arising in cartilage. Yet even here there is evidence of locally arrested development in the widely open fontanelles. The anterior fontanelle is as widely open as that of an infant; the lateral ones are not quite closed, and there is a small membranous gap between the upper and lateral portions of the occipital bone where they abut on the mastoid. The mastoid foramen is also widely open. The cartilage bones, on the contrary, are imperfectly developed; the bony units of the basis cranii remain, to a large extent, independent. There is no shortening of the basis cranii, and no premature synostosis; even the line of junction between the basi-sphenoid and presphenoid can still be distinguished. The contrast between membrane bones and cartilage bones is well seen in the occipital, where the ill-developed basi-occipital and condylar masses resemble those of a very young child, while the upper portion of the bone is thick and firm. The root of the nose is broad and flattened, but not drawn in. Dentition is backward. None of the milk-teeth have been shed, though the permanent teeth can be seen in the jaws, some of them in abnormal situations. The lower jaw is disfigured on the left side by a large periosteal abscess in connection with a decayed temporary molar. Many of the milk-teeth are worn and decayed. 1905.

The patient, a girl aged 12 years, was the sixth child in a family of nine. The other members of the family were normal. This child showed no evident abnormality at birth, but signs of defective development became apparent after six months. She had never walked nor talked, and in her twelfth year she was 33 inches in height, and weighed 32 pounds. The external appearance was characteristic of cretinism; the body was very hairy, and fatty tumours were present above the clavicles. Her temperature was subnormal. The child came under observation in 1893, when thyroid treatment for cretinism had recently been introduced. She was fed with half a sheep's thyroid three times a week. After ten days she became febrile and restless, and the thyroid administration was suspended. The fever continued, and the child died of broncho-pneumonia some ten days later. The thyroid gland was found after death to be replaced by a little fatty tissue. The specimen is in the Museum of the Royal Free Hospital.

Presented by James Berry, F.R.C.S.

MULTIPLE MYELOMATOSIS.

289f. A humerus bisected longitudinally to show myelomatous deposits in the cavity of the shaft. The bone-marrow is replaced by a soft whitish growth, mottled in places by hæmorrhages. The new formation has here and there eroded the inner face of the shaft, and at one point has penetrated it, but without forming any external tumour. Some cancellous bone still remains in the head of the humerus, but even this appears infiltrated with the growth.   1905.

Microscopic Examination showed the new formation to have "the general characters of a sarcoma. It is composed of practically one variety of rounded cell, which presents certain resemblances to the neutrophile myelocyte. In the protoplasm there can be shown a large number of oxyphil granules, which vary considerably in size, but the smallest are distinctly larger than the neutrophile granules" (Prof. R. Muir).

From a man, aged 50, who suffered from rheumatoid symptoms for two years before his death. A few months after the onset of the articular affection the patient's back began to bend, and his attitude became a habitual stoop. He grew progressively weaker, and died after a copious hæmorrhage from the intestines. For the last six months of life, at least, Bence-Jones proteid was constantly present in the urine. At the autopsy the whole osseous system was found to be invaded by a tumour-growth similar to that seen in the specimen. The neoplasm was strictly limited to the osseous system, and appeared to have arisen independently in many places at once.

See *Histological Records*, i. 289f.

For full account, see *Medico-Chirurgical Society's Transactions*, 1903, p. 395.

Presented by F. Parkes Weber, M.D.

MYXO-SARCOMA.

435b. Section through the right half of a lower jaw, showing an endosteal new growth. The inner wall of the bone is intact, but its cavity is expanded by a new formation, which had destroyed the outer surface and fungated in that direction. The cut surface of the tumour consists chiefly of myxomatous tissue containing a good deal of calcareous material. 1905.

Microscopic Examination shows the growth to be chiefly myxomatous, but in places, where it is invading muscular tissue, it has the structure of a round-celled sarcoma.

Removed by operation from a man aged 31, who, in the year 1887, had suffered from a "gumboil" on the right side of the lower jaw. This subsided after the extraction of a tooth, but a swelling recurred, and grew till 1890. At this date an operation was performed, by which a tumour was removed from the body of the mandible. This was described as presenting the appearances of a "loose connective-tissue tumour." For 13 years subsequently the patient remained in good health, when the swelling recurred in conjunction with an abscess below the last molar tooth on the right side.

See *Histological Records*, i. 435b (A and B); *Male Surgical Register*, vol. i. (1904), pt. i., No. 1047.

PERIOSTEAL SARCOMA.

440a. A left scapula, with part of the clavicle, surrounded by masses of malignant growth. A longitudinal section has been made through the tumour, showing that the bone is intact, the growth having originated in the periosteum. All the fossæ of the bone are filled by the neoplasm, which has invaded, and, for the most part, destroyed the muscles of the region. 1905.

Microscopic Examination shows the growth to be a round-celled sarcoma.

From a man aged 25, who had noticed a swelling of his shoulder for five weeks before admission to the Hospital. He refused operation in the first instance, and was discharged, but was admitted again a month later and underwent amputation of the arm and scapula with part of the clavicle.

See *Histological Records,* i. 440a ; *Male Surgical Register,* vol. i. (1904), pt. i., No. 867.

PERIOSTEAL SARCOMA.

453c. Section through a knee-joint, showing a new growth arising from the periosteum of the femur on its posterior surface. The growth followed an excision of the knee-joint for tuberculous disease. The cut surface shows complete bony union between the femur and tibia. The popliteal space is occupied by a mass of new growth extending to, but not involving, the skin. The articulation of the fibula with the tibia remains, and immediately behind it is a cavity leading to a chronic sinus, lined by a grey slough, and opening on the outer aspect of the joint. A transverse scar at the level of the femoro-tibial ankylosis indicates the incision made previously for the excision of the joint. 1905.

Microscopic Examination shows the growth to be a spindle-celled sarcoma, containing a good deal of fibrous tissue.

From a woman, aged 41 years, who had suffered from tuberculous disease of the knee-joint for five years. One year before the date of the operation by which the leg was amputated, an excision of the joint had been performed, but a discharging sinus remained, and the swelling about the joint had increased.

See *Histological Records,* i. 453c ; *Female Surgical Register,* vol. iv. (1904), pt. ii., No. 1657.

CARCINOMA.

456a. Part of a skull and brain, showing a malignant growth which has destroyed the vertex of the skull. A coronal section has been made through scalp, skull, and brain, revealing extensive destruction of bone in the neighbourhood of the sagittal suture. In this region the vault is replaced by a dense new growth, which involves the cortex of the brain on either side of the longitudinal fissure, and raises the scalp from its natural contact with the cranium. The skin of the scalp is involved, but nowhere completely penetrated. The skull is abnormally thick.

1905.

Microscopic Examination shows the growth to be of alveolar structure, apparently a carcinoma, and of a type which in places is columnar-celled.

From a woman, who said that four months before her admission to the Royal Free Hospital she had knocked her head against a beam. A swelling appeared the following day, and had steadily increased in size. She died two months later, and the autopsy revealed secondary growths in the lungs, kidneys, glands of the neck, sternum, anterior abdominal wall, and the erector spinæ muscle. In view of the histological characters of the tumour, it is possible that the growth here seen was also secondary to some undetected carcinoma of columnar epithelial structures.

See *Histological Records*, i. 456a.

Received in exchange from the Museum of the Royal Free Hospital.

ENDOTHELIOMA.

538a. Section of a left upper jaw occupied by a large solid tumour. The growth is rounded, and limited by a well-defined capsule. It measures nearly 4 inches from front to back, and 2½ inches from above downwards. It occupies chiefly the outer portion of the jaw, and, although there is no evidence of ordinary infiltration, a considerable part of the bone has been destroyed. Much of the hard palate has gone, though the alveolar margin, with a few teeth, remains. The growth projects above into the left nasal passages, which are blocked, and reaches as high as the level of the orbit. Its consistency is firm and elastic, and it is seen to be intersected by fibrous bands. At one spot a small cavity appears to have been formed by softening. 1905.

Microscopic Examination shows the tumour to consist of minute cavities lined by irregular or cubical cells, many of which have undergone mucoid degeneration. Many of the spaces contain mucoid material, and appear to have originated in the degeneration of cells. There is an abundant fibrous stroma, but no cartilage is present. The growth appears to be an endothelioma, allied to the form seen in mixed parotid and mixed palatine tumours. It is not clear that it possesses more than limited malignancy.

The jaw was removed by operation from a Chinese woman aged 47 years, at a Mission Hospital in Formosa. She stated that four or five years previously a small lump appeared on the side of the face, about an inch to the left, and a little above the left nostril. This lump had steadily increased in size, but had caused little pain. The teeth on that side had gradually become loose, and the left nostril had been blocked for some months. The orbit was narrowed, but the eye did not protrude. On the facial aspect the growth formed a prominent mass as large as a cricket ball, and it bulged into the mouth for about three-quarters of an inch, extending to the middle line of the palate and back into the soft palate. The skin was freely movable over the tumour. There was no enlargement of the neighbouring lymphatic glands, and no evidence of any metastatic growths. The entire upper jaw was removed, and the patient made a rapid recovery.

See *Histological Records*, i. 538a.

Presented by Dr. James L. Maxwell.

SERIES II.

DISEASES OF JOINTS.

CHARCOT'S DISEASE.

691h. An elbow-joint, showing the lesions typical of Charcot's disease. The articular cartilages are worn away, and the articulating surfaces of the bones are in parts polished and in parts rough from the exposure of their cancellous spaces. There is little lipping of the cartilages, but large masses of periarticular overgrowth are seen in connection with some of the muscles round the joint; these are reddish in colour, and contain calcareous deposits; the largest masses are seen in relation with the brachialis anticus, the flexors arising from the internal condyle, and the insertion of the biceps.   There is also a large supracondylar exostosis on the inner margin of the humerus.   The synovial membrane of the joint is throughout greatly thickened, and in parts fibrillated.   1905.

From a man aged 50, who, sixteen years before, had begun to experience weakness of the right arm, followed eight years later by similar weakness of the left.   For six weeks the right elbow and both wrists had been swollen but painless.   The patient was a typically tabetic subject, and had contracted syphilis twenty-eight years before the date of his admission to this hospital, where he died.   At the autopsy the elbow-joint was found to be distended with fluid blood.

See *Male Medical Register*, vol. iv. (1904), No. 167; and *Medical Post-Mortem Register* (1904), No. 171.

SERIES IV.

DISLOCATIONS.

DISLOCATION OF ASTRAGALUS.

1053c.   A right foot showing dislocation of the astragalus.   The bone is dislocated forwards and outwards, and rotated upon its longitudinal axis. As a result the head lies upon the dorsum of the cuboid and outer part of the scaphoid bones, while the superior articular surface faces to the left.   The bone is firmly fixed by adhesions in its new position.   1905.

From a woman aged 65, who fell from a stool nineteen weeks before admission to the Hospital.   Attempts at reduction were made at the time, but failed.   On admission the relations of the malleoli to the astragalus appeared normal, the dislocation being regarded as subastragaloid.   Further attempts at reduction proving unsuccessful, Syme's amputation was performed.

See *Female Surgical Register*, vol. iv. (1896), No. 2215.

SERIES VII.

DISEASES AND INJURIES OF THE PERICARDIUM AND HEART.

PYO-PERICARDITIS.

1233e.   The thoracic viscera of a child, showing an empyema on the right side, and purulent pericarditis associated with collapse and bronchiectasis of the left lung.   The pericardium, which is displayed through an incision in the left lung, is much distended, and both layers are covered with thick shaggy lymph.   The left lung is much collapsed, and in the upper part shows a remarkable degree of bronchiectasis. The posterior part of the right lung is covered with thickened pleura, upon which there is much thick lymph. Apart from some degree of collapse the right lung appears to be normal. The condition was due to infection by the pneumococcus.   1905.

Microscopic Examination.—The lung is completely collapsed and the bronchi dilated, their walls being much thickened. In many places the mucous membrane has disappeared, its place being taken by granulation tissue.

From a female child aged 2½ years, admitted to the Hospital in a moribund condition. She had suffered for some two months with cough and progressive wasting. The child had been much neglected, and the history was vague. *Post-mortem* much pus was found in the pericardium and in both pleuræ, and there were several small collections of thick pus amongst the coils of the intestines.

See *Histological Records*, vii. 1233e; *Female Medical Register.* vol. v. (1904), No. 75; *Medical Post-Mortem Register*, vol. xxxi. (1904), p. 77.

GUMMA.

1280b.   A heart showing infiltration by gummatous deposits. The right ventricle has been laid open from the front, and shows in its upper part a large whitish tumour, which has destroyed the ventricular muscle over a considerable area, and forms a rounded projection into the cavity of the ventricle. The section has passed through the main mass of the gumma, which extends as far as the base of the pulmonary valve. There are in addition several small outlying masses, some of which may be seen on the anterior surface of the left ventricle. The heart is dilated, and the anterior wall of the right ventricle is thin.   1905.

Microscopic Examination shows the deposit to consist of necrotic material surrounded by a zone of round-celled infiltration. The coronary arteries show an endarteritis indistinguishable from that of syphilis.

From a policeman aged 36 years, who fell dead on his beat. For three months before his death he had complained of attacks of sharp pain about the heart, but these had never been severe enough to incapacitate him. He had been a soldier but was not known to have suffered from syphilis.

See *Histological Records*, vii. 1280b.

Presented by Mr. H. Duncan.

SERIES XI.

DISEASES AND INJURIES OF THE PLEURA BRONCHIAL TUBES AND LUNGS.

TUBERCULOUS EMPHYSEMA.

1690e.   The thoracic viscera of an infant affected by tuberculosis. The upper and middle lobes of the right lung and the upper lobe of the left lung show numerous caseating tubercles, associated with many of which are bullæ due to acute over-distension of the air-spaces. The lower lobes are partially consolidated, and present numbers of tubercles especially along their superior margins. The lymphatic glands about the bifurcation of the trachea are large and caseous. There is a caseous deposit at the extreme apex of the heart, and two other larger ones in the substance of the left ventricle. Pericardial adhesions were present at the apex.

1905.

Microscopic Examination shows caseous foci surrounded by zones of small-celled infiltration, with intervening areas of apparently normal lung tissue.

From a male infant of 8 months, who had been the subject of otorrhœa and wasting for some weeks. A mastoid abscess appeared, for the relief of which an operation was performed, but the child gradually sank. The autopsy showed a generalised tuberculosis, with ulceration of the intestines and caseation of the mesenteric lymphatic glands.

See *Histological Records,* xi. 1690e; *Male Surgical Register,* vol. iv.(1903), No. 387; *Surgical Post-Mortem Register* (1903), p. 36.

ACUTE PNEUMONIA.

1700a. Section through a left lung, showing acute lobar pneumonia. The lower lobe is completely consolidated and is in the stage of grey hepatisation. The cut surface is a uniform grey colour, and shows the granular surface characteristic of pneumonia. On the pleural surface is a thin layer of recent fibrinous exudation. The upper lobe is intensely engorged, but was still crepitant in the fresh state. 1905.

Microscopically the condition is typical of lobar pneumonia.

From a man, aged 28 years, who died on the ninth day of his illness, having shown the classical signs and symptoms of acute lobar pneumonia. The immediate cause of death was a purulent meningitis from the pus of which the pneumococcus was cultivated.

See *Histological Records,* xi. 1700a; *Male Medical Register,* vol. i. (1905), No. 11; and *Medical Post-Mortem Register,* vol. xxxii. p. 30.

PYO-PNEUMOTHORAX.

1704a$_1$. The right lung and pleura from a case of pyo-pneumothorax occurring in the course of pulmonary tuberculosis. The lung is seen as a shrunken mass, about the size of a man's fist. The two layers of the pleura are widely separated, and their surfaces are covered with thick purulent lymph. A glass rod has been passed into the rupture in the lung, which is situated at its hinder part, about the level of the middle lobe, and which communicates with a small cavity. The shrunken lung shows, on the cut surface, numerous tuberculous foci. 1905.

Microscopic Examination.—The lung shows complete collapse with numerous tuberculous foci.

From a man aged 28, who had suffered from cough for eight months, and had a severe hæmoptysis three weeks before admission to the Hospital. Three days before admission he had sudden severe pain in the right side, with violent cough and dyspnœa. On admission he showed the signs typical of pneumothorax. Pus and air were on two occasions withdrawn from his chest, but he died 3½ weeks after the occurrence of the rupture. *Post-mortem* three pints of thick pus were found in the right pleural cavity, the left lung was emphysematous, but otherwise healthy.

See *Histological Records,* xi. 1704a$_1$; *Male Medical Register,* vol. iv. (1904), No. 195; and *Medical Post-Mortem Register,* vol. xxxi. (1904), p. 289.

ACUTE TUBERCULOSIS.

1717. The lungs of a child, showing acute tuberculosis. They are densely and uniformly infiltrated with tubercles in an early stage of caseation. In places these have coalesced into larger caseous areas. Between the tubercles the lung tissue is deeply congested; there is no evidence of pleurisy. The glands at the bifurcation of the trachea are caseous. 1905.

Microscopic Examination.—There is a patchy tuberculous consolidation, caseous areas alternating with areas of almost normal lung tissue.

From a breast-fed infant of five months, who had been ailing for one month with wasting and diarrhœa, with frequent bloody stools. *Post-mortem* tubercles were found in every organ, with ulceration throughout the intestine.

See *Histological Records*, xi., 1717; *Female Medical Register*, vol. v. (1904), No. 171; and *Medical Post-Mortem Register*, vol. xxxi. (1904), p. 300.

CHRONIC PULMONARY TUBERCULOSIS.

1723a. Section through a left lung affected with chronic pulmonary tuberculosis. In the upper lobe, which is somewhat contracted, are two quiescent cavities, lined with a smooth membrane, and communicating with one another by a small rounded opening; at the extreme apex the wall of the larger cavity is much thinned, consisting of little but the pleura. The lower lobe is densely infiltrated with grey and yellow tubercles, coalescing in the upper portion into larger patches in which minute cavities are in process of formation. The visceral layer of the pleura is opaque and thickened over the upper lobe, and a few thick adhesions are to be seen at the extreme apex. There is also some thickening of the pleura over the lower lobe, especially at its upper part. Patches of sub-pleural emphysema are scattered over the lower lobe.   1905.

Microscopic Examination.—The lung shows typical tuberculosis.

From a man aged 21, who had an attack of pleurisy one year before his death, and for seven months had suffered from symptoms of progressive phthisis and tuberculous laryngitis. *Post-mortem* recent tubercles were found in both lungs, in the larynx, intestines and kidneys.

See *Histological Records*, xi. 1723a; *Male Medical Register*, vol. ii. (1905), No. 8; *Medical Post-Mortem Register*, vol. xxxii. (1905), p. 24.

TUBERCULOSIS IN AN INFANT.

1723b. The right lung of an infant, showing advanced tuberculous disease. The greater part of the upper lobe is occupied by a large cavity with ragged walls. Numerous miliary tubercles are present throughout the remainder of the lung. There is some opacity of the visceral pleura over the upper lobe, but no marked thickening. The bronchial glands are caseous.   1905.

Microscopic Examination shows extensive caseation of the lung around the cavity.

From a child aged 5½ months, who had been losing flesh and strength since weaning at the age of 3 weeks. Diarrhœa and vomiting had been present intermittently, and for a month the child had suffered from cough. General miliary tuberculosis was found at the autopsy.

See *Histological Records*, xi. 1723b; *Female Medical Register*, vol. v. (1904), No. 196; *Medical Post-Mortem Register*, vol. xxxi., p. 298.

SERIES XII.

DISEASES OF THE NOSE, MOUTH, TONGUE, PALATE, AND FAUCES.

EPITHELIOMA.

1777c.   A lower lip showing extensive cancerous invasion.   The tumour involves the outer and upper aspects of the lip, and has begun to invade the inner surface.   It presents the appearance of a warty growth ulcerated in parts, and shows along its lower border an everted edge.

1905.

Microscopic Examination shows the growth to be a squamous-celled carcinoma.
From a man aged 58.   Eight years previously a wart had been removed from a part of the lower lip corresponding with the middle of the present growth.   He remained well until nine months before the second operation, when an ulcer appeared, which subsequently extended to its present dimensions.
See *Histological Records*, xii. 1777c; and *Male Surgical Register*, vol. iv. (1900), No. 70.

PAPILLOMA.

1785a₄.   Longitudinal section of a tongue, showing a large papillomatous growth.   The tip of the tongue is natural, but the bulk of the dorsal surface is the seat of a warty growth.   The tumour is marked by deep fissures, and is composed of many lobes, covered by a thick layer of epithelium.   There is no infiltration of the deeper tissues of the organ.

1905.

Microscopic Examination shows the growth to be a papilloma presenting no evidence of malignancy.
Removed by operation from a man of. 50.   The patient contracted syphilis twenty-eight years previously, and had suffered from leucoplakia for years.   The growth was first observed six months before the date of operation.   On examination the parts of the tongue unaffected by the growth showed large areas of leucoplakia.   The dorsal aspect of the organ was almost entirely covered by a large mushroom-shaped growth, which sprang from the left half only, but overhung the right.
See *Histological Records*, xii. 1785a₄.
Presented by C. Gordon Watson, F.R.C.S.

SERIES XIV.

DISEASES OF THE SALIVARY GLANDS.

SUBMAXILLARY GLAND WITH CALCULUS.

1826b.   A submaxillary salivary gland in which is lying a calculus, embedded in the substance of the gland just internal to the constriction caused by the mylohyoid muscle.

1905.

From a man aged 30, who had suffered from intermittent swelling of his left submaxillary gland for a period of eighteen months. A small calculus was removed from Wharton's duct without relief to the symptoms, and on further examination the second calculus was found and the gland removed.

Presented by H. J. Waring, F.R.C.S.

SERIES XVII.

DISEASES AND INJURIES OF THE STOMACH.

CONGENITAL HYPERTROPHIC STENOSIS OF PYLORUS.

1907a₁. Section through the stomach and duodenum of an infant, show-ing the condition known as congenital hypertrophic stenosis of the pylorus. There is marked hypertrophy of the muscular sphincter of the pylorus, ending abruptly at the duodenal, but shelving off gradually at the gastric end. The mucous membrane is thrown into a well-marked longitudinal fold by the contraction of the thickened muscle. The stomach is somewhat dilated, and its muscular coat shows considerable hypertrophy.   1905.

Microscopic Examination shows that the increased thickness of the pylorus is due entirely to increase in its muscular elements.

From a child aged 7 weeks, who had vomited persistently since the age of 3 weeks. The pyloric thickening was not palpable during life.

See *Histological Records*, xvii. 1907a₁; *East London Hospital for Children Post-Mortem Register*, vol. iv., No. 157.

Presented by H. Morley Fletcher, M.D.

GASTRIC ULCER.

1914b. Portion of a stomach in which is a simple ulcer, showing erosion of a blood-vessel. The ulcer is punched out, with sharply defined and somewhat overhanging edges; the mucous membrane surrounding it is thickened. On the serous surface there is slight thickening of the peritoneum. A bristle is passed into a small vessel at the base of the ulcer, from which fatal hæmorrhage had occurred.   1905.

From a man aged 50, who had been a hard drinker, and had suffered from some pain after food for a short time before admission to the Hospital. He had profuse hæmatemesis, and died two days later.

See *Male Medical Register*, vol. ii. (1905), No. 106; and *Medical Post-Mortem Register* (1905), No. 90.

CARCINOMA.

1933a. A stomach, the anterior wall of which has been removed to show a carcinoma involving the pyloric region. At its cardiac extremity the growth projects into the cavity of the stomach as a semilunar elevation, embracing two-thirds of the circumference of the wall. From this point onwards the viscus is converted into a narrowed tube, marked by irre-gular excrescences on its walls or by ulcerated excavations in them, and terminating in the diminished aperture of the pylorus. On the posterior wall of the stomach, close to the commencement of the growth, is an opening made during life for the purpose of gastro-intestinal anastomosis. A portion of the liver, firmly adherent to the peritoneal surface of the tumour, is shown in the upper part of the specimen. 1905.

Microscopic Examination shows the growth to be a columnar-celled carcinoma, which has more or less lapsed into the spheroidal-celled type.

From a man aged 53, who for twelve months had suffered from pain in the epigastrium, radiating to the left scapula. For six months he had been extremely constipated, and had lost flesh, and for eight days had vomited frequently after food. A posterior gastro-jejunostomy was performed, but the patient died the following day. The autopsy showed no secondary growths.

See *Histological Records*, xvii. 1933a; *Male Surgical Register*, vol. v. (1905), No. 1121; also *Surgical Post-Mortem Register* (1905), p. 64.

SERIES XVIII.

DISEASES AND INJURIES OF THE INTESTINES.

FIBROUS STRICTURE OF DUODENUM.

2017b. Part of a liver with the duodenum and pylorus, showing a tight fibrous stricture of the duodenum. The gall-bladder contains many gall-stones, and is densely adherent to the liver and surrounding structures so that only its tip is visible. The front margin of the right lobe of the liver is turned up, and adherent to its upper surface. The duodenum is drawn in and narrowed, by adhesions to the gall bladder, at a point some two inches beyond the pylorus. In the recent state the stricture almost completely occluded the lumen of the gut. The muscular coats of the proximal portion of the duodenum and of the stomach are hypertrophied. 1905.

From a woman aged 68 years, who began to suffer from pain after food nine weeks before her death. About the same time she began to vomit profusely at intervals of several days. The stomach was found much dilated after death.

See *Female Surgical Register*, vol. iv. (1904), pt. i., No. 340, and *Surgical Post-Mortem Register* (1904), p. 41.

MALIGNANT STRICTURE OF DUODENUM.

2021b. Portion of a duodenum, showing constriction caused by a localised cancerous growth. The tumour is at the junction of the second and third parts of the duodenum, and extends over about an inch of its length. It has invaded the bowel in its whole circumference, causing extreme narrowing. Between the growth and the pylorus the duodenum is greatly dilated, especially its second part. The stomach wall shows some hypertrophy. 1905.

Microscopic Examination.—The growth is a columnar-celled carcinoma.

From a woman aged 28 years, who gave a history of three months' vomiting and loss of flesh. Whilst in the Hospital stomach washings of 3½ pints were made. She suffered from several severe attacks of tetany.

See *Histological Records*, xviii. 2021b; *Female Medical Register*, vol. i. (1904), Nos. 114 and 114a; *Medical Post-Mortem Register*, vol. xxxi. (1904), p. 74.

CARCINOMA.

2021c.   Portion of a sigmoid flexure excised for cancerous stricture. The lumen of the gut is almost completely occluded by a firm white malignant growth which has caused an annular constriction. The surface of the growth is ulcerated in its lower part.   1905.

Microscopic Examination.—The growth is a columnar-celled carcinoma.

Removed by operation from a woman aged 56, who was admitted to the Hospital for intestinal obstruction of one week's duration. She had suffered more or less from constipation for a year. The obstruction was relieved by operation, and one week later the gut was resected. The woman left the Hospital in good health, but with a fæcal fistula.

See *Histological Records*, xviii. 2021c ; *Female Surgical Register*, vol. iii. (1905), No. 395.

SERIES XIX.

DISEASES OF THE RECTUM AND ANUS.

CARCINOMA OF ANUS.

2069d.   An anus showing cancerous invasion of the skin at the orifice. The growth, which originated higher up in the rectum, has spread downwards, infiltrating the wall of the gut and the tissues adjacent. The lower part of the rectum is narrowed, smooth and rigid, but the anus itself is the seat of a diffuse warty growth which extends for some distance over the skin.   1905.

Microscopic Examination.—The growth is a columnar-celled carcinoma.

From a man aged 24 years, who, eighteen months before admission to the Hospital, began to suffer from irritation round the anus, in which region the skin shortly became hard and warty. For eight months before admission he had been troubled with incontinence of fæces and had lost flesh. He developed secondary growths in the liver and, later, obstruction of the gut, for which an inguinal colotomy was performed. *Post-mortem* the pelvis was found to be filled by a mass of growth which appeared to have originated at the junction of the second and third portions of the rectum.

See *Histological Records*, xix. 2069d ; *Male Surgical Register*, vol. iii. (1903), No. 532 ; *Surgical Post-Mortem Register* (1903), p. 47.

SERIES XXI.

DISEASES AND INJURIES OF THE LIVER.

CIRRHOSIS AND PERIHEPATITIS.

2193e.   Portion of a liver showing cirrhosis and perihepatitis. The capsule is greatly thickened by the deposit of a whitish hyaline membrane, with many pits upon it giving it a "worm-eaten" appearance. This membrane can be stripped off the true capsule of the liver. The cut surface of the organ shows typical cirrhotic changes.   1905.

Microscopic Examination shows marked fibrosis of the multilobular type with much fatty change in the liver-cells. The adventitious membrane on the surface consists of dense fibrous tissue, practically devoid of cells.

From a man aged 32, who was admitted comatose to the Hospital and died a week later without recovering consciousness. A history of continuous drinking for two years was obtained from his friends. *Post-mortem* general chronic peritonitis was found, with several ounces of free fluid in the belly. The liver weighed 70 ounces, and the spleen 33 ounces.

See *Histological Records*, xxi. 2193e; *Male Medical Register*, vol. i. (1905), No. 6; and *Medical Post-Mortem Register*, vol. xxxii., p. 49.

TUBERCULOUS CHOLANGITIS.

2196a₅. Portion of a child's liver, showing tuberculous deposits in relation with the bile-ducts. Under the capsule—which is thickened and in places adherent—many small tuberculous foci are seen. These have coalesced in many places to form larger caseous areas. On the cut surface many of these foci are seen to be deeply bile-stained. 1905.

Microscopic examination shows caseous foci surrounded by zones of tuberculous infiltration containing giant-cells.

From a boy aged 2 years, who died after two months' illness with tubercles in all the viscera—the immediate cause of death being tuberculous meningitis.

See *Histological Records*, xxi. 2196a₅; *Female Medical Register*, vol. iv. (1905), No. 134; and *Medical Post-Mortem Register*, vol. xxxii., p. 96.

HYDATID CYST RUPTURING INTO COMMON BILE DUCT.

2235d. A portion of liver in which are two hydatid cysts, one of which communicates with the common bile duct. The larger cyst, the position of which is indicated on the upper surface of the organ by a puckered scar, has been opened from below, and is seen to communicate with the common bile duct, in the dilated cavity of which several daughter cysts are lying. The papilla of Vater is distended with cysts which are protruding into the lumen of the duodenum. The smaller cyst is on the upper surface of the liver at the highest part of the right lobe. The gall-bladder is natural, and at its fundus has been joined by operation to the jejunum. 1905.

From a man aged 26, who had suffered for seven weeks from paroxysms of epigastric pain with vomiting. He had one attack of pain in the Hospital, during which he became jaundiced for the first time. An operation was performed, and the bile passages were thought to be clear. The patient became collapsed after the operation and died three days later. *Post-mortem* both cysts were found distended with daughter cysts.

See *Male Surgical Register*, vol. i. (1904), No. 1907; and *Surgical Post-Mortem Register* (1904), p. 153.

ACTINOMYCOSIS OF LIVER.

2239e. Part of the right lobe of a liver in which is an actinomycotic abscess. On the under surface a distinct bulging is seen, over which the capsule is thickened and shows a few adhesions. There is also some bulging of the upper surface. On the cut surface this bulging is seen to correspond with a large multilocular abscess, the walls of which are lined with thickened yellowish exudation.   On one of the cut surfaces a small area of yellowish colour and honeycombed structure is seen near the main abscess.   1905.

Microscopic Examination.—A section through a part of the abscess shows that its cavity is lined by a layer of granulation tissue and polynuclear leucocytes. The liver cells are compressed and for the most part degenerated ; Glisson's capsule is thickened, and strands of fibrous tissue traverse the remnant of the liver.

From a man aged 38, who had noticed a swelling in the right hypochondrium for five weeks prior to his admission to the Hospital. This had gradually extended and, on its being incised, a large quantity of thick pus was obtained in which many actinomyces-granules were found. Several operations were performed, but the sinuses never healed and the man slowly sank till his death six weeks after his admission. During the last fortnight of his life he suffered with jaundice and frequent rigors.   *Post-mortem* another abscess was found in the left lobe of the liver, and a recent infarct in the spleen.

Actinomyces and streptococci were found in the pus from the abscess.

See *Histological Records*, xxi. 2239e ; *Male Surgical Register*, vol. iii. (1904), No. 1256 ; and *Surgical Post-Mortem Register* (1904), p. 115.

SERIES XXII.
DISEASES OF THE GALL-BLADDER.

TUBERCULOSIS OF GALL-BLADDER.

2245a.   A gall-bladder and part of a liver from a case of tuberculous peritonitis.   The wall of the gall-bladder is thickened, and tubercles of various sizes are thickly deposited upon it.   The gall-bladder was adherent to the liver along its whole length.   1905.

From a boy aged 1½ years, who had suffered for six months with wasting, frequent offensive stools, and swelling of the belly.   *Post-mortem* general tuberculous peritonitis was found.

See *Male Medical Register*, vol. iii. (1904), No. 55 ; *Medical Post-Mortem Register*, vol. xxxi. (1904), p. 44.

SERIES XXIV.
DISEASES OF LYMPHATIC GLANDS AND VESSELS.

TUBERCULOSIS.

2281.   A mass of enlarged mesenteric glands showing advanced caseous tubercle.   A portion of the duodenum and pancreas may be seen, firmly adherent to the glandular mass.   On the peritoneal covering of the glands are many small tubercles.   1905.

From a boy of 14 years, who had been losing flesh for many months, and had for three months suffered much from diarrhœa and sickness, associated with distension of the belly.   He presented the clinical features of chronic tuberculous peritonitis. The autopsy revealed a generalised tuberculosis, the oldest lesion being a healed focus at the apex of one lung. The abdominal viscera showed advanced tuberculous lesions, including extensive ulceration of the intestines.

See *Male Medical Register*, vol. i. (1904), pt. i., No. 86; and *Medical Port-Mortem Register*, vol. xxxi. (1904), p. 101.

SECONDARY CARCINOMA.

2287b. Part of the pectoral muscles with infiltrated lymphatic glands, from a case of cancer of the breast. The glands appear as large, whitish, discrete tumours in the areolar tissue under the muscle.   1905.

Microscopic Examination shows the growth to be a spheroidal-celled carcinoma. Removed by operation from a woman aged 55 years, who had observed a lump in her left breast for eighteen months.

See *Histological Records*, xxiv. 2287b; and *Female Surgical Register*, vol. ii. (1905), No. 161.

MELANOTIC SARCOMA.

2294c. Two enlarged lymphatic glands infiltrated with melanotic sarcoma. Each gland is completely encapsulated, and consists of deeply pigmented tissue mottled by a few lighter areas.   1905.

Microscopic Examination shows the growth to be composed chiefly of spindle-shaped cells. It contains many necrotic areas, and a patchy deposit of brown pigment.

From a woman, aged 34 years, who for nine months had noticed a swelling in her left groin. The swelling had slowly increased in size, but resulted in no affection of the general health. No primary focus was discovered to account for the condition, except a slightly pigmented area on the left labium majus. This area was excised at the operation for removal of the glands, but the histology of it is unknown.

See *Histological Records*, xxiv. 2294c; *Female Surgical Register*, vol. i. (1904), pt. ii., No. 2983.

SERIES XXVI.

DISEASES OF THE THYMUS AND THYROID GLANDS.

MEDIASTINAL TUMOUR.

2309a₁. Median vertical section through a superior mediastinum occupied by a malignant growth. A portion of the sternum is seen in the specimen, pushed forward by the neoplasm, which has formed a tumour just underneath the skin. The growth has displaced the trachea backwards and slightly to the right, and is seen to be infiltrating and partially blocking the left bronchus. In the lower portion of the specimen part of the pericardium is shown with some deposits of new growth in it. The aorta makes its way through the mass without any narrowing.   1905.

Microscopic Examination.—The growth is composed of rounded cells irregular in size and shape, with a fibrous stroma separating them into more or less distinct groups. It is probably an endothelioma.

From a man aged 54, who had been ailing for six months with pain in the left arm and shoulder, and progressive loss of flesh. He had noticed a lump in the left side of his neck for six weeks before admission to the Hospital, and the swelling in the chest for four weeks. He lived five weeks in the Hospital, his chief distress arising from bronchitis. On examination large hard masses were found above the left clavicle and in the left axilla, and a smooth rounded tumour in the first two left intercostal spaces. The breath sounds were weakened all over the left lung. At the *post-mortem* the lungs and pericardium were found studded with nodules, and the left lung was collapsed.

See *Histological Records*, xxvi. 2309a₁ ; *Male Medical Register*, vol. i. (1904), No. 97 ; and *Medical Post-Mortem Register*, vol. xxxi. (1904), p. 83.

HYPERTROPHY.

2311c. A thyroid gland removed by operation. It shows a great and proportional enlargement of both lateral lobes and isthmus. There is no sign of any inflammatory process or new growth, and no cysts are present. 1905.

Microscopically the overgrowth was found to consist of normal thyroid tissue.

The patient was a single woman of 22 years. The swelling appeared at the age of 14, and had gradually progressed in size. For three years she had suffered from palpitation of the heart and dyspnœa on exertion. She presented no exophthalmos or fibrillary tremor, nor any undue rapidity of pulse, though the rhythm of the heart was irregular. At the operation a small central lobule ¾ inch in diameter was isolated from the isthmus and left in position. The patient recovered without any bad symptoms, and left the Hospital on the eighteenth day after operation.

See *Histological Records*, xxvi. 2311c ; and *Female Surgical Register*, vol. v. (1904), pt. ii., No. 2281.

SARCOMA.

2318e. A larynx, trachea, and adjoining parts showing a sarcomatous tumour of the thyroid gland, with a large mass of secondary growth, involving the mediastinal lymphatic glands. The primary growth is in the right lobe of the thyroid gland, and forms a smooth rounded tumour situated on the right and anterior aspects of the trachea in its upper third. To the left of this mass is seen a bilobed projection, representing the left lobe of the thyroid gland in process of involvement by the growth. At the lower end of the specimen is the arch of the aorta, displaced to the left by a large secondary mass occupying the posterior mediastinum. Upon this mass lies the superior vena cava, indicated by a glass rod ; the innominate artery disappears into the mass and divides within it. On the posterior surface the œsophagus is seen, laid open from behind. Its course is distorted by the irregular outline of the growth, which in places forms rounded projections into the lumen of the tube. 1905.

Microscopic Examination of the secondary mass shows the growth to be a mixed-celled sarcoma. In some parts the cells are uniformly spindle-shaped, while in others flat epithelioid cells predominate.

From a woman aged 60, who had noticed a swelling in the region of her thyroid gland for four months, and had for three months been subject to dysphagia and dyspnœa. She died suddenly on the fifth day after her admission to the Hospital, apparently from heart-failure. At the autopsy secondary deposits were found in the pleura and lungs, but none elsewhere.

See *Histological Records*, xxvi. 2318e ; and *Female Surgical Register*, vol. i. (1904), pt ii. No. 2165 ; also *Surgical Post-Mortem Register* (1904), p. 176.

SERIES XXVIII.

DISEASES AND INJURIES OF THE KIDNEYS, THEIR PELVES, AND THE URETERS.

RED GRANULAR KIDNEY.

2335g. Half of a kidney, showing the variety of chronic interstitial nephritis resulting in the "small red kidney." The cortex is of a brownish-red colour, mottled by lighter areas. The capsule has been removed, leaving the granular surface typical of the condition. The cortex is diminished in depth and the pelvic fat excessive. An aberrant renal artery is seen entering the kidney at the upper extremity of its inner aspect.   1905.

Microscopic Examination shows a marked intertubular fibrous over-growth, distorting the tubules and crowding them together. The capsules of the Malpighian tufts are generally thickened, and in places the tufts themselves are reduced to knobs of fibrous tissue. The renal arterioles present a pronounced thickening of their middle and outer coats.

From a man aged 45 who had suffered from cough and swelling of the legs for ten months before his admission to the Hospital. He died a month later from gradual heart failure, and the autopsy showed great hypertrophy of the left ventricle, without valvular disease. The arterial system showed a slight but widespread degeneration of the intima. The great-toe joint was the seat of uratic deposit.

See *Histological Records*, xxviii. 2335g; *Male Medical Register*, vol. i. (1904), pt. i., p. 114; and *Medical Post-Mortem Register*, vol. xxxi., p. 257.

TUBERCULOSIS.

2341a₂. Urinary organs showing advanced tuberculous disease. The left kidney is riddled with tuberculous abscesses, and many small tuberculous foci are to be seen beneath the capsule. The right kidney shows the same condition but in a less advanced stage. Both ureters show tuberculous deposits, and the mucous membrane of the bladder is thickened and presents small areas of ulceration. In the prostate there is one large mass of caseous material and several smaller ones.   1905.

Microscopic Examination.—The kidneys show typical tuberculous deposits.

From a man aged 21, who gave a history of frequent micturition for two years, with constant pain in the back. He often passed blood in his urine, and suffered at intervals from severe paroxysms of pain resembling renal colic. The urine contained tubercle bacilli in large numbers. *Post-mortem* the apex of the right lung showed tuberculous lesions, both old and recent, and the mesenteric glands were caseous in the region of the kidneys.

See *Histological Records*, xxviii. 2341a₂; *Male Medical Register*, vol. iv. (1905), No. 28; and *Medical Post-Mortem Register*, vol. xxxii. (1905), p. 50.

CYST.

2378c. Section of a kidney the lower extremity of which is occupied by a large thin-walled cyst. The cyst is not altogether solitary, for several crater-like depressions are present on the surface which represent the site of cortical cysts destroyed by the removal of the capsule. The kidney is not apparently granular, but its cortex is diminished.   1905.

From a man aged 62, who was admitted to the Hospital for intestinal obstruction, due to new growth of the sigmoid flexure, and died shortly after an operation for its relief. *Post-mortem* the other kidney was found to be natural. The condition of the kidney is not known to have caused any symptoms during life.

See *Male Surgical Register*, vol. i. (1902), No. 3439; also *Surgical Post-Mortem Register* (1902), p. 232.

CYSTIC DEGENERATION.

2384. Half of a left kidney, showing an advanced condition of cystic degeneration. The kidney substance has been almost entirely replaced by cysts, and can only be traced in small scattered islands. Many of the larger cysts are filled with colloid material. The kidney weighed 38 oz. The right kidney was in the same condition, and weighed 22 oz.   1905.

Microscopic Examination of the least affected portions of the kidney reveals a patchy round-celled infiltration amongst the renal tubules, which in places appear to be destroyed by the pressure. There is little or no fibrosis.

From a man aged 61, who died of a pontine hæmorrhage. He showed some general arterial sclerosis. His heart weighed 14 oz., and gave evidence of left ventricular hypertrophy.

See *Histological Records*, xxviii. 2384.

Presented by Mr. T. M. Hine.

SECONDARY SARCOMA.

2390d₈. Part of a kidney, showing many nodules of new growth. The deposits are white in colour, and are distributed throughout the organ, being most abundant in the cortex ; a large mass involves the pelvis.

1905.

Microscopic Examination shows the growth to be a small round-celled sarcoma. The renal tubules are separated, and in places destroyed by densely-packed round cells.

From a boy of 12, who had suffered for four months from attacks of dyspnœa and cough of increasing severity. In one of these attacks he died, and the autopsy showed a large mass of new growth in the thorax, involving the pericardium. Metastatic deposits were also present in the intestine and mesenteric glands.

See *Histological Records*, xxviii. 2390d₃; *Male Medical Register*, vol. i. (1905), No. 61 ; and *Medical Post-Mortem Register*, vol. xxxii., p. 51.

PRIMARY CARCINOMA.

2390h₅. A kidney, the substance of which is almost entirely replaced by new growth. The outline and general plan of the organ remain distinct. The perinephric tissue is extensively infiltrated, and forms a thick fibrous case. The whole of the kidney is involved by a dense white growth, with the exception of three or four darker areas, representing the remains of pyramids. The pelvis is occupied by a large plug of similar white growth, the boundaries of which are distinctly defined from the surrounding infiltration which has replaced the kidney proper.   1905.

Microscopic Examination shows the growth to be a carcinoma of spheroidal-celled type, with a well-marked fibrous stroma.

From a man aged 53, who had suffered from constant pain in the region of the left kidney for fifteen weeks, without colic. One month prior to the onset of the pain he had hæmaturia lasting four weeks, but no blood had been present in the urine since the pain began. The kidney was explored, and then removed by operation, but the patient died on the following day. The lungs and liver were found to contain numerous metastatic deposits.

See *Histological Records*, xxviii. 2390b₂; *Male Surgical Register*, vol. ii. (1905), No. 399; *Surgical Post-Mortem Register*, 1905, p. 25.

SERIES XXX.

DISEASES AND INJURIES OF THE BRAIN AND ITS MEMBRANES.

HÆMORRHAGIC PACHYMENINGITIS.

2449d. A dura mater, showing a copious extravasation of blood on its inner surface. The clot is evidently of some standing: it adheres firmly to the dura, and on its inner aspect presents in places a thin whitish membrane. 1905.

Microscopic Examination shows no evidence of inflammation of the dura mater. The clot on the inner surface of the membrane is in process of organisation.

From a child aged 8 months, who had suffered from convulsions for fourteen days prior to admission to Hospital. When admitted the patient was semi-comatose and febrile. The head was retracted, and vomiting was frequent till death about six weeks from the onset of the illness. The autopsy showed a septic broncho-pneumonia, with subserous petechiæ on the pleuræ, and the whole surface of the brain was covered with soft clot.

See *Histological Records*, xxx. 2449d; and *East London Hospital for Children Post-Mortem Register*, vol. ii. p. 248.

Presented by H. Morley Fletcher, M.D.

ACROMEGALY.

2504b. Half of the base of a skull from a case of acromegaly, with the soft parts *in situ*. The bones are somewhat massive, and the frontal sinus is of unusual size for a woman. In the position of the pituitary body is a large soft growth, which has greatly enlarged the sella turcica, and which projected upwards into the third ventricle of the brain: the upper part of the growth has in part been destroyed. 1905.

Microscopic Examination.—The growth appears to be an adenoma of the pituitary body.

The patient was a woman, 32 years of age, who had suffered from the disease for several years. She attended the Hospital as an out-patient, and died quite suddenly.

See *Histological Records*, xxx. 2504b; *Surgical Post-Mortem Register* (1903) p. 193.

ACROMEGALY.

2504c. The other half of the preceding specimen, macerated and dried. It shows the great increase in the size of the sella turcica produced by the pressure of the growth. The olivary eminence has disappeared, the sella sloping directly backwards from the optic groove. The posterior clinoid processes are very thin, and there has been considerable absorption of the body of the sphenoid.   1905.

For references, see under the preceding description.

SERIES XXXIII.

DISEASES AND INJURIES OF THE EYE AND ITS APPENDAGES.

ORBITAL EXOSTOSIS SPRINGING FROM THE FRONTAL SINUS.

2569a. A bony tumour removed from the left orbit. It consists of a firm thin plate of bone with nodular prominences, and is coated by a layer of soft tissue.   1905.

Microscopic Examination.—The hard tissue is true membrane-bone with numerous osteoblasts; no cartilage is present. The soft tissue coating it is a mucous membrane identical with that of the nose, and covered by stratified columnar epithelium.

From a woman aged 39 years. For twelve months she had suffered from constant headache and lachrymation, and for six months from gradually increasing proptosis of the left eye. A hard nodular tumour was felt at the upper margin of the orbit, pushing the globe downwards and forwards, and causing great limitation of upward movement. An incision was made along the brow, and through this the growth was removed. A probe could then be passed through the seat of attachment into the frontal sinus, where the tumour doubtless originated. No disease could, however, be found either in the nose or in any of the accessory sinuses.

See *Histological Records*, xxxiii. 2569a; *Ophthalmic Ward Notes* (1905), No. 136.

CARCINOMA OF CONJUNCTIVA.

2578b. Section of an eye, showing a small growth springing from the conjunctiva at the outer side of the sclero-corneal junction. The growth has a warty appearance, and does not infiltrate the proper structures of the eye, though adherent to the sclerotic.   1905.

Microscopic Examination shows the tumour to be a squamous-celled carcinoma, with cell-nests. There is very little infiltration.

From a man aged 64 years. The growth had only been noticed for a month. There was no glandular affection.

See *Histological Records*, xxxiii. 2578b; *Ophthalmic Ward Notes* (1903), No. 1220.

MELANOTIC SARCOMA OF CONJUNCTIVA.

2578c. The outer half of an eye, with its appendages, showing a pigmented new growth occupying the space between the globe and the upper lid, and protruding forward between the lids. The tumour is assumed to have originated in the conjunctiva: the iris and choroid are natural; the only structure of the globe which is infiltrated is the cornea, and this only in its outermost layers, just beneath Bowman's membrane.   1905.

Microscopic Examination.—The growth is a melanotic sarcoma, composed chiefly of large round cells, only a few of which are pigmented.

From a woman aged 62 years. The mass came down from beneath the upper lid, and obscured the sight about four months previous to her admission to the Hospital. The patient asserted that a small "blister" had appeared just above the cornea four years before, and had gradually increased in size. Vision was not quite lost: on pulling down the lower lid the patient could count fingers. The pupil also reacted to light. There was a very slight detachment of the retina. A complete exenteration of the orbit was performed. There was no evidence while in Hospital of any recurrence, or of any secondary growth elsewhere. Eighteen months later the patient was still in good health.

See *Histological Records,* xxxiii. 2578c; *Ophthalmic Ward Notes* (1904), No. 354.

CILIARY STAPHYLOMA.

2584a. Oblique section through an eye, presenting an enormous staphyloma of·the ciliary region. The cornea is not bulged, though it is opaque and shows pigment in its substance. The staphyloma is situated above and to the outer side of the cornea. It measures 15 mm. in diameter, and projects about 7 mm.; the oblique diameter of the eye to the summit of the projection is 35 mm. The sclerotic in the ciliary region is thinned and atrophic, and there is evidence of old choroiditis. An iridectomy seems to have been performed below. The retina is not detached.   1905.

Microscopic Examination shows only an atrophic condition of the thinned sclerotic.

From a woman aged 35 years, who had suffered from smallpox in infancy, and had probably had a perforating ulcer of the cornea.

Presented by Frank Broadbent, Esq.

ADHESION OF RETINA TO CORNEAL WOUND.

2592b. Vertical section through a left eye, showing the results of an old injury. The cornea is opaque, except above and below, owing to the presence of a dense transverse scar. The anterior chamber is almost obliterated, and the lens has entirely disappeared. A deeply pigmented cyclitic membrane stretches across the eye in the ciliary region; this is penetrated by a whitish cord, which represents the detached retina, extending from the back of the eye to the corneal scar, to which it is firmly adherent. The greater part of the globe is occupied by an albuminous fluid which has been coagulated by the preservative.   1905.

Microscopic Examination shows that the degenerated remains of the retina are in actual contact with the corneal scar.

Removed from a boy 7 years of age. Three years previously he had been struck in the eye by a piece of glass, which had produced total blindness. Excision was performed because the other eye showed signs of sympathetic irritation.

See *Histological Records,* xxxiii. 2592b; *Ophthalmic Ward Notes* (1904), No. 3290.

ADHESION OF CAPSULE TO WOUND AFTER EXTRACTION OF LENS.

2593e. Vertical section of a right eye, showing an untoward sequel of an extraction for cataract. The scar of the incision is seen at the upper part of the sclero-corneal junction, just trespassing on the cornea. Iridectomy has been performed. The capsule of the lens has become caught up and adherent to the extraction wound : the iris is atrophic and adherent below to the cornea : the iridic angle is obliterated. 1905.

Microscopic Examination shows the adhesions between capsule and cornea, and also flattening and congestion of the ciliary processes on the affected side.

From a man aged 68, who suffered from a unilateral cataract of the common senile type. The ordinary extraction was performed, but the eye remained irritable for three months, when plastic iritis developed in the opposite eye. The case was considered to be one of sympathetic ophthalmia, and the exciting eye was therefore removed. The left eye recovered after some months with half vision.

See *Histological Records*, xxxiii. 2593e ; *Ophthalmic Ward Notes* (1905), No. 191.

TUBERCULOSIS OF IRIS.

2604a. Horizontal section through a left eye, with conglomerate tubercle of the iris. A whitish growth springs from the ciliary region and iris, and fills almost the whole of the anterior chamber, displacing the lens backward. The disease has not affected the structures of the posterior chamber. No individual tubercles can be seen : the process takes the form of a diffuse plastic inflammation. 1905.

Microscopic Examination shows the white mass to be inflammatory in nature. Scanty giant cells are present here and there, but the structure is not characteristic of ordinary tubercle. In places the tissue is necrotic, and commencing to caseate. No tubercle bacilli could be demonstrated.

From a girl aged 14 years, admitted to the Hospital for joint trouble, which was diagnosed as tuberculous. She developed plastic iritis while in the Hospital, and this rapidly advanced till the whole anterior chamber was blocked by the exudation. The eye was removed on account of the pain and because vision had been lost. A week later a nodule, as large as a hazel-nut, appeared in the orbit and was removed, but after another three weeks the patient died of tuberculous meningitis and general miliary tuberculosis. Old tuberculous lesions were found in the elbow, kidney, uterus, Fallopian tube, and intestine.

See *Histological Records*, xxxiii. 2604a; *Ophthalmic Ward Notes* (1903), No. 1667 ; *Female Medical Register*, vol. i. (1903), No. 22 ; *Medical Post-Mortem Register* (1903), p. 28.

IRIS BOMBÉ.

2605b₁. Horizontal section through a right eye, showing the results of chronic inflammation of the whole uveal tract. The pupillary margin of the iris is fixed to the capsule of the lens by a complete annular adhesion, and the iris is bulged forward into the anterior chamber. The retina is completely detached everywhere, except in the macular region, where a small fibrous nodule anchors it to the choroid. Elsewhere bands of adhesion may be seen connecting the detached retina and the choroid. The space between the two was filled, in the recent state, with cholesterin crystals. The retina itself is thickened, and shows numerous small hæmorrhages. 1905.

Microscopic Examination shows the iris to be thinned and atrophic. The ciliary processes are in a similar condition. The retina is thickened by chronic inflammation, especially towards the ora serrata, where there are numerous dilated blood-channels The nodule in the macular region consists of very dense fibrous tissue.

Removed, as a painful blind eye, from a boy of 7 years. There was no history of injury, and the child was otherwise healthy. The eye was enlarged, being of about the usual size of a normal adult eye. It had been blind for three years, and painful for most of that time.

See *Histological Records*, xxxiii. 2605b₁; *Ophthalmic Ward Notes* (1903), No. 1067.

LEUCO-SARCOMA OF CHOROID.

2629d. Horizontal section of an eye, showing a small white growth between the retina and sclerotic, to the outer side of the disc. There is no detachment of the retina. Although the growth is small, it has already assumed the "cottage-loaf" form.   1905. ·

Microscopic Examination.—The tumour is a spindle-celled sarcoma, with numerous dilated lymph-spaces, giving it an almost cavernous appearance. No pigment is present.

From a man 60 years of age. The growth is known to have been present for at least a year, and was at first regarded as a cyst. With the ophthalmoscope a prominent nodular swelling was seen on the outer side of the disc, covered by the retina : beneath the retina vessels were seen running over the tumour, which appeared to be choroidal. The growth was white and somewhat translucent. There was no recurrence a year after removal.

See *Histological Records*, xxxiii. 2629d.

SARCOMA OF CHOROID.

2629e. Section of an eye, in which a slightly pigmented sarcoma springs from the choroid on its outer side. The growth shows the characteristic "cottage-loaf" form, resulting from fungation through the inner limiting membrane of the choroid. It has caused complete detachment of the retina.   1905.

Microscopic Examination.—The growth is a spindle-celled sarcoma, honeycombed with dilated lymphatic spaces, with scanty pigment here and there.

From a woman aged 31 years. She gave a history of loss of sight in the right eye for twelve months. She was well fifteen months after excision.

See *Histological Records*, xxxiii. 2629e ; *Ophthalmic Ward Notes* (1904), No. 484.

MELANOTIC SARCOMA.

2629f. Section of an eye, long blind, in which a sarcoma has originated. The anterior chamber is very shallow, and the iridic angle obliterated, owing to chronic cyclitis. From the choroid, close to the disc, an oval tumour projects into the posterior chamber, and has caused complete retinal detachment. It appears to have broken through the choroid at an early period. The basal part of the growth is pigmented ; the apical portion, which is very soft, shows no pigment.   1905.

Microscopic Examination.—The growth is a sarcoma, in places spindle-celled, in places round-celled, but everywhere honeycombed by small lymph-spaces. Not much pigment is visible microscopically.

From a man aged 39 years. The eye had been blind since he was thirteen years old, when some operation had been performed on it. For the past eighteen months the eye had been painful, and it was therefore removed. The presence of the tumour was not suspected till after removal.

See *Histological Records*, xxxiii. 2629f ; *Ophthalmic Ward Notes* (1905), No. 70.

MELANOTIC SARCOMA.

2629g. The inner half of a right eye, showing a melanotic sarcoma bulging into the posterior chamber beneath the retina. It has not yet broken through the inner limiting membrane of the choroid. There is a considerable detachment of the retina away from the tumour at the lower part of the eye. 1905.

Microscopic Examination.—The tumour is a mixed round- and spindle-celled sarcoma, with much pigment and many dilated lymphatic spaces.

From a man aged 57 years, who gave a history of failing sight in his right eye for six months. He could still count fingers in a certain position.

See *Histological Records*, xxxiii. 2629g ; *Ophthalmic Ward Notes* (1905), No. 284.

RUPTURED GLOBE AND DISLOCATION OF LENS.

2640b. The front of a right eye, in which, as the result of a blow, the sclerotic has been ruptured, and the lens dislocated upwards beneath the conjunctiva. The rent in the sclera is situated 4 mm. above the sclerocorneal junction. The anterior chamber contains blood-clot, and the iris is displaced backwards over the upper third of its extent. Here the edge of the lens can be seen through the cornea, but its greater part lies beneath the conjunctiva. 1905.

From a man aged 42, who was struck in the eye by a potato two weeks before the eye was removed.

See *Ophthalmic Ward Notes* (1901), No. 1846.

FOREIGN BODY IN THE VITREOUS.

2651e. Horizontal section through an eye injured by a fragment of stone. In the lower part of the cornea, at its junction with the sclera, is a linear white scar, marking the spot where the foreign body entered the eye. The prolapsed iris has been removed. There is a traumatic cataract, and the substance of the lens is protruding through its capsule, both in front and behind. Beneath the lens, resting on the ciliary processes, is the wedge-shaped piece of flint which caused the injury. 1905.

From a man aged 21 years. The accident occurred while he was breaking stones without spectacles. Iridectomy was performed three days later, but as signs of inflammation persisted, the eye was removed fourteen days after the injury, when the foreign body—the presence of which had been strongly suspected—was found in the situation shown.

See *Ophthalmic Ward Notes* (1903), No. 2255.

RETINAL HÆMORRHAGE FROM THROMBOSIS.

2653a. Horizontal section of a left eye, showing numerous retinal hæmorrhages scattered diffusely over every part of the fundus. The condition is probably associated with thrombosis of the retinal veins. The retina is thickened, and pale lines border the blood-vessels. There are a few hæmorrhages in the vitreous also, just behind the lens. The lens presents a small central opacity. 1905.

Microscopic Examination.—The retina is thickened by diffuse blood extravasation. Near the disc is a group of veins, showing a fibrinous coagulum not yet organised, but containing a few cells.

From a woman aged 64 years. Four months previously she had suddenly lost the sight of her left eye. There was no evidence of cardiac or renal disease. The eye was painful, and showed increased tension. It was therefore removed.

See *Histological Records*, xxxiii. 2653a ; *Ophthalmic Ward Notes* (1901), No. 2086.

CYCLITIS AND RETINAL DETACHMENT.

2654b. Horizontal section of a highly myopic eye, upon which the operation of needling the lens had been performed four years previously. The eye is large, exceeding the normal adult measurements by 3 mm. in length and 2 mm. in width. The lens has disappeared, only the remains of the capsule being visible. A condition of cyclitis appears to have been set up, with much proliferation of pigment in the ciliary region. The iris has become folded forward on itself all the way round, so that the pupil is very large, and is surrounded by a densely black ring, representing the uveal pigment of the back of the iris. Outside this black ring the iris is adherent to the cornea, with obliteration of the iridic angle. The vitreous humour has been completely absorbed, and in the process of shrinking has dragged the retina from its natural position. The detached retina forms a cord, which gradually widens as it passes forward from the disc to the lens capsule, to which it is adherent. The retina has further undergone cystic degeneration; one well-marked cyst is visible, and others are present on the under surface of the cord-like mass. The space between the choroid and the detached retina was occupied, in the fresh condition, by a blood-stained mucoid fluid. 1905.

Microscopic Examination.—The iris is seen to be folded upon itself, the uveal layer being continued round the margin of the pupil on to the front of the iris. The retina is thickened, folded, and in a state of chronic inflammation.

From a girl aged 15 years, who presented fifteen diopters of myopia in each eye. Four years previously two needling operations had been performed to break up the lens. Three and a half years later the retina was found to be detached. The eye became painful, and was removed six months later. The left eye, upon which a similar needling operation had been performed, had much improved vision in consequence.

See *Histological Records*, xxxiii. 2654b; *Ophthalmic Ward Notes* (1902), No. 2110.

RETINITIS PROLIFERANS.

2655a. Horizontal section of a right eye, showing the condition known as "retinitis proliferans," following an old injury. The cornea and lens are natural, but the iridic angle is obliterated, and there are some posterior synechiæ. The retina is completely detached, and is gathered up into a thickened, funnel-shaped mass, adherent to the capsule of the lens, and covered in front by a white layer of scar tissue. Fibrous bands here and there unite the detached mass with the choroid. 1905.

Microscopic Examination.—The detached mass of retina is greatly thickened and thrown into folds. The thickening is chiefly due to an extensive new formation of fibrous tissue in the retinal substance, with a general proliferation of its supporting structures. There is no evidence of any increase in its nervous elements. The mass is bounded in front by dense scar tissue.

From a boy aged 13 years. Nine years previously he had received a blow, followed by a "black eye," and soon afterwards by an internal squint. Four years after the injury he was admitted to the Hospital. He then presented a white mass projecting from the fundus in the lower and outer quadrant, with vessels running over it. The eye was soft, and there was no perception of light. The condition was diagnosed as retinitis proliferans. Five years later the eye became painful, and was excised.

See *Histological Records*, xxxiii. 2655a; *Ophthalmic Ward Notes* (1897), No. 94 and (1902) No. 224.

EARLY GLIOMA.

2663b₁. Horizontal section through the left eye of a child, showing a comparatively early stage of retinal glioma. The growth springs from the nasal side of the retina, and protrudes into the cavity of the eye, with very little detachment of the retina on that side. On the temporal side there is some slight detachment. The growth is white, and shows no degeneration. It does not extend to the optic nerve, and all the other structures of the eye are natural.   1905.

Microscopic Examination shows the growth to be a typical retinal glioma, with
· the cells characteristically arranged round the numerous blood-vessels. The
optic nerve was healthy.
From a girl aged 6 years and 3 months. A "brass-plate" reflex had first been
noticed at six years of age. She could just count fingers with the affected eye.
See *Histological Records.* xxxiii. 2663b₁ ; *Ophthalmic Ward Notes* (1905), No. 248.

GLIOMA.

2663c₁. Section through a child's eye, showing an advanced stage of retinal glioma. The retina is detached, and is diffusely involved by the growth, which, however, by no means fills the eye. The other structures of the globe are natural.   1905.

Microscopic Examination.—The growth has the characters of a "glioma" in its
later stages, having lost the perivascular arrangement of the cells.
The history of the case is unknown.

BILATERAL GLIOMA.

2663d₁. Section through the right eye of an infant, showing an advanced retinal glioma. The entire retina is affected, and the growth almost fills the globe. The other structures of the eye are healthy, and the optic nerve is not invaded.   1905.

Microscopic Examination.—The growth has the ordinary characters of retinal
glioma, being built up of small rounded cells having a honeycombed arrangement, and grouped round the blood-vessels. The optic nerve showed no
infiltration.
Removed from a male child aged 11 months. For two and a half months
the mother had noticed a "brass-plate" reflex from the pupil. Eighteen
months after removal of the eye a similar condition was found in the left eye.
Operation was advised but refused, but after another seven months, the child
having become totally blind and having suffered from fits for four months, the
left eye was removed, and is preserved in the following specimen, No. 2663d₂.
The left orbit later became the seat of recurrent growth, and the child died
about nine months after the excision of the second eye.
See *Histological Records*, xxxiii. 2663d₁ and 2663d₂ ; *Ophthalmic Ward Notes*
(1902), No. 1231 and (1904) No. 1690.

BILATERAL GLIOMA.

2663d₂. Section through the left eye of the child from whom the preceding specimen was removed. It shows an advanced stage of retinal glioma, in which most of the growth has softened and broken down into a grumous material which has disappeared in the preparation of the specimen. The eye is seen to be much enlarged as compared with its fellow, the measurements being actually greater than those of an adult eye. The sclera is thinned and the cornea opaque save at the margin. The iridic angle is obliterated, and the iris is adherent and atrophied. The retina is completely detached, and forms a hæmorrhagic mass with areas of caseation. The optic nerve is thickened and much infiltrated with gliomatous growth. The growth also extends into the choroid, around the optic disc. 1905.

Microscopic Examination shows the growth to be of the same character as that in the preceding specimen, but with much hæmorrhage and degeneration. The most recent growth is that in the choroid ; the optic nerve is practically replaced by new growth.

The history and references will be found under the preceding specimen, No. 2663d₁. The absence of any infiltration of the optic nerve in the first eye removed renders it probable that the disease originated independently in the two eyes.

ADVANCED GLIOMA.

2666b. Horizontal section of a left eye, the cavity of which is completely filled with gliomatous growth. The point of origin of the growth cannot be determined, nor can the position of the retina be seen. The anterior chamber is very shallow, and the iridic angle is obliterated. The tumour is moulded to the back of the lens, and is of a marbled white colour.

1905.

Microscopic Examination.—The growth has the ordinary characters of retinal glioma, though in many parts the perivascular arrangement of the cells is obscured. The optic nerve is densely infiltrated with growth near the globe, but at 12 mm. from the globe proved healthy.

From a male child aged 3 years. A "brass-plate" reflex had been noticed in the left eye for three months. On admission to the Hospital the tension was + 2 ; the eye was totally blind, and the white mass of the tumour could be seen applied to the back of the lens.

See *Histological Records*, xxxiii. 2666b; *Ophthalmic Ward Notes* (1904) No. 3054.

SERIES XXXIX.

DISEASES OF THE PROSTATE GLAND.

ENUCLEATION OF PROSTATE.

2848c. A prostate gland, greatly enlarged, which has been enucleated entire. All the three lobes of the gland are enlarged, the middle lobe forming a large pale projection of the size and shape of a testicle at the posterior extremity of the specimen. A glass rod has been passed through the urethra. 1905.

Microscopic Examination shows a combination of dense fibrosis, with patches of adenomatous overgrowth.

Removed by operation from a man aged 69, who had suffered from difficult micturition for five years. Catheterisation being impossible, the prostate was removed through the bladder, and the patient left the Hospital cured, being able to discharge his urine by the urethra.

See *Histological Records*, xxxix. 2848c ; and *Male Surgical Register*, vol. ii. (1905), No. 762.

SERIES XL.

DISEASES OF THE PENIS.

SQUAMOUS-CELLED CARCINOMA.

2897b. A penis which is the seat of a cancerous growth. On the dorsal surface of the foreskin there is an irregular warty tumour, the edges of which are markedly everted. The growth was very hard. The glans appears not to be infiltrated, but before removal a distinct hard cord of lymphatic infiltration could be traced along the dorsum of the penis.

1905.

Microscopic Examination.—The growth is a typical squamous-celled carcinoma.

Removed by operation from a man aged 50, who had noticed some ulceration of his foreskin for about a year. He had suffered severely from gonorrhœa twenty years previously, and since then had never been free from urethral discharge. The glands in the groin were infiltrated and were removed at the time of the amputation.

See *Histological Records*, xl. 2897b ; and *Male Surgical Register*, vol. iv. (1905), No. 985.

SERIES XLI.

DISEASES OF THE OVARIES.

"CLUSTER-CYST" OF OVARY.

2904b₁. A lobulated ovarian cyst, two portions of which are connected with the ovary by pedicles. These pedicles have undergone torsion, which has led to extravasation of blood into the cavities. Adherent to the cyst are a portion of omentum and the vermiform appendix. The latter in the recent state contained 3 or 4 drachms of pus. 1905.

Microscopic Examination.—The largest lobe of the tumour is composed partially of ovarian stroma. The other lobes are cystic. The wall is lined by columnar epithelium, which forms small papillary projections into the lumen.

Removed by operation from a lady of 32, who had for twelve months suffered from symptoms of pelvic inflammation. The opposite ovary was also cystic, and had attained the size of a cocoa-nut. The patient made an uninterrupted recovery.

See *Histological Records*, xli. 2904b₁.

Presented by W. S. A. Griffith, M.D.

HÆMATOMA OF OVARY.

2910c. An ovary and part of the Fallopian tube. The central part of the ovary contains a hæmatoma; the tissues around are infiltrated with blood. At the periphery several Graafian follicles are visible. 1905.

Microscopic Examination.—The sections show blood extravasations into the ovarian stroma. No chorionic villi or other evidences of gestation are seen.

Removed by operation from an unmarried girl of 19, who was seized by a sudden attack of acute pain in the right iliac fossa accompanied by vomiting. The pulse frequently rose to 112, but the temperature remained normal. There was no hæmorrhage from the vagina. A tender elastic swelling was detected in the right posterior quadrant of the pelvis. Abdominal section was performed, and the swelling proved to be the enlarged right ovary; this ruptured during removal and about 1 oz. of dark fluid blood escaped.

See *Histological Records*, xli. 2910c; and *Female Surgical Register*, vol. i. (1905), No. 345; also *Lancet*, vol. i. (1905), p. 1196.

CYSTIC TERATOMA.

2917e. An ovary greatly enlarged by the growth of a cystic teratoma. The organ is replaced by a cystic tumour, the cavity of which is filled with hair. At the lower part of the cyst-wall is a small solid mass, covered by skin from which hair is growing abundantly (the embryoma). At the upper part of the specimen is seen the Fallopian tube. 1905

Microscopic Examination.—The embryoma contains a canal lined by mucous membrane, indistinguishable from that of the large intestine; hair follicles, sebaceous glands, nervous tissue and unstriped muscle are also present, with many large giant-cells. No hair follicles are present over the greater part of the cyst-wall, which is lined by a sort of granulation tissue in which small hairs have become accidentally included.

Removed per vaginam from a woman of 49, who had suffered from menorrhagia for some years previous to the menopause, which occurred ten months before admission to the Hospital. The patient sought relief because of prolapsus uteri, and the tumour was discovered during the routine examination.

See *Histological Records*, xli. 2917e; *Female Medical Register*, vol. vi. (1904), No. 263; *Obstetrical Society's Transactions* (1904).

SERIES XLII.

DISEASES OF THE UTERINE APPENDAGES.

CYST OF THE PAROVARIUM.

2923d. Portion of a large unilocular cyst on the inner wall of which are seen a number of small warty growths. The Fallopian tube, tortuous and greatly elongated, runs over the surface; the ostium is flattened and spread out on the surface of the tumour; its position is indicated by a coloured glass rod and one of its fimbriæ extends on to the surface of a pedunculated warty growth the size of a goose's egg, which is attached to the outer surface of the cyst wall. The ovary and part of the broad ligament have been removed with the cyst. The cyst contained clear watery fluid.

1905.

Microscopic Examination.—The warty growths are composed of cellular connective tissue covered by polymorphous epithelium.

Removed by operation from a woman aged 21 years, who suffered from abdominal enlargement without any other symptoms.

See *Histological Records*, xlii. 2923d ; *Female Surgical Register*, vol. v. (1905), No. 609.

DOUBLE PYOSALPINX.

2936c. Fallopian tubes and ovaries showing a condition of double pyosalpinx. The tubes are enormously thickened and the right is distended with inspissated pus. The peritoneal surfaces show many adhesions, and are reddened from long-standing inflammation. The fimbriated ends are completely sealed and obscured by adhesions. The ovaries show early cystic degeneration, and are densely adherent to the tubes, the whole forming a closely matted tumour.　　　　1905.

Microscopic Examination.—The walls of the tube are very much thickened, containing much fibrous tissue, and are very vascular. The epithelium is degenerate and, in many places, shed.

From a woman aged 47, who had suffered from more or less continuous abdominal pain for twelve years. She had borne three living children and had had three miscarriages, the last six years before admission. Latterly she suffered from menorrhagia. A fibroid and double pyosalpinx were diagnosed and the uterus and appendages removed by abdominal section. Recovery was complete.

See *Histological Records*, xlii. 2936c ; and *Female Medical Register*, vol. vi. (1904), No. 38.

HYDRO-SALPINX WITH TORSION OF PEDICLE.

2937. An ovary and Fallopian tube showing a hydro-salpinx which has undergone torsion. The tube is distended, its lumen increasing in diameter from the uterine attachment to the fimbriated termination. A window has been cut in the sac at its dilated extremity. Torsion of the pedicle has occurred near to the uterine attachment ; the tube has undergone three complete rotations. The wall of the hydro-salpinx is discoloured from effused blood.　　　　1905.

Removed by operation from an unmarried girl of 18, who three days previously had suffered from a sudden attack of severe abdominal pain, at first localised in the right iliac fossa, later becoming more diffuse. This was followed by vomiting and abdominal distension. A diagnosis of appendicitis was made.

See *Obstetrical Society's Transactions* (1905), p. 5.

Presented by Norman Maclaren, F.R.C.S.

SERIES XLIII.

DISEASES OF THE UTERUS.

MUCOUS POLYPUS.

2967c.   A uterus from the cervix of which a mucous polypus is hanging. The uterus is enlarged, and contains a small fibroid at the fundus. 1905.

Microscopic Examination.—The growth is covered by stratified squamous epithelium, and shows numerous spaces lined with columnar epithelium in a loose fibrous tissue matrix.

From an Italian woman aged 53, who died suddenly of fatty heart and aortic regurgitation, on the day of her admission to the Hospital. No history was obtainable.

See *Histological Records*, xliii. 2967c ; *Female Medical Register*, vol. vi. (1904), No. 334 ; *Medical Post-Mortem Register*, vol. xxxi., p. 144.

FIBRO-MYOMA SHOWING EARLY NECROTIC DEGENERATION.

2996e.   A uterus, containing a large fibro-myoma. At one side of the lower part of the specimen is the uterine cavity ; the anterior wall is occupied by a large interstitial fibro-myoma, which has undergone the form of degeneration described as "necrobiosis." The tissues of the tumour are softened, and in the recent state were stained a uniform red colour.   1905.

Microscopic Examination.—The tumour is unusually vascular, in places the tissues are very degenerate, and nuclear staining is lost ; patches of small-celled infiltration are seen.

Removed by abdominal section from a woman 38 years of age. Enlargement of the abdomen had been noticed for eighteen months previous to the operation. Ten months before operation the patient became pregnant for the first time, and was delivered at full term of a healthy male child ; a fortnight after delivery she was suddenly seized with a severe attack of abdominal pain, the temperature rose to 101° F. and the pulse frequency was increased. On examination a tumour, very tender to the touch, was discovered rising from the pelvis and reaching nearly to the costal arch. After operation the symptoms subsided, and the patient made an uninterrupted recovery.

See *Histological Records*, xliii. 2996e ; *Obstetrical Society's Transactions*, vol. xlvi., p. 274.

Presented by Alban Doran, F.R.C.S.

DEGENERATING FIBRO-MYOMA.

2996f.   A fibro-myoma of the uterus which has undergone extensive mucoid degeneration. In the lower part of the specimen is an area of white fibrous-looking tissue which is still firm and solid ; the rest of the tumour has become converted into a jelly-like mass by a process of mucoid degeneration.   1905.

Microscopic Examination shows that the degenerative change commences as a mucoid transformation of the interstitial material between the muscle cells.

Where most advanced, all resemblance to fibro-myoma tissue is lost. The growth is very vascular.

Removed by operation from a woman of 36 in the fifth month of her ninth pregnancy. For two months previous to admission into Hospital, she had suffered from severe abdominal pain. On admission the abdomen was very tender, the temperature was raised to 100.6° F. and the pulse frequency was 110. The uterus was enlarged, its size corresponding with that of the fifth month of gestation, and to its left could be felt a tumour the size of a child's head. The abdomen was opened, and the tumour found to be a sub-peritoneal fibroid, lying between the two layers of the left broad ligament. The tumour was enucleated and the patient made a good recovery, but aborted the day after the operation.

See *Histological Records*, xliii. 2996f; *Female Medical Register*, vol. vi. (1905), No. 113.

DEGENERATING FIBRO-MYOMA.

2996g. Half of a uterus. The posterior wall contains a solitary interstitial fibro-myoma which has undergone degenerative change.   In the recent state the tissues of the fibro-myoma were soft and semi-fluid, and stained a bright pink colour.   The cavity of the uterus, measuring five inches in length, is encroached upon by the growth of the tumour.   1905.

Microscopic Examination of the tumour shows that in the greater part of its extent it has undergone necrotic change, having lost all nuclear staining. In places it is infiltrated with polynuclear leucocytes.

From a single woman, aged 29 years, who had suffered from metrorrhagia for twelve months. Two weeks before her admission to the Hospital she had been attacked by stabbing pains in the lower part of the abdomen, which were relieved by recumbency. The uterus was removed by operation, and the patient made a good recovery.

See *Female Surgical Register*, vol. i. (1905), 1249; and *Histological Records*, xliii. 2996g.

FIBRO-MYOMA OF THE UTERUS WITH CARCINOMA OF THE CERVIX.

3004c. A uterus with a large interstitial fibro-myoma, together with a carcinoma of the cervix.   The cavity of the uterus is compressed by the fibroid which is growing in the substance of the posterior and upper wall. The cervical portion of the uterus is elongated, and its lips thickened and ulcerated by carcinomatous infiltration.   1905.

Microscopic Examination.—The large tumour is an ordinary fibro-myoma; the growth in the cervix is a squamous-celled carcinoma.

Removed by abdominal section from a woman aged 42, who had suffered from almost continuous vaginal bleeding for six months. The discharge had been offensive for two months, and for four months she had been getting noticeably thinner. She recovered completely from the operation.

See *Histological Records*, xliii. 3004c; *Female Surgical Register* (1904), vol. ii., No. 1819; *Female Medical Register*, vol. vi. (1904), No. 478.

GRAPE-LIKE SARCOMA OF CERVIX.

3009c. A large tumour removed from the enlarged anterior lip of a cervix uteri. It occupied· and greatly distended the vagina. The central part of the mass is composed of a firm whitish tissue; from it spring a number of branching processes, many of which exhibit semi-translucent cyst-like dilatations. In the recent state some of these were as large as a cherry, and the mass somewhat resembled a bunch of grapes. Some of the smaller ·cysts spring directly from the surface of the larger ones. In the lower part of the mass there has been a considerable extravasation of blood.

1905.

Microscopic Examination shows the central mass to be an oval and spindle-celled sarcoma with a considerable amount of fibrous stroma. The swollen grape-like bodies are much less cellular, and resemble a loose fibrous tissue in a condition of extreme œdema. No mucin could be found in the fresh fluid expressed from them. They are covered with a thin layer of stratified squamous epithelium.

From a married woman aged 39 years,who had borne seven children,the last eight years previously. Four years before the operation her menses had become more profuse. Eighteen months before the operation a polypus had been removed from the cervix, but a year later several polypi were found in the same situation. On admission to the Hospital a ragged mass was found occupying the vagina and filling the pelvis. It was attached by a broad pedicle to the anterior lip of the cervix, and was removed by the ecraseur. The uterus was firmly fixed and could not be removed.

See *Histological Records*, xliii. 3009c; *Female Medical Register*, vol. vi. (1904), No. 472; *Obstetrical Society's Transactions* (1905).

SERIES XLIV.

DISEASES OF THE VAGINA AND EXTERNAL ORGANS OF GENERATION IN THE FEMALE.

VAGINAL POLYPUS.

3029a. A lobulated tumour which grew from the mucous membrane of the vagina. It possesses a broad base of vaginal mucosa, to which are attached, by narrow pedicles, four lobes; the largest of these is deeply congested with effused blood.　　　　1905.

Microscopic Examination.—The tumour consists of loose fibrous tissue through which are scattered many cells of irregular size and shape. It contains large blood channels lined by endothelium; its surface is covered by stratified squamous epithelium.

Removed by operation from the anterior vaginal wall of a primi-gravida aged 20, in whom gestation had advanced to the eighth month. The only symptom of which she complained was that something protruded from the vulva.

See *Histological Records*, xliv. 3029a.

Presented by Dr. C. Hubert Roberts.

DISEASES OF THE MAMMARY GLANDS.

SARCOMA.

3163e$_2$. Section of a breast occupied by a large malignant growth. On the cut surface it is seen that the whole of the breast-tissue has been replaced by the growth, which is whitish in colour, and dotted with paler necrotic areas. In some places the original capsule of the gland still limits the tumour. In other places the skin is involved, and presents nodules of varying size.   1905.

Microscopic Examination.—The tumour is a sarcoma, composed of cells, mostly rounded, but irregular in shape and size. There are considerable areas of necrosis.

Removed by operation from a woman aged 46 years. She had first noticed a small swelling in the left breast nine months before admission to the Hospital. It had rapidly increased and become painful; at times there was some discharge from the nipple. On admission she was found to be in a condition of mental stupor. The breast was removed, but the patient died within twenty-four hours. Secondary deposits were found to be present in the brain, in the pancreas, and in the supra-renals. The axillary glands were involved.

See *Histological Records*, xlviii. 3163e$_2$; *Female Surgical Register*, vol. v. (1905), No. 541 ; *Surgical Post-Mortem Register* (1905), p. 33.

FUNGATING CARCINOMA.

3180. A female breast, showing a nodular cancerous growth involving the skin in many places, and excavated by ulceration. One ulcer is very large and deep, with thick, everted edges.   1905.

Microscopic Examination.—A secondarily-infected gland from the axilla showed the growth to be a spheroidal-celled carcinoma undergoing mucoid degeneration.

Removed by operation from a woman aged 52 years. The patient attributed the disease to a blow upon the breast received five months before. She poulticed the swelling until the skin gave way, and persisted in this treatment, in spite of medical advice, until the date of admission.

See *Histological Records*, xlviii. 3180 ; and *Female Surgical Register*, vol. iii., pt. i. (1904), No. 822.

CARCINOMA.

3184e. Section through a breast, showing a rounded and sharply-defined cancerous growth, into which much hæmorrhage has occurred. The growth is situated just below the nipple, which is not retracted.   1905.

Microscopic Examination.—The growth is a spheroidal-celled carcinoma.

From a woman aged 59, who had received a blow on her breast four months previous to her coming to the Hospital. Since then she had noticed a rapidly-growing lump in her breast and much "bruising."

See *Histological Records*, xlviii. 3184e ; *Female Surgical Register*, vol. ii. (1902), No. 2655.

SERIES LVII.

DRAWINGS AND PHOTOGRAPHS OF DISEASED OR INJURED PARTS.

CONTRACTURES.

67c. Two photographs illustrating extreme and generalised contractures.

1905.

The subject was a lad of 16 years, who had for eight years suffered from progressive muscular weakness. The joints affected were not ankylosed, their distortion depending upon unequal contractures of the muscles governing them. The condition was believed to be the sequel of a generalised muscular dystrophy.

See *Male Surgical Register*, vol. ii. (1905), No. 1581.

XANTHOMA DIABETICORUM.

840a. A drawing to illustrate an eruption occurring in the course of acute diabetes mellitus. 1905.

The patient was a man aged 23, who had suffered from polyuria, thirst, and loss of flesh for two months prior to his admission to the Hospital. A few days after his admission a symmetrical eruption appeared over the elbows, and rapidly involved the neck, back, loins, and buttocks. The patient died in a state of coma after an illness of about five months' duration.

See *Male Medical Register*, vol. i. (1905), No. 68; and *Medical Post-Mortem Register*, vol. xxxii., No. 56.

Presented by Sir Dyce Duckworth.

TERATOLOGICAL CATALOGUE.

CONGENITAL ABSENCE OF NASAL CAVITIES AND EXTERNAL AUDITORY MEATUS.

3433a. Median vertical section through a fœtal head, showing various deformities. The eyelids are adherent in their outer halves. The nose is very much flattened, and hardly rises above the surface of the face; the anterior nares are completely absent. The left ear is imperfectly developed, owing to the irregular fusion of its constituent tubercles, and the external auditory meatus is absent. The cut surface shows total absence of the nasal cavities, save for a single small median cavity, completely closed in on all sides, at the extreme front. The posterior nares are represented by a shallow pit. 1905.

From a child born dead at full time. A dissection of the right ear showed that there had been no invagination to form the external auditory meatus; the middle ear appeared normal in size and situation, as was the attic, but the antrum was entirely absent. The outer wall of the tympanum was formed by a well-defined membrane with a smooth inner surface, the outer coming into contact with the parotid gland. Of the ossicles the malleus was normal, but the incus was very small, and its posterior crus short and peg-shaped. The stapes was absent. The internal ear appeared normal, and the seventh and eighth nerves were well developed.

Presented by W. S. A. Griffith, M.D.

MALFORMATION.

3474b. An atlas showing imperfect development of the posterior arch. The laminæ are unusually delicate, and taper rapidly to their extremities, where a thin bridge of bone completes the neural arch. There is no actual union of the laminæ behind, although they come into close contact. 1905.

From the dissecting-room.

MALFORMATION.

3488b. A sacrum in which the spinal canal is left completely open by an arrested development of the laminæ and spinous processes of its constituent vertebræ. 1905.

From a disused burial-ground on the site of Christ's Hospital.

CONGENITAL ABSENCE OF GALL-BLADDER.

3623a₁. A liver showing complete absence of the gall-bladder. The hepatic duct is seen running from the hilum of the liver, and the papilla marking its opening into the duodenum is very well marked. There is no trace of a gall-bladder, but a small branch, cut off short in the specimen, is given off from the hepatic duct in the situation of the cystic duct, which it probably represents.   1905.

From a child aged 3, who died of mitral disease.
See *Female Medical Register*, vol. iii. (1903), No. 32 ; and *Medical Post-Mortem Register*, vol. xxx., p. 56.

CONGENITAL INTERRUPTION OF ILEUM.

3635e. A portion of small intestine from an infant, showing a congenital interruption of the ileum. The gut ends blindly at a spot two feet above the ileo-cæcal valve, and begins again after an interruption of about an inch. There is no sign of any connection between the two blind ends. The upper part of the intestine is dilated and the lower collapsed. 1905.

From a female infant, admitted to the Hospital on the fourth day of her life. She had been born at full term, of 7 lbs. weight. She had passed meconium in small amount on the first day, but none since. Vomiting began on the second day, and was constant until death on the eighth day. The vomit was profuse, occurring at intervals of about one hour, and was frequently bile-stained. *Post mortem* there was no other discoverable abnormality.
See *Female Medical Register*, vol. i. (1905), No. 1 ; and *Medical Post-Mortem Register*, vol. xxxii. (1905), p. 58.

ECTOPIA VESICÆ ET INTESTINI.

3667b. The lower part of the trunk of a newly-born male child, showing extroversion of both intestine and urinary bladder. From a point a short distance above the insertion of the umbilical cord, the dermal, muscular and bony elements of the anterior abdominal and pelvic walls are deficient. Over the upper smooth portion of the defective area the right hypogastric artery is seen passing to the cord. This smooth portion, which seems alone to represent the abdominal wall proper, is bounded below by a narrow transverse ridge of skin. Below the ridge is another smooth surface, forming on either side a triangle, the blunt apex of which meets with its fellow in the middle line. At the lower angle of the base of each of these triangles is the aperture of the corresponding ureter, indicated by a bristle. This area, therefore, at least in part, represents the bladder. Below this the surface is velvety, consisting of intestinal mucous membrane set with villi. The mucosa here forms two conspicuous projections—a pointed, trunk-like one above, and a broader, irregular one below. The upper, trunk-like process is a prolapse of the small intestine through an expanded Meckel's diverticulum. Meconium could be expressed from its apex in the fresh condition. The lower projection simulates, in form and situation, a penis and scrotum ; this, however, is mere simulation, for the penis and scrotum are completely cleft, and the two halves are seen in the groin on either side. There is no trace of large intestine or anus, and the lower projection represents the extroverted mucosa of a sort of cloaca, which leads upwards, in the anal region, to the cavity of a short length of gut terminating blindly above the brim of the pelvis. Three circular infoldings are seen in a transverse row on the lower projection: it is the central one of these which simulates a penis: their nature is not apparent. The testes are undescended.   1905.

The history of the case is unknown.

ANATOMICAL CATALOGUE.

MUSCULAR ATTACHMENTS.

321a.   A set of human bones marked to show the attachments of the principal muscles.   1905.

These bones are of historical interest, as probably the first which were ever marked in this way. They were prepared by Mr. Cornelius Hanbury, when a student at St. Bartholomew's Hospital during the winter session of 1848–49. The circumstances are detailed by him in a letter to the *Lancet*, vol. i. (1905), p. 1297.

Presented by Cornelius Hanbury, Esq.

III.

HISTOLOGICAL RECORDS OF MUSEUM SPECIMENS.

I. **289f.** Section of the bone marrow of the sternum from the case of multiple myelomatosis preserved in No. 289f.

I. **435b.** Sections of the jaw tumour preserved in No. 435b. (*a*) is a section of the main myxomatous portion. (*b*) is a section showing the structure of a round-celled sarcoma, where the muscle is being invaded by the growth.

I. **440a.** Section of the round-celled sarcoma of the scapula preserved in No. 440a.

I. **453c.** Section of the spindle-celled sarcoma of the femur preserved in No. 453c.

I. **456a.** Section of the malignant growth from the vertex of the skull in Specimen No. 456a. It appears to be a columnar-celled carcinoma.

I. **538a.** Section of the new growth of the upper jaw preserved in No. 538a. It appears to be an endothelioma.

VII. **1233e.** Section of the lung from the case of purulent pericarditis preserved in No. 1233e. It shows collapse and bronchiectasis.

VII. **1280b.** (*a*) Section of the gumma of the heart preserved in No. 1280b. (*β*) Section of a coronary artery from the same case, showing an endarteritis indistinguishable from that associated with syphilis. (*γ*) Section of a branch of the same artery showing an identical lesion.

XI. **1690e.** Section of the tuberculous lung with acute emphysema preserved in Specimen No. 1690e.

XI. **1700a.** Section of the pneumonic lung preserved in No. 1700a. It shows grey hepatization.

XI. **1704a.** Section of the tuberculous lung from the case of pyo-pneumothorax preserved in No. 1704a. It shows complete collapse, with scattered tubercles.

XL. **1717.** Section of the specimen of acute pulmonary tuberculosis preserved in No. 1717.

XI. **1723a.** Section of the specimen of chronic tubercle of the lung preserved in No. 1723a.

XI. **1723b.** Section of the caseous tissue about the cavity in the infant's lung in Specimen No. 1723b.

XII. **1777c.** Section of the squamous-celled carcinoma of the lip in Specimen No. 1777c.

XII. **1785a₄.** Section of the papilloma of the tongue preserved in No. 1785a₄.

XVII. **1907a₁.** Section of the pylorus from the case of congenital hypertrophic stenosis in No. 1907a₁.

XVII. **1933a.** Section of the carcinoma of the stomach in Specimen No. 1933a.

XVIII. **2021b.** Section of the malignant growth of the duodenum in Specimen No. 2021b. It is a columnar-celled carcinoma.

XVIII. **2021c.** Section of the malignant growth of the colon in Specimen No. 2021c. It is a columnar-celled carcinoma.

XIX. **2069d.** Section of columnar-celled carcinoma involving the anus in Specimen No. 2069d.

XXI. **2193e.** Section of the cirrhotic liver with perihepatitis preserved in Specimen No. 2193e.

XXI. **2196a₅.** Section of the specimen of tuberculous cholangitis in No. 2196a₅.

XXI. **2239e.** Section of the actinomycotic abscess of the liver in Specimen No. 2239e.

XXIV. **2287b.** Section of the lymphatic glands from the axilla preserved in Specimen No. 2287b. They are infiltrated by spheroidal-celled carcinoma.

XXIV. **2294c.** Section of one of the lymphatic glands in Specimen No. 2294c. It is infiltrated with melanotic sarcoma.

XXVI. **2309a₁.** Section of the mediastinal new growth in Specimen No. 2309a₁. It appears to be an endothelioma.

XXVI. **2311c.** Section of the hypertrophied thyroid gland in Specimen No. 2311c.

XXVI. **2318e.** Section of the primary tumour of the thyroid gland in Specimen No. 2318e. It is a mixed-celled sarcoma.

xxviii. **2335g.** Section of the granular kidney preserved in No. 2335g. It shows the ordinary changes of chronic interstitial nephritis.

xxviii. **2341a$_2$.** Section of one of the tuberculous kidneys in No. 2341a$_2$.

xxviii. **2384.** Section of the cystic kidney preserved in No. 2384. It is taken from the most solid portion of the organ.

xxviii. **2390d$_2$.** Section of the secondary growth in the kidney preserved in No. 2390d$_2$. It is a small round-celled sarcoma.

xxviii. **2390h$_5$.** Section of the primary carcinoma of the kidney preserved in Specimen No. 2390h$_5$.

xxx. **2449d.** Section of the specimen of hæmorrhagic pachymeningitis preserved in No. 2449d.

xxx. **2504b.** Section of the pituitary tumour from the case of acromegaly preserved in Specimen No. 2504b. It appears to be an adenomatous growth.

xxxiii. **2569a.** Section of the bony orbital tumour preserved in No. 2569a. It shows membrane bone covered by nasal mucous membrane.

xxxiii. **2578b.** Section of the squamous-celled carcinoma of the conjunctiva preserved in No. 2578b.

xxxiii. **2578c.** Section of the eye and lids from No. 2578c, showing a melanotic sarcoma of the conjunctiva.

xxxiii. **2592b.** Section of the injured eye preserved in No. 2592b. It shows adhesion of the retina to the corneal wound.

xxxiii. **2593e.** Section of the eye preserved in No. 2593e, showing adhesion of the lens-capsule to the wound after extraction.

xxxiii. **2604a.** Section of the specimen of tuberculous iritis preserved in No. 2604a.

xxxiii. **2605b$_1$.** Section of the specimen of iris bombé and detached retina preserved in No. 2605b$_1$.

xxxiii. **2629d.** Section of the leuco-sarcoma of the choroid preserved in No. 2629d.

xxxiii. **2629e.** Section of the choroidal sarcoma preserved in No. 2629e.

xxxiii. **2629f.** Section of the choroidal sarcoma preserved in No. 2629f.

xxxiii. **2629g.** Section of the melanotic sarcoma of the choroid in No. 2629g.

xxxiii. **2653a.** Section of the hæmorrhagic retina preserved in No. 2653a. It shows some small thrombosed veins near the disc.

xxxiii. **2654b.** Section of the detached retina in No. 2654b. It shows thickening and chronic inflammation of the retina, and folding back of the iris upon itself.

xxxiii. **2655a.** Section of the case of retinitis proliferans preserved in No. 2655a. It shows a mass of thickened retina, in a state of chronic inflammation and fibroid proliferation.

xxxiii. **2663b$_1$.** Section of the specimen of retinal glioma preserved in No. 2663b$_1$. It shows the characters of that growth in very typical fashion.

xxxiii. **2663c$_1$.** Section of the retinal glioma preserved in No. 2663c$_1$. It shows the disease in an advanced form.

xxxiii. **2663d$_1$.** Section of retinal glioma from the right eye of an infant.

xxxiii. **2663d$_2$.** Sections from the left eye of the same child two years later. (*a*) is a section of the disc and detached retina, showing degenerate gliomatous growth. (*b*) is a section of the infiltrated optic nerve.

xxxiii. **2666b.** Sections from the case of retinal glioma preserved in No. 2666b. (*a*) is a section of the main growth filling the eye. (*b*) shows the optic nerve in two situations. The more deeply stained section is from close to the globe, the more lightly stained is at a greater distance, where the infiltration has almost ceased.

xxxix. **2848c.** Section of the enlarged prostate gland preserved in No. 2848c. It shows adenomatous overgrowth and fibrosis.

xl. **2897b.** Section of the tumour of the penis in No. 2897b. It is a squamous-celled carcinoma.

xl. **2904b$_1$.** Section of the "cluster-cyst" of the ovary preserved in No. 2904b$_1$. The cyst-wall is lined by columnar epithelium forming papillary projections into the cavity.

xli. **2910c.** Section of the hæmatoma of the ovary preserved in No. 2910c. There are no chorionic villi or other evidences of gestation.

xli. **2917e.** Section of the cystic teratoma of the ovary preserved in No. 2917e. It shows a canal lined by mucous membrane indistinguishable from that of the large intestine; also hair-follicles, sebaceous glands, nervous and unstriped muscular tissues.

xlii. **2923d.** Section of the parovarian cyst preserved in No. 2923d. It shows a cellular connective-tissue covered by polymorphous epithelium.

xlii. **2936c.** Section of the pyo-salpinx preserved in No. 2936c. The walls of the tube are greatly thickened and contain much fibrous tissue. The epithelium lining them is degenerate.

xliii. **2967c.** Section of the mucous polypus of the cervix preserved in No. 2967c. The tumour is covered with squamous epithelium, and contains spaces lined by columnar epithelium.

xliii. **2996e.** Section of the fibro-myoma of the uterus preserved in No. 2996e.

xliii. **2996f.** Section of the degenerating fibro-myoma of the uterus preserved in No. 2996f.

xliii. **2996g.** Section of the degenerating fibro-myoma of the uterus preserved in No. 2996g.

xliii. **3004c.** (α) Section of the fibro-myoma of the uterus preserved in No. 3004e. (β) Section of the growth in the cervix uteri of the same specimen. It is a squamous-celled carcinoma.

xliii. **3009c.** (α) Section of the central mass of the grape-like sarcoma of the cervix uteri preserved in No. 3009c. It is a spindle-celled sarcoma. (β) Section of one of the grape-like bodies. It gives the appearance of a loose fibrous tissue in a condition of extreme œdema.

xliv. **3029a.** Section of the vaginal polypus preserved in No. 3029a. It shows a loose fibrous tissue traversed by large blood-channels and covered by stratified squamous epithelium.

xlviii. **3163e$_2$.** Section of the sarcoma of the breast preserved in specimen No. 3163e$_2$.

xlviii. **3180.** Section of the spheroidal-celled carcinoma of the breast preserved in No. 3180.

xlviii. **3184e.** Section of the spheroidal-celled carcinoma of the breast preserved in No. 3184e.

BOOKS ADDED TO THE LIBRARY.
1905.

	Presented by

Caton, Richard, M.D. The Harveian Oration, delivered before the Royal College of Physicians on June 21, 1904 . . . .
    I. I-em-Hotep and Ancient Egyptian Medicine . . . .
    II. Prevention of Valvular Disease. Lond. 1904 . . . .
	THE ORATOR.

Howes, John (M.S. 1582). Being "a brief note of the order and manner of the proceedings in the first erection of" The Three Royal Hospitals of Christ, Bridewell, and St. Thomas the Apostle. Reproduced. Lond. 1904 .	SEPTIMUS VAUGHAN MORGAN, Esq.
Grant, Frederick James, F.R.C.S. From our Dead Selves to Higher Things. A Course of Human Experience and Progressive Development. Lond. 1904	THE AUTHOR.
Grant, Frederick James, F.R.C.S. Modern Natural Theology, with the Testimony of Christian Evidences. Lond. 1904	THE AUTHOR.
Andrewes, F. W., M.D. Lessons in Disinfection and Sterilisation. Lond. 1903	THE AUTHOR.
Edwards, F. Swinford, F.R.C.S. Carcinoma of the Rectum : its Diagnosis and Treatment. Lond. 1905 . .	THE AUTHOR.
Hamer, W. H., M.D. Manual of Hygiene. Lond. 1902 . . .	THE AUTHOR.
Paton, D. Noel, M.D. Essentials of Human Physiology (2nd Edition). Edinburgh, 1905	W. BALFOUR GOURLAY, Esq.
Pick, T. Pickering, F.R.C.S., and Howden, Robert, M.B. Gray's Anatomy, Descriptive and Surgical (16th Edition). Lond. 1905 . . .	THE PUBLISHERS.

Presented by

Klein, E. E., M.D., F.R.S. Experiments and Observations on the Vitality of the Bacillus of Typhoid Fever, and of Sewage Microbes in Oysters and other Shellfish. Investigations on behalf of the Worshipful Company of Fishmongers. Lond. 1905 . . . } THE AUTHOR.

Rawling, Louis Bathe, F.R.C.S. Landmarks and Surface Markings of the Human Body (2nd Edition). Lond. 1905 . . . . . . } THE AUTHOR.

Report of the Inter-Departmental Committee on Physical Deterioration. Lond. 1904 . . . . . } BRITISH MEDICAL TEMPERANCE ASSOCIATION.

An Atlas of Illustrations of Clinical Medicine, Surgery, and Pathology, compiled for the New Sydenham Society (Fasciculi 21, 22, 23, 24) . } NEW SYDENHAM SOCIETY.

von Bergmann, Prof. E., M.D., von Bruns, Prof. P., M.D., von Mikulicz, Prof. J., M.D. A System of Practical Surgery. Translated and Edited by William T. Bull, M.D., and Walton Martin, M.D. Vols. 1–5. New York, 1904 .

Cabot, Richard C., M.D. A Guide to the Clinical Examination of the Blood for Diagnostic Purposes (5th Revised Edition). Lond. 1904 . . .

Green, T. Henry, M.D. An Introduction to Pathology and Morbid Anatomy. Revised and Enlarged by W. Cecil Bosanquet, M.D. (10th Edition). Lond. 1905 . . . . .

Hektoen, Ludwig, M.D., and Riesman, David, M.D. A Text-book of Pathology. Lond. 1902 . . .

Hutchison, Robert, M.D. Lectures on Diseases of Children. Lond. 1904 .

Hutchison, Robert, M.D., and Rainy, Harry, M.A. Clinical Methods: A Guide to the Practical Study of Medicine (3rd Edition). Lond. 1905 .

Kelly, Howard A., M.D., and Hurdon, E., M.D. The Vermiform Appendix and its Diseases. Lond. 1905 . .

Lewers, Arthur H. N., M.D. A Practical Text-book of the Diseases of Women (6th Edition). Lond. 1903

} THE LIBRARY COMMITTEE.

Presented by

Osler, William, M.D. The Principles and Practice of Medicine (5th Edition). Lond. 1905 . . . . .

Osler, William, M.D. The Principles and Practice of Medicine (6th Edition). Lond. 1905 . . . . .

Rose, William, M.B., and Carless, Albert, M.S. A Manual of Surgery for Students and Practitioners (6th Edition). Lond. 1905 . . .

Starling, Ernest H., M.D. Elements of Human Physiology (7th Edition). Lond. 1905 . . . .

Taylor, Frederick, M.D. A Manual of the Practice of Medicine (7th Edition). Lond. 1904 . . . . .

THE LIBRARY COMMITTEE.

SUMMARY OF SCHOLARSHIPS AND PRIZES

Obtainable by Students at St. Bartholomew's Hospital.

AT ENTRANCE :—

Senior Entrance Scholarship in Science	£75	0	0
Senior Entrance Scholarship in Science	75	0	0
Junior Entrance Scholarship in Science	150	0	0
Preliminary Scientific Exhibition .	50	0	0
Jeaffreson Exhibition .	20	0	0
Shuter Scholarship	50	0	0

AT END OF FIRST YEAR :—

Junior Scholarship in Anatomy and Biology (First) .	30	0	0
Junior Scholarship in Anatomy and Biology (Second) .	20	0	0
Junior Scholarship in Chemistry and Physics and Histology (First) .	25	0	0
Junior Scholarship in Chemistry and Physics and Histology (Second)	15	0	0
Treasurer's Prize .	5		0

AT END OF SECOND YEAR :—

Senior Scholarship	50	0	0
Foster Prize	5	0	0
Harvey Prize	6	6	0
Wix Prize .	5	0	0
Hichens Prize	6	0	0

AT END OF THIRD AND LATER YEARS :—

Lawrence Scholarship and Gold Medal .	45	0	0
Kirkes Scholarship and Gold Medal	30	0	0
Brackenbury Medical Scholarship .	39	0	0
Brackenbury Surgical Scholarship	39	0	0
Sir George Burrows Prize .	10	10	0
Skynner Prize .	13	13	0
Bentley Prize .	5	5	0
Matthews Duncan Prize and Gold Medal	20	0	0
Willett Medal for Operative Surgery .	3	3	0
Walsham Prize in Surgical Pathology	7	7	0
Luther Holden Scholarship .	105	0	0

The total value of the Scholarships and Prizes
awarded annually is about £890.

EXAMINATIONS, 1903-1904.

Lawrence Scholarship and Gold Medal—
  C. M. H. HOWELL.

Brackenbury Medical Scholarship—
  A. R. NELIGAN.

Brackenbury Surgical Scholarship—
  A. F. HAMILTON.

Matthews Duncan Prizes—
  C. W. HUTT. }
  J. K. WILLIS. } Æq.

Senior Scholarship in Anatomy, Physiology, and Chemistry—
  P. L. GIUSEPPI.

Senior Entrance Scholarships in Science—
  1. G. C. E. SIMPSON.
  2. F. W. W. GRIFFIN. }
   J. J. PATERSON. } Æq.

Junior Entrance Scholarship in Science—
  T. L. BOMFORD.

Preliminary Scientific Exhibition—
  H. H. KING.

Jeaffreson Exhibition—
  A. J. S. FULLER.

Shuter Scholarship—
  T. S. HELE.

*Kirkes Scholarship and Gold Medal—*E. E. MAPLES.

*Bentley Prize—*J. R. R. TRIST.

*Hichens Prize—*H. D. DAVIS.

*Wix Prize—*C. A. STIDSTON.

*Harvey Prize—*H. BLAKEWAY.

Sir George Burrows Prize—
  E. H. SHAW. }
  K. S. WISE. } Æq.

*Skynner Prize—*K. S. WISE.

PRACTICAL ANATOMY.

JUNIOR.	SENIOR.
*Treasurer's Prize—*1. A. J. S. FULLER.	*Foster Prize—*1. M. FAWKES.
2. T. L. BOMFORD.	2. G. H. DIVE.
3. W. W. WELLS.	3. H. O. WILLIAMS.
4. R. B. PRICE.	4. E. R. JONES.
5. N. E. DAVIS.	
6. F. E. SEARLE.	
7. H. H. KING.	
8. J. RAMSAY.	

Junior Scholarships in Anatomy and Biology (1904)—
  1. T. L. BOMFORD. }
   H. H. KING. } Æq.

Junior Scholarships in Chemistry and Histology (1903)—
  1. P. HAMILL.   2. R. L. DOWNER.

EXAMINATIONS, 1904-1905.

Lawrence Scholarship and Gold Medal—
E. H. SHAW.

Brackenbury Medical Scholarship—
C. W. HUTT.

Brackenbury Surgical Scholarship—
H. W. WILSON.

Matthews Duncan Medal—
G. O. E. SIMPSON.

Matthews Duncan Prize—
P. L. GIUSEPPI. } Æq.
E. H. SHAW.

Senior Scholarship in Anatomy, Physiology, and Chemistry—
E. M. WOODMAN.

Senior Entrance Scholarships in Science—
1. E. P. CUMBERBATCH.   2. G. GRAHAM.

Junior Entrance Scholarship in Science—
T. S. LUKIS.

Preliminary Scientific Exhibition—
G. R. LYNN.

Jeaffreson Exhibition—
K. C. BOMFORD.

*Shuter Scholarship—*R. B. SEYMOUR SEWELL.

Kirkes Scholarship and Gold Medal—
J. K. WILLIS. } Æq.
J. G. WATKINS.

*Willett Medal—*H. W. WILSON.

*Walsham Prize—*E. H. SHAW.

*Bentley Prize—*P. L. Giuseppi.

*Hichens Prize—*F. W. W. GRIFFIN.

*Wix Prize—*W. B. GRANDAGE.

*Harvey Prize—*A. E. GOW.   *Certificate—*A. J. S. FULLER.

*Sir George Burrows Prize—*J. G. GIBB.

*Skynner Prize—*J. G. GIBB.

PRACTICAL ANATOMY.

JUNIOR.	SENIOR.
*Treasurer's Prize—*1. T. S. LUKIS.	*Foster Prize—*1. T. L. BOMFORD.
2. G. R. LYNN.	2. F. C. SEARLE.
3. R. R. SMITH.	3. R. B. PRICE.
4. A. P. FRY.	4. A. L. CANDLER.
5. A. L. WEAKLEY.	

Junior Scholarships in Anatomy and Biology (1905)—
A. P. FRY. } Æq.
R. R. SMITH.

Junior Scholarships in Chemistry and Histology (1904)—
1. T. L. BOMFORD.   2. H. H. KING.

ST. BARTHOLOMEW'S HOSPITAL & COLLEGE.

THE MEDICAL AND SURGICAL STAFF.

Consulting Physicians—Sir William Selby Church, Bart., K.C.B., Dr. Hensley, Sir Lauder Brunton, F.R.S., Dr. Gee, Sir Dyce Duckworth.·

Consulting Surgeons—Sir Thomas Smith, Bart., K.C.V.O., Mr. Willett, Mr. Butlin, Prof. Marsh, Mr. Langton.

Consulting Ophthalmic Surgeon—Mr. Henry Power.

Physicians—Dr. Norman Moore, Dr. S. West, Dr. Ormerod, Dr. Herringham, Dr. Tooth, C.M.G.

Surgeons—Mr. Cripps, Mr. Bruce Clarke, Mr. Bowlby, C.M.G., Mr. Lockwood, Mr. D'Arcy Power.

Assistant-Physicians—Dr. A. E. Garrod, Dr. Calvert, Dr. Morley Fletcher, Dr. J. H. Drysdale, Dr. Horton-Smith Hartley.

Assistant-Surgeons—Mr. Waring, Mr. M'Adam Eccles, Mr. Bailey, Mr. Harmer, Mr. Rawling.

Physician-Accoucheur—Dr. Champneys.

Assistant-Physician-Accoucheur—Dr. Griffith.

Ophthalmic Surgeons—Mr. Jessop, Mr. Holmes Spicer.

Aural Surgeon—Mr. Cumberbatch.

Pathologist—Dr. F. W. Andrewes.

Dental Surgeons—Mr. Paterson, Mr. Ackery.

Assistant-Dental Surgeons—Mr. Ackland, Dr. Austen.

Administrators of Anæsthetics—Mr. Gill, Dr. Edgar Willett.

Junior Administrators—Mr. Cross, Mr. Boyle.

Medical Registrars—Dr. Horder, ——.

Surgical Registrar—Mr. Gask.

Medical Officer in charge of the Electrical Department—Dr. Lewis Jones.

Casualty Physicians—Dr. Branson, Dr. Howell.

LECTURES AND DEMONSTRATIONS.

Medicine—Dr. Norman Moore, Dr. West.

Clinical Medicine—Dr. Norman Moore, Dr. S. West, Dr. Ormerod, Dr. Herringham, Dr. Tooth.

Practical Medicine—Dr. J. H. Drysdale, Dr. Hartley.

Junior Demonstrator—Dr. W. Langdon Brown.

Surgery—Mr. Bowlby, C.M.G., Mr. Bruce Clarke.

Clinical Surgery—Mr. Harrison Cripps, Mr. Bruce Clarke, Mr. Bowlby, Mr. Lockwood, Mr. D'Arcy Power.

Practical Surgery—Mr. Bailey, Mr. Rawling.

Junior Demonstrator—Mr. Gask.

Operative Surgery—Mr. Bailey, Mr. M'Adam Eccles, Mr. Harmer.

Midwifery and the Diseases of Women and Children—Dr. Champneys.

Practical Midwifery—Dr. Williamson.

Pathology—Dr. F. W. Andrewes.

Bacteriology (Advanced)—Dr. E. E. Klein.

Chemical Pathology—Dr. Garrod, Dr. Hurtley.

Morbid Anatomy—Dr. Horder, ——.

Practical Pathology—Mr. Rose, Dr. Thursfield.

Junior Demonstrators—Mr. Jennings, Dr. Riviere.

Post-mortems—Dr. Horder, ——, Mr. Gask.

Ophthalmic Medicine and Surgery—Mr. Jessop.

Diseases of the Eye—Mr. Jessop, Mr. Spicer.

Ophthalmoscopic Demonstrations—Mr. Spicer.

Diseases of the Ear—Mr. Cumberbatch.

Diseases of the Larynx—Mr. Harmer.

Orthopædic Surgery—Mr. M'Adam Eccles.

Diseases of the Skin—Dr. Ormerod.

Diseases of Children—Dr. Garrod, Dr. Morley Fletcher.

Medical Electricity and Electro-Therapeutics—Dr. Lewis Jones.

Mental Diseases and Insanity—Dr. Claye Shaw.

Dental Surgery—Mr. Paterson, Mr. Ackery.

Anæsthetics—Mr. Gill, Mr. Edgar Willett, Mr. Cross, Mr. Boyle.

Forensic Medicine—Dr. Herringham.

Practical Toxicology—Dr. Chattaway, Dr. Hurtley.

Descriptive and Surgical Anatomy—Mr. Waring, Mr. M'Adam Eccles.

Practical Anatomy—Mr. Rawling.

Junior Demonstrators—Mr. West, Mr. Scott, Mr. Watson, Mr. Faulder.

General Anatomy and Physiology—Dr. J. S. Edkins.

Practical Physiology—Dr. J. S. Edkins, Dr. Langdon Brown, Mr. Paterson.

Materia Medica, Pharmacology and Therapeutics—Dr. Calvert.

Pharmacology—Dr. Bainbridge.

Biology and Comparative Anatomy—Dr. Shore.

Practical Biology—Dr. Shore.

Junior Demonstrators—Mr. Griffin, Mr. Bomford.

Chemistry and Practical Chemistry—Dr. F. D. Chattaway, Dr. Hurtley.

Physics and Practical Physics—Mr. F. W. Womack.

Botany—Rev. George Henslow, M.A.

Public Health—Dr. Newman.

Practical Hygiene and Public Health—Dr. Warry.

Museum Curator—Dr. F. W. Andrewes.

Junior Curator—Dr. Branson.

Dean of the School—T. W. SHORE, M.D., B.Sc. Lond.

COLLEGIATE ESTABLISHMENT.
Warden—Mr. G. E. GASK.

Students can reside within the Hospital walls, subject to the College regulations.

Further information may be obtained from Mr. G. E. GASK, F.R.C.S. Eng.

ST. BARTHOLOMEW'S HOSPITAL REPORTS.

VOLUME XLI.

INDEX.

	PAGE
ABDOMINAL wall, cellulitis of, with diphtheritic infection	235
Abernethian Society, proceedings of the	237
Abscess, cerebral, secondary to orbital periostitis	211
,, ,, secondary to old fracture of skull	214
Actinomycosis of the cæcum, vermiform appendix, and right iliac fossa (H. J. Waring, M.S., F.R.C.S.)	197
Adrenalin, risks attending injection of	119
Albuminous expectoration, following paracentesis of the chest (Dr. Horton-Smith Hartley)	77
Albuminous expectoration, apart from paracentesis of chest	108
.. .. ætiology of	104
chemical examination of	82
,, ,, literature of	86
,, ,, table of cases of	87
Alcoholic neuritis (Norman Moore, M.D.)	5
Aneurysm of the aorta, communicating with the superior vena cava and left innominate vein (J. H. Drysdale, M.D.)	71
Aorta, aneurysm of, communicating with superior vena cava	71
Appendix, vermiform, actinomycosis of	197
Ascites, treatment of, by deprivation of salt	25
Auden, G. A., M.D., a series of fatal cases of jaundice in the newborn, occurring in successive pregnancies	139
BACTERIA, share of, in the causation of gall-stones	11
Blood-clotting, tendency to, during life	1

PAGE

Brown, W. Langdon, M.D., on cardiac dropsy in children   .   115
Burfield, J., two cases of diphtheritic infection of operation
     wounds   233

Cæcum, actinomycosis of   197
Cancer of bowel, gastro-jejunostomy for   177
Cardiac dropsy in children (W. Langdon Brown, M.D.) .   .   115
Cellulitis following diphtheritic infection   .   .   .   233
Cervical nerves, sensory areas of   39
Children, pulmonary fibrosis in   123
     ,,   cardiac dropsy in   115
Choroid, tuberculosis of the   183
Cockles, poisoning by   146
Colic, biliary, following typhoid fever   9
Congenital occlusion of the small intestine (C. M. H. Howell,
     M.B.)   135
Congenital occlusion of alimentary canal   .   .   .   137
Cranio-cerebral surgery, cases of (J. B. Rawling, F.R.C.S.)   .   211

Deformities of the liver   15
Diphtheria, infection of operation wounds with   .   .   233
Dorsal nerves, sensory areas of   47
Drysdale, J. H., M.D., a case of aneurysm of the aorta, com-
     municating directly with the superior vena cava and with
     the left innominate vein   71
Duckworth, Sir Dyce, M.D., LL.D., clinical notes respecting a
     tendency to blood-clotting during life   .   .   .   1
Duckworth, Sir Dyce, M.D., LL.D., and Dr. Champneys,
     cases from the wards of (H. U. Gould, M.B.)   .   .   143
Duodenal constriction, gastro-jejunostomy for   .   170, 171, 172
Dyspepsia, severe, gastro-jejunostomy for   .   .   .   173

Endocarditis, malignant   144
Examinations, 1903–1905   294
Expectoration, albuminous, following paracentesis of the
     chest   77
Eye, excision of, in intra-ocular tuberculosis .   .   .   193
Eye, tuberculosis of the   183

PAGE

FIBROSIS of the lung in childhood (Clive Riviere, M.D.) . 123

Forbes, J. Graham, M.D., intra-medullary teratoma of the spinal cord 221

Four cases of cranio-cerebral surgery (L. B. Rawling, F.R.C.S.) 211

GALL-BLADDER, disease of, as cause of Riedel's lobe . 18, 21

Gall-stones, causes of formation of 10

  ,,   ,,   passed after an attack of typhoid fever . . 9

Gastric ulcer, perforation of, simulated by rupture of a pelvic abscess 157

Gastric ulcer, ruptured during labour 155

  ,,   ,,   gastro-jejunostomy for 176

Gastritis, chronic, gastro-jejunostomy for . . . 178, 179

Gastro-jejunostomy (D'Arcy Power, F.R.C.S.) . . . 169

Gould, H. U., M.B., cases from the wards of Sir Dyce Duckworth and Dr. Champneys 143

HADFIELD, C. F., and W. P. Herringham, M.D., cases of ascites treated by deprivation of salt 25

Hartley, *see* Horton-Smith Hartley.

Hawes, C. S., three cases of primary malignant disease of the liver 161

Herringham, W. P., M.D., cases of Riedel's lobe, with remarks on the various deformities of the liver 15

Herringham, W. P., M.D., and C. F. Hadfield, cases of ascites treated by deprivation of salt 25

Holden, Luther, F.R.C.S., the late, *In Memoriam* . . . xxxi

Horder, T. J., M.D., a case of complete transposition of viscera in an adult 111

Horton-Smith Hartley, P., M.D., albuminous expectoration following paracentesis of the chest 77

Hottentots, primary malignant disease of the liver in . . 161

Howell, C. M. H., M.D., a case of congenital occlusion of the small intestine 135

Hyperinosis 1

ILIAC fossa, actinomycosis in 197

Innominate vein, communication of an aortic aneurysm with . 71

PAGE

Intestine, congenital occlusion of the small . . . 135
Intra-medullary teratoma of the spinal cord (J. Graham Forbes,
    M.D.) 221
Intra-ocular tuberculosis (W. H. Jessop, F.R.C.S.) . . 183
Iris, tuberculosis of the 190
Iritis, tubercular 191

JAUNDICE, series of fatal cases of, in the newborn, occurring
    in successive pregnancies (G. A. Auden, M.D.) . . 139
Jessop, W. H., F.R.C.S., intra-ocular tuberculosis . . . 183

LABOUR, rupture of a gastric ulcer during 155
Langton, John, F.R.C.S., *In Memoriam* Luther Holden . . xxxi
Library, books added to the 289
Liver, deformities of the 15
   „ primary malignant disease of, three cases (C. S. Hawes) . 161
   „ Riedel's lobe of 15
   „ of tight-lacing 19
Lumbar nerves, sensory areas of 56
Lung, acute œdema of, as a cause of albuminous expectoration 105
   „ fibrosis of, in childhood 123

MALIGNANT disease, primary, of liver 161
Meconium, presence of, below a congenital occlusion of the
    small intestine 136
Moore, Norman, M.D., alcoholic neuritis 5
Murmur, due to communication of an aortic aneurysm with the
    superior vena cava 72
Muscular fibres in teratoma of spinal cord 224
Museum, specimens revised and added to the . . . 243

NEURITIS, alcoholic 5
Newborn infants, fatal form of jaundice in 139

ŒDEMA of lung, as a cause of albuminous expectoration . . 105
Operation wounds, diphtheritic infection of 233
Orbit, periostites of the, followed by a cerebral abscess . . 211
Ovariotomy 152

PAGE

PARACENTESIS of chest, albuminous expectoration after . . 77
Pelvic abscess, rupture of, simulating perforation of a gastric
  ulcer 157
Pelvic inflammation, simple stricture of rectum following . 158
Pernicious anæmia, albuminous expectoration in a case of . 78
Phlebitis, after gastro-jejunostomy 172
Pleuritic effusion, diagnosis of, from consolidation of lung . 152
Pneumonia, rapidly fatal 147
  „ without physical signs 147
Post-colic gastro-jejunostomy 170
Power, D'Arcy, F.R.C.S., a year's gastro-jejunostomies . . 169
Prizes and scholarships, summary of 293
  „ „ award of 294
Pulmonary fibrosis, complications of 129
  .. „ diagnosis of 130
  „ in childhood 123
  .. „ prognosis of 131
  „ „ signs of 127
Pyloric adhesions, gastro-jejunostomy for 181
  „ obstruction, gastro-jejunostomy for 177

RAWLING, L. B., F.R.C.S., four cases of cranio-cerebral surgery 211
Rectum, simple stricture of, following pelvic inflammation . 158
Rheumatic fever, hæmaturia in 148
  „ „ with pericarditis and dilatation of heart . 148
Riedel's lobe of liver 15
Rigors in typhoid fever, significance of 150
Riviere, Clive, M.D., pulmonary fibrosis in childhood . . 123
Round worm, pyrexia and vomiting relieved by passage of . 148

SACRAL nerves, sensory areas of 63
Salt, deprivation of, in treatment of ascites 25
Scalp, cellulitis of, followed by diphtheritic infection . . 233
Scholarships and prizes, summary of 293
Segmental spinal sensory areas, clinically considered (H. H.
  Tooth, M.D.) 37
Sensory spinal areas 37
Skull, fractures of 214, 217, 218
Spinal cord, teratoma of, intra-medullary 221
  „ tumours of, classification of 225

PAGE

Spinal cord, tumours of, bibliography of   230

Stomach, dilated, gastro-jejunostomy for   .   . 173, 174, 175

,,   chronic ulcer of, gastro-jejunostomy for (*see also*

        gastric ulcer)   176

TERATOMA, intra-medullary, of spinal cord   221

Thrombosis during life, causes of 2

Tight-lacing, deformity of liver caused by   .   .   . 19

Tooth, H. H., M.D., the segmental spinal sensory areas

     clinically considered   37

Transposition of viscera, complete, in an adult (T. J. Horder,

     M.D.) 111

Trephining for fracture of skull 214, 217

Trunk, segmental, sensory areas of the 51

Tuberculin, value of, in treatment and diagnosis   .   . 193

Tuberculosis, intra-ocular   183

Two cases of diphtheritic infection of operation wounds

     (J. Burfield) 233

Typhoid fever, biliary colic following   9

,,   ,,   occurrence of a rigor in 150

ULCER of stomach, *see* gastric ulcer.

VENA cava superior, communication of an aortic aneurysm with 71

Vermiform appendix, actinomycosis of 197

Viscera, complete transposition of 111

WARING, H. J., F.R.C.S., actinomycosis of the cæcum, vermi-

     form appendix, and right iliac fossa   .   .   . 197

West, Samuel, M.D., a case of typhoid fever followed by biliary

     colic and the passage of gall-stones 9

GENERAL INDEX

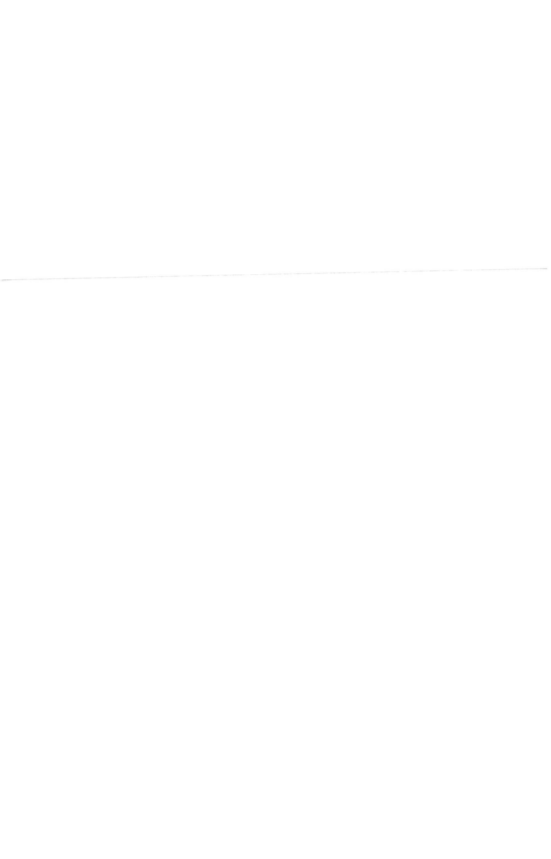

A GENERAL INDEX

TO THE

SECOND TWENTY VOLUMES

(VOLS. XXI–XL)

OF THE

ST. BARTHOLOMEW'S HOSPITAL REPORTS

FROM

1885—1904

COMPILED BY

W. McADAM ECCLES, M.S., F.R.C.S.

LONDON

SMITH, ELDER & CO., 15 WATERLOO PLACE

1906

Printed by BALLANTYNE, HANSON & CO.
At the Ballantyne Press

PREFACE.

In 1885, Sir William Church compiled and published a General Index to the first twenty volumes of the Hospital Reports. This has proved of immense value.

I have endeavoured to repeat for Vols. xxi.–xl. what he so ably performed for Vols. i.–xx.

I have to acknowledge my great indebtedness to Dr. C. Medlicott, without whose generous assistance this index would never, I fear, have seen its completion.

As far as possible the arrangement of the previous index has been followed, except that under an author's name his papers have been given in alphabetical and not in chronological order, it having been pointed out that this was the more convenient method. Doubtless there are omissions and errors, but it is hoped that they will but slightly detract from the usefulness of the pages.

W. McAdam Eccles.

January 1906.

LIST OF ILLUSTRATIONS.

VOL. XXI. (1885).

	PAGE
Sections of the medulla oblongata and spinal cord	142
Diagram illustrating the production of the respiratory sounds .	192
Illustration of an apparatus for producing expansion and contraction of the lungs without the admission of fresh air	194
Diagrams illustrating the production of unnatural respiratory sounds	199, 202
Diagram illustrating the movement of the air in the lungs and trachea .	204
Illustration of the artificial thorax	207
,, ,, a sliding frame for the artificial thorax	208
,, ,, ,, ,, ,, ,, ,, with lung *in situ*	208
Diagrams illustrating paper on the temperature after death (*Womack*) .	255

VOL. XXII. (1886).

Rickety curvature of the legs, before and after treatment by osteotomy .	241
Sarcoma of the ribs	249
Sketch of cooling and warming apparatus (*Brunton* and *Cash*) . .	275
Diagrams of the temperatures of pigeons and guinea-pigs treated by aconite	276–280, 282–285
Sketch of apparatus used in experimenting on the absorption of gas by the intestines (*Brunton* and *Cash* on Carminatives) . . .	290, 291

VOL. XXIII. (1887).

Diagram of the physical signs of the chest of Fanny P. (pneumothorax of the right side)	37
Illustrations of twenty foreign bodies removed from the rectum . .	81
Diagrams illustrating the amount of pulsation in case of aortic aneurysm (*Martin*)	84, 88
Four sections of the spinal cord	142
Section of the medulla at the lower third of the olive	145
Diagram representing the confluence of the mitral and aortic orifices after boiling	162
Diagram illustrating a vertical section of the aorta and the auriculo-ventricular ring	163
Diagrams illustrating the different directions and degrees of obliquity taken by the different fibres of the heart	166
Diagrams showing the rate of cooling after death	194, 197
Multiple polypi of the lower bowel (lithograph) . . *To face page*	228
Temperature charts of three patients treated by continuous warm baths . . . . *To face page*	266

VOL. XXIV. (1888).

PAGE

Diagrams showing the position of some chronic ulcers of the tongue
(*Butlin*) 84, 85, 86
Diagram showing sections of the spinal cord in a case of disseminated
sclerosis (*Ormerod*) 158
Dislocation of the shoulder-joint (*Evill*) 164
Case of uterine dilators (*Godson*) 171
The end of a walking-stick which entered the brain through the orbit . 181
Punctured fracture of the orbital plate of the frontal bone . . . 185
A hat-peg which entered the orbit and became impacted . . . 194
A piece of glass removed from an eyeball 202
Section of the eyeball, showing the position of the piece of glass in
the eye 202
Charts showing the amounts of urea, uric acid, and acidity, with the
temperature, in a case of gout 218, 220, 222
Seven illustrations of sinus over the sacrum and coccyx . . . 231,
233, 236, 237, 238, 239
Outline of the brain of the cat in a normal and abnormal condition . 244
The same seen in longitudinal section 244

VOL. XXV. (1889).

Three illustrations to show the condition of the neck in case of goître
(*Berry* and *Jessop*) . . . . . *To face page* 100
Section of a portion of the goître 101
Two illustrations to show wasting of the muscles of the lower extremi-
ties in a case of progressive muscular atrophy 146
Microscopic appearance of a portion of a deposit of actinomyces in
the liver 162
Portions of the above more highly magnified 163

VOL. XXVI. (1890).

Diagram to illustrate the acidity and the amounts of urea and uric
acid present in urine 46
Vertical section through frontal region of the brain, to show the
situation of softening 63
Lithograph of fibromatous growth in the skin of the neck *To face page* 148
Microscopical section of growth in the skin of the neck . . . 151
Mortality chart of cholera and influenza 207
Temperature charts of influenza 212, 242
Drawing of stud and piece of trimming removed from the nose . . 273

VOL. XXVII. (1891).

Plate illustrating paper on nasal obstruction (*Walsham*) . *To face page* 32
Bladder, showing a calculus imbedded in its walls . . . 121, 123
Diagram of the relative position of the nerve nuclei beneath floor of
the fourth ventricle (after *Gowers*) 147
Diagram showing the relation of age to gastric ulcer in male and
female cases (*Habershon*) 152
Diagrams showing the absolute liability of each age to gastric ulcer
in male and female cases 153
Plate illustrating cases of unusual forms of carcinoma of the breast
(*Masterman*) . . . . *To face page* 204

PAGE

Diagrammatic representation of the brain of bonnet-monkey, showing
the position of the motor and sensory centres 226
Diagrammatic representation showing the localisation of the motor
centres (after *Horsley*) 228
The outer surface of the left half of the brain of the orang-outan
(after *Horsley*) 229
Diagram showing the distribution of the middle cerebral artery (after
Ross) 230
Diagram of the outer surface of the left hemisphere, showing the dis-
tribution of the vessels (from *Ross*, after *Seller* and *Duret*) . . 231
Representation of a " barley hale " which passed down the trachea . 251

VOL. XXVIII. (1892).

Section of the lower end of the femur, showing a cavity containing an
old sequestrum 10
Gelatinous naso-pharyngeal polypus 70
Liver in a case of cirrhosis 169
Spleen from the same case 169
Section of cirrhosed liver, showing the thickened capsule of Glisson
and increased fibrous tissue 171
Diagrammatic figures showing areas of loss of sensation to heat and
cold 212, 214, 215, 218
Sections through the kidney in a case of sprouting endocardial growths 223
Section through the liver in a case of sprouting endocardial growths . 225
Diagram of the systemic and pulmonary circulations 258
Temperature charts of cases of general spastic rigidity . . . 266, 273
Typo-etchings of a case of general spastic rigidity . . . 269, 270
Outline sketch ,, ,, ,, ... 274
Tracings of the blood-pressure of a rabbit under the influence of com-
mercial amyl nitrite 283
Tracings of the blood-pressure of a rabbit under the influence of amyl
nitrite and iso-butyl nitrite 284
Tracings of the blood-pressure of a rabbit under influence of Bertone's
ether 285
Tracings of the blood-pressure of a rabbit under the influence of pure
amyl nitrite 285

VOL. XXIX. (1893).

Interior of operating theatre attached to Martha ward . *To face page* 1
Operating table . . . . ,, ,, 2
Tables for dressings and instruments . . . . ,, ,, 3
Irrigator 3
Sterilisers . . . . *To face page* 4
Instrument case 5
Uterus with ovaries, one of which is cystic and papillomatous, the other
papillomatous . . . . *To face page* 26
An unusual form of nodule upon the joints of the fingers . . . 158
Torsion of the spermatic cord, causing strangulation of the epididymis. 164
,, ,, ,, ,, ,, causing strangulation of the testis and
epididymis in a dog 168
Rodent ulcer 194
Outline drawings of sections of the pons 218
,, ,, ,, ,, medulla . . . . . 219—221
Diagrammatic outlines of the pupil 297
,, drawings of blood extravasated into the layers of the
cornea 298, 299
,, drawing of fundus of an eye 301

                                                                              PAGE
Diagrams of the visual fields of the eyes 301, 302
Diagrammatic drawing of an ossified choroid 303
      ,,   ,,   the legs in pseudo-hypertrophic paralysis   . 329

VOL. XXX. (1894).

Sections of grain   116
Absence of pectoral muscles   126
Tracing, showing the action of amyl nitrites   190
     ,,   ,,   ,,   effect of hydroxylamine hydrochlorate .   .   . 191
Bipolar electrode   207
The left side of brain, to show seat of lesion   213
Abdomen, showing situation of wound in right iliac colotomy   .   . 219

VOL. XXXI. (1895).

Diagram showing age of onset of epilepsy   64
Primary sarcoma of vagina in child 124, 125

VOL. XXXII. (1896).

Temperature charts illustrating cases (*Church*) 8, 14
     ,,   ,,   ,,   ,, (*Herringham*)   .   .   . 108–113
Skin grafting   171
Charts illustrating leucocytosis of scarlet fever   241–259
     ,,   ,,   treatment of anæmia by oxygen   .   .   . 322–332
     ,,   ,,   ætiology of chorea   388–393
Some cases of deformity 400–402
Microphotographs of degenerate nerves in alcoholic paralysis   .   . 412

VOL. XXXIV. (1898).

Fig. 1. Skiagram of a healthy thorax (*H. Walsham*)   .   *To face page*   29
Fig. 2. Skiagram of the lungs of a fœtus that had never breathed
    (*H. Walsham*)   .   .   .   .   .   .   *To face page*   29
Fig. 3. Skiagram of the chest, from a case of chronic pulmonary tuber-
    culosis (*H. Walsham*) .   .   .   .   .   *To face page*   30
Fig. 4. Skiagram of the chest, from a case of tubercular consolidation
    of the right apex (*H. Walsham*)   .   .   .   *To face page*   30
Fig. 5. Skiagram of the chest, from a case which presented the physical
    signs of enlarged bronchial glands (*H. Walsham*)   *To face page*   31
Fig. 6. Skiagram of the chest, from a case of fibroid phthisis of the left
    lung (*H. Walsham*)   .   .   .   .   .   *To face page*   31
Fig. 7. Skiagram of the chest, from a case of aneurism of the transverse
    aorta (*H. Walsham*)   .   .   .   .   .   *To face page*   31
Fig. 7. Amputation of the breast, showing the skin incisions employed
    in Halsted's method (*Butlin*)   64
Fig. 8. Amputation of the breast, showing later stages of Halsted's
    method (*Butlin*)   65
Fig. 9. Photograph of a patient, to show the range of movement of
    which the arm is capable after Halsted's operation of amputation
    of the breast (*Butlin*)   67
Fig. 10. Diagram of the field of vision of the right eye of a patient who
    had partial hemianopia after a fracture of the base of the skull
    (*H. G. Wood-Hill*)   259

VOL. XXXV. (1899).

PAGE

Dr. A. A. Kanthack . . . . *Frontispiece*
A case of Graves' disease, with extreme emaciation (*Herringham*)—
 Before the illness . . . . *To face page* 125
 On admission . . . . ,, ,, 126
 In July 1898 . . . . ,, ,, 127
Section through the cornea and iris, from a case of hypopyon
 (*Turner*) . . . . *To face page* 142
Talipes spasticus—
 Left foot (*Joseph Griffiths*) . . . . . ,, ,, 181
 Section of left foot . . . . ,, ,, 181
 Section of right foot . . . . ,, ,, 181
 Section of the right foot of a normal fœtus at full time ,, ,, 182
 Casts of the feet of a child with talipes spasticus (*Kent Hughes*)
 To face page 182
Diagram of the appearances seen in a case of gangrenous appendicitis
 (*Willett* and *Cholmeley*) 212

VOL. XXXVI. (1900).

Sir James Paget, Bart., F.R.S. . . . . *Frontispiece*
Facsimile of Sir James Paget's handwriting 18
Drawings of a peculiar form of spinal deformity (*Herbert Mundy*) . 56, 57
Perimeter charts from a case of diabetes insipidus (*Bousfield*) . . 240, 241

VOL. XXXVII. (1901).

Perimeter chart of case (*Bull*) 187
Diagram showing seat of primary carcinomatous tumours of the breast . 304
Perimeter chart of case (*Jessop*) 316
A new form of cataract knife 318
A new form of instrument for the performance of "after-cataract" . 319

VOL. XXXVIII. (1902).

A case of intracapsular fracture—dislocation of the head of the humerus
 (*Preston Maxwell*) 35
Two diagrams of apparatus to illustrate the causation of the first sound
 of the heart (*Inchley*) 92, 96
Five photographs from a case of erythema iris (*Gardner* and *Scott*) 135–139
Two plates showing the minute details of cases of glioma of the retina
 (*Jessop*) . . . . *To face page* 168

VOL. XXXIX. (1903).

The late William Johnson Walsham, M.B., C.M., F.R.C.S. . *Frontispiece*
 (*From a block kindly lent by the "British Medical Journal."*)
Plate I. Sketch map of Gold Coast Colony, showing the route of the
 Boundary Commission on the western frontier, and also the dis-
 tribution of filariasis . . . . *To face page* 171
Plate II., Fig. 1. Photograph of a leprous boy, native of Soko, in the
 Ivory Coast Colony. Fig. 2. Photograph of a leper of Debango, in
 the north of the Ivory Coast Colony . . . . *To face page* 177
Plate III., Fig. 1. Photograph of a case of leucoderma in a native
 woman of the Gold Coast. Fig. 2. Photograph of a case of uni-
 lateral goundou in a native of Enchy, in the Gold Coast
 Colony . . . . *To face page* 179

PAGE

Plate IV. Two drawings of congenital nævoid hypertrophy of the lower lip in a native woman of Soumbala, in the Ivory Coast Colony . . . . *To face page* 180

Plate V. Sketch map of West Africa, showing the route of the Boundary Commission and the distribution of filariasis . . *To face page* 183

Plate VI. Photograph of a native of Kwitta, with enlargement and curvature of both tibiæ . . . . *To face page* 193

VOL. XL. (1904).

Plate I. Sections of spinal cord, showing combined degeneration (*Ormerod*)—

Fig. 1. Cervical region . . . . . . *To face page* 30

Fig. 2. Mid-dorsal region . . . . . . ,,   ,, 30

Fig. 3. Lumbar region . . . . . . ,,   ,, 30

Plate II. Tuberculosis of the female breast (*S. R. Scott*) . *To face page* 100

Diagram showing position of the abscesses in case of appendicitis (*Compton*) 145

GENERAL INDEX.

(VOLS. XXI.–XL.)

	VOL.	PAGE
Abdomen, case of injury to and disease of (*Mayo, Willett,* and *Hawes*)	XXXVII.	273
contusions of (*Mayo, Willett,* and *Hawes*)	XXXVII.	273
hydatids in, drained through bladder	XXV.	261
incision of, for tubercular peritonitis	XXIX.	81
Abdominal abscesses	XXI.	242
cyst, a remarkable case of (*Sir Thomas Smith*)	XXXIV.	1
section, action of the recti muscles in	XXVIII.	17
,, dressings in	XXVIII.	22
,, for ovariotomy	XXIX.	1
,, ,, ,, after-treatment of	XXIX.	20
,, ,, ,, closure of wound	XXIX.	18
,, ,, ,, death-rate after	XXIX.	22
,, ,, ,, dressings in	XXIX.	19
,, ,, ,, instruments for	XXIX.	4
,, ,, ,, sutures in	XXIX.	19
,, ,, ,, rupture of small intestine	XXXIV.	276
,, hernia through cicatrix of	XXVIII.	23
,, incision in	XXVIII.	17, 20
,, mortality after	XXIX.	22
,, preparation of patient for	XXVIII.	17
,, sutures in	XXVIII.	21
,, table of cases admitted into Martha (*Cripps*)	XXXV.	25
,, treatment of distended bowels in	XXVIII.	20
tumour, post-mortem in a case of	XXV.	252
tumours, discussion on	XXV.	279
,, of	XXXII.	43
wall, abscess of (*Marsh*)	XXXIV.	244
Abductors of vocal cords, paralysis of	XXII.	209
Abnormal synovial cysts in connection with the joints	XXI.	177
use of the great omentum	XXX.	89
Abscess, acute of the tongue	XXV.	257
and cancer of lower jaw	XXIII.	151
,, new growth, diagnosis between (*Marsh*)	XXXIV.	251
associated with epithelioma of mouth	XXIII.	151
cerebral, from a fall, with optic neuritis	XXI.	228
,, with epilepsy	XXIII.	188
cervical, from caries	XXVII.	244
cheek, from unsound wisdom tooth (*Marsh*)	XXXIV.	254
complicating cancer of pelvic glands	XXIII.	152
,, malignant disease of cervical glands	XXIII.	153
,, ,, ,, larynx	XXIII.	153
,, ,, ,, testis	XXIII.	152
connection with ribs (*Marsh*)	XXXIV.	242
diagnosis of acute (*Marsh*)	XXXIV.	241
gall-bladder	XXVIII.	125
,, , gall-stones causing	XXVIII.	123, 126
hemiplegia from cerebral	XXI.	23

2

	VOL.	PAGE
Abscess, iliac, imitated by carcinoma of sigmoid flexure (*Marsh*)	XXXIV.	253
in axilla, giving exit to foreign body from lung	XXVII.	251
ischio-rectal, following foreign body in rectum, treatment of	XXIII.	80
„ T-shaped incision	XXIII.	80
jaw, lower	XXVII.	63
mediastinal	XXVIII.	94
of antrum	XXXIV.	237
„ bone	XXVIII.	8
„ brain (*S. L. O. Young*)	XL.	53
„ breast, simulating carcinoma	XXIII.	149
„ liver, with parametritis	XXI.	173
„ lower jaw	XXVII.	63
„ mediastinum, and intra-thoracic growths	XXVIII.	94
„ septum nasi	XXIII.	128
parotid, in typhoid fever	XXI.	112, 114
pelvic, from injury (*Marsh*)	XXXIV.	255
peri-urethral, cases of (*Mayo, Willett*, and *Hawes*)	XXXVII.	281
points of interest in connection with various forms of (*Marsh*)	XXXIV.	241
post-mammary (*Marsh*)	XXXIV.	249
"shirt-stud" „	XXXIV.	244
sub-gluteal „	XXXIV.	246
sub-pectoral „	XXXIV.	246
sub-periosteal „	XXXIV.	250
thigh, after typhoid fever	XXI.	115
Abscesses, abdominal	XXI.	242
metastatic, of lung following appendicitis	XL.	143
peritoneal, secondary to appendicitis	XL.	143
pyæmic, formation of in osteo-periostitis	XXIX.	271
Absence of both pectoral muscles	XXX.	125
of kidney, a case of (*D'Arcy Power*)	XXXV.	48
Accessory nasal sinuses, chronic purulent catarrh of	XXX.	237
Accidents in the cricket-field (*J. F. Steedman*)	XXXVI.	221
Acid, amount of, in the urine of gout	XXIV.	218, 220, 222
nitro-hydrochloric, its use in uric acid headache	XXIII.	201
uric, a cause of headache (*Haig*)	XXIII.	201
„ its excretion in gout	XXIV.	217
„ the action of some drugs on	XXIV.	217
Aconite, action on guinea-pigs	XXII.	281
„ pigeons	XXII.	275
and cold, action on guinea-pigs	XXII.	282
„ „ pigeons	XXII.	277
„ heat, action on guinea-pigs	XXII.	284
„ „ pigeons	XXII.	279
modifications in the action of, produced by changes in the body-temperature (*Brunton* and *Cash*)	XXII.	271
in rheumatism	XXIV.	23
Acromegaly, overgrowth resembling	XXXII.	405
Actinomycosis, clinical and post-mortem note of a case of	XXV.	159
diagnosis of	XXV.	164
discrepancy in descriptions of	XXV.	164
hominis, a case of (*Waring*)	XXVII.	173
of thoracic wall (*Sir Dyce Duckworth*)	XXXI.	23
Action and reaction, in pathology and therapeutics (*F. P. Weber*)	XXXIX.	139
Acute insanity, its early symptoms	XXIX.	109
Adams (*James*), immunity of puerperal women from infection of diphtheria	XXX.	140

	VOL.	PAGE

Aden, epidemic of plague at, points of interest in˙ (*J. E. Sandilands*) . . . . XXXVI. 61
Adenoid polypi of the lower bowel . . . . XXIII. 225
   vegetations . . . . XXV. 272
      ,,   alteration of voice in . . . . XXVII. 27
      ,,   and enlarged tonsils . . . . XXVII. 25
      ,,   diagnosis of . . . . . XXVII. 27
      ,,   expression of face in . . . . XXVII. 27
      ,,   in naso-pharynx . . . . . XXI. 152
      ,,   ,, vault of pharynx . . . . XXIII. 134
      ,,   symptoms of . . . . . XXVII. 26
      ,,   treatment of . . . . . XXVII. 28
Adenoids and tonsils, operations on (*W. J. Walsham*) . XXXIV. 271
Adenomata, fibro- of breast, removed during the year 1900 . XXXVII. 298
   of the palate . . . . XXII. 330
Adhesion of inferior turbinated body to septum . . XXIII. 133
Adhesions in chronic nasal catarrh . . . . XXVII. 18
   in ovarian operations . . . . . . XXIX. 13
Addisonii morbus, case of . . . . . . XXIV. 253
   nitrite of amyl in . . . . XXIV. 254, 256
   nitro-glycerine in . . . . XXIV. 255, 258
   treatment of . . . . XXIV. 258
Adolescence, general paralysis of (*Weber*) . . . XXXIV. 312
Adrenals, cases of hæmorrhage into (*Talbot*) . . . XXXVI. 207
Adults, gangrene round the mouth in . . . . XXVII. 205
Æther, subcutaneous injection of . . . . . XXV. 182
Africa, West, filariasis in . . . . . . XXXIX. 182
   Gold Coast (*see*).
   goundou in . . . . XXXIX. 179
   guinea-worm, native treatment of in . . . XXXIX. 194
   gynæcology, native, in . . . . . . XXXIX. 204
   leprosy in . . . . XXXIX. 177
   madura foot in . . . . XXXIX. 178
   midwifery, native, in . . . . . . XXXIX. 204
   native method of treatment in (*J. G. Forbes*) . XXXIX. 189
After-treatment of intestinal obstruction . . . XXV. 175
   of ovariotomy . . . . XXIX. 20
   ,, tracheotomy . . . . . XXI. 79 ; XXVIII. 160
Age, in intra-thoracic growths . . . . . XXVIII. 75
   ,, intussusception . . . . XXVIII. 97
Agoraphobia, its cause . . . . XXI. 5
Ague, a cause of paroxysmal hæmaturia . . . XXII. 139
   brassfounders' . . . . XXV. 77
   connection with glycosuria . . . . . XXV. 9
Air, ground, its connection with summer diarrhœa . XXVI. 6
   inhalations in phthisis of hot . . . . XXVI. 91
   its relation to subsoil water . . . . XXVI. 5, 6
   of theatre, report on . . . . . . XXIX. 100
   tubes, cicatricial stricture of . . . . XXV. 223
Albumin, its action when injected subcutaneously . XXIII. 173
Albuminous expectoration . . . . . . XXII. 99
Albuminuria, absence of, in malignant diphtheria . XXIII. 17
   after meals . . . . XXVI. 26
   ,, measles . . . . XXVI. 26
   chronic, in children . . . . . . XXVI. 29
   from gastro-intestinal disturbance . . . XXVI. 28
   in children (*Herringham*) . . . . . XXVI. 25
   ,, diphtheria . . . . XXVIII. 194
   ,, influenza . . . . XXVI. 203
   ,, the apparently healthy (*Levison*) . . XXXV. 169

	VOL.	PAGE
Albuminuria in the new-born	XXVI.	27
prognosis in (*Lewis Jones*)	XXVI.	307
the induction of false	XXIII.	173
toxic, in adults	XXVI.	27
Alcohol, causing neuritis	XXII. 182, 183	
connection with paralysis	XXII. 171, 181	
its use	XXII.	360
Alcoholic cirrhosis (*Weber*)	XXXIV.	321
,,　　(*Yeld*)	XXXIV.	215
hæmatemesis (*Gee*)	XXXVIII.	1
neuritis, three cases of multiple peripheral in women (*Sir Dyce Duckworth*)	XXIII.	253
paralysis, pathology of	XXXII.	407
Alcoholism, treated by hypnotism	XXV.	126
Alexander (*J. Finlay*), notes on a case of operation for the radical cure of a right inguinal hernia, followed by acute gangrenous appendicitis second operation on the ninth day—recovery	XL.	153
Alkalies, their use in diabetes mellitus	XXV.	10
Altitude, effects of, on Graves' disease	XXIX.	186
Alum-whey in typhoid fever	XXI.	117
Amputation at hip	XXXI. 32, 40	
,, ,, when needed	XXIV.	336
,, shoulder	XXI. 183 ; XXIV. 205 ; XXIX. 93 ; XXXIV. 231	
for arrested pulsation in brachial artery	XXV.	259
,, ,, ,, popliteal artery	XXV.	259
,, elephantiasis of leg	XXXII.	183
,, fracture of patella	XXXVII.	272
,, senile gangrene at age of 45	XXXIX.	236
,, ,, tuberculosis of knee	XXXIV.	289
of arm	XXIV. 205, 207 ; XXXVII. 283	
,, breast	XXIV. 287, 297 ; XXIX. 96 ; XXX. 233 ; XXXVII. 217	
,, finger, spastic condition of muscles after	XXIV.	293
,, foot	XXX.	229
,, forearm	XXIV. 285, 299 ; XXV. 259 ; XXIX. 93 ; XXXVII. 217	
,, hand	XXXVII.	218
,, leg	XXX. 229 ; XXXIV. 289 ; XXXV. 43 ; XXXVII. 217, 218	
,, limbs	XXXIV.	289
,, penis	XXV. 198 ; XXIX. 98	
,, thigh	XXI. 178, 179 ; XXIV. 279, 303 ; XXV. 259 ; XXIX. 93 ; XXX. 229 ; XXXI. 34, 35, 40 ; XXXIV. 235, 291 ; XXXV. 43, 45 ; XXXVI. 46, 47 ; XXXVII. 218, 272.	
,, toes	XXIV.	303
,, turbinal bones	XXVII.	19
Syme's	XXX.	229
through knee	XXXI. 35, 42	
Amyl-nitrite, effects in paralysis of sympathetic nerve	XXIX.	104
hydroxylamine hydrochlorate as a substitute for	XXX.	189
in morbus Addisonii	XXIX.	104
Anæmia, loudness of murmur in	XXVII.	37
of the brain, in the insane	XXI.	12
treated by oxygen inhalations	XXXII.	321
Anæsthesia, from chloroform, mechanical factor in (*Gill*)	XXXI.	155
,, ,, notes on (*Gill*)	XXX.	17
,, ,, stomachic phenomena during (*Gill*)	XXXIV.	107
,, ,, three cases illustrating exceptions from recent practice (*Gill*)	XXXVI.	147
,, hypnotism	XXV.	119

	VOL.	PAGE
Anæsthesia in abdominal section	XXIX.	7
in tetanus	XXVII.	212, 214
palatal and laryngeal, in disseminated sclerosis .	XXXII.	173
Anæsthetics, discussion on	XXIV.	316
Anatomy, biography of	XXII.	367
morbid, of gout	XXIII.	291
of great omentum (*McAdam Eccles*)	XXX.	81
topographical, of the spinal cord . . .	XXI.	137
Andrew (*James*), obituary notice (*Sir W. S. Church*) .	XXXIII.	xxix
Andrewes (*F. W.*), a case of enlarged and dislocated spleen .	XXVI.	131
cases from Dr. Andrew's wards illustrating some of the nervous phenomena of typhoid fever . . .	XXV.	127
descriptive list of specimens added to the Museum	XXXVI.	275
diphtheria bacillus, in a series of sore throats among nurses	XXXII.	145
on glycogen	XXI.	239
„ pneumonia	XXVI.	305
„ puerperal eclampsia	XXII.	358
„ the growth and work of the Pathological Department	XXXIV.	193
„ ulcerative endocarditis	XXV.	273
and **Herringham** (*W. P.*), two cases of cerebellar disease in cats with staggering	XXIV.	241
and **Fletcher** (*Morley*), descriptive list of additions to Museum	XXXIV.	331
Andrews (*L.*), on the relation of diet to medicine . . .	XXVI.	313
Aneurysm, aorta, abdominal . . XXI. 215, 220; XXV. 249; XXVII		257
„ „ and innominate artery . .	XXII.	235
„ „ and innominate artery, operation in	XXII.	235
„ „ and innominate artery, post mortem of	XXII.	237
aortic, and intra-thoracic growths	XXVIII.	94
„ cases of (*T. G. Styan*)	XXI.	211
„ difficulties in diagnosis of	XL.	3
„ table of dietary in	XXIII.	85
ascending part of aorta, sac taking natural position of the heart (*S. Gee*)	XXX.	1
associated with tuberculosis, cases of	XXIII.	246
axillary artery	XXVII.	253
carotid artery, internal	XXII.	194
„ „ „ sacculated in two cases . .	XXII.	194
„ „ „ vegetations, calcification of in one case . .	XXII.	194
„ „ „ „ on cardiac valves in both . .	XXII.	194
cerebral, associated with endocarditis in the young (*P. Kidd*)	XXII.	187
„ its connection with embolism	XXII.	187
„ two cases of (*P. Kidd*)	XXII. 190,	192
cirsoid (a fibro-angeioma) case of	XXXVI.	49
cure of popliteal	XXVII.	255
„ pulmonary	XXI.	57
diagnosis from tumour	XXVIII.	94
„ of	XL.	3
diet in aortic	XXIII.	85
dissecting arch of aorta at junction with descending portion	XXI.	215
„ freedom from atheroma at place of rupture .	XXI.	216
embolism, a probable cause of	XXII.	187
endocarditis, associated with cerebral	XXII.	187

	VOL.	PAGE
Aneurysm, erosion of ribs by	XXX.	3
,, vertebræ by	XXI. 219 ; XXVII.	259
facts connected with pulmonary	XXI.	52
hæmoptysis, remittent, from ruptured (*S. West*)	XXI.	54
injection with solution of iron into sac of	XXVII.	254
,, ,, ,, tannin into sac of	XXVII.	257
innominate artery	XXVII.	253
,, ,, and aorta	XXIII.	235
,, ,, ,, practically cured by ligature of right common carotid	XXIII.	237
Macewen's treatment of	XXVII. 254,	256
palatine artery	XXII.	322
popliteal artery cured	XXVII.	255
,, ,, (right) ligature of for	XXXIV.	301
,, ,, ligature of superficial femoral for	XXXV.	43
,, ,, treated by injection	XXVII.	253
,, ,, ,, pressure	XXVII.	253
pulmonary	XXI. 52, 54,	55
,, cure of	XXI.	57
ribs, eroded by	XXX.	3
subclavian artery	XXVII. 41,	45
,, ,, rupturing into lung	XXVII.	42
,, ,, with cerebral embolism and malignant endocarditis	XXVII.	41
,, ,, (left) with embolism right middle cerebral artery	XXVII.	44
thoracic aorta	XXI. 219, 253 ; XXIII.	83
,, ,, sac taking natural position of heart (*S. Gee*)	XXX.	1
,, ,, great infrequency of this form of disease	XXX.	1
treated by injection of iron into sac of	XXVII.	254
,, ,, ,, tannin into sac of	XXVII.	258
,, ,, Macewen's plan	XXVII. 254,	256
,, ,, pressure, unsuccessful	XXVII.	253
,, ,, Tufnell's plan	XXI. 220, 222 ; XXIII. 84 ; XXVII.	254
ulcerative endocarditis, a cause of embolic	XXII.	190
value of Tufnell's plan of treating	XXI. 223 ; XXIII.	84
vertebræ eroded in	XXI.	219
,, ,, ,, with hole in body of third lumbar by, but not opening the spinal canal	XXV.	251
Angina externa, or Ludovici	XXVI. 275,	282
Ludovici, case of	XXVII.	178
Anginal symptoms in influenza	XXVI.	199
Angioma, cerebral	XXIII.	180
Anglo-French Boundary Commission on the western frontier of the Gold Coast Colony (1902-1903), medical report of (*J. G. Forbes*)	XXXIX.	171
Animals and plants, their relationship	XXIV.	65
Ankle-joint, synovial cyst in connection with	XXI.	187
syphilitic disease of	XXVI.	84
tuberculous disease of	XXIV.	277
Annals in the life of a country doctor (*Webb*)	XXXIV.	231
Antipyrin in diabetes mellitus	XXV.	7
Antiseptic inhalations	XXV.	40
measures in midwifery	XXIII.	45
treatment of phthisis	XXV.	49
Antiseptics, the best in the lying-in room	XXIII.	53
Antistreptococcic serum in treatment of septicæmia	XXXII.	23

		VOL.	PAGE
Antitoxin, Aronson's, cases of diphtheria treated by	.	xxxii.	369
cases of diphtheria treated by, cause of death and prognosis in (*Kanthack* and *May*)	.	xxxii.	335
diphtheria, experiment with	.	xxx.	150
,, paralysis after, treatment of (*Hayward*)	.	xxxi.	101
Antrum, abscess of	.	xxxiv.	237
malignant polypus of	.	xxvii.	81
mastoid, communication with tympanum	.	xxvii.	346
,, exploration of	.	xxxv.	45
purulent catarrh of	.	xxx.	240
pus in	.	xxix.	346
tumour of, with rodent ulcer	.	xxiv.	284
Anus, fissure of (*Goodsall*)	.	xxviii.	205
,, causes	.	xxviii.	206
,, constipation in	.	xxviii.	206
,, fistula in	.	xxviii.	207
,, frequency of	.	xxviii.	206
,, position of	.	xxviii.	206
,, sex in	.	xxviii.	206
,, signs of	.	xxviii.	210
,, stretching	.	xxviii.	208
,, symptoms	.	xxviii.	206
,, syphilitic and non-syphilitic	.	xxviii.	205
,, treatment of	.	xxviii.	207
Aorta, aneurysm of (*see* Aneurysm).			
Aortic and mitral orifices confluent	.	xxiii.	162
,, ,, morbus cordis, cases of	.	xxii. 119, 125, 127	
incompetence with phthisis	.	xxiii.	248
valves, degeneration of, in gout	.	xxiii.	293
Apex, phthisical disease of left, with vomiting	.	xxiv.	131
Aphasia	.	xxxii.	50
and allied conditions	.	xxv.	263
case of	.	xxvi.	114
in a child (*Parkes Weber*)	.	xxxiv.	310
Aphorisms, from Dr. Gee's ward (*T. J. Horder*)	.	xxxii.	29
Apoplexy in a young woman	.	xxvi.	296
Apothecaries, list of	.	xxii.	55
shop, account of	.	xxii.	1
,, expenses of	.	xxii.	17
Appendages, uterine, removal of	.	xxix.	46, 56
,, ,, for convulsions	.	xxix.	48
,, ,, ,, dysmenorrhœa	.	xxix.	48
,, ,, ,, dyspareunia	.	xxix.	48
,, ,, ,, fibroids	.	xxix.	47
,, ,, ,, hystero-epilepsy	.	xxix.	48
,, ,, ,, neuroses	.	xxix.	48
,, ,, ,, threatened insanity	.	xxix.	48
Appendicitis, acute, perforating (*D'Arcy Power*)	.	xxxviii.	23
cases of (*Mayo, Willett,* and *Hawes*)	.	xxxvii.	273
,, ,, in Mr. Butlin's wards	.	xxxiv.	71
,, ,, Mr. Willett's	.	xxxv. 205 ; xxxvi.	46
gangrenous, following operation for radical cure of right inguinal hernia	.	xl.	153
notes on a case of, with multiple abscesses in the peritoneal cavity, and metastatic abscesses in the left lung (*Alwyn T. Compton*)	.	xl.	143
some difficulties in the diagnosis of (*Izard*)	.	xxxix.	41
Appendix, vermiform, hernia, femoral of	.	xxvii. 179, 180	
,, ,, (*McAdam Eccles*)	.	xxxii.	93
,, in sac of femoral hernia	.	xxvii.	179

	VOL.	PAGE
Appendix, vermiform, removal of	XXVII.	180
,, ,, ,, (*Harrison Cripps*) . .	XXXV.	31
,, and cæcum in sac of left femoral hernia	XXVII.	180
Aronson's antitoxin, cases of diphtheria treated . . .	XXXII.	369
Arrest of development in lower jaw	XXXII.	403
Arteries, cases of ligature of (*D'Arcy Power*) . . .	XXXV.	43
Arteritis, in relation to enteric fever (*Auden*) . . .	XXXV.	55
Artery, axillary, aneurysm of	XXVII.	253
,, ligature of	XXXIV.	231
,, rupture of	XXXIV.	235
basilar, fibrous emboli in	XXVIII.	222
brachial, arrest of pulsation in	XXV.	258
carotid, common, ligature of	XXII.	235
,, internal, wound of, ligature of . . .	XXVII.	55
,, its position in goitre	XXV.	102
cerebral left anterior, embolism of	XXVIII.	222
,, right ,, ,, ,, . . .	XXVIII.	222
,, aneurysm of	XXII.	187
coronary, right, embolism of	XXXII.	8
femoral, deep, ligature of (*Sir T. Smith*) . .	XXX.	223
,, occlusion of, in enteric fever . . .	XXXV.	60
,, superficial, ligature of (*Sir T. Smith*) . .	XXX.	223
iliac, external, ligature of, for secondary hæmorrhage		
(*W. D. Harmer*)	XXXV.	269
innominate, aneurysm of	XXII. 235 ; XXVII.	255
,, ,, operation in	XXII.	235
lingual, ligature of (*D'Arcy Power*)	XXXVI.	49
,, ,, ,, in removing epithelioma of tongue .	XXXIV.	272
meningeal, middle, ligature of posterior branch of .	XXXIV.	269
palatine, aneurysm of	XXII.	322
popliteal, ligature of	XXXIV.	301
,, (upper part), ligature of (*Sir T. Smith*) .	XXX.	223
,, rupture of	XXXIV.	235
retinal, case of obliteration of a branch of . . .	XXXVII.	316
right middle cerebral, embolism of, in aneurysm of left		
subclavian	XXVII.	44
right Sylvian, main trunk of firmly blocked, subclavian		
aneurysm	XXVII.	41
subclavian (left), aneurysm of	XXVII.	44
,, ,, aneurysm of	XXVII.	4
Arthritic conditions, &c., observations on (*Sir Dyce Duckworth*)	XXXV.	13
Arthritis, absence of, in rheumatic fever . . .	XXIV.	21
chronic in Graves' disease	XXVII.	143
rheumatoid	XXXV. 13 ; XXXVI.	176
strumous	XXV.	271
Arthrodesis, operation for (*D'Arcy Power*) . . .	XXXV.	44
Arytænoid cartilage, necrosis of, in typhoid fever .	XXV.	133
Asafœtida, its action on the absorption of intestinal gas .	XXII.	292
Ascending antero-lateral tract	XXIII.	141
Ashes of animals, difference in composition of . .	XXII.	272
Association of suppuration with malignant disease .	XXIII.	147
Asthenia and nasal obstruction	XXIX.	250
Astragalectomy	XXVIII.	201
operation for	XXVIII.	201
Astragalus, removal of (*D'Arcy Power*) . . .	XXXV.	44
Astringents in hæmoptysis	XXVII.	95
Ataxia, locomotor, with abnormal symptoms . .	XXI.	97
motor, due to injury of the back . . .	XXII.	101
Ataxy, locomotor, in children	XXIX.	261
syphilitic (*J. Graham Forbes*)	XXXVIII.	81

	VOL.	PAGE
Atkinson (*Stanley B.*), forensic physiology	XXXIX.	127
Atresia vaginæ	XXXIV.	232
Atrophy, muscular, and gangrene of lungs after typhoid fever	XXIII.	109
„ hereditary, of the legs	XXV.	145
„ of arm and shoulder	XXIII.	104
„ „ arm (upper)	XXIII.	106
„ peroneal type	XXIII.	100
„ progressive	XXIII. 92; XXVIII.	211
„ varieties of	XXIII.	89
myopathic	XXIII.	104
of choroid	XXIX.	300
„ liver (acute)	XXXII.	425
„ the optic nerve in insular sclerosis	XXII.	308
optic, primary, with diabetes insipidus (*Stanley Bousfield*)	XXXVI.	235
symmetrical, affecting the hands of young people	XXIX.	307
„ „ „ „ cases of	XXIX.	308
Atropine, introduction and consumption of	XXII.	52
Auden (*G. A.*), arteritis in relation to enteric fever	XXXV.	55
the focus of tuberculous infection in children	XXXV.	79
Aural catarrh, in Graves' disease	XXXVII.	143
pyæmia	XXX.	247
Auricle, right, malformation of	XXII.	99
supernumerary	XXIV.	284
Auriculo-ventricular orifices, relationship of muscular fibres to	XXIII.	164
„ their functions	XXIII.	161
valves, their action	XXIII.	167
Auscultation, theory of the breathing sounds in (*S. Gee*)	XXVI.	103
Average number of casualty patients at St. Bartholomew's Hospital	XXVI.	194
Axilla, abscess in, giving exit to foreign body from trachea	XXVII.	251
Bacilli, putrefactive, inhalations of	XXV.	66
Bacillus coli communis causing cystitis after typhoid fever (*T. J. Horder*)	XXXIII.	85
of fowl tuberculosis	XXVI.	2
„ pneumonia (*Klein*)	XXVIII.	176
„ tubercle (*Koch's*)	XXVI.	1
„ „ in tumours of the larynx	XXI.	40, 93
„ „ present in old specimens of lung disease (*Harris*)	XXI.	45
„ typhoid fever (*see* Typhoid Fever Bacillus)	XXVIII.	289
„ „ „ cultivation of	XXVIII.	292
Back, injury of, producing ataxia	XXII.	101
Back-to-back houses, their insalubrity	XXVI.	8
Bacteria, biology of (*Hankin*)	XXIII.	352
influence of light on	XXVI.	10, 11
their relationship to disease	XXIV.	79
Bacteriological examination of membrane from fauces in diphtheria	XXX.	142
examination of diphtheritic membrane from post-mortem room	XXX.	146
examination of membrane from tracheotomy in diphtheria	XXX.	140
investigations in diphtheria (*Kanthack* and *White*)	XXXI.	87
Bacteriology of acute broncho-pneumonia (*P. Horton-Smith* (*Hartley*))	XXXIII.	25
of perforated gastric ulcer	XXXVII.	52
„ pneumonia	XXVIII.	177
„ suppurative pylephlebitis (*Langdon Brown*)	XXXVII.	113
the relation of, to malignant endocarditis (*Ware*)	XXXV.	253

	VOL.	PAGE
Baker (*W. Morrant*), brief note on the relief of pain in cases of cancer of the tongue	XXIX.	85
cases from his wards	XXIV.	205
obituary notice of	XXXII.	xxxix
on abnormal synovial cysts in connection with joints	XXI.	177
„ perforating wounds of the orbit	XXIV.	179
., whitlow	XXV.	185
„ submaxillary cellulitis; syn. cynanche cellulitis of Gregory; angina externa; angina Ludovici; cynanche sublingualis rheumatico-typhoides	XXVI.	275
Bailey (*R. Cozens*), intra-cranial complications of chronic middle ear disease	XXXVII.	287
the treatment of senile gangrene	XXX.	69
two cases of intestinal resection	XXXIII.	55
Bainbridge (*F. A.*), some neuroses of children	XXXVII.	343
Balsam of Peru, subcutaneously in phthisis	XXVI.	89
Bandages, methods of applying after removal of goitre	XXV.	100
Bark, consumption of	XXII.	47
Barley hale passing into trachea	XXVII.	251
Baths, arrangement for, &c., at the hospital	XXII.	18
Batten (*F. E.*), notes on three cases of progressive muscular atrophy, associated with loss of sensation to heat and cold	XXVIII.	211
on a clinical pulse-manometer	XXIX.	350
tuberculosis, infection of lymphatic glands in children	XXXI.	183
and **Fletcher** (*Morley*), a case of myasthenia gravis, with autopsy	XXXVI.	213
with **Horne** (*W. J.*), disseminated sclerosis with palatal and laryngeal anæsthesia	XXXII.	173
Batteries, electric	XXVIII.	245
Battey's operation	XXIX.	47
Bed-sores, absence of, in spastic paralysis	XXVIII.	269, 279
in paraplegia	XXVII.	242
Bell's paralysis, associated with herpes zoster	XXXIX.	167
Bell-sound, its value in pneumothorax	XXIII.	44
Benzoate of soda, inhalations of	XXV.	53
Bernheim, the suggestive therapeutics of	XXV.	124
Berry (*James*), on hæmorrhage	XXII.	355
two cases of cholecystotomy; removal of a hundred and thirty and of sixty-four calculi	XXVIII.	47
and **Calvert** (*J.*), a case of one-sided traumatic epileptiform convulsions relieved by trephining	XXVI.	69
and **Jessop** (*W. H.*), successful removal of a large goitre	XXV.	97
Bibliography of erythema multiforme	XXIV.	53
of erythema nodosum	XXIV.	53
„ hæmaturia	XXII.	148
„ postero-lateral sclerosis of cord	XXIX.	212
„ the writings of W. J. Walsham	XXXIX.	41
Bickersteth (*E.*), case from Mr. Smith's ward, multiple polypi of the rectum, occurring in a mother and child	XXVI.	299
Bile, flow of, from the cavity of an hydatid of liver	XXIX.	336, 338
pressure of, in the biliary ducts	XXIX.	340
Bile-ducts and gall-bladder, some remarks on the surgery of (*W. J. Walsham*)	XXXVII.	321
rupture of hydatid of liver into	XL.	5
Bilharzia hæmatobia, in West Africa	XXXIX.	178
length of life in man	XXI.	91
ova and embryo, cases of	XXI.	90

	VOL.	PAGE
Bilharzia hæmatobia, situations of the ova . . .	XXI.	92
use of santonin in the treatment of . . .	XXI.	92
vesical calculi due to	XXI.	91
Biography of anatomy, the (*R. Farrar*) . . .	XXII.	367
Biology, arrangements for the teaching of . . .	XXII.	154
in relation to medicine	XXIV.	65
of bacteria	XXIII.	352
Bird (*Robert*), five cases of volvulus of the sigmoid flexure .	XXXVI.	199
Birth, nerve injury at	XXXII.	404
Bladder, abdominal hydatids drained through . . .	XXV.	261
calculus in	XXV.	230, 232, 233
drainage of, through perinæum	XXVII.	120
epithelioma of	XXIV. 211; XXV. 230, 234
extroversion of	XXVII.	170
fistulous opening of, into intestine . . .	XXIV.	258
hæmaturia from	XXV.	229
malignant disease of	XXXII. 200, 205
multiple mucous polypi	XXIII.	236
rupture of	XXVII. 49, 51
„ „ in fractured pelvis	XXXII.	199
tumour in	XXIV. 292; XXV. 280
„ villous	XXV. 230, 233; XXXII. 207
urinary, with imbedded calculi . . .	XXVII.	117
with fistulous openings into intestine . . .	XXIV.	258
Bleeders, joint-disease in	XXVI. 77, 81
Blindness, eclipse, cases of (*W. H. Jessop*) . . .	XXXVI.	250
following optic neuritis	XXI. 225, 228
verbal, cause of	XXVI.	114
Blood, aëration of, defective in nasal obstruction . .	XXIX.	243
bullock's, defibrinated, in splenic leukæmia . .	XXII.	245
cells, effect of cold on	XXII.	143
changes in, in Raynaud's disease (*A. Haig*) . .	XXVIII.	37
condition of, in coal-gas poisoning . . .	XXI.	78
„ „ „ malignant diphtheria . . .	XXIII.	17
„ „ „ phthisis	XXVII.	92
corpuscles, diapedesis of, in hæmoptysis . .	XXVII.	85
„ white, the number of in diabetes (*S. H. Habershon*)	XXVI.	153
defibrinated, enemata of	XXII.	245
quantity of uric acid in (*A. Haig*) . . .	XXVI.	33
specific gravity of, in health and disease (*J. Lloyd*) .	XXIV.	314
spitting of, in phthisis	XXVII.	84
„ the significance of (*V. D. Harris*) . .	XXII.	199
Blood-casts, in phthisis	XXX.	253
Blood-letting, its utility in various diseases . . .	XXI.	243
Blood-tumours of the septum nasi . .	XXIII. 128; XXVII. 21
Blood-vessels, diseases of	XXXII.	39
operations on (*D'Arcy Power*) . .	XXXV. 43; XXXVI. 48
pulmonary, innervation of	XXV.	33
Bloody urine, as the only sign of infantile scurvy . .	XXV.	85
Body, equilibrium of, how maintained . . .	XXIII.	69
rate of cooling, after death . . .	XXI. 252; XXIII. 193
temperature of, modifying the action of aconite . .	XXII.	271
Bone, abscess of	XXVIII.	8
diagnosis of inflammatory enlargement of (*Marsh*) .	XXVIII.	11
diagnosis of new growths in (*Marsh*) . . .	XXVIII. 7, 11
inferior turbinated, hypertrophy of . . .	XXIII.	130
„ „ necrosis of	XXIII.	133
necrosis of	XXVIII.	10
operations for club-foot	XXVIII.	200

	VOL.	PAGE
Bone, parietal, compound fracture of	XXVII.	183
pieces of, removed from bladder	XXVII.	129
„ „ through perinæum	XXVII.	129
suppuration in	XXVIII.	8
turbinate, removal of in Graves' disease	XXVIII.	28
Bones, metacarpal, with bosses, in lead-poisoning	XXI.	169
operations on (*D'Arcy Power*)	XXXV.	44
turbinal, hypertrophy of	XXIX.	249
Bonnet-monkey, structure of brain in	XXVII.	226
Book of the foundation of St. Bartholomew's, the (*Norman Moore*)	XXI.	31
Boro-glyceride, as a remedy in pruritis	XXI.	119
in cystitis	XXI.	120
Bosses on the metacarpal bones in lead-poisoning	XXI.	169
Bougard's paste, cases suitable for treatment by (*Butlin*)	XXIII.	61
composition of	XXIII.	57
method of applying, in cancer of breast	XXIII.	58
on the use of, in cancer of the breast	XXIII.	57
severe constitutional disturbance, after use of	XXIII.	60
Bougies, metallic, for dilating the os uteri	XXIV.	170
Bousfield (*Stanley*), two cases of diabetes insipidus, with primary optic atrophy	XXXVI.	235
Bowel, lower, multiple polypi in	XXIII.	220
rupture of	XXVIII.	117
Bowes (*T. Armstrong*), the complications of suppurative otitis media	XXXIV.	127
a case of membranous colitis	XXXVI.	225
Bowlby (*A. A.*), cases illustrating the clinical course and structure of duct-cancer or villous carcinomas of the breast	XXIV.	263
cases illustrating syphilitic disease of joints	XXVI.	83
on hip disease	XXIV.	323
„ the treatment of wounds	XXVI.	303
some cases of joint-disease in bleeders	XXVI.	77
Bowman (*H. M.*), congenital absence of both pectoral muscles	XXX.	125
Bradford (*Rose*), results of experiments on the innervation of the blood-vessels of the lungs	XXV.	33
Braid, his methods of hypnotism	XXV.	118
Brain, abscess of the (*S. L. O. Young*)	XL.	53
cases of concussion of (*Mayo, Willett,* and *Hawes*)	XXXVII.	279
concussion of, followed by double optic neuritis and paralysis of external rectus	XXIII.	217
electrical excitation of	XXV.	29
ganglia of, occupied by cyst	XXVI.	112
gummata in the	XXIX.	215
gunshot wound of	XXIX.	228
influence of hereditary syphilis on (*J. Graham Forbes*)	XXXVIII.	41
laceration of, without fracture of skull	XXVII.	186, 187
latent defect of	XXIX.	253
lesion, on right side of	XXIX.	253
non-progressive disease of (*Parkes Weber*)	XXXIV.	309
sarcoma of	XXVI.	112
structure of, in bonnet-monkey	XXVII.	226
syphilitic gummata in	XXIX.	215, 217
and meninges, congenital and traumatic cysts of (*L. B. Rawling*)	XL.	97
and spinal cord, physiology of	XXV.	28
Brassfounders' disease (*Samuel Gee*)	XXV.	77
Bread, relative digestibility of white and brown (*Sir Lauder Brunton* and *F. W. Tunnicliffe*)	XXXIII.	157

	VOL.	PAGE
Breast, abscess of (*Howard Marsh*)	XXXIV.	249
,, ,, simulating carcinoma . . .	XXIII.	149
amputation of (*H. T. Butlin*)	XXXIV.	49
,, ,, (*W. J. Wolsham*)	XXXIV,	273
analysis of tumours of, removed during 1900 (*H. Morley*		
Fletcher and *E. H. Shaw*)	XXXVII.	295
cancer of	XXVII.	61
,, ,, caseating	XXVII.	195
,, ,, colloid	XXVII.	194
,, ,, treated by caustics	XXIII.	57
carcinoma of (*E. W. G. Masterman*)	XXVII.	193
,, ,, simulating abscess	XXIII.	149
carcinomata of, removed during the year 1900 (*H.*		
Morley Fletcher and *E. H. Shaw*)	XXXVII.	300
chronic mastitis of	XXXVII.	307
colloid carcinoma of	XXXVII.	302
duct-cancer of	XXVII.	199
,, ,, or villous carcinoma of	XXIV.	263
encephaloid cancer of	XXVII.	202
female, tuberculosis of the (*S. R. Scott*) . . .	XL.	97
fibro-adenomata of, removed during 1900 . . .	XXXVII.	298
hæmorrhagic cancer of	XXVII. 169, 196	
malignant growth developed in floor of ulcer of .	XXIII.	159
microscopic pathology of carcinoma of	XXVII.	193
multiple tumours of	XXXVII.	308
operations on (*D'Arcy Power*)	XXXV.	49
peculiar tumour of	XXVII.	201
result of primary operations for cancer of (*H. T. Butlin*)	XXXVII.	263
results of operations in cancer of (*H. T. Butlin* and		
J. P. Maxwell)	XXXIV.	49
swelling beneath	XXIV.	277
tuberculosis of the female (*S. R. Scott*) . . .	XL.	97
tumours of . . . . . XXIV. 286, 293, 296, 298, 304, 308		
two cases of cancer of, treated by caustics . .	XXIII.	57
unusual forms of cancer of	XXVII.	193
Breath sounds in health and disease	XXI.	191
Breathing, difficulty of, in intra-thoracic growths .	XXVIII.	91
nasal, in nasal obstruction	XXIX.	235
Bright's disease (*see* Nephritis).		
as a cause of sudden death (*T. J. Horder*) . .	XXXV.	155
Brinton (*R. D.*), on blood-letting	XXI.	243
British Isles, geographical distribution of mortality in	XXXIX.	95
Broad ligament, cysts in	XXIX. 11, 27, 28	
,, ,, ,, communicating with rectum .	XXIX.	34
,, ,, ,, enucleation of	XXIX.	38
Bronchi and trachea, simple stricture in . . .	XXV.	225
Bronchial hæmorrhage	XXVII. 81, 82	
Bronchitis in influenza	XXVI.	202
Broncho-pneumonia (acute) bacteriology of (*Horton-Smith*		
Hartley))	XXXIII.	25
Brown (*R.*), the treatment of primary hæmorrhage .	XXIX.	352
Brown (*W. Langdon*), local paralysis in posterior basic		
meningitis	XL.	37
on pylephlebitis	XXXVII.	53
Browne (*Oswald*), on Peter Mere Latham, as a clinical teacher	XXIV.	321
on the study of medicine	XXIX.	350
Bruce-Clarke (*W.*), latent calculus of the bladder; an		
account of six cases in which a calculus was in		
the wall of the bladder	XXVII.	117
remarks on the diagnosis and treatment of such cases .	XXVII.	117

	VOL.	PAGE
Bruce-Clarke (*W.*), the rarer sequelæ of gonorrhæa	XXII.	261
the relation of the testes to prostatic atrophy	XXXV.	249
with **Herringham** (*W. P.*), on idiopathic dilatation of sigmoid flexure	XXXI.	57
Brunton (*Sir Lauder*), hydroxylamine hydrochlorate, as a substitute for nitrate of amyl, or nitro-glycerine	XXX.	189
on a case of staphylococcic infection	XXXIX.	227
notes of a case of hemiplegia	XXVII.	225
and **Tunnicliffe** (*F. W.*), on the relative digestibility of white and brown bread	XXXIII.	157
with **Tunnicliffe** (*F. W.*), acute atrophy of liver	XXXII.	425
Bubo, parotid, in typhoid fever	XXI.	112
Bulbar paralysis without anatomical change, a case of, with autopsy (*F. E. Batten* and *H. Morley Fletcher*)	XXXVI.	213
Bull (*G. V.*), cases of head injury admitted to Mr. Willett's wards, October 1900 to March 1901	XXXVII.	181
Bullar (*J. F.*), on the breath sounds in health and disease	XXI.	191
some uncommon ophthalmic cases	XXIX.	297
Bullock's blood, defibrinated, in splenic leukæmia	XXII.	245
Bullous eruption following poisoned wound	XXIX.	313
Burnett (*F. M.*), treatment of anæmia with oxygen inhalations	XXXII.	321
Burns and scalds, cases of (*Mayo, Willett,* and *Hawes*)	XXXVII.	275
Burrows (*Sir George*), memoir of	XXIII.	xxxiii
Bursa, under annular ligament	XXIV.	286
Butlin (*H. T.*), a year's surgery at St. Bartholomew's Hospital	XXIX.	89
a second year's surgery at St. Bartholomew's Hospital	XXX.	227
introductory address to the Abernethian Society	XXIX.	249
on some diseases of the larynx	XXI.	145
„ the operative surgery of malignant disease of the scrotum, illustrated by the further history of cases which have been treated at the Hospital	XXV.	193
„ the results of operations for primary cancer of the breast, performed during the years 1895, 1896, and 1897	XXXVII.	263
„ the results of Halsted's operations for cancer of breast	XXXVII.	264
„ the treatment by removal of some chronic ulcers of the tongue	XXIV.	83
sarcoma of bones of thigh and leg	XXXI.	31
two cases of cancer of the breast treated by caustics	XXIII.	57
and **Douglas** (*A. R. J.*), on appendicitis	XXXIV.	71
„ **Maxwell** (*J. P.*), on the results of operations for cancer of the breast	XXXIV.	49
Cæcum and appendix, in sac of left femoral hernia	XXVII.	180
and colon, ulceration of	XXIII.	215
Calcareous masses from lung (*West*)	XXXI.	253
Calculi, biliary, removal of	XXVIII.	47
in cases of bilharzia	XXI.	89, 91
prostatic, a cause of vesical	XXVII.	131
renal, multiple	XXVII.	170
Calculus, case of impacted urethral	XXXVI.	47
encysted	XXVII.	118, 122, 123
„ suprapubic lithotomy for	XXVII.	124, 128
in wall of bladder	XXVII.	117
latent, its diagnosis and treatment	XXVII.	117
prostatic	XXVII.	130
renal	XXI. 122, 126; XXV.	231, 236
„ removed by operation	XXV.	236
vesical	XXV.	230, 232, 233

		VOL.	PAGE
Calculus, vesical, case of		XXXVL.	48
„ uric acid		XXV.	233
„ phosphatic		XXV.	233
urethral		XXXIV.	234
Calculous pyelitis, nephrectomy for		XXI.	121
Calvert (*J.*), a case of tracheal obstruction, causing expiratory dyspnœa and emphysema		XXIX.	323
on hydatid disease of the heart		XXXIX.	207
„ intra-pleural pressure and manner of contraction of the lung in pleural effusion		XXVIII.	131
„ peripheral neuritis		XXIII.	356
and **Berry** (*J.*), a case of traumatic one-sided epileptiform convulsions relieved by trephining		XXVI.	69
Calves of the legs, enlargement of		XXIII.	106
Campbell (*Harry*), gradations of health and disease		XXX.	155
physiological aspects of disease		XXXI.	169
the reserve force of the heart		XXXVIII.	144
„ „ forces of the animal organism		XXXVIII.	143
Cancrum oris and gangrene of the fauces		XXV.	75
phagedænic and gangrenous		XXV. 76 ; XXVII.	209
Cancer, and infective endocarditis		XXVIII.	228
„ tuberculosis (*Forbes*)		XXXV.	183
cells, their motivity		XXV.	110
„ „ nature		XXV.	110
chimney sweep's		XXV.	193
duct, or villous carcinoma		XXIV. 263, 266, 269	
of bowel (lower)		XXIII.	229
„ „		XXVII. 116, 117	
„ breast, encephaloid		XXVII.	202
„ „ Halsted's operation for		XXXIV.	64
„ „ results of operations for (*Butlin*)		XXXVII.	263
„ „ „ „ „ (*Butlin* and *Marwell*)	XXXIV.	49	
„ „ treated by caustics		XXIII.	57
„ bronchi (main), primary		XXXIII.	117
„ colon simulating abscess (*Marsh*)		XXXIV.	253
„ heart		XXIV.	263
„ jaw (upper) with abscess		XXIII.	151
„ liver and gall-bladder with gall-stones		XXVII.	228
„ lung, primary		XXXII.	121
„ lungs, body of		XXXIII.	117
„ „ root of		XXXIII.	117
„ œsophagus, summary of sixty-one cases of (*Forbes*)		XXXV.	194
„ omentum, in intestinal obstruction		XXVIII.	120
„ pancreas, primary		XXX. 5 ; XXXVII.	337
„ pelvic glands, abscess complicating		XXIII.	152
„ pleura		XXXIII.	117
„ „ (secondary)		XXXIII.	126
„ tongue, relief of pain in		XXIX.	85
„ „ removal of		XXIX. 87 ; XXXIV. 272	
Cancerous stricture, intestinal obstruction from		XXVIII. 113, 116	
Carbolic acid, as an inhalation		XXV.	54, 65
introduction and consumption of		XXII.	53
its use in the removal of goître		XXV.	103
Carcinoma, caseating		XXVII.	193
colloid		XXVII.	194
encephaloid of lungs		XXVII. 196 ; XXVII. 80	
„ „ stomach		XXVIII.	80
hæmorrhagic		XXVIII. 169, 196	
medullary, tabular analysis of		XXVIII.	89

		VOL.	PAGE
Carcinoma, medullary, of lung		XXVIII.	88
metastatic of choroid (*W. H. Jessop*)		XXXV.	240
of breast, Halsted's operation for	XXXIV. 63;	XXXVII.	264
,, ,, recurrent		XXIV.	286, 309
,, ,, simulating abscess		XXIII.	149
,, ,, treated by caustics		XXIII.	57
,, ,, unusual forms of		XXVII.	193
,, cervical glands, conjoined with suppuration		XXIII.	150
,, colon, sigmoid flexure, imitating iliac abscess		XXXIV.	253
,, duodenum		XXXVII.	338
,, gall-bladder		XXVIII.	228
,, liver		XXXI.	106
,, ,, simulating abscess		XXIII.	148
,, lung		XXVIII.	84
,, œsophagus	XXVIII. 79; XXXV. 195;	XXXIX.	223, 224
,, palate		XXII.	351
,, pelvic glands with abscess		XXIII.	152
,, pylorus, pylorectomy for	XXXIV. 275;	XL.	133
,, sigmoid flexure of colon		XXXIV.	253
,, stomach, encephaloid		XXVII.	80
,, thyroid gland		XXVIII.	79, 80
,, vertebræ		XXVIII.	80
recurrent in breast		XXIV.	286, 309
scirrhous, of breast, excision of		XXXIV.	273
sclerosing tuberculosis simulating scirrhous		XL.	107
unusual forms of, in breast (*Masterman*)		XXVII.	193
Carcinomata of breast removed during the year 1900 (*Morley Fletcher* and *E. H. Shaw*)		XXXVII.	300
of palate		XXII.	351
Carcinomatous growth in intestinal obstruction, inguinal colotomy for		XXXIV.	277
growth of pyloric end of stomach		XXXIV.	276
tumour of groin		XXXII.	194
tumours, inguinal colotomy in ten cases of		XXXVII.	44
ulcer of right breast		XXIV.	301
Cardiac cases in influenza		XXVI.	261
failure, hypodermic injection of strychnia in (*Habershon*)		XXII.	115
first sound, on the causation of (*Inchley*)		XXXVIII.	91
hypertrophy, œdema, and renal disease (*Holmes*, with *Kanthack*)		XXXII.	261
irregularity, in Graves' disease		XXIX.	184
malformations, and other congenital defects (*Garrod*)		XXX.	53
murmur, hæmic, notes on (*Garrod*)		XXVII.	33
murmurs, audible, without touching the chest (*Moore*)		XXVI.	165
reserve force (*Harry Campbell*)		XXXVIII.	144
Cargill's detergent fluid, formula of		XXIII.	128
respirator, in nasal disease		XXIII.	128
Caries of cervical vertebræ		XXVII.	242, 245
spinal (*Gardner*)		XXIII.	357
Carminatives, their action on the absorption of gas by the intestines		XXII.	279
Carotid artery, its position in goître		XXV.	102
ligature of internal		XXVII.	56
Cartilage, articular, changes in, in gout		XXIII.	291
arytænoid, in typhoid fever, necrosis of		XXV.	133
Cash (*T.*) and **Brunton** (*L.*) on absorption of gas by the intestines, and the action of carminatives upon it		XXII.	279
on modifications in the action of aconite, produced by changes in the body temperature		XXII.	271

	VOL.	PAGE
Casualty Department, notes from	XXVI.	263
patients, average number of, at St. Bartholomew's Hospital	XXVI.	194
patients, diagnosis of disease in	XXVI.	310
variola, as seen in the	XXI.	131
Catalepsy in the insane	XXI.	20
Cataract, extraction without iridectomy (*Jessop*) . . .	XXXVII.	317
secondary (*H. Power*)	XXXIV.	5
Catarrh, aural, in Graves' disease	XXVII.	143
chronic purulent, of the accessory nasal sinuses . .	XXX.	237
in influenza	XXVI.	198
naso-pharyngeal	XXVII.	15
Cats, cerebellar disease in	XXIV.	241
experiments on, for the absorption of intestinal gas .	XXII.	293
Cause of death, in cases of diphtheria treated by antitoxin (*Kanthack* and *May*)	XXXII.	335
in hemiplegia	XXVI.	114
Caustics, in the treatment of cancer of the breast . . .	XXIII.	57
Cautery, Paquelin's, epulis of lower jaw treated by . .	XXII.	239
Cautley, (*E.*), aphasia and allied conditions	XXV.	263
cases from Sir William Savory's wards	XXV.	229
report on influenza	XXVI.	234
etiology of croupous pneumonia	XXVIII.	173
irregularity of the heart	XXIX.	283
on headache	XXVII.	287
Cavities in the lung, effect on the respiratory sounds .	XXI.	201
Cell memory (*Claye Shaw*)	XXXI.	239
Cells, ethmoidal, case of suppuration in	XXXVI.	53
„ purulent catarrh of	XXX.	243
Cellulitis, submaxillary	XXVI.	275
„ its dangers	XXVI.	281
„ „ treatment	XXVI.	281
Cellulose, its nature, and occurrence in animals . . .	XXIV.	73
Cephaloceles	XL.	75
Cerebellar disease in a child	XXIV.	247
„ „ cats	XXIV.	241
„ „ kittens	XXIII.	70
„ staggering in, two cases of (*Herringham* and *Andrewes*)	XXIV.	241
„ symptoms of	XXIII.	67, 68
Cerebellum, a case of tumour of (*Herringham*) . . .	XXIII.	65
description of abnormal, in a cat	XXIV.	245
disease of, in kittens	XXIII.	70
psammoma in	XXIII.	65
tumour of	XXIII.	65
„ „ tubercular	XXIII.	186
Cerebral abscess, hemiplegia from	XXI.	230
„ with epilepsy	XXIII.	188
aneurysm, associated in young persons with endo-carditis (*Kidd*)	XXII.	187
angioma	XXIII.	180
complications of middle ear disease (*Bailey*) . .	XXXVII.	287
concussion, cases of (*Mayo*, *Willett*, and *Hawes*) .	XXXVII.	279
disease, irregularity of heart in	XXIX.	287
embolism	XXXVII.	41, 285
hæmorrhage	XXVII.	285
„ in a child (*Weber*)	XXXIV.	311
„ „ young woman	XXVI.	296
symptoms, localising, produced by cortical meningitis in course of general tuberculosis	XXX.	211

3

	VOL.	PAGE
Cerebral symptoms, with pericæcal suppuration . . .	XXX.	63
Cerebro-spinal system, tumours of the (*Murray*) . .	XXIII.	350
Cerebrum, syphilitic disease of (*Forbes*). . . .	XXXVIII.	41
Cervical glands, malignant disease of, with abscess . .	XXIII.	150, 153
rib	XXIV.	290
Cervix, inflammation and congestion of the (*Drage*) . .	XXIII.	365
Champneys.(*F. H.*), on the removal of the uterine appendages	XXIX.	46
Chaplin (*T. A.*), notes on the influenza epidemic at the City		
of London Hospital for Diseases of the Chest .	XXVI.	259
Cheek, epithelioma of	XXIV.	283
sinus of, due to unsound wisdom tooth (*Marsh*) . .	XXXIV.	254
Chemistry, arrangements for the teaching of . . .	XXII.	155
Chest, deformities of, from nasal obstruction . . .	XXIX.	247
recession of, in croup	XXIV.	145
the X-rays, in diseases of (*H. Walsham*). . .	XXXIV.	29
three hundred hydatids, discharged from . .	XXV.	221
Chilblain, suppurating	XXIII.	259
Child, aphasia in (*Weber*).	XXXIV.	310
Children, albuminuria in (*Herringham*)	XXVI.	25
head-banging in	XXII.	97
,, shaking in	XXII.	96
locomotor ataxy in (*Norman Moore*) . . .	XXIX.	261
nephritis, acute, in	XXVI.	27
partial paralysis in	XXIX.	261
some neuroses of (*F. A. Bainbridge*) . . .	XXXVII.	343
sudden death in young (*Thursfield*) . . .	XXXVIII.	129
tuberculous infection, the focus of, in (*Auden*) .	XXXV.	79
,, ,, of lymphatic glands, in (*F. E.*		
Batten)	XXXI.	183
Chimney-sweep's cancer	XXV.	193
Chloral hydrate, introduction and consumption of . .	XXII.	51
Chlorine gas, as an inhalation	XXV.	50, 52
Chloroform, anæsthesia	XXX.	17
,, mechanical factor in (*Gill*) . .	XXXI.	155
,, notes on (*Gill*)	XXX.	17
,, stomachic phenomena during (*Gill*). .	XXXIV.	107
,, three cases illustrating exceptions		
from recent practice (*Gill*) .	XXXVI.	147
in tetanus	XXVII.	212, 214
Chlorophyll, its activity dependent on potassium . .	XXIV.	74
its parallelism with hæmoglobin . . .	XXIV.	73
Cholecystitis, a case of (*W. J. Walsham*) . .	XXXVII.	340
Cholecystotomy, cases of XXVIII. 47; XXXV. 39; XXXVI. 43; XXXVII. 328		
operation for	XXXIII.	49, 52
Choledocho-lithotomy, a case of (*W. J. Walsham*) .	XXXVII.	334
Cholelithiasis, cases of (*W. J. Walsham*) . .	XXXVII.	328
Cholera, on the etiology of (*Klein*)	XXI.	260
Cholmeley (*H. P.*), cases from Mr. Willett's wards .	XXIII.	255
(*M. A.*), and Willett (*A.*), cases of appendicitis .	XXXV.	205
Chorea, artifical production of	XXIV.	62
as a cause of endocarditis	XXIV.	55
cured by typhoid fever	XXII.	224
due to embolism	XXIV.	61
endocarditis, a result of	XXIV.	55
etiology of (*Morley Fletcher*)	XXXII.	383
gravidarum, induction of labour in (*Sir Dyce Duckworth*)	XXXIX.	7
,, observations on	XXXIX.	1
insaniens, cases of	XXII.	89
,, and rheumatism	XXII.	93
,, with pregnancy	XXII.	91

	VOL.	PAGE
Chorea, its relation to rheumatism	XXVI. 265 ; XXXII.	52
post-mortem examinations in	XXIV. 56, 57,	59
symptoms intermediate between it and tetany	XXVI.	65
the pathogeny of (*Sir Dyce Duckworth*)	XXXVII.	9
typhoid fever curing	XXII.	224
with stomatitis, parotides, and rheumatoid pyæmia	XXII.	89
Choroid, atrophy of	XXIX.	300
metastatic carcinoma of (*Jessop*)	XXXV.	240
ossification of	XXIX.	303
sarcoma of (*Jessop*)	XXXV.	239
Church (*Sir W. S.*), an examination of nearly seven hundred cases of acute rheumatism	XXIII.	269
cases from his wards	XXI. 211 ; XXVI. 289 ; XXXII.	1
note on the Six Gifts of Theophilus Philanthropos	XXI.	231
obituary notice of James Andrew	XXX.	1
on the prevalence of diphtheria and throat-disease within Hospital during the year 1890	XXVII.	261
our Hospital Pharmacopœia and Apothecary's Shop	XXII.	1
two cases of hydatid disease	XXIX.	335
Churchill (*J. H.*), notes on the serum reaction in typhoid fever	XXXIV.	205
Cicatrix, hernia through, after abdominal section	XXIX.	21
„ „ of incision	XXVIII.	23
Circulation, Michal Foster, on the pulmonary	XXVIII.	259
Cirrhosis (*Gow*)	XXIV.	315
alcoholic (*Yeld*)	XXXIV.	215
of liver, a case of (*Weber*)	XXXIV.	321
„ „ in child of eleven (*Hall*)	XXVIII.	167
„ „ its connection with gout	XXIII. 293,	295
„ „ with obscure and fatal symptoms	XXVI.	57
„ „ „ obstruction of superior vena cava (*Sir Dyce Duckworth* and *A. E. Garrod*)	XXXII.	71
„ lung	XXVIII.	2
„ „ due to tubercle	XXVIII.	4
Cirsoid aneurysm, case of	XXXVI.	49
Clarke (*W. Bruce*), (*see also* Bruce-Clarke (*W.*)).		
cases from his wards (*L. Noon*)	XL.	125
on the value of the cystoscope	XXVI.	308
some remarks on nine cases of intestinal obstruction	XXVIII.	113
some thoughts on the progress of medical science	XXIX.	351
the relation of the testes to prostatic atrophy	XXXV.	249
and **Herringham** (*W. P.*), on idiopathic dilatation of sigmoid flexure	XXXI.	57
Claye-Shaw (*T.*) (*see* Shaw (*T. Claye*)), on cell memory	XXXI.	239
destructive impulses in the insane,	XXI.	1
on the expression of emotion	XXXVI.	243
the sexes in lunacy	XXIV.	1
Clergyman, umbrella for, at the burying ground of the Hospital	XXII.	36
Cleft palate, operations on (*W. J. Walsham*)	XXXIV.	271
Clinical aphorisms from Dr. Gee's wards	XXXII.	29
Cloves, oil of	XXII.	292
Club-foot, bone operations for	XXVIII.	200
congenital, treatment of (*see also* Talipes)	XXVIII.	199
Coal-gas poisoning, artificial respiration in	XXI.	74
coma in	XXI.	76
condition of the blood in	XXI.	78
„ pupils in	XXI.	77
inhalation of oxygen in	XXI.	74, 78
medico-legal aspect of	XXI.	77

	VOL.	PAGE
Coal-gas poisoning, percentage of coal gas to produce symptoms	XXI.	75
three cases of (*Morton*)	XXI.	73
Cocaine, a cause of glaucoma	XXII.	307
action of on the eye	XXI. 237 ; XXII.	305
anæsthetic properties of	XXII.	307
in nasal obstruction	XXIII.	120
„ ophthalmic practice	XXII.	305
its effect on the intra-ocular muscles	XXII.	307
Coccyx, excision of (*Walsham*)	XXXIV.	293
injury to	XXIV.	285
and sacrum, sinuses over (*Goodsall*)	XXIV.	229
Cod-liver oil, introduction and consumption of	XXII.	49
Cœliac affection, age of occurrence of	XXIV.	18
fæces, their colour and consistency in the	XXIV.	17
on the (*Gee*)	XXIV.	17
symptoms of	XXIV.	18
treatment of	XXIV.	18
Colby (*J. G. E.*), cases from Mr. Willett's wards	XXV.	257
cases from Sir Dyce Duckworth's wards	XXVIII.	151
on hæmoglobin, and its derivates	XXII.	361
with **Butlin** (*H. T.*), sarcoma of bones of thigh and leg	XXXI.	31
Colchester and Essex Hospital, cases from	XXVII.	239
influenza at	XXVI.	252
Cold, cases of peripheral neuritis from	XXII.	179
effects of, in paroxysmal hæmaturia	XXII.	137
„ „ on the bloodvessels	XXII.	143
loss of sensation to	XXVIII.	211
use of, in Graves' disease	XXVIII.	25
Coleman (*Alfred*), memoir of	XXXVIII.	xxxiii
Colic and enteritis, simulating intestinal obstruction	XXXII.	61
gall-stone, case of	XL.	136
lead colic, mistaken diagnosis in	XXXIX.	52
menstrual	XXII.	95
Colitis, a case of membranous (*T. A. Bowes*)	XXXVI.	225
Collapse, and rigor, in typhoid fever	XXXII.	107
Colles' fracture, cases of (*Mayo, Willett,* and *Hawes*)	XXXVII.	271
Collins (*W. J.*), on cocaine	XXI.	237
on physiognomy and phrenology — what are they worth ?	XXI.	244
the title of doctor	XXII.	363
three years' surgery at London Temperance Hospital	XXIX.	352
Collyns (*R. J.*), on optic neuritis	XXI.	238
Colon, cancer of, simulating an iliac abscess (*Marsh*)	XXXIV.	253
ulceration of	XXIII.	213
Colotomy, cases of (*D'Arcy Power*)	XXXV.	40
inguinal	XXVIII.	117
right iliac, for intestinal obstruction (*D. H. Goodsall*)	XXX.	215
Coma, in coal-gas poisoning	XXI.	76
its definition, causes, &c.	XXI.	249
„ varieties	XXIV.	318
Combes (*R.*), on quacks and quackery	XXI.	248
Compton (*Alwyne T.*), notes on a case of appendicitis with multiple abscesses in the peritoneal cavity, and metastatic abscesses in the left lung	XL.	143
Conception, occurrence of, in regard to menstruation	XXIV.	172
Concussion, cases of cerebral (*Mayo, Willett,* and *Hawes*)	XXXVII.	279
of brain, followed by double optic neuritis and paralysis of right external rectus	XXIII.	217

	VOL.	PAGE
Congenital absence of both pectoral muscles	XXX.	125
„ „ radius	XXXII.	400
cysts of brain and meninges	XL.	75
defects, associated with cardiac malformations XXX, 53 ; XXXV.		147
disease of heart, associated with pulmonary tuberculosis	XXIII.	239
„ „ „ the tendency to phthisis in . .	XXIII.	240
hygroma, cystic, of neck	XXIV.	277
morbus cordis	XXVIII.	151
Conjunctiva, translucent cyst of (*Jessop*) . . .	XXXV.	237
vaccinia of (*Jessop*)	XXXV.	232
Conjunctivitis, membranous (diphtheritic) cases of (*Jessop*)	XXXV.	232
Consolidation of the lung, its effect on the respiratory sounds	XXI.	200
Constipation, its effect on gout	XXIV.	227
Consultations, cases shown at	XXIV.	273
Consumption, its relation to the dwelling-house (*see* Phthisis)	XXVI.	1
Contagion in influenza	XXVI.	204
infection and predisposition (*Kanthack*) . . .	XXIX.	351
Contusion of kidneys, a case of (*Mayo, Willett,* and *Hawes*) .	XXXVII.	282
Contusions of abdomen, cases of (*Mayo, Willett,* and *Hawes*) .	XXXVII.	273
Convulsions, epileptiform, relieved by trephining (*Calvert* and *Berry*)	XXVI.	69
following head injury	XL.	138
in spastic paralysis	XXVIII.	271
removal of the uterine appendages for . . .	XXIX.	48
traumatic, one-sided	XXVI.	74
Cook (*E. G.*), report on influenza, at the Royal Free Hospital	XXVI.	241
on rheumatic hyperpyrexia	XXVII.	286
Cooling of the body after death	XXIII.	193
Copaiba rash, simulating variola	XXI.	136
Cornea, extravasation of blood into	XXIX.	298
herpes of, cases of (*Jessop*)	XXXV.	238
Corneal limbus, growths at (*Jessop*)	XXXVI.	258
Corpus spongiosum, indurated nodule in . . .	XXIV.	284
Corpuscles, white, numbers in diabetes	XXVI.	153
Corrosive sublimate, as an antiseptic	XXIII.	53
Cortical tubercular meningitis in the course of general tuberculosis, producing localising cerebral symptoms .	XXX.	211
Cough, in intra-thoracic growths	XXVIII.	91
Cozens (*C.*), and **Rudolph Smith** (*T.*), two cases of impaction of a vegetable foreign body, one in the submaxillary, the other in the sublingual salivary duct, leading to obstruction of the duct, and formation of an abscess in the gland	XXXIII.	105
Crace-Calvert (*G. A.*), and **Harris** (*V. D.*), the human pancreatic ferments in disease	XXIX.	125
Cramp, agonising, in the muscles of the neck . . .	XXII.	218
Cranial nerves, segmental value of	XXV.	45
Creasote, as an inhalation	XXV.	54, 55
Cretinism, sporadic, treated by thyroid extract (*Murrell*) .	XXIX.	101
Cricket accidents (*J. F. Steedman*)	XXXVI.	221
Cripps (*W. Harrison*), abdominal section for ovariotomy, &c., in the Women's Ward at St. Bartholomew's Hospital	XXIX.	1
case of hysteropexy	XXXV.	35
cases of laparotomies	XXXV.	23
case of nephrectomy	XXXV.	35
ovariotomy and hysterectomy in Martha Ward . .	XXXIX.	143

	VOL.	PAGE
Cripps (*W. Harrison*), table of the cases of abdominal section in Martha (Women's) Ward, St. Bartholomew's Hospital, 1898	XXXV.	23
the incision in abdominal section	XXVIII.	17
Croton-chloral hydrate, introduction and consumption of	XXII.	52
Crouch (*C. P.*), Bavarian and similar splints	XXII.	365
on adenoid vegetations	XXV.	272
,, mesmerism	XXI.	245
and Rolleston (*H. D.*), a case of intestinal obstruction	XXV.	169
Croup, in its relation to tracheotomy (*Hamer*)	XXIV.	141
its definition	XXIV.	141
recession of chest in	XXIV.	145
Croupous pneumonia	XXVIII.	173
Crowd accidents (*Hunt*)	XXXVIII.	179
Crura cerebri, homologies of	XXV.	41
Cuboid, and os calcis, removal of portions of	XXVIII.	202
Cupping, fees for	XXII.	27
wet, the use of, in the insane	XXII.	106
Cutaneous disease, a case of erythema iris (*Gardner* and *Scott*)	XXXVIII.	135
two cases of tinea favosa capitis (*Sir Dyce Duckworth*)	XXXVIII.	155
Cut throat, cases of (*Mayo, Willett,* and *Hawes*)	XXXVII.	279
Cyanosis, condition of serum in	XXII.	144
Cynanche cellulitis, or sublingualis rheumatico-typhoides (*see* Angina)	XXVI.	275
Cyst, a case of abdominal (*Sir Thomas Smith*)	XXXIV.	1
between the eyes	XXIV.	306
dermoid presacral, a case of (*D'Arcy Power*)	XXXVII.	42
hydatid, rupturing into bile-ducts (*see* Hydatid Cyst)	XL.	5
hygroma, congenital, of neck	XXIV.	277
in axilla	XXIV.	304
,, the basic ganglia	XXVI.	112
of broad ligament (*see* Broad Ligament Cyst).		
ovarian (*see* Ovarian Cyst).		
,, burrowing beneath broad ligament	XXIX.	11
synovial, in connection with ankle-joint,	XXI.	187
,, ,, ,, ,, elbow-joint	XXI.	184
,, ,, ,, ,, hip-joint	XXI.	186
thyroid, removal of, followed by ulceration opening into trachea	XXIII.	218
translucent, of conjunctiva (*Jessop*)	XXXV.	237
urachal (*Doran*)	XXXIV.	33
Cysts, abnormal synovial, in connection with joints	XXI.	177
congenital and traumatic, of brain and meninges	XL.	75
dentigerous, of the palate	XXII.	320
hydatid (*see* Hydatid Cyst), drained through bladder	XXV.	261
,, suppurating, in thorax	XXV.	214
,, three hundred discharged from thorax	XXV.	221
urachal, observations on (*Alban Doran*), with Stanley's case of patent urachus	XXXIV.	33
Cystic disease of ovaries	XXIX.	24
,, ,, the kidneys and liver (*J. Forbes*)	XXXIII.	181
hygroma of neck, congenital	XXIV.	277
tumour of lower jaw	XXII.	238
Cystitis, acute	XXV.	232
,, following typhoid fever, and due to bacillus coli communis (*T. J. Horder*)	XXXIII.	85
boro-glyceride in	XXI.	120
in influenza	XXVI.	203
Cystoscope, its value	XXVI.	308

	VOL.	PAGE
Dalal (*R. D.*), a short account of the second epidemic of plague at Bhiwudi, Thana district	XXXV.	119
Damp-course, its want in houses	XXVI.	5
Davenport (*C. J.*), resorption-diabetes of lactation . .	XXIV.	175
Davidson (*H.*), cases from Mr. Willett's wards . .	XXIII.	255
Davies (*A.*), on the structure and function of the auriculo-ventricular orifices	XXIII.	161
Death, Bright's disease, a cause of sudden (*Horder*) . .	XXXV.	155
causes of, in diphtheria . . . . . :	XXVIII.	193
in puncture of hydatids	XXVIII.	236
rate of cooling of body after	XXI. 252 ; XXIII.	193
sudden, in infants (*Thursfield*)	XXXVIII.	129
„ some remarks on (*Horder*)	XXXV.	153
Decubitus, sacral, in paraplegia	XXI.	140
Deep femoral, superficial femoral, and popliteal arteries, with their corresponding veins, ligature of . . .	XXX.	224
Deformities of the chest, in nasal obstruction . . .	XXIX.	247
„ „ feet and toes, operations for (*Walsham*) .	XXXIV.	296
Deformity, cases of (*Heath*)	XXXII.	400
„ „ spinal, with myopathy (*Mundy*) .	XXXVI.	55
Degeneration, subacute, combined, of spinal cord (*Ormerod*)	XL.	23
Deglutition pneumonia after tracheotomy. . . .	XXI.	80
Delirium, and its allied conditions	XXV.	279
in typhoid fever	XXV.	128, 129
meaning of the word (*S. Gee*)	XXXIII.	8
with jaundice, a case of	XXIII.	184
Delusions, in spastic paralysis	XXVIII.	275
Demonstrations and lectures, list of	XXXIX.	303
Dentist appointed to Hospital	XXII.	44
Department, Casualty, notes from the	XXVI.	263
„ patients, diagnosis of disease in .	XXVI.	310
„ variola, as seen in the . . .	XXI.	131
Diseases of the Larynx	XXI.	145
„ „ „ Throat and Nose, cases of malignant disease from the	XXXIX.	219
Dispensing	XXII.	16
Electrical, cases treated in	XXVIII.	251
„ foundation of	XXII.	29
„ notes from	XXVIII.	245
„ report from	XXII.	57
„ „ of the year's work in (*H. Lewis Jones*) .	XXXIII.	169
Dermatitis, herpetiformis, description of . . .	XXIX. 313,	318
„ three cases of	XXIX.	313
„ treatment of	XXIX, 316,	319
multiple, gangrenous, in enteric fever . . .	XXVII.	189
Dermoid cyst, presacral, a case of (*D'Arcy Power*) . .	XXXVII.	42
De Santi (*P.*), the indications for opening the mastoid in chronic suppurative otitis media	XXXV.	103
Development, arrest of in lower jaw	XXXII.	403
of great omentum (*McAdam Eccles*) . . .	XXX.	81
Deviation of tongue and soft palate, a case of (*Weber*) . .	XXXIV.	307
Deviations of the septum, in nasal obstruction . . .	XXIII.	122
Diabetes and glycosuria	XXXII.	53
insipidus, cases of, with primary optic atrophy (*Stanley Bousfield*)	XXXVI.	235
mellitus, condition of the liver in	XXV.	8
„ connection with gout	XXV.	7
„ effect of fever on	XXV.	14
„ use of alkalies in , , , , ,	XXV.	10

	VOL.	PAGE
Diabetes mellitus, use of opium in	XXV.	7
number of the white corpuscles of the blood in (*Habershon*)	XXVI.	153
of lactation	XXIV.	175
recent research in (*Tylden*)	XXVII.	71
Diagnosis, between abscess and new growth (*Marsh*) . .	XXXIV.	25
differential, new growths and inflammatory enlargements of bones (*Marsh*)	XXVIII.	7
difficulties presenting in tumour of mediastinum (*Sir Dyce Duckworth*)	XXXIII.	7
facial (*Lewis Jones*)	XXV.	277
of acute abscess (*Marsh*)	XXXIV.	241
,, appendicitis, difficulties in (*Izard*) . . .	XXXIX.	41
,, diphtheria (*Hayward*)	XXX.	139
,, intestinal obstruction	XXV.	172
,, intra-cranial pressure	XXVIII.	65
,, intra-thoracic growths, from aortic aneurysm .	XXVIII.	94
,, ,, ,, ,, ,, pericardical effusion	XXVIII.	94
,, suppuration, associated with malignant disease .	XXIII.	155
value of the ophthalmoscope in medical (*Napier*) .	XXIV.	337
,, ,, melanuria, in	XXXVIII.	25
Diarrhœa, alba	XXIV.	17
and dysentery	XXXII.	43
chylosa	XXIV.	17
discussion on (house-physicians')	XXII.	359
infantile (*Lankester*)	XXI.	242
in Graves' disease	XXVII.	141
summer, its connection with ground air . .	XXVI.	6
Diet, after abdominal operations	XXV.	175
influence in uric acid headache	XXIII.	204, 206
its relation to medicine	XXVI.	313
Dietetic values of food-stuffs prepared by plants (*Rev. G. Henslow*)	XXX.	113
Diets of Hospital	XXII.	8
Digestibility, relative, of white and brown bread (*T. Lauder Brunton* and *F. W. Tunnicliffe*)	XXXIII.	157
Digestion, in invertebrata	XXIV.	67
Diphtheria, albuminuria in	XXVIII.	194
antitoxin, experiments with . XXX. 150; XXXI. 101; XXXII. 369		
,, in treatment of paralysis after (*Hayward*)	XXXI.	101
bacillus in series of sore throats among nurses .	XXXII.	145
,, of	XXVII.	277
bacteriological investigations in (*Kanthack* and *White*) .	XXXI.	87
causes of death in	XXVIII.	193
contraction of the field of vision after . . .	XXII.	308
cubic space for patients in wards	XXVII.	277
diagnosis of (*Hayward*)	XXX.	139
diffusibility of poison of.	XXVII.	274
early sequelæ of severe faucial, and their treatment (*G. C. Garratt*)	XL.	41
hæmorrhagic, malignant	XXIII.	13, 17
heart disease, aortic reflux, complicating . .	XXV.	1
,, disturbance of, as sequel of severe faucial .	XL.	42
immunity of puerperal women from infection of .	XXX.	151
increase in London	XXVII.	262
incubation period of	XXVII.	273
in Hope Ward	XXVII.	266
in-patients, number attacked with	XXVII.	264
malignant, absence of albuminuria in . . .	XXIII.	17
,, ,, pyrexia in	XXIII.	17

	VOL.	PAGE
Diphtheria, malignant, causes of death in	XXIII.	17
„ condition of blood in	XXIII.	17
„ „ „ spleen in	XXIII.	17
„ hæmorrhages in	XXIII.	13, 17
membrane from fauces examined bacteriologically	XXX.	142
method of removing membrane from trachea in	XXI.	84
nurses, number affected by	XXVII.	264
on (*Hamer*)	XXV.	274
paralysis after	XXVII.	263, 287
„ „ antitoxin treatment of (*Hayward*)	XXXI.	101
rules for nursing	XXVII.	278
slow pulse in	XXVIII.	193
some points in (*Herringham*)	XXIX.	351
spread of, to nurses	XXVII.	275
suppression of urine in	XXVIII.	193
tracheotomy in	XXVI.	173
treated by antitoxin, prognosis and causes of death	XXXII.	335
treatment by antitoxin (*Herringham*)	XXXI.	73
value of patellar reflex in	XXX.	151
vomiting, a bad symptom in (*Gee*)	XXV.	69
with heart-disease	XXV.	1
within the Hospital	XXVII.	261
Diphtheritic membrane, solvents of	XXX.	149
paralysis, history of	XXX.	129
Diplococcus pneumoniæ	XXVIII.	174
Diplopia, in Graves' disease	XXVII.	147
„ insular sclerosis	XXII.	308
Disease, acute, effect of in the insane	XXIII.	29
and health, gradations of (*Campbell*)	XXX.	151
brassfounders', a case of (*Gee*)	XXV.	77
Bright's, as a cause of sudden death (*Horder*)	XXXV.	155
desirability of expectoration in certain forms of lung	XXI.	120
disuse of limbs, after severe	XXV.	201
„ „ „ treatment of	XXV.	210
ear, cases of (*Mayo, Willett,* and *Hawes*)	XXXVII.	280
eye, notes on cases of (*Jessop*)	XXXV.	231
hydatid, of arm	XXXII.	187
„ „ heart (*Calvert*)	XXXIX.	208
influence of environment on development of	XXXIX.	78
influenza, a zymotic	XXVI.	204
its relation to nerve-physiology (*T. W. Shore*)	XXV.	27
malignant, cases of, from Department for Diseases of the Throat and Nose	XXXIX.	219
„ of cervical glands with abscess	XXIII.	150, 153
microzymes, their relation to	XXIV.	79
physiological aspects of (*Campbell*)	XXXI.	169
the coincidence of tuberculosis and malignant (*Forbes*)	XXXV.	183
use of Leiter's tubes in Graves'	XXVIII.	25
Diseases, calling for isolation	XXIV.	25
geographical distribution of, on the Continent	XXXIX.	102
of great omentum	XXX.	105
„ infancy, puberty, and maturity	XXII.	353
spinal, syphilis, a cause of (*Forbes*)	XXXVIII.	78
which may present misleading or seemingly unimportant symptoms (*Sir Dyce Duckworth*)	XL.	1
Disinfection, the scientific aspect of (*Klein*)	XXV.	275
Dislocation of foot	XXXIV.	234
„ humerus	XXXIV. 235 ; XXXVIII.	33
„ jaw	XXXIV.	235
„ lens, spontaneous	XXIX.	304

		VOL.	PAGE
Dislocation of nasal septum	. . . . .	XXIII.	124
„ radius and ulna	. . . .	XXIV.	308
„ shoulder, without rupture of capsule	. .	XXIV.	163
„ spine, with fracture	. . .	XXI.	140
„ thumb, compound	. . .	XXXIV.	269
„ „ metarcarpo-phalangeal	. .	XXXV.	45
„ wrist, compound	. . . .	XXXVII.	283
Dispensing Department	. . . .	XXII.	16
Disseminated sclerosis, syphilitic (*Forbes*)	. .	XXXVIII.	83
with palatal and laryngeal anæsthesia	. .	XXXII.	173
Disuse of limbs, after severe disease	. .	XXV.	201
„ „ „ treatment of	. .	XXV.	210
Diverticulum of Meckel, intussusception of	. .	XXVII.	171
Dobel's solution, formula of	. . . .	XXIII.	120
Doctor, the title of	. . .	XXII.	365
Duran (*Alban*), Stanley's case of patent urachus, with observations on urachal cysts	. . .	XXXIV.	33
Douglas (*James*), dissection of a heart	. . .	XXVI.	165
(*A. R. J.*), and **Butlin** (*H. T.*), on cases of appendicitis	XXXIV.	71
Drage (*L.*), on inflammation and congestion of the cervix	.	XXIII.	355
„ tracheotomy	. . . .	XXII.	354
Drainage of lung	. . . .	XXVIII.	5
„ peritoneum	. . . .	XXIX.	171
tube, retention and extraction of a	. .	XXII.	236
„ use of, in ovariotomy	. .	XXII.	235
Dressers, directions to	. . . .	XXIX.	91
Dressings, carbolic acid, danger of in removal of goitre	XXV.	103
in abdominal section	. . .	XXVIII. 22; XXIX.	19
report on	. . . .	XXIX.	100
Dropsy, general, with chronic peritonitis	. .	XXVII.	247
of pregnancy	. . .	XXVI.	115
sudden disappearance of renal (*Weber*)	. .	XXXIV.	303
Drugs, action of certain, in gout	. .	XXIV.	217
„ „ on insomnia	. . .	XXV.	153
causes of failure in their action	. .	XXII.	271
failure of their action in gout	. .	XXIV.	226
production of gout by	. . .	XXIV.	225
scepticism as to the use of	. .	XXVII.	81
Drunkenness, in insanity	. . .	XXIX.	114
Drysdale (*J. H.*), with **Garrod** (*A. E.*), and **Kanthack** (*A. A.*), on the green stools of typhoid fever, with some remarks on green stools in general	. .	XXXIII.	13
with **Kanthack,** ulceration of larynx in typhoid fever	.	XXXI.	113
Duckworth (*Sir Dyce*), clinical contributions to practical medicine	. . .	XXI.	105
a case of mediastinal tumour, presenting difficulties in diagnosis	. . .	XXXIII.	7
a fatal case of rheumatism, associated with hæmorrhagic erythema, with remarks on rheumatic purpura	.	XXVII.	1
note on taches bleuâtres	. . .	XXIX.	331
„ the occurrence of subcutaneous fibroid nodules in gouty persons	. . .	XL.	15
„ some anomalies of the papular eruption in enteric fever	. . .	XXV.	5
notes of two cases of heart-disease (aortic reflux) which recovered respectively from severe enteric fever and diphtheria	. . .	XXV.	1
observations on chorea gravidarum	. . .	XXXIX.	1

VOL. PAGE

Duckworth (*Sir Dyce*), observations on Heberden's nodes, Dupuytren's contraction, and some other arthritic conditions . . . . XXXV. 13
observations on rheumatoid arthritis . . . . XXXV. 13
on actinomycosis of thoracic wall . . . . . XXXI. 23
on malignant (hæmorrhagic) diphtheria . . . XXIII. 13
remarks on some diseases which may present misleading or seemingly unimportant symptoms . . . XL. 1
the pathogeny of chorea . . . . . . XXXVII. 9
three cases of multiple peripheral (alcoholic) neuritis in women . . . . XXII. 253
two cases of tinea favosa capitis, recovery under treatment with izal . . . . XXXVIII. 155
and **Garrod** (*A. E.*), hepatic cirrhosis, with obstruction in superior vena cava . . . . . . XXXII. 71
and **Tooth** (*H. H.*), two cases of general spastic rigidity XXVIII. 263
Duct, sublingual, foreign body in . . . . . XXXIII. 105
submaxillary, foreign body in . . . . . XXXIII. 105
vitelline, patent . . . . XXVII. 171
Duct-cancers of the breast . . . . XXIV. 263 ; XXVII. 194
Duncan (*J. Matthews*), a case of progressive suppurative parametritis . . . . XXIV. 39
concerning medical education . . . . XXIII. 345
memoir of . . . . XXVI., xxxiii
Dunn (*W. E. N.*), double empyema with recovery . . XXXII. 213
Duodenal ulcer, gastro-enterostomy for (*D'Arcy Power*) . XL. 71
perforated, cases of (*D'Arcy Power*) . . . XXXVII. 46
perforating, treated by operation (*D'Arcy Power*) . XXXVIII. 14
Duodenum, case of rupture of first part (*D'Arcy Power*) . XXXV. 41
perforating ulcer of, treated by operation (*D'Arcy Power*) XXXVIII. 14
Dupuytren's contraction, &c., observations on (*Sir Dyce Duckworth*) . . . . XXXV. 13
relation of gout and rheumatism to (*Hedges*) . . XXXII. 119
Dura mater, fibrous tumour of . . . . . XXVII. 171
Duration of life, on (*Hamer*) . . . . . . XXVI. 307
„ pregnancy, difficulty in determining by means menstruation ; its medico-legal importance (*C. Godson*) . . XXIV. 167, 169
„ „ on (*Graham*) . . . . . XXV. 177
Dysmenorrhœa, cured by dilatation of the os uteri . . XXIV. 170
notes of a case of (*C. Godson*) . . . . . XXIV. 167
spasmodic, with sterility . . . . . XXIV. 170
Dyspareunia, removal of uterine appendages for . . . XXIX. 49
Dyspepsia, on (*Habershon*) . . . . . . XXIII. 350
Dysphagia, in spastic paralysis . . . . . XXVIII. 265
Dyspnœa, hysterical . . . . XXII. 216
Dwelling-house, conditions tending to the promotion of phthisis . . . . XXVI. 13
necessity for adequate space round . . . XXVI. 7
„ „ light in . . . . . XXVI. 10
relation to tubercular consumption . . . XXVI. 1
size, and position of windows in . . . . XXVI. 9

Ear, affections of, and eye, in influenza . . . . XXVI. 202
disease middle, cases of (*Mayo, Willett*, and *Hawes*) . XXXVII. 280
„ „ mastoid suppuration . XXIX. 343
intra-cranial complications of chronic disease of (*Bailey*) XXXVII. 287
middle, changes in, due to nasal obstruction . . XXVII. 15
some functions of the middle (*Lawrence*) . . XXXV. 113
the complications of disease of the middle (*Bowes*) . XXXIV. 127
Eberth's bacillus in typhoid fever . . . . XL. 19

			VOL.	PAGE
Eclampsia of pregnancy	. . . . . .	.	XXVI.	115
puerperal	. . . . . .	.	XXII.	358
Eccles, (*McAdam*) an analysis of twenty-eight cases of intus-	susception . . .	.	XXVIII.	97
,,	,,　of a second series of forty cases	of intussusception . .	.	XXXIII.	139
,,	,,　of a third list of twenty-eight	cases of intussusception .	XXXVII.	189
,,	,,　of ninety-six cases of intussus-	ception . . .	XXXVII.	203
,,	development, anatomy, physiology, and	pathology of the great omentum .	.	XXX.	81
,,	hernia of vermiform appendix .	.	.	XXXII.	93
,,	on retention of urine in women	.	.	XXIX.	350
,,	strangulation of small intestine, in fossa	inter-sigmoidea	.	XXXI	177
,,	temperature in relation to injuries of the	head . . .	.	XXIX.	225
,,	,,　on the two sides of the body	XXIX.	231
,,	and **Waring** (*H. J.*), cases from Mr.	Langton's wards	.	XXVII.	177
Eclipse blindness, cases of (*Jessop*)	. . . . .	.	XXXVI.	260
Edinburgh Infirmary, notes on surgical cases in (*Edgar Willett*)	. . . .	.	XXXVII.	215
Effusion, pericardial, and intra-thoracic growths .	.	.	XXVIII.	94
pleural, and intra-thoracic growths	.	.	.	XXVIII.	95
,,　manner of contraction of lung in	.	.	.	XXVIII.	131
Effusions, pleural (*Gow*) .	.	.	.	XXIII.	357
Egg-albumin, its action, injected subcutaneously	.	XXIII.	173
Ehrlich's reaction, in typhoid fever	.	.	.	XXXII.	217
test for typhoidal urine	.	.	.	.	XXVI.	290
Elbow, injury to	.	.	.	.	XXIV.	308
joint, synovial cyst in connection with	.	.	.	XXI.	184
,,　syphilitic disease of	.	.	.	.	XXVI.	86
Electric batteries, &c.	.	.	.	.	XXVIII.	245
light, effects of on eye (*Jessop*)	.	.	.	XXXVII.	311
Electrical condition of muscles in sclerosis	.	.	.	XXI.	95, 96
,,　　　,,　spastic paralysis	.	XXVIII.	267, 278
reactions in Laudry's paralysis	.	.	.	XXVIII.	137
Electrical Department, cases treated in	.	.	.	XXVIII.	251
foundation of .	.	.	.	.	XXII.	29
notes from (*Lewis Jones*)	.	.	.	.	XXVIII.	245
report from	.	.	.	.	XXII.	57
,,　of the work in (*Lewis Jones*)	.	.	.	XXXIII.	169
Electricity, at the Hospital, .	.	.	.	XXII.	25, 28
in infantile paralysis	.	.	.	.	XXVIII.	252
nature of, used for fibro-myomata of uterus .	.	.	XXIV.	129
results of, in fibro-myomata of uterus	.	.	.	XXIV.	129
statical machine for	.	.	.	.	XXVIII.	247
strictures treated by	.	.	.	.	XXVIII.	256
switches for	.	.	.	.	XXVIII.	250
the induction coil	.	.	.	.	XXVIII.	249
treatment by, of enuresis	.	.	.	.	XXVIII.	255
,,　fibro-myomata of uterus	.	.	.	XXIV.	89
,,　hemiplegia .	.	.	.	XXVIII.	255
,,　injury to nerves .	.	.	.	XXVIII.	254
,,　nævus .	.	.	.	.	XXVIII.	251
,,　neuralgia	.	.	.	.	XXVIII.	255
,,　sciatica	.	.	.	.	XXVIII.	254
,,　tinnitus aurium	.	.	.	XXVIII.	254

	VOL.	PAGE
Electrodes, distinction of positive from negative	XXVIII.	248
Electrolysis, of hairs	XXVIII.	256
treatment of nævus by	XXX.	205
Elephantiasis	XXIV.	305
of one leg, in a boy	XXXII.	181
Emaciation, in Graves' disease	XXXV.	126
in intra-thoracic growths	XXVIII.	92
in spastic paralysis	XXVIII. 263, 279	
Embolism, a cause of aneurysm	XXII.	187
and its results	XXVIII.	229
capillary, a cause of chorea	XXIV.	61
cerebral	XXVII. 41, 285	
of right middle cerebral artery	XXVII.	44
of right coronary artery	XXXII.	7
Emergencies, surgical (*Mayo, Willett*, and *Hawes*)	XXXVII.	269
Emetics, in hæmoptysis	XXVII.	85
Emotion, on the expression of (*Claye Shaw*)	XXXVI.	243
Emphysema, gangrenous	XXVII.	213
its connection with gout	XXIII.	292
on (*Gabriel*)	XXIII.	354
Empyema, and taches bleuâtres (*Sir Dyce Duckworth*)	XXIX.	333
double, with recovery (*Dunn*)	XXXII.	213
fetid	XXXII.	83
of gall-bladder	XXXII.	189
Enchondrosis of the septum nasi	XXIII.	126
Endocardial growths, a page in the life-history of (*Hollis*)	XXVIII.	221
Endocarditis, a result of chorea (*Herringham*)	XXIV.	55
associated in young persons with cerebral aneurysm (*Kidd*)	XXII.	187
infective, and cancer	XXVIII.	228
its frequency in acute rheumatism	XXIII. 269, 273, 275	
malignant	XXVII.	41
„ (streptococci)	XXXII.	1
relation of, to micro-organisms (*Ware*)	XXXV.	253
ulcerative, a cause of aneurysm	XXII.	189
„ (*Harris*)	XXIX.	352
Endocardium, sprouting growths on	XXVIII.	221
Endothelioma, a case of (*D'Arcy Power*)	XXXVII.	44
Enemata, of defibrinated blood	XXII.	245
vomiting (*Weber*)	XXXIV.	314
Enteric fever, arteritis in relation to (*Auden*)	XXXV.	55
pericarditis in (*Norman Moore*)	XL.	19
(*see* Fever, Typhoid).		
Enteritis and colic, simulating intestinal obstruction	XXXII.	61
Entero-vesical fistula	XXIV.	307
Enuresis, treatment of, by electricity	XXVIII.	255
Environment, influence of, on development of disease	XXXIX.	78
of medicine and surgery	XXIX.	352
Epidemic of influenza, 1890	XXVI.	193
of typhoid, Maidstone, points of interest in (*W. E. Lee*)	XXXIII.	93
Epididymis, strangulation of (*Nash*)	XXIX.	163
Epilepsy and nasal obstruction	XXIX.	250
compared with insanity	XXIII. 20, 30	
condition of the cerebral circulation in	XXV.	33
historically considered	XXVII.	283
Jacksonian	XXIII.	188
observations on	XXXI.	63
on (*Fletcher*)	XXVII.	283
with cerebral abscess	XXIII.	188
Epileptics, suicide in	XXI.	3, 7

	VOL.	PAGE
Epileptiform convulsions, relieved by trephining.(*Calvert* and *Berry*)	XXVI.	69
Epiphysis of femur, fracture of	XXIV.	288
Epistaxis in influenza	XXVI.	206
Epithelioma, effect of irritation in	XXV.	113
its connection with horns and warts	XXV. 106,	107
melanotic	XXVI.	309
on (*Francis*)	XXVI.	309
pathology of	XXV.	105
recurrent beneath jaw	XXIV.	287
of ala of nose	XXI.	151
„ bladder, cure of	XXIV. 211 ;	XXV. 230, 234
„ cheek	XXIV.	283
„ labium	XXVII.	137
„ larynx	XXXIX.	221
„ mouth, with abscess	XXIII.	151
„ pelvis of kidney	XXI. 127,	129
„ penis	XXIV.	302
„ scrotum	XXV.	193
„ tongue	XXIV.	288
„ upper jaw	XXIV.	311
Epitheliomatous ulcer of leg	XXIV.	285
Epulis of lower jaw	XXII.	239
„ „ „ treated by Paquelin's cautery	XXII.	239
Equilibrium of body, how maintained	XXIII.	69
maintained by lumbar muscles	XXIV.	242
Erection of inferior turbinated body	XXIII.	129
„ theatre in the Hospital	XXII.	40
Erectores spinæ, their function	XXIII.	69
Ergot, in hæmoptysis	XXVII.	93
its introduction and consumption	XXII.	50
Erysipelas, its varieties	XXIV.	321
on (*Lyndon*)	XXIV.	321
Erythema, hæmorrhagic, a case of	XXII.	225
„ in rheumatism (*Duckworth*)	XXVII.	1
iris, a case of (*Gardner* and *Scott*)	XXXVIII.	135
multiforme, bibliography of	XXIV.	53
„ cases of	XXIV.	46
„ in rheumatism	XXVII.	45
„ its relation to rheumatism (*Garrod*)	XXIV.	43
nodosum, associated with purpura (*Duckworth*)	XXVII.	2
„ bibliography of	XXIV.	53
„ cases of	XXIV.	50
„ its relation to rheumatism (*Garrod*)	XXIV.	43
Erythemata, connected with rheumatism	XXIV.	53
Essex and Colchester Hospital, cases from	XXVII.	239
notes and observations from	XXIV.	253
Ether, Bertoni's	XXVIII.	287
Ether rash	XXXII.	79
Ethmoidal cells, case of suppuration in	XXXVI.	53
sinuses, purulent catarrh of	XXX.	243
Etiology of acute infective periostitis	XXIX.	265
„ cholera (*Klein*)	XXI.	260
„ chorea (*Fletcher*)	XXXII.	383
„ croupous pneumonia	XXVIII.	173
„ infectious diseases (*T. F. Raven*)	XXXVII.	205
„ inter-thoracic growths	XXVIII.	75
„ primary pleurisy (*Hedges*)	XXXVI.	75
„ pylethrombosis	XXXVII.	60
„ Raynaud's disease	XXVIII.	33

	VOL.	PAGE
Etiology of suppurative pylephlebitis	XXXVII.	95
„ typhoid fever	XXVIII.	289
Eustachian tube, outgrowths from	XXIII.	136
Evill (*C.*), on a case of dislocation of the shoulder, without		
rupture of the capsule	XXIV.	163
on the man of the future	XXIV.	338
Evolution of predispositions or tendencies	XXIV.	76, 78
Examination of the nasal chambers for obstruction . .	XXIII.	120
Excision of chronic ulcers of the tongue	XXIV.	83
„ coccyx	XXXIV.	293
„ hip, statistics of	XXIV.	335
„ knee, with sinus	XXIV.	304
„ scapula, a case of	XXIV.	205, 207
Excretion of uric acid, influenced by some drugs (*Haig*) .	XXIV.	217
„ „ in gout	XXIV.	217
Exercise, in paralysis of right sympathetic, effects of .	XXIX.	104
Exophthalmic goître, a case of (*Herringham*) . .	XXXV.	125
Exophthalmos, some rare clinical points in . .	XXIX.	181
Expectoration, albuminous	XXII.	99
its desirability in certain forms of lung disease .	XXI.	120
stinking	XXXII.	34
Expression of emotion, an essay on the (*Claye Shaw*) .	XXXVI.	243
Extirpation of the labyrinth, two cases of (*C. E. West*) .	XL.	93
Extra-uterine gestation	XXIX.	350
Extravasation of urine, cases of (*Mayo, Willett*, and *Hawes*) .	XXXVII.	281
Eye, affections of, in influenza	XXVI.	202
cataract extraction, without iridectomy (*Jessop*) .	XXXVII.	317
effect of exposure to electric light (*Jessop*) .	XXXVII.	311
effects of gunshot wounds of orbit (*Jessop*) . .	XXXVII.	312
double sub-conjunctival hæmorrhage caused by com-		
pression of the chest (*Hunt*)	XXXVIII.	179
hæmorrhage into retinal macula (*Jessop*) . .	XXXV.	241, 247
notes on cases of diseases of (*Jessop*) . .	XXXV.	231
obliteration of retinal artery (*Jessop*) . . .	XXXVII.	314
ophthalmic cases and notes (*Jessop*) . . .	XXXVI.	253
optic atrophy, in diabetes insipidus (*Stanley Bousfield*) .	XXXVI.	235
secondary cataract (*Henry Power*)	XXXIV.	5
some points in the pathology and prognosis of glioma		
of the retina (*Jessop*)	XXXVIII.	159
unusual symptoms with fractured base (*Willett* and		
Wood-Hill)	XXXIV.	257
value of the pupil, as an aid to diagnosis . .	XXV.	38
Eyes, conjugate deviation of (*Gee*)	XXVI.	106
Eyeball, foreign bodies in (*Jessop*)	XXXV.	245
glass in	XXIV.	201
Eyelids, swelling of, in Graves' disease	XXVII.	142
Face, palsy of, cases of	XXII.	172
Facial diagnosis, on (*Lewis Jones*)	XXV.	277
paralysis, in Graves' disease	XXVII.	138
„ of syphilitic origin, a case of (*Weber*) .	XXXIV.	308
Fæcal impaction in rectum	XXVII.	250
mass retained in rectum	XXVII.	58
vomiting (*Weber*)	XXXIV.	314
Fæces, incontinence of	XXIV.	260
present in the urine	XXIV.	258
their colour and consistency, in the cœliac affection	XXIV.	17
Failure, cardiac, on the hypodermic injection of strychnia		
in cases of (*Habershon*)	XXII.	115
of the action of certain drugs in gout . . .	XXIV.	226

	VOL.	PAGE
Fallopian tubes, distension of	XXIX.	51
tumours of	XXIX.	50
Faradisation, in typhoid fever	XXI.	107
Faria (*Abbé*), his practice of magnetism	XXV.	117
Farrar (*R.*), on general paralysis of the insane	XXIV.	317
the biography of anatomy	XXII.	367
Farre (*Frederic J.*), memoir of	XXII.	xxxiii
Fasciæ, operations on (*Walsham*)	XXXIV.	294
Fat, free, in urine	XXI.	117
Fatal hæmoptysis	XXVII.	85
in a case of gangrene of lung, treated by operation	XXV.	225
Fauces, gangrene of, and cancrum oris (*Gee*)	XXV.	75
,, ,, in diphtheria, membrane from, examined bacteriologically	XXX.	142
Features, expression of, in the insane	XXIV.	11
Feet, swelling of, in Graves' disease	XXVII.	143
Femoral artery, ligature of (*D'Arcy Power*)	XXXV.	43
secondary hæmorrhage from	XXXV.	269
sloughing of (*Harmer*)	XXXV.	269
superficial, ligature of	XXX.	224
deep, ligature of	XXX.	224
Femur, diffuse idiopathic osteomyelitis of	XXIII.	223
epiphysis of, fracture of	XXIV.	288
osteitis of, following typhoid fever	XXIII.	220
,, ,, lower end	XXIV.	306
osteomyelitis of, invading knee-joint	XXIII.	223
osteotomy, for mal-union of	XXI.	65
re-fracture of (*Lankester*)	XXI.	68
sarcoma of	XXIV.	305
Ferguson (*G. B.*), on the nature and origin of rodent ulcer	XXI.	101
Ferment, glycolytic	XXVII.	72
Ferments, the pancreatic, in disease (*Hurris* and *Crace-Calvert*)	XXIX.	125
Fetid empyema	XXXII.	83
Fever, menstrual	XXII.	93
puerperal, precautions against propagation of	XXIII.	52
,, septicæmia in	XXIII.	46
,, sources of infection in	XXIII.	51
,, what it is	XXIII.	45
rheumatic, in a child of seven months	XXII.	215
,, with numerous nodules	XXII.	213
,, ,, pericarditis	XXII.	213
,, without arthritis	XXIV.	21
scarlet (*see* Scarlatina).		
typhoid, abscesses in	XXI.	115
,, acute cystitis in	XXXIII.	85
,, alum-whey, use of in	XXI.	115
,, arteritis, in relation to	XXXV.	55
,, arytænoid cartilage, necrosis of an, in	XXV.	133
,, bacillary phthisis supervening	XXI.	115
,, bacillus of	XXVIII.	289
,, ,, coli communis in	XXXIII.	85
,, causes of death in	XXVIII.	298
,, ,, ,, ulceration of bowel	XXVIII.	298
,, collapse in	XXXII.	107
,, cultures of typhoid bacilli used in serum reaction	XXXIV.	206
,, curing chorea	XXII.	224
,, death from strangulation of intestine in	XXIV.	153
,, delirium in	XXV.	128

			VOL.	PAGE
Fever, typhoid, delirium of collapse in	.	.	xxv.	130, 133, 134
,,	,, resembling acute mania in	.	xxv.	129
,,	dermatitis, multiple, gangrenous in	.	xxvii.	189
,,	discussion on	.	xxvii.	282
,,	Eberth's bacillus, in	.	xl.	19
,,	effect of diabetes mellitus on	.	xxv.	14
,,	Ehrlich's reaction in	.	xxxii.	217
,,	etiology of	.	xxviii.	289
,,	experimental production of	.	xxviii.	294
,,	faradisation in	.	xxi.	107
,,	followed by acute cystitis, due to bacillus coli communis	.	xxxiii.	85
,,	,, ,, bacillary phthisis	.	xxi.	115
,,	,, ., gangrene of lung	.	xxiii.	109
,,	,, ,, muscular atrophy and gangrene		xxiii.	109
,,	gangrene of skin in	.	xxvii.	189
,,	green stools of	.	xxi. 110; xxxiii.	13
,,	hæmaturia in	.	xxi.	105
,,	hæmorrhage in	.	xxi. 109; xxxi.	297
,,	hæmorrhagic	.	xxxi.	259
,,	heart disease, aortic reflux	.	xxv.	1
,,	in a child with retraction of head	.	xxii.	224
,,	is typhoid fever always begotten of	.	xxviii.	289
,,	laryngismus stridulus in	.	xxv.	138
,,	leading to the formation of an adhesion		xxiv.	152, 154
,,	loss of power in hand in	.	xxiii.	109
,,	loss of speech in	.	xxi.	106
,,	lumbrici, passage of many, in	.	xxi.	109
,,	Maidstone epidemic	.	xxxiii.	93
,,	malt extract, use of in	.	xxi.	117
,,	mania, during convalescence from	.	xxv.	131
,,	mental symptoms in	.	xxv.	127
,,	multiple gangrenous dermatitis in	.	xxvii.	189
,,	muscular paralysis in	.	xxv.	138
,,	,, rigidity in	.	xxv.	134, 136, 137
,,	,, tremor and twitchings in	.	xxv.	133
,,	necrosis of larynx in	.	xxv.	133
,,	nervous affection after	.	xxiii.	115, 116
,,	,, phenomena in	.	xxv.	127
,,	noma in	.	xxv.	133
,,	notes on the papular eruption of	.	xxv.	5
,,	osteitis of femur, after	.	xxiii.	220
,,	parotid abscess in	.	xxi.	112, 114
,,	,, bubo in	.	xxi.	112
,,	passage of lumbrici in	.	xxi.	109
,,	perforation of bowel in	.	xxv. 138; xxxix.	133
,,	pericarditis in	.	xl.	19
,,	periostitis following	.	xxi.	107
,,	purpura in	.	xxvii.	189, 191
,,	retention of urine in	.	xxv.	139
,,	retraction of head in	.	xxii.	224
,,	rigidity, and jactitation in	.	xxv.	134
,,	rigor in	.	xxxii.	107
,,	rules for nursing	.	xxvii.	279
,,	simulating meningitis	.	xxii.	224
,,	stools, green in	.	xxi. 110; xxxiii.	13
,,	sweating in	.	xxv.	139
,,	tables of temperature in	.	xxxii.	15
,,	tâche cérébrale	.	xxv.	139
,,	ulceration of larynx in	.	xxxi.	113

34   *General Index.*

	VOL.	PAGE
Fever, typhoid, use of alum-whey in	XXI.	115
,, ,, malt extract in	XXI.	117
,, with heart disease	XXV.	1
,, ,, low temperature, during convalescence	XXII.	220
,, ,, mottled rash	XXII.	219
,, ,, pregnancy	XXII.	221
,, ,, relapse	XXII.	219, 220
,, ,, severe abdominal pain during convalescence	XXII.	220
,, ,, special symptoms	XXI.	111
,, ,, squint	XXII.	224
Fibroid (*see* Fibromyoma).		
Fibroids of uterus, hysterectomy for	XXIX.	38
removal of uterine appendages in case of	XXIX.	47
Fibromatous growth in the skin of neck	XXVI.	147
Fibro-adenomata of breast, removed during the year 1901	XXXVII.	298
Fibro-myomata of the uterus, nature of electricity used for	XXIV.	120
,, ,, treatment by electricity	XXIV.	89
Fibrosis of heart wall, as result of syphilis	XXXIX.	11
Fifth nerve, ascending root of	XXIX.	215
trunk lesion of	XXIX.	215
,, ,, microscopical appearances in	XXIX.	217
Filariasis in West Africa	XXXIX.	182
Fingers, nodules on the joints of	XXIX.	157
Fissure of anus, constipation in	XXVIII.	206
symptoms of	XXVIII.	206
syphilitic and non-syphilitic	XXVIII.	205
,, age in	XXVIII.	210
,, cases of	XXVIII.	209
,, signs of	XXVIII.	210
Fistula, entero-vesical	XXIV.	307
in fissure of anus	XXVIII.	207
Fistulous opening into intestine	XXIV.	258
tracks, over sacrum and coccyx	XXIV.	229
Flat-foot and hallux valgus	XXIV.	303
gonorrhoeal	XXII.	261
Fletcher (*H. Morley*), a case of pseudo-hypertrophic paralysis in an adult	XXIX.	327
descriptive list of specimens added to the Museum	XXXVI.	275
etiology of chorea	XXXII.	383
on epilepsy	XXVII.	283
on periarteritis nodosa	XXIX.	352
and **Andrewes** (*F. W.*), descriptive list of additions to Museum	XXXIV.	331
and **Batten** (*F. E.*), a case of myasthenia gravis, with autopsy	XXXVI.	213
and **Shaw** (*E. H.*), analysis of tumours of mammary gland removed during 1900	XXXVII.	295
and **Shaw** (*E. H.*), carcinomata of mammary gland removed during 1900	XXXVII.	300
Fluids, injection of, in intussusception of bowel	XXVIII.	100, 115
Fœtal veins, persistence of, a cause of varicocele	XXIII.	137
Food-stuffs, prepared by plants, dietetic value of	XXX.	113
Foramina, abnormal, of heart and valves	XXVI.	314
Forbes (*J. Graham*), cystic disease of the kidneys and liver	XXXIII.	181
general paralysis, due to syphilis	XXXVIII.	68
medical report of the Anglo-French Commission on the western frontier of the Gold Coast Colony (1902–1903)	XXXIX.	171
native methods of treatment in West Africa	XXXIX.	189

	VOL.	PAGE
Forbes (*J. Graham*), remarks on carcinoma of the œsophagus	XXXV.	195
spinal cord, syphilitic disease of	XXXVIII.	78
syphilis, a cause of general paralysis	XXXVIII.	68
„ „ spinal disease	XXXVIII.	78
syphilitic locomotor ataxy	XXXVIII.	81
„ desseminated sclerosis . . . , . .	XXXVIII.	83
the coincidence of malignant disease and tuberculosis, with some reference to carcinoma of the œsophagus	XXXV.	183
the influence of hereditary syphilis on the nervous system	XXXVIII.	37
Foreign body down the trachea, its subsequent exit through abscess in axilla (*Good*)	XXVII.	251
in nose	XXVI.	271
„ nostril	XXVII.	57
„ sublingual duct	XXXIII.	105
„ submaxillary duct	XXXIII.	105
bodies in the eyeball (*Jessop*)	XXXV.	245
„ „ rectum, twenty cases of (*Goodsall*) .	XXIII.	71
„ „ vitreous, use of magnet in . . .	XXII.	311
Forensic physiology (*Stanley B. Atkinson*) . . .	XXXIX.	127
Formula of Dobell's solution	XXIII.	120
Fossa intersigmoidea, strangulation of small intestine in (*McAdam Eccles*), ...	XXXI.	177
Foster (*Michael*), on the pulmonary circulation . . .	XXVIII.	259
Foulerton (*A. G. R.*), on the pathology of horns occurring in man ; warts, and epitheliomata	XXV.	105
Foundation of St. Bartholomew's, The Book of the (*Norman Moore*)	XXI.	xxxix
Fracture, Colles'	XXXVII. 269, 271
compound	XXIII.	347
in necrosis	XXVIII.	11
of epiphysis of femur	XXIV.	288
„ femur, compound	XXVII.	211
„ „ intercondyloid	XXXIV.	269
„ „ neck of	XXXII.	63
„ „ osteotomy for mal-union of . .	XXI.	65
„ fibula	XXXVII.	270
„ humerus	XXXVIII.	33
„ „ compound	XXIV.	164
„ ilium	XXVII.	51
„ jaw	XXXIV.	237
„ leg, compound	XXIX. 99 ; XXXVII. 283
„ lower jaw	XXXVII.	269
„ olecranon	XXXVII.	269
„ patella . . XXI. 68 ; XXVII. 211 ; XXX. 230 ; XXXVII. 272
„ pelvis	XXXVI.	41
„ „ with rupture of bladder	XXXII.	199
„ phalanges	XXXVI.	222
„ ribs . . . . . . XXVII. 50 ; XXXVII. 269
„ „ in the insane . . . . XXVI. 15 ; XXVII. 50
„ „ sarcomatous tumour following . . .	XXII.	247
„ skull, XXV. 241 ; XXVII. 183, 185 ; XXIX. 226, 227, 229 ; XXXIV. 257, 269 ; XXXV. 44 ; XXXVII. 182, 184, 187
„ spine	XXI.	259
„ „ with dislocation	XXI.	140
„ thumb	XXXVI.	223
„ tibia, ununited	XXIV.	288
operations for mal-united . . XXIV. 288 ; XXXIV. 292, 293
Pott's, old-standing . . XXIV. 295 ; XXXIV. 292 ; XXXVII. 269
through roof of orbit . . . . . . XXIV. 182, 185
ununited of tibia	XXXIV.	288

	VOL.	PAGE
Fragilitas ossium	XXXIV.	238
Francis (*A. G.*), on epithelioma	XXVI.	309
two cases of lymphangioma of the tongue, with some remarks on macroglossia	XXIX.	143
Frequency of endocarditis, in acute rheumatism .	XXIII. 269, 273, 275	
relative of hæmoptysis, in the different sexes . .	XXI.	52
Fright, followed by somnambulism	XXI.	63
Frontal sinuses, purulent catarrh of	XXX.	244
Fugitive œdema, of obscure origin	XXX.	195
Gabriel (*M.*), on empyema	XXIII.	354
Gall-bladder, a case of rupture of (*Walsham*) . .	XXXVII.	341
abscess of (*Norman Moore*) . . .	XXVIII. 123, 125	
cancer of, and liver, with gall-stones . .	XXVIII.	228
distension of, causing an abdominal tumour .	XXV.	252
„ „ with clear fluid . . .	XXVIII.	47
empyema of	XXXII.	189
gall-stones, causing abscess of . .	XXVIII. 123, 126	
operations on	XXXVI.	43
stones in distended	XXV.	252
suppuration of	XXVIII.	51
and bile-ducts, some remarks on the surgery of	XXXVII.	321
Gall-stone colic, case of	XL.	136
Gall-stones, and cancer of gall-bladder, and liver .	XXVIII.	228
causing abscess of gall-bladder . .	XXVIII. 123, 126	
impacted in intestine	XXVIII.	113
„ „ „ removed by laparotomy .	XXVIII.	118
Galvano-cautery, in amputation of turbinal bones .	XXVII.	19
in erection of turbinal bones . . .	XXVII.	17
„ hypertrophy of turbinal bones . .	XXVII.	18
Ganglia of brain, occupied by cyst . . .	XXVI.	112
Ganglion, treatment of (*D'Arcy Power*) . .	XXXV.	50
Ganglionic swelling over external malleolus . .	XXI.	187
Gangrene, emphysematous	XXVII.	212
its causes	XXI.	246
of fauces, and cancrum oris . . .	XXV.	75
„ lung, after typhoid fever . . .	XXIII. 109, 113	
„ „ treated by operation . .	XXV.	253
„ skin, in enteric fever . . .	XXVII.	189
„ testis	XXIX.	172
„ toes	XXIV.	280
senile	XXX.	69
„ in a man aged forty-five . .	XXXIX.	235
spreading around the mouth . . .	XXVII.	205
„ „ „ „ treatment of . .	XXVII.	210
traumatic, of leg	XXXII.	192
and phagedæna, distinction between . .	XXV.	76
Gardner (*H. Willoughby*), a case of erythema iris .	XXXVIII.	135
on spinal caries	XXIII.	357
on treatment of heart disease . . .	XXIV.	337
Garratt (*G. C.*), general tuberculosis, with cortical meningitis, producing localising cerebral symptoms .	XXX.	211
the early sequelæ of severe faucial diphtheria, and their treatment	XL.	41
Garrod (*A. E.*), a case of paralysis of the abductors of the vocal cords, with lesions of several cranial nerves .	XXII.	209
association of cardiac malformations with other congenital defects .	XXX.	53
notes on the common hæmic cardiac murmur . .	XXVII.	33
on an unusual form of nodule upon the joints of the fingers	XXIX.	157

	VOL.	PAGE
Garrod (*A. E.*), on hysteria	XXII.	364
on the relationship of erythema multiforme and nodosum to rheumatism	XXIV.	43
some cases of sclerosis of the spinal cord . . .	XXI.	93
the diagnostic value of melanuria	XXXVIII.	25
and **Duckworth** (*Sir Dyce*), hepatic cirrhosis, with obstruction in superior vena cava	XXXII.	71
with **Kanthack** (*A. A.*), and **Drysdale** (*J. H.*), on the green stools of typhoid fever, with some remarks on green stools in general	XXXIII.	13
Gas, absorption of, by the intestines	XXII.	279
Gastric surgery, some cases of (*D'Arcy Power*) . .	XXXIX.	19
ulcer, cases of leaking perforated (*D'Arcy Power*) . .	XXXVII.	50
,, ,, ,, ,, ,, (*Mayo, Willett, and Hawes*) . .	XXXVII.	277
,, ,, treated by operation (*D'Arcy Power*) . .	XXXVIII.	5
,, leaking, case of, treated by operation (*D'Arcy Power*)	XXXVIII.	6
,, perforated, cases of, bacteriology of . . .	XXXVII.	52
,, prognosis of simple (*Habershon*)	XXVII.	149
Gastro-enterostomy, cases of	XXXIX.	24
for duodenal ulcer	XL.	71
Gastro-intestinal disturbance, a cause of albuminuria .	XXVI.	28
in influenza	XXVI.	97
Gastro-jejunostomy, four cases of (*D'Arcy Power*) . .	XL.	67
Gay (*J.*), on suppuration of the kidney	XXIII.	345
Gee (*S.*), a case of brassfounder's disease . . .	XXV.	77
bloody urine as the only sign of infantile scurvy .	XXV.	85
case of hemiopia, followed by hemianæsthesia and hemiplegia	XXVI.	109
cases from his wards	XXIII.	179
chronic solidification of base of lung . . .	XXVIII.	1
clinical aphorisms from his wards (*T. J. Horder*) .	XXXII.	29
conjugate deviation of the eyes, with examination post-mortem	XXVI.	106
hæmatemesis, due to alcohol	XXXVIII.	1
hereditary infantile spastic paraplegia . . .	XXV.	81
meaning of the word "delirium"	XXXIII.	3
memoir of Francis Harris, M.D.	XXI.	xxxiii
miscellanies	XXII.	89
on aneurysm of ascending aorta, taking natural position of heart	XXX.	1
on gangrene of the fauces, and cancrum oris . .	XXV.	75
on the cœliac affection	XXIV.	17
repeated vomiting, a bad prognostic in diphtheria .	XXV.	69
rheumatic fever, without arthritis	XXIV.	21
the tripod of life	XXXIII.	1
theory of the breathing sounds heard by auscultation .	XXVI.	103
General paralysis, due to syphilis (*J. Graham Forbes*) .	XXXVIII.	68
of adolescence (*Weber*)	XXXIV.	312
,, the insane, cases resembling	XXI.	23
Genito-urinary system, cases of injury to, and disease of (*Mayo, Willett, and Hawes*)	XXXVII.	281
Geographical distribution of diseases on the Continent .	XXXIX.	102
,, ,, mortality in the British Isles .	XXXIX.	95
German Hospital, some cases from (*Parkes Weber*) . .	XXXIV.	303
Germiculture, on (*Jessop*)	XXI.	252
Gestation, extra-uterine, some points on (*Griffith*) . .	XXIX.	350
length of	XXV.	177
Giant cells, their formation	XXIV.	69

			VOL.	PAGE
Gill (*R*), chloroform anæsthesia			XXX.	17
,,	,,	mechanical factor in	XXXI.	155
	,,	notes on	XXX.	17
	,,	stomachic phenomena during	XXXIV.	107
,,	,,	three cases illustrating exceptions from recent practice	XXXVI.	147
Gland, lachrymal, a case of tubercle of (*Jessop*)			XXXV.	23
mammary, analysis of tumours removed during 1900 (*Morley Fletcher* and *E. H. Shaw*)			XXXVII.	295
,, carcinomata of, removed during 1900 (*Morley Fletcher* and *E. H. Shaw*)			XXXVII.	300
,, chronic mastitis of			XXXVII.	307
,, colloid carcinoma of			XXXVII.	302
,, multiple tumours of			XXXVII.	308
parotid, inflammation of, in punctured wound of intestine			XXVII.	177
submaxillary, inflammation of, in punctured wound of intestine			XXVII.	177
Glands, cervical, malignant disease of, with abscess			XXIII.	150, 153
lymphatic, in rodent ulcer			XXIX.	191
,, removal of (*Walsham*)			XXXIV.	298
mediastinal, lymphadenoma of			XXIII.	101
,, primary lympho-sarcoma of			XXIII.	231
mesenteric, suppuration in			XXXVII.	110
pelvic, abscess complicating cancer of			XXIII.	152
removal of, results of			XXIX.	95
Glandular affections, in influenza			XXVI.	203
Glass in eyeball			XXIV.	201
Glaucoma, caused by cocaine			XXII.	307
removal of eye for			XXXIV.	238
Glioma of the aqueduct of Sylvius, a case of (*Herringham*)			XXXVI.	31
of the retina (*Jessop*)			XXXVI.	253
,, ,, prognosis, after operation in			XXXIX.	213
,, ,, some points in the pathology of (*Jessop*)			XXXVIII.	159
Glycerine, nitro-, hydroxylamine hydrochlorate as a substitute for			XXX.	189
introduction and consumption of			XXII.	53
Glycogen, its synthesis, and its utilisation			XXI.	239
Glycolytic ferment			XXVII.	72
Glycosuria, and diabetes			XXXII.	53
connection with ague			XXV.	9
from pressure of clot			XXVIII.	156
Godson (*C.*), on the difficulty in determining by means of menstruation the duration of pregnancy, with notes of a case of spasmodic dysmenorrhœa			XXIV.	167
Goître, cases of removal of			XXXVI.	49
exophthalmic			XXVII. 133 ; XXVIII. 25	
,, a case of (*Herringham*)			XXXV.	125
,, aural catarrh in			XXVII.	143
,, chronic arthritis in			XXVII.	143
,, diarrhœa in			XXVII.	141
,, diplopia in			XXVII.	147
,, facial paralysis in			XXVII.	138
,, v. Gräfe's sign in			XXVII. 133, 134, 138, 139	
,, lid symptoms in			XXVII.	133
,, nine cases of			XXVII.	133
,, ophthalmoplegia in			XXVII.	138
,, swelling of eyelids in			XXVII.	142
,, ,, ,, feet in			XXVII.	143
,, tinnitus in			XXVII.	138
,, trembling in			XXVII.	142

	VOL.	PAGE
Goître, removal of, danger of carbolic acid dressings in	xxv.	103
,, ,, ,, wounding recurrent laryngeal nerve in operation for . .	xxv.	103
,, methods of applying bandages after	xxv.	103
,, mortality of	xxv.	104
,, position of incision through the skin in	xxv.	102
,, ,, jugular vein, and carotid artery in	xxv.	102
,, steps in the operation for . . .	xxv.	102
,, successful (*Jessop* and *Berry*) . .	xxv.	97
,, suture used in	xxv.	103
Gold Coast Colony, filariasis in (*J. G. Forbes*) . .	xxxix.	182
goundou in	xxxix.	179
guinea-worm, native treatment of, in . .	xxxix.	194
gynæcology, native, in	xxxix.	204
leprosy in	xxxix.	177
madura foot in	xxxix.	178
Medical Report of the Anglo-French Boundary Commissioners	xxxix.	171
midwifery, native, in	xxxix.	204
native method of treatment in . . .	xxxix.	189
Gonorrhœa, a cause of flat-foot	xxii.	262
connection with acute suppuration of joints .	xxii.	263
discussion on	xxii.	366
rarer sequelæ of	xxii.	261
Gonorrhœal rheumatism	xxii.	261
Good (*F.*), passage of a foreign body down the trachea, and its subsequent exit through an abscess in the axilla	xxvii.	251
Goodsall (*D. H.*), fissure, non-syphilitic, and syphilitic, of rectum and anus	xxviii.	205
right iliac colotomy in intestinal obstruction .	xxx.	215
six cases of sinus over the sacrum and coccyx .	xxiv.	229
twenty cases of foreign bodies in the rectum .	xxiii.	71
Goundou, in West Africa	xxxix.	179
Gout, amount of acid in the urine of . . .	xxiv.	218, 220, 222
cartilage, articular, changes of, in . . .	xxiii.	291
condition of the liver in	xxv.	9
degeneration of aortic valves in . . .	xxiii.	293
effect of constipation on	xxiv.	227
heredity of	xxvi.	268
its connection with chronic interstitial nephritis .	xxiii.	292, 293
,, ,, cirrhosis of the liver .	xxiii.	293, 295
,, ,, diabetes mellitus (*Haig*) .	xxv.	7, 12
,, ,, emphysema . .	xxiii.	292
its treatment	xxvi.	270
observations on the morbid anatomy of (*Norman Moore*)	xxiii.	291, 293, 295
on the excretion of uric acid in (*Haig*) . .	xxiv.	217
production of, by drugs	xxiv.	225
relation of Dupuytren's contraction to rheumatism and (*Hedges*)	xxxii.	119
the action of some drugs in	xxiv.	217
urate of soda in joints	xxiii.	291
Gouty persons, occurrence of subcutaneous fibroid nodules in	xl.	15
Gow (*W. J.*), on cirrhosis	xxiv.	315
,, pleural effusions	xxiii.	357
,, primary sarcoma of the vagina . .	xxvii.	97
,, suppression of urine	xxv.	272
Gradations of health and disease (*H. Campbell*) . .	xxx.	151
v. Gräfe's sign in exophthalmic goitre . .	xxvii.	133, 134, 138, 139

	VOL.	PAGE
Graham (*A. R.*), on the duration of pregnancy	XXV.	177
Graves' disease, a case of	XXXV.	125
a rare form of œdema in	XXIX.	187
and cardiac irregularity	XXIX.	184
„ myxœdema	XXIX.	182
case of larval	XXXIX.	168
diarrhœa in	XXVII.	141
diplopia in	XXVII.	147
emaciation in	XXXV.	126
eyelids, swelling of, in	XXVII.	142
facial paralysis in	XXVII.	138
feet, swelling of, in	XXVII.	143
nine cases of	XXVII.	133
removal of turbinate bones in	XXVIII.	28
rhythmical jerking in	XXIX.	185
sense of smell in	XXIX. 181,	185
some rare clinical points in	XXIX.	181
surgical interference in	XXVIII.	26
swelling of eyelids in	XXVII.	142
„ feet in	XXVII.	143
thyroidectomy in	XXVIII.	27
thyroid extract in	XXIX.	182
tracheotomy in	XXVIII.	28
use of Leiter's tubes in	XXVIII.	25
with spasms	XXIX.	185
Great omentum, development, anatomy, physiology, and pathology of the (*McAdam Eccles*)	XXX.	81
diseases of	XXX.	105
displacement of	XXX.	93
injuries of	XXX.	91
normal physiological functions of the	XXX.	88
Green stools in general, some remarks on (*Garrod, Kanthack, Drysdale*)	XXXIII.	13
of typhoid fever (*Garrod, Kanthack, Drysdale*) XXI. 110;	XXXIII.	13
Griffith (*W. S. A.*), note on the renal affection of pregnancy and parturition	XXVI.	115
on gynæcological case-taking	XXVI.	120
some antiseptic measures in midwifery	XXIII.	45
„ points on extra-uterine gestation	XXIX.	350
Ground-air, its connection with summer diarrhœa	XXVI.	6
„ relation to subsoil water	XXVI.	5, 6
Growth, fibromatous, in the skin of neck	XXVI.	147
in gums and palate	XXIV.	293
„ rectum	XXXII.	21
malignant, developed in floor of ulcer of breast	XXIII.	159
new and abscess, diagnosis between	XXXIV.	251
Growths at limbus corneæ (*Jessop*)	XXXVI.	258
cartilaginous and bony, of palate	XXII.	323
effect of post-nasal	XXIX.	236
endocardial sprouting (*Hollis*)	XXVIII.	221
intra-thoracic (*Harris*)	XXVIII.	73
new, in bone (*Marsh*)	XXVIII.	7
„ of lung and pleura (*Samuel West*)	XXXIII.	109
polypoid and warty, of palate	XXII.	324
vascular, of palate	XXII.	320
Guinea-pig, action of aconite on	XXII.	281
„ „ and cold on	XXII.	282
„ „ „ heat „	XXII.	284
Guinea-worm, native treatment of, in West Africa (*Forbes*)	XXXIX.	194
Gumma, of the heart	XXXIX.	10

	VOL.	PAGE
Gummata, in the brain	XXIX.	215
„ liver, and kidneys	XXIX.	217
of the septum nasi	XXIII.	128
on the septum of nose	XXVII.	21
Gums, growth in palate and	XXIV.	293
Gunshot wound of the brain	XXIX.	228
„ „ orbit (*Jessop*)	XXXVII.	312
Gynæcological case-taking (*Griffith*)	XXVI.	120
Gynæcology, native, in West Africa (*Forbes*) . . .	XXXIX.	204
table of cases admitted into Martha Ward, during 1898		
(*Harrison Cripps*)	XXXV.	23
Habershon (*S. H.*), medical discussion on abdominal tumours	XXV.	279
observations on the variation of number of the white		
corpuscles, in diabetic patients	XXVI.	153
on dyspepsia	XXIII.	350
„ the hypodermic injection of strychnia, in cases of		
cardiac failure	XXII.	115
„ the prognosis of simple gastric ulcer . . .	XXVII. 149,	159
report on influenza	XXVI.	239
the after-treatment of tracheotomy	XXI.	79
vomiting in phthisis, with special reference to the		
association of this symptom with left apex-disease	XXIV.	131
Hæmangioma, of the tongue	XXIX.	149
Hæmatemesis	XXIV.	315
due to alcohol (*Gee*)	XXXVIII.	1
Hæmatinuria	XXII.	153
Hæmatoma, of the septum nasi	XXIII.	128
Hæmatosalpinx	XXIX.	51
Hæmaturia, bibliography of	XXII.	148
cases of	XXXII.	210
causes of	XXII.	145
connection with syphilis	XXII.	141
effects of cold in	XXII.	137
„ „ mental worry in	XXII.	137
from bladder	XXV.	229
„ prostate	XXV.	229
„ urethra	XXV.	229
illustrated by cases	XXV.	229
in enteric fever	XXI.	105
its seats	XXV.	229
malaria, a cause of	XXII.	139
parasitic, two cases of (*Norman Moore*) . . .	XXI.	89
paroxysmal (*Herringham*) . . .	XXII. 133, 137, 138,	140
purpura in	XXII.	137
quinine in	XXII.	140
Raynaud's disease in	XXII.	138
renal	XXV.	230
two cases of parasitic	XXI.	89
urticaria in	XXII.	137
value of post-mortem examination in . . .	XXII.	144
Hæmoglobin, and its derivatives	XXII.	363
its parallelism with chlorophyll	XXIV.	73
„ presence dependent on iron	XXIV.	74
Hæmoglobinuria	XXII.	133
Hæmophilia, joint-disease in	XXVI.	77
Hæmoptysis, astringents in	XXVII.	95
causes of	XXVII. 84,	91
condition of arteries in	XXVII. 92,	93
diapedesis of blood corpuscles in	XXVII	85

	VOL.	PAGE
Hæmoptysis, due to pulmonary aneurysm	XXI.	52
due to ulceration of the walls of the pulmonary vessels	XXI.	53, 58
emetics in	XXVII.	86
fatal	XXVII.	85
,, in a case of gangrene of lung, treated by operation	XXV.	225
in influenza	XXVI.	201
,, phthisis	XXII.	200
intermittent	XXI.	54, 56, 57
its significance	XXII.	199
pathology of	XXI.	51
profuse, non-fatal	XXI.	51
relative frequency of, in the different sexes	XXI.	52
remittent	XXI.	53
salt in	XXVII.	96
suffocative	XXI.	53
treatment of	XXVII.	81, 85, 90
use of ergot in	XXVII.	93
venesection in	XXVII.	87
Hæmorrhage, bronchial	XXVII.	81, 82
cerebral	XXVII.	285
,, in a boy of eight	XXIII.	181
,, ,, case of tumour	XXIII.	179
,, ,, child	XXXIV.	311
,, ,, young woman	XXVI.	296
double, sub-conjunctival, caused by compression of the chest	XXXVII.	179
from kidney, after injury	XXV.	239
in influenza	XXVI.	200
,, malignant diphtheria	XXIII.	17
,, surgery	XXII.	355
,, typhoid fever	XXI.	109
into spinal cord	XXI.	140
its connection with gout	XXIII.	293, 295
,, effect in insanity	XXIII.	29
meningeal	XXVIII.	153
pulmonary	XXVII.	83
retinal	XXXV.	241, 247
secondary, from femoral artery	XXXV.	269
subarachnoid	XXVIII.	152, 153, 155
Hæmorrhages, in malignant diphtheria	XXIII.	17
Hæmorrhagic erythema, a case of	XXII.	225
,, associated with a fatal case of rheumatism (*Sir Dyce Duckworth*)	XXVII.	1
in malignant diphtheria	XXIII.	13, 17
in typhoid fever (*West*)	XXXI.	259
Haig (*A.*), a case of Raynaud's disease, and some points in its pathology	XXVIII.	29
excretion of uric acid in a case of gout, with notes of the action of some drugs	XXIV.	217
some clinical features of the uric acid headache	XXIII.	201
some investigations regarding the quantity of uric acid in the blood, and various tissues of the body, with remarks on the causes which increase or diminish it	XXVI.	33
the use of salicylate of soda in diabetes mellitus, and its connection with gout	XXV.	7, 12
variola, as seen in the Casualty Department	XXI.	131
Hairs, treated by electrolysis	XXVIII.	256
Halsted's operations for cancer of breast	XXXIV. 63; XXXVII.	264

	VOL.	PAGE
Hall (*A. J.*), cirrhosis of liver, in a child of eleven	XXVIII.	167
Hallux valgus	XXIV.	303
with flat-foot, and hammer-toe	XXIV.	303
Hamer (*W. H.*), on croup, in its relation to tracheotomy	XXIV.	41
on diphtheria	XXV.	274
„ duration of life	XXVI.	307
Hand, loss of power in, with atrophy, following typhoid fever	XXIII.	109
punctured wound of	XXVII.	213
weakening, and wasting of	XXIII. 92, 93, 94	
Hands, method of cleansing	XXIX.	91
symmetrical atrophy of, in young people	XXIX.	307
„ „ „ cases of	XXIX.	308
Hankin (*D.*), on the biology of bacteria	XXIII.	352
Hare, the virtues of the foot of	XXII.	4
Harelip, and cleft palate, operations on (*W. J. Walsham*)	XXXIV. 238, 271	
Harmer (*W. D.*), a case of ligature of external iliac artery for secondary hæmorrhage	XXXV.	269
sloughing of femoral artery	XXXV.	269
Harris (*Francis*), memoir of	XXI.	xxxiii
(*V. D.*), cases of spontaneous pneumothorax	XXIII.	33
intra-thoracic growths	XXVIII.	73
on endocarditis, and ulcerative endocarditis	XXIX.	352
„ the presence of the tubercle bacillus in old specimens of diseased lungs	XXI.	45
„ the significance of blood-spitting	XXII.	199
„ the antiseptic treatment of phthisis	xxv. 49 ; xxvi. Part ii. 87	
treatment of hæmoptysis	XXVII.	81
and **Crace-Calvert** (*G. A.*), the human pancreatic ferments in disease	XXIX.	125
Hartley (*P.*), (*see* Horton-Smith (*P.*)).		
Harvey, additional notes of (*Munk*)	XXIII.	1
Haviland (*G. D.*), on hepatic tumours	XXIII.	356
Hawes (*C. S.*), surgical emergencies	XXXVII.	269
and **Willett** and **Mayo,** case of contusion of kidneys	XXXVII.	282
„ „ cases of diseases of joints	XXXVII.	281
„ „ „ „ fractured leg	XXXVII.	270
„ „ „ hernia	XXXVII.	277
„ „ „ injury to head	XXXVII.	271
„ „ „ „ „ and disease of the genito-urinary system	XXXVII.	281
„ middle ear disease, cases of	XXXVII.	280
„ perforated gastric ulcer, cases of	XXXVII.	277
„ „ surgical smashes	XXXVII.	282
Hayward (*J. A.*), antitoxin treatment of paralysis after diphtheria	XXXI.	101
diagnosis of diphtheria	XXX.	139
paralysis, after antitoxin treatment for diphtheria	XXXI.	101
report on influenza	XXVI.	231
Head-banging, in children	XXII.	97
Head, convulsions following injury to	XL.	138
four cases of severe injury to	XXVII.	183
injury, cases of, admitted to Mr. Willett's wards (*Bull*)	XXXVII.	181
injury to the, mania after (*Mayo, Willett,* and *Hawes*)	XXI.	166
injuries of the, temperature in (*McAdam Eccles*)	XXIX.	225
„ „ „ on the two sides of the body (*McAdam Eccles*)	XXIX.	231

		VOL.	PAGE
Head, protrusion of, from spasm of the muscles of the neck		xxiv.	249
retraction of, in typhoid fever		xxii.	224
shaking, in children		xxii.	96
Headache		xxvii. 287 ; xxxii. 49	
in intra-thoracic growths		xxviii.	92
the uric acid		xxiii.	201
,, effect of diet on		xxiii. 204, 206	
,, its factors		xxiii.	207
,, theory of its production		xxiii.	206
,, treated by nitro-hydrochloric acid		xxiii.	201
,, use of strychnia in		xxiii.	206
Health and disease, gradations of (*H. Campbell*)		xxx.	151
Heart, abnormal foramina in		xxvi.	314
aneurysm of ascending aorta, taking natural position of (*Gee*)		xxx.	1
causation of the first sound of (*Inchley*)		xxxviii.	91
congenital valvular defects, on left side of (*Parkes Weber*)		xxxv.	147
dilatation of, in hæmic murmurs		xxvii.	39
disease, complicating labour		xxvi.	311
disease of, congenital, associated with pulmonary tuberculosis (*Kidd*)		xxiii.	239
,, ,, the tendency to phthisis in		xxiii.	240
,, rheumatic		xxiii. 273, 275, 277	
dissection of a (*J. H. Douglas*)		xxvi.	165
disturbance of, as sequel of severe faucial diphtheria		xl.	42
gumma of the		xxxix.	10
hydatid disease of the (*James Calvert*)		xxxix.	208
hypertrophy of, œdema, and renal disease		xxxii.	261
intermission of action of		xxix.	284
irregularity of		xxix.	283
,, cases of		xxix.	289
,, in cerebral disease		xxix.	287
,, ,, hysteria		xxix.	286
,, ,, morbid conditions of the		xxix.	288
,, ,, old people		xxix.	293
,, ,, rhythm		xxix.	284
,, ,, various diseases		xxix.	285
regular irregularity of		xxix.	284
,, cases of		xxix.	294
structure of the orifices of the		xxiii.	164
syphilis of the (*Herringham*)		xxxix.	9
the reserve force of the (*Harry Campbell*)		xxxviii.	144
treatment of disease of the (*Gardner*)		xxiv.	337
wall, fibrosis of, as result of syphilis		xxxix.	11
weak, or irregular action of, in the insane		xxi.	12, 16
Heart-disease, aortic reflux		xxv.	1
,, complicating diphtheria		xxv.	1
,, enteric fever		xxv.	1
,, pregnancy		xxv.	181
Heat, loss of sensation to		xxviii.	211
its effects on paralysis of sympathetic nerve		xxix.	104
and aconite, their action on guinea-pigs		xxii.	284
,, ,, pigeons		xxii.	279
Heath (*A.*), cases of deformity		xxxii.	400
Heaton (*G.*), on tumours of the bladder		xxv.	280
Heberden's nodes, &c. observations on (*Sir Dyce Duckworth*)		xxxv.	13
Hedges (*C. E.*), relation of gout and rheumatism to Dupuytren's contraction		xxxii.	119
the etiology, immediate and remote prognosis of primary pleurisy with serous effusion		xxxvi.	75

	VOL.	PAGE
Hemi-anæsthesia .	XXV.	31
cause of .	XXVI.	114
and hemiplegia following hemianopia .	XXVI.	109
Hemianopia .	XXV. 30; XXVI.	109
Hemiatrophy, a case of lingual (*Weber*)	XXXIV.	307
Hemiopia, case of (*Gee*) .	XXVI.	109
its cause .	XXVI.	113
Hemiplegia, absence of knee-jerk .	XXVII.	47
and hemi-anæsthesia, following hemianopia .	XXVI.	109
from cerebral abscess .	XXI.	230
functional and organic .	XXI.	238
its cause .	XXVI.	114
notes of a case of .	XXVII.	225
treatment by electricity .	XXVIII.	255
Henslow (*Rev. G.*), dietetic values of food-stuffs prepared by plants	XXX.	113
Hepatic cirrhosis, with obstruction in superior vena cava (*Sir Dyce Duckworth* and *Garrod*) .	XXXII.	71
tumours (*Haviland*) .	XXIII.	356
Hepburn (*M. L.*), heredity of gout .	XXVI.	268
mal des montagnes .	XXXI.	191
Hereditary infantile spastic paraplegia (*Gee*) .	XXV.	81
influences .	XXII.	361
progressive muscular atrophy, commencing in legs .	XXV.	141
syphilis, influence of, upon the nervous system .	XXXVIII.	37
Heredity of gout .	XXVI.	268
„ phthisis .	XXVI.	263
Hernia, Bassini's operation for .	XXIX. 95; XXX. 232; XXXVI.	50
chicken bone in sac of femoral .	XL.	137
femoral, complicated .	XL.	137
„ hydrocele of sac of .	XXXV.	45
„ irreducible .	XXXVII.	278
„ of cæcum .	XXVII. 180,	181
„ „ vermiform appendix .	XXVII.	179
„ strangulated XXIX. 98; XXXIV. 234; XXXV. 45; XXXVI.		50
inguinal .	XXXV.	96
„ double, with laparotomy .	XXXI.	177
„ followed by gangrenous appendicitis .	XL.	153
„ irreducible .	XXIV. 291; XXXVII.	278
„ strangulated .	XXXIV. 234; XXXV. 45; XXXVI.	50
Kocher's operation for .	XXXV. 46; XXXVI.	50
obturator, strangulated .	XXVII.	67
„ symptoms of .	XXVII.	65
of vermiform appendix .	XXXII.	93
on (*Lockwood*) .	XXVI.	312
operations for .	XXIX. 95; XXX. 232; XXXV. 46; XXXVI.	49
radical cure of .	XXX. 232; XXXV. 45; XXXVI. 49; XL.	153
rectal, a rare form of .	XXVII.	59
symptoms of obstruction, hernial sac opened with negative result .	XXVIII.	119
testis .	XXIV.	291
trance, after operation for .	XXI.	166
through cicatrix after abdominal incision .	XXVIII. 23; XXIX.	21
traumatic .	XXVII.	51
umbilical, cases of .	XXVIII.	113
„ irreducible .	XXXVII.	278
„ of 30 years' standing .	XXVIII.	119
„ strangulated .	XXXVI.	50
ventral .	XXXV.	45
vermiform appendix .	XXVII. 179; XXXII.	93
Herniotomy .	XXVII. 179,	180

	VOL.	PAGE
Herpes, of cornea, cases of (*Jessop*)	xxxv.	238
zoster, associated with Bell's paralysis	xxxix.	167
,, symmetrical	xxi.	119
Herringham (*W. P.*), a case of acute pemphigus . . .	xl.	33
,, lead poisoning, with bosses on the metacarpal bones . .	xxi.	169
,, mental disturbance, after operation	xxi.	165
,, tumour of the cerebellum, with remarks on cerebellar staggering	xxiii.	65
,, Graves' disease, with extreme emaciation	xxxv.	125
chorea, as a cause, rather than a result of endocarditis	xxiv.	55
of purpura, as it occurs in sarcoma, lymphadenoma, and tubercle	xxxviii.	117
on a minute glioma of the aqueduct of Sylvius, with some remarks on the causation of opisthotonos .	xxxvi.	31
on chronic peritonitis, with especial reference to that form which is caused by tubercle	xxix.	63
on paralysis agitans	xxv.	271
,, paroxysmal hæmaturia	xxii.	133
,, some points in diphtheria	xxix.	351
,, syphilis of the heart	xxxix.	9
primary cancer of pancreas	xxx.	5
renal albuminuria, in children	xxvi.	25
treatment of diphtheria by antitoxin	xxxi.	73
and **Andrewes** (*F. W.*), two cases of cerebellar disease in cats, with staggering	xxiv.	241
and **Clarke** (*Bruce*) on idiopathic dilatation of sigmoid flexure	xxxi.	57
Hip, amputation of, when needed	xxiv.	336
excision of	xxix.	98
statistics of	xxiv.	335, 336
Hip-joint, pain about the, various causes of . . .	xl.	4
synovial cyst, in connection with	xxi.	186
Histological records of Museum specimens . . .	xxxii.	513
History of diphtheritic paralysis (*Macan*) . . .	xxx.	129
,, hypnotism	xxv.	116
,, symphysiotomy	xxx.	27
Hogarth, thanks of the Governors to, for paintings .	xxii.	34
Holden (*G. H. R.*), concerning tracheotomy . . .	xxviii.	157
Hollis (*W. A.*), a page in the life-history of sprouting endocardial growths	xxviii.	221
Holmes (*H.*), with **Kanthack** (*A. A.*), cardiac hypertrophy, œdema, and renal disease	xxxii.	261
Homicide and insanity	xxix.	119
in imbeciles	xxi.	4
,, the insane	xxi.	2
,, ,, melancholic	xxi.	7
Hope Ward, diphtheria in	xxvii.	266
Horder, (*T. J.*), a case of chronic and streptococcus pyæmia, in which the serum treatment produced no benefit .	xxxiii.	89
a case of typhoid fever, followed by acute cystitis, due to bacillus coli communis	xxxiii.	85
cases in surgical wards	xxxii.	181
chronic Bright's disease, as a cause of sudden death, with some remarks upon sudden death generally .	xxxv.	153
clinical aphorisms from Dr. Gee's wards . . .	xxxii.	29
life and work of Percivall Pott	xxx.	163

	VOL.	PAGE
Horne (*W. J.*), case of fugitive œdema, ending fatally . .	**xxx.**	195
and **Power** (*D'Arcy*), cases of malignant disease from the Department for Diseases of the Throat and Nose	**xxxix.**	219
with **Batten** (*F.*), disseminated sclerosis, with palatal and laryngeal anæsthesia	**xxxii.**	173
Horns, occurring in man (*Foulerton*)	**xxv.**	105
connection [of epithelioma with warts and horns (*Foulerton*)	**xxv.** 106, 107
on glans penis	**xxv.**	107
papillary	**xxv.**	106
pathology of	**xxv.**	105
varieties of	**xxv.**	106
Horton-Smith (*P.*), on the bacteriology of acute broncho-pneumonia (*see* Hartley)	**xxxiii.**	25
Horton-Smith prize essay, the, on pylephlebitis (*Langdon Brown*)	**xxxvii.**	53
Hospital, Essex and Colchester, cases from . . .	**xxvii.**	239
German, some cases from	**xxxiv.**	303
St. Bartholomew's, admission of patients to . .	**xxii.**	35
„ barber at	**xxii.**	41
baths at	**xxii.**	18
bugs in	**xxii.**	18
burial-fees at	**xxii.**	34
burying-ground for . . .	**xxii.**	35
church in, repaired . . .	**xxii.**	39
clergyman, umbrella for . .	**xxii.**	36
condition of, during eighteenth century	**xxii.**	30
convalescent	**xxii.**	44
dentist to, appointed . .	**xxii.**	44
diets of	**xxii.**	8
diphtheria within the . .	**xxvii.**	261
directions to the Staff of . .	**xxii.**	34
discipline in	**xxii.**	10
duties of Matron of . . .	**xxii.**	41
electricity at	**xxii.**	25, 28
erection of theatre in . .	**xxii.**	40
museum of	**xxii.**	32
ophthalmic cases at . . .	**xxii.**	33
pharmacopœias of . . .	**xxii.**	1
post-mortems at . . .	**xxii.**	37
prescribing at	**xxii.**	38
re-building of	**xxii.** 22, 32, 39
report of special committee, on apothecaries' shop at . .	**xxii.**	30
rooms for hydrophobic patients at .	**xxii.**	41
sisters' fees at	**xxii.**	36
small-pox at, the arrangements for .	**xxii.**	37
„ umbrella for clergyman . .	**xxii.**	36
„ water-closets at . .	**xxii.**	43
Victoria Park, influenza at . . .	**xxvi.**	259
Hospitals, isolation, the provision of	**xxiv.**	25
Hot air inhalations in phthisis	**xxvi.**	91
House (*see* Dwelling-house).		
House-physicians' discussion on diarrhœa	**xxii.**	359
House-surgeons' discussion on gonorrhœa . . .	**xxii.**	366
first mention of	**xxii.**	40
Hughes (*W. Kent*), a new kind of talipes . . .	**xxxv.**	181
Huggins (*S. P.*), **Walsham** (*W. J.*), and **Smith** (*G.*), report of operation cases	**xxxiv.**	263

	VOL.	PAGE
Humerus, case of intracapsular fracture dislocation of (*Maxwell*)	XXXVIII.	33
swelling of	XXIV.	290
Humphrey (*Sir George Murray*), In Memoriam . .	XXXII.	xxxi
Humphreys, on scarlet fever	XXVII.	281
Hunt, (*E. H.*), notes on a case of double sub-conjunctival hæmorrhage, caused by compression of the chest .	XXXVIII.	179
Hydatid cyst in liver and kidney	XXVII.	165, 240
„ „ treatment of	XXVII.	164
„ in omentum	XXVII.	241
„ „ thorax	XXVII.	239
cysts, drained through bladder	XXV.	261
„ suppurating, in thorax	XXV.	214
„ three hundred discharged from thorax .	XXV.	221
disease of the arm	XXXII.	187
„ „ heart	XXXIX.	207
fluid, causing urticaria	XXVIII.	236
„ nature of	XXVIII.	236
of liver	XXVII.	240
„ „ rupturing into bile-ducts . . .	XL.	5
„ pelvis, case of	XXXVI.	45
tumours, two cases of : one of the liver, one of the kidney	XXVII.	163
Hydatids, of the liver	XXIX.	335, 336, 338
„ „ post-mortem appearances in .	XXIX.	337
in abdomen, drained through bladder . .	XXV.	261
operation for	XXVIII.	241
puncture of, causing death	XXVIII.	236
surgical treatment of	XXVIII.	235
thoracic	XXVIII.	238
suppurating in thorax	XXV.	214
three hundred discharged from chest . .	XXV.	221
Hydrocele in child of 8 years	XXXV.	96
operations for (*D'Arcy Power*) . . .	XXXV.	47
radical operation for (*Walsham*) . .	XXXIV.	285
Hydrocephalus, acute external and internal . .	XXXIX.	39
"primary" internal, in an adult (*Weber*) . .	XXXII.	307
Hydrogen, sulphuretted, injections of in phthisis . .	XXV.	66
„ its action when absorbed from intestine	XXII.	301
Hydrophobic patients, rooms for at the hospital . .	XXIII.	41
Hydrosalpinx	XXIX.	51
Hydroxylamine hydrochlorate, as a substitute for nitrate of amyl, or nitroglycerine	XXX.	189
Hygroma, congenital, cystic of neck . . .	XXIV.	277
Hyperpyrexia, in acute rheumatism . . .	XXIII.	288
rheumatic	XXVII.	286
Hypertrophy of heart, œdema, and renal disease . .	XXXII.	261
„ „ inferior turbinated body . .	XXIII.	130
„ pharyngeal tonsil . .	XXIII.	135
„ septum nasi	XXIII.	127
„ „ narium with œdema . .	XXVII.	25
„ tongue	XXIX.	154
„ „ turbinal bodies . . .	XXVII.	16
„ „ „ bones . . .	XXVII.	18
Hypnotic suggestion, treatment by . . .	XXV.	118
Hypnotics, on (*Turnbull*)	XXV.	280
Hypnotism, as a means of producing anæsthesia . .	XXV.	119
on (*Liebault*)	XXV.	120
in insanity	XXVIII.	61
in the treatment of alcoholism . . .	XXV.	126
its history	XXV.	116
its phenomena	XXV.	116

	VOL.	PAGE
Hypnotism, phenomena of	XXVII.	284
Hypodermic injection of strychnia in cardiac failure (*Habershon*)	XXII.	115
Hypopyon, on (*P. E. Turner*)	XXXV.	131
Hysterectomy, cases of (*Harrison Cripps*)	XXXV.	23
for fibroids of uterus	XXIX.	38
,, myoma ,, ,,	XXIX.	39, 40
and ovariotomy, in Martha Ward	XXXIX.	143
Hysteria	XXVII. 285 ; XXXII.	47
cardiac, irregularity in	XXIX.	286
importance, and treatment of (*Garrod*)	XXII.	364
Hysterical dyspnœa	XXII.	216
intestinal obstruction (*Weber*)	XXXIV.	314
Hystero-epilepsy, and removal of uterine appendages for	XXIX.	48
Hysteropexy, case of (*Harrison Cripps*)	XXXV.	85
Icterus gravis, a case of	XXIII.	180
Idiopathic dilatation of sigmoid flexure (*Herringham* and *Bruce Clarke*)	XXXI.	57
Ileo-cæcal valve, tuberculous stricture of	XL.	128
Iliac region, swelling in the left	XXIV.	297
right colotomy in intestinal obstruction (*Goodsall*)	XXX.	215
Imbeciles, homicide among	XXI.	4
suicide among	XXI.	4
Impulses, destructive, on the forecast of, in the insane (*Claye Shaw*)	XXI.	1
Inchley (*O.*), on the causation of the first sound of the heart	XXXVIII.	91
Incision, abdominal, hernia through cicatrix, after	XXIX.	21
,, ,, ,, ,, of	XXVIII.	23
in ovariotomy	XXIX.	8
position of, through the skin, in removal of goitre	XXV.	102
the, in abdominal section, its direction	XXVIII.	17
,, ,, ,, ,, mode of making	XXVIII.	18
Incontinence of fæces	XXIV.	260
Increased intra-cranial pressure, surgical treatment of (*C. A. Morton*)	XXXIII.	63
India, a short account of the second epidemic of plague at Bhiwudi (*Dalàl*)	XXXV.	119
Indications for symphysiotomy	XXX.	42, 48
Induction of labour, in chorea gravidarum	XXXIX.	7
Infancy, puberty, and maturity, diseases of	XXII.	353 .
Infantile diarrhœa (*Lankester*)	XXI.	242
paralysis, electricity in	XXVIII.	252
spastic paraplegia, hereditary (*Gee*)	XXV.	81
Infants, bloody urine in scurvy of	XXV.	85
sudden death in (*Thursfield*)	XXXVIII.	129
Infarcts in kidney	XXVII.	42, 46
Infection, contagion, and predisposition, on (*Kanthack*)	XXIX.	351
Infectious diseases	XXXII.	50
some aspects of the etiology of (*T. F. Raven*)	XXXVII.	205
Infective endocarditis	XXVIII.	228
granulomata of tongue	XXIX.	156
lesions in lobar pneumonia	XXXII.	309
Inferior turbinated body, adhesion of, to septum	XXIII.	133
,, bone, necrosis of	XXIII.	133
Influenza, a zymotic disease	XXVI.	204
affections of eye and ear in	XXVI.	202
albuminuria in	XXVI.	203
at Victoria Park Hospital	XXVI.	259
case of, in a doctor	XXVI.	252
catarrhal form of	XXVI.	198

		VOL.	PAGE
Influenza, character of its defervescence	. . . .	XXVI.	261
,, ,, ,, fastigium	. . . .	XXVI.	260
,, ,, the pyrogenetic stage	. . .	XXVI.	259
complications of	. . . . . .	XXVI.	202
contagion in	. . . .	XXVI.	204
cystitis in	. . . .	XXVI.	203
epidemic of 1890	. . . . . .	XXVI.	193
epistaxis in	. . . .	XXVI.	200
gastro-intestinal irritation in	. . . .	XXVI.	197
glandular affections in	. . . . .	XXVI.	203
greater prevalence among men	. . .	XXVI.	195
hæmoptysis in	. . . . . .	XXVI.	201
hæmorrhage in	. . . . . .	XXVI.	200
in cardiac cases	. . . . . .	XXVI.	261
its definition	. . . .	XXVI.	196
,, effect on the nursing staff	. . . .	XXVII.	261
,, effects on phthisis	. . . .	XXVI. 209, 260	
,, ,, ,, pregnancy	. . . .	XXVI.	203
,, ,, ,, the healthy and diseased	. . .	XXVI.	259
joint affections in	. . . . .	XXVI.	199
menorrhagia in	. . . . . .	XXVI.	200
mode of onset	. . . . . .	XXVI.	196
mortality in	. . . .	XXVI. 207, 208	
neuralgic form of	. . . . . .	XXVI.	198
orchitis in	. . . .	XXVI.	203
outbreak at Colchester	. . . . .	XXVI.	252
parotitis in	. . . .	XXVI.	203
percentage of population of London attacked	.	XXVI.	195
pleurisy in	. . . .	XXVI.	202
pneumonia in	. . . .	XXVI.	202
presence of rash in	. . . . . .	XXVI.	201
purpura in	. . . .	XXVI.	201
relapses of	. . . .	XXVI.	199
report by Habershon	. . . . .	XXVI.	239
,, ,, Hayward	. . . . .	XXVI.	231
,, ,, Knight	. . . . .	XXVI.	223
,, ,, E. T. Moore	. . . . .	XXVI.	224
,, ,, the matron of St. Bartholomew's Hospital		XXVI.	235
,, ,, ,, ,, the Royal Free Hospital	.	XXVI.	247
,, ,, ,, resident officers of St. Bartholomew's Hospital	.	XXVI.	210
,, ,, ,, ,, officer of the Royal Free Hospital	XXVI.	241
,, ,, Wallace of Colchester	. . .	XXVI.	251
resembling angina pectoris	. . . .	XXVI.	199
sequelæ of	. . . . . .	XXVI. 253, 262	
temperature in	. . . . . .	XXVI.	200
treatment of	. . . .	XXVI.	209
Inhalations, antiseptic	. . . . . .	XXV.	40, 54
of hot air in phthisis	. . . . .	XXVI.	91
,, putrefactive bacilli	. . . . .	XXV.	66
through respirators	. . . . .	XXV.	54
Injection, hypodermic, of strychnia in cardiac failure	.	XXII.	115
of defibrinated bullock's blood in splenic leukæmia	.	XXII.	245
Injections, direct, of lung tissue	. . . .	XXV.	67
of sulphuretted hydrogen gas in phthisis	. .	XXV.	66
Injury to elbow	. . . .	XXIV.	308
,, head, mania after	. . . . .	XXI.	166
,, kidney, hæmorrhage from, after	. .	XXV.	239
,, nerve, at birth	. . . . . .	XXXII.	404
,, nerves, treatment by electricity	. . .	XXVIII.	254

	VOL.	PAGE
Injuries and diseases of the spinal column	XXI.	258
of abdomen (*D'Arcy Power*)	XXVII.	28
,, the great omentum	XXX.	91
,, ,, head, temperature in relation to (*McAdam Eccles*)	XXIX.	225
in and about joints	XXI.	251
to head, cases of (*Ball*)	XXXVII.	181
Innes (*C. B.*), on variola	XXII.	356
In-patients, number attacked with diphtheria . . .	XXVII.	264
Insane, catalepsy in the	XXI.	20
destructive impulses in the	XXI.	I. 16
effects of previous training on	XXIV.	7
fractured ribs in	XXVI.	15
general paralysis of, cases resembling . . .	XXI.	23
,, ,, ,, on (*Farrar*) . . .	XXIV.	317
heart disease in the	XXI.	12
homicide in the	XXI.	2
suicide among	XXI.	4
women, difficulty of amusing	XXIV.	8
,, foulness of their language . . .	XXIV.	4
,, impulsiveness of	XXIV.	6
,, occupation for	XXIV.	2
,, tendency to cover the head . . .	XXIV.	13
Insanity, abortion of attacks of	XXIX.	111
acute, its early symptoms	XXIX.	109
affection of speech in	XXIII.	31
among females	XXIX.	112
and drunkenness	XXIX.	114
,, homicide	XXIX.	119
,, letter-writing	XXIX.	123
bad effects of non-restraint in certain cases . . .	XXIV.	14
causes of an attack	XXIII. 25 ; XXIX. 110
compared with epilepsy	XXIII.	20, 30
confessions of patients in	XXIX.	121
effect of acute disease in	XXIII.	29
,, ,, new Lunacy Act	XXIX.	116
,, ,, operation on the skull in . . .	XXVIII.	68
expression of the features in	XXIV.	11
following fracture of base of skull	XXVII.	185
hæmorrhage in	XXIII.	29
history of fresh attacks	XXIII.	19
hypnotism in	XXVIII.	61
lymphatic system in	XXVIII.	63
mesmerism in	XXVIII.	61
motor stages of	XXIX.	115
non-restraint, its bad effect in certain cases of . .	XXIV.	14
neurasthenia	XXIX.	118
on its commencement and end	XXIII.	19
pathology of	XXVIII.	58
poisoning	XXIX.	122
removal of uterine appendages for threatened . .	XXIX.	48
sexual excitement	XXIX.	119
suddenness of its cure	XXIII.	27
,, ,, ,, onset	XXIII.	22
suicide in	XXIX.	118
tendency to deny	XXIX.	118
the sexual element in women in	XXIV.	10
trephining the skull in	XXVIII.	55
with remitted or intermittent symptoms . . .	XXIII.	30

		VOL.	PAGE
Insanity, with sexual complications	. . . .	XXII.	103
worry, a cause of	. . . . .	XXVIII.	60
Insomnia, action of drugs on	. . . .	XXV.	153
causes of	. . . .	XXV.	152
treatment of	. . . . . .	XXV.	151
,,　,, by drugs	. . . . . .	XXV.	156
Instruments for abdominal section	. . . .	XXIX.	4
preparation of, for operations	. . .	XXIX.	91
Insular sclerosis, atrophy of optic nerve in	. . .	XXII.	308
Intestinal obstruction, a case of	. . . .	XXV.	169
,,　cases of (*Mayo, Willett,* and *Hawes*)	.	XXXVII.	275
,,　diagnosis of	. . . .	XXV.	172
,,　from cancerous stricture	. .	XXVIII.	113, 116
,,　,, doubtful cause	.	XXVIII.	121
,,　,, impacted gall-stone	. .	XXVIII.	113
,,　,, intussusception	. .	XXVIII.	97, 113
,,　hysterical (*Weber*)	. . .	XXXIV.	314
,,　nine cases of	. . .	XXVIII.	113
,,　operation for	. . .	XXV.	171
..　,, after-treatment	. .	XXV.	174
,,　right iliac colotomy in (*Goodsall*)	.	XXX.	215
,,　simulated by enteritis and colic	.	XXXII.	61
,,　treatment of	. . .	XXIV.	320
resection, two cases of (*R. C. Bailey*)	. .	XXXIII.	55
Intestine, fistulous opening into bladder	. . .	XXIV.	258
melanotic sarcoma of	. . . . .	XL.	131
perforation of the, in typhoid fever	XXV. 138; XXXIX.		133
punctured wound of, with inflammation of parotid gland	XXVII.		117
,,　,, with inflammation of submaxillary gland	. . . .	XXVII.	177
rupture of small, case of	. . . .	XXXVI.	41
strangulation of	. . . . .	XXIV.	152
,,　,, in fossa intersigmoidea	. .	XXXI.	177
Intestines, absorption of gas by	. . . .	XXII. 279,	301
Intra-capsular fracture, dislocation of humerus (*Maxwell*)	.	XXXVII.	33
Intra-cranial cases, two (*C. E. West*)	. . .	XXXIX.	37
complications of chronic disease of ear (*Bailey*)	.	XXXVII.	287
disease with optic neuritis	. . . .	XXI.	223
pressure, diagnosis of	. . . . .	XXVIII.	65
,,　increased, surgical treatment of (*C. A. Morton*)	XXXIII.		63
,,　signs of	. . . . .	XXVIII.	55
Intra-nasal obstruction	. . . . . .	XXIII.	122
obstructions	. . . . . .	XXVII.	16
Intra-pleural pressure	. . . . .	XXVIII.	131
Intra-thoracic growths, alteration of voice in	. .	XXVIII.	92
,,　and abscess of mediastinum	.	XXVIII.	94
,,　,, aneurysm	. . .	XXVIII.	94
,,　,, pleuritic effusion	.	XXVIII.	95
,,　complications of	. .	XXVIII.	93
,,　consolidation of lung in	.	XXVIII.	95
,,　cough in	. . . .	XXVIII.	91
,,　diagnosis of	. . .	XXVIII.	91
,,　,, from aortic aneurysm	.	XXVIII.	94
,,　,, pericardial effusion	XXVIII.		94
,,　difficulty of breathing in	. .	XXVIII.	91
,,　divisions of	. . .	XXVIII.	74
,,　duration of	. . .	XXVIII.	91
,,　emaciation in	. . .	XXVIII.	92
,,　enlarged veins in	. .	XXVIII.	92
,,　etiology of	. . .	XXVIII.	75

					VOL.	PAGE
Intra-thoracic growths, frequency of	.	.	.	.	XXVIII.	74
,,	headache in	.	.	.	XXVIII.	92
,,	inequality of pupils in	.	.	XXVIII.	92
,,	influence of age in	.	.	XXVIII.	75
..	,, ,, sex in	.	.	XXVIII.	75
,,	irregularity of pulse in	.	.	XXVIII.	92
,,	on (*Hamer*)	.	.	.	XXVIII.	73
,,	outset of	.	.	.	XXVIII.	92
,,	pain in	.	.	.	XXVIII.	91
,,	pathology of	.	.	.	XXVIII.	89, 90
,,	pericardial effusion in	.	.	XXVIII.	94
,,	physical signs of	.	.	XXVIII.	92
,,	pleural effusions in	.	.	XXVIII.	95
,,	predisposing causes of	.	.	XXVIII.	75
,,	sputum in	.	.	.	XXVIII.	91
,,	statistics of	.	.	.	XXVIII.	76
,,	symptoms of	.	.	.	XXVIII.	91
,,	temperature in	.	.	XXVIII.	93
	pressure	.	.	.	.	XXVIII.	259
Intussusception of bowel, a table of twenty-eight cases of (*McAdam Eccles*)				.	XXXVII.	196
age in	.	.	.	.	.	XXXVIII.	97
an analysis of twenty-eight cases of (*McAdam Eccles*)	.	XXVIII.	97
an analysis of forty cases of (*McAdam Eccles*)	.	XXXIX.	139
an analysis of a third list of twenty-eight cases of (*McAdam Eccles*)	.	.	.	XXXVII.	189
an analysis of ninety-six cases of (*McAdam Eccles*)	.	XXXVII.	203
cardinal symptoms of	.	.	.	XXVIII.	98
cases of (*D'Arcy Power*)	.	.	.	XXXVII.	82
causes of	.	.	.	.	XXVIII.	98
day of admission, and mortality of	.	.	XXVIII.	98
from intestinal obstruction	.	.	.	XXVIII.	97, 113
injection of fluids in	.	.	.	XXVIII.	100, 115
laparotomy for	.	.	.	XXVIII.	101, 102, 114, 115
mortality of	.	.	.	.	XXVIII.	98
of a Meckel's diverticulum	.	.	.	XXVII.	171
sex in	.	.	.	.	XXVIII.	97
signs of	.	.	.	.	XXVIII.	98
treatment of	.	.	.	.	XXVIII.	99
Invertebrata, digestion in	.	.	.	.	XXIV.	67
Iodine, as an inhalation	.	.	.	.	XXV.	54, 65
standard solution of, for pancreatic ferments	.	XXIX.	127
Iodoform, introduction and consumption of	.	.	XXII.	46, 53
Irregularity of the heart	.	.	.	.	XXIX.	283
Iris, malformation of	.	.	.	.	XXIX.	297
Iritis, sympathetic	.	.	.	.	XXIX.	302
Irrigator	.	.	.	.	.	XXIX.	3
Irritation, its effect in epithelioma	.	.	.	XXV.	113
Iron, perchloride of, injected into the sac of an aneurysm	.	XXVII.	254
Ischio-rectal abscess following foreign body in the rectum, treatment of	.	.	.	.	XXIII.	80
T-shaped incision in	.	.	.	XXIII.	80
Islington waters	.	.	.	.	.	XXII.	18
Isolation, diseases calling for	.	.	.	XXIV.	25
hospitals, air-space per patient needed	.	.	XXIV.	35
,,	character of accommodation required	.	XXIV.	33
,,	extent of, required	.	.	.	XXIV.	32
,,	number of beds in a ward in	.	.	XXIV.	36
,,	sites for	.	.	.	.	XXIV.	33, 89

	VOL.	PAGE
Izal, treatment of tinea favosa capitis by	xxxviii.	155
Izard (*A. W.*), some difficulties in the diagnosis of appendicitis	xxxix.	41
Jacksonian epilepsy	xxiii.	188
Jaundice	xxxii.	44
protracted	xxviii.	127
with delirium	xxiii.	184
Jaw, lower, abscess of	xxvii.	63
„ arrest of development in	xxxii.	403
„ cystic tumour of	xxii.	238
„ epulis of	xxii.	239
„ necrosis of	xxvii.	179
„ removal of half	xxii.	238
upper, abscess in cancer of	xxiii.	151
„ epithelioma of	xxiv.	311
„ necrosis of	xxvii.	205
„ „ „ from syphilis . . .	xxvi.	85
„ recurrent epithelioma beneath . . .	xxiv.	287
„ sarcoma of	xxiv.	310
„ swelling of	xxiv.	279
Jerking, rhythmical, in Graves' disease . . .	xxix.	185
Jessop (*W. H. H.*), a case of tubercle of lachrymal gland .	xxxv.	231
cases of eclipse blindness	xxxvi.	260
cataract extraction, without iridectomy . .	xxxvii.	317
conjunctivitis, diphtheritic	xxxv.	232
cyst of conjunctiva	xxxv.	237
eclipse blindness	xxxvi.	260
electric light, effect of on eye	xxxvii.	311
foreign bodies in eye-ball	xxxv.	245
germiculture	xxi.	252
glioma of the retina	xxxvi.	253
„ „ prognosis after operation in .	xxxix.	213
growths at limbus corneæ	xxxvi.	258
gunshot wounds of orbit, effects on eye . .	xxxvii.	312
hæmorrhage into macula	xxxv.	241
herpes of cornea, cases of	xxxv.	238
metastatic carcinoma of choroid	xxxv.	240
notes on cases of diseases of the eye . . .	xxxv.	231
obliteration of retinal artery	xxxvii.	314
on germiculture	xxi.	252
„ the prognosis, after operation, in glioma of the retina	xxix.	213
ophthalmic cases and notes . . .	xxxv. 231 ;	xxxvii. 309
„ notes and cases . . .	xxii. 305 ;	xxxvi. 253
papillitis, double	xxxvi.	263
removal of lens in high myopia	xxxv.	242
sarcoma of choroid	xxxv.	239
section of optic nerve, physiological effects of .	xxxvii.	309
the pathology of glioma of the retina . . .	xxxviii.	159
„ prognosis, some points in retina . .	xxxviii.	159
vaccinia of conjunctiva	xxxv.	237
and **Berry** (*J.*), successful removal of a large goitre,		
with remarks	xxv.	97
Johnson (*G. L.*), on the Medical School of Vienna . .	xxv.	275
Joint affections in influenza	xxvi.	199
disease, hæmophilia in	xxvi.	77
elbow, synovial cyst in connection with . .	xxi.	184
hæmophilia in disease of	xxvi.	77
hip, pain about the, various causes of . . .	xl.	4
„ synovial cyst in connection with . . .	xxi.	186

	VOL.	PAGE
Joint, knee, idiopathic osteo-myelitis of femur, invading	XXIII.	223
syphilitic disease of	XXVI.	83
Joints, abnormal synovial cysts in connection with the	XXI.	177
acute suppuration of, a sequela of gonorrhœa	XXII.	263
cases of disease of (*Mayo, Willett*, and *Hawes*)	XXXVII.	281
in bleeders	XXVI.	77, 81
injuries in and about	XXI.	251
nodules on finger, on an unusual form of (*Garrod*)	XXIX.	157
operations on (*Walsham*)	XXXIV.	286
„ „ (*D'Arcy Power*)	XXXV.	45
results of opening of	XXIX.	93
syphilitic disease of	XXVI.	83
urate of soda in, in gout	XXIII.	291
Jones (*Lewis*), notes from the Electrical Department	XXVIII.	245
on facial diagnosis	XXV.	277
on symmetrical atrophy affecting the hands in young people	XXIX.	307
report of the year's work in the Electrical Department	XXXIII.	169
treatment of nævus by electrolysis	XXX.	205
Jones (*Lloyd*), on the specific gravity of blood in health and disease	XXIV.	314
prognosis in albuminuria	XXVI.	307
Jowers (*R. F.*), cases from Mr. Smith's wards	XXIII.	231
Kanthack (*A. A.*), bacteriological investigations in diphtheria	XXXI.	87
descriptive list of specimens added to the Museum during 1896	XXII.	451
memoir of	XXXV.	5
on infection, contagion, and predisposition	XXIX.	35
and **Mayo**, prognosis and causes of death in diphtheria treated by antitoxin	XXXII.	335
with **Drysdale** (*J. H.*), ulceration of larynx in typhoid fever	XXXI.	113
„ **Garrod** (*A. E.*), and **Drysdale** (*J. H.*), on the green stools of typhoid fever, with some remarks on green stools in general	XXXIII.	13
„ **Holmes**, cardiac hypertrophy, œdema, and renal diseases	XXXII.	261
„ **Lance**, secondary infective lesions in lobar pneumonia	XXXII.	309
„ **Lloyd**, primary malignant disease of liver	XXXI.	105
Kent Hughes (*W.*), a new kind of talipes	XXXV.	181
Kidd (*P.*), note on tuberculous tumours of the larynx	XXI.	37
the association of pulmonary tuberculosis with disease of the heart	XXIII.	239
two cases of cerebral aneurysm in young persons associated with endocarditis, with remarks on the connection between aneurysm and embolism	XXII.	187
Kidney, absence of, a case of (*D'Arcy Power*)	XXXV.	48
affections of, in parturition (*Griffith*)	XXVI.	115
case of contusion of (*Mayo, Willett*, and *Hawes*)	XXXVII.	282
epithelioma of pelvis of	XXI.	125
exploration of	XXIV. 283 ; XXXIV.	281
hæmorrhage from, after injury	XXV.	239
hydatid of, and of liver	XXVII.	165, 240
infarcts in	XXVII.	42, 46
on chronic Bright's disease of (*Horder*)	XXXV.	155
operations on (*D'Arcy Power*)	XXXV.	47
removal of	XXI.	121
rupture „	XXXII.	196

		VOL.	PAGE
Kidney, rupture of (*D'Arcy Power*)		XXXVII.	29
stone from		XXI.	126
,, in	XXIV. 283 ;	XXV. 231,	236
Kidneys, chronic interstitial nephritis, and its connection			
with gout		XXIII. 292,	293
cystic disease of, and liver (*J. G. Forbes*) . .		XXXIII.	181
gummata in, and in liver		XXIX. 216,	217
parenchymatous nephritis, and its connection with			
urate of soda		XXIII. 293,	294
suppuration of, on (*Gay*)		XXIII.	345
King's evil, cure of		XXVII.	282
Kirsopp (*T.*), on disablement during treatment . .		XXVI.	306
Kittens, disease of the cerebellum in . . .		XXIII.	70
Klein (*E.*), on the etiology of cholera . . .		XXI.	260
the scientific aspect of disinfection . . .		XXV.	275
Klein's bacillus pneumoniæ . . , . .		XXVIII	176
Knee, disease of, and tubercle in other parts of the body		XXIV.	308
,, ,, old, with outward displacement . .		XXIV.	283
,, ,, syphilitic	XXVI.	83, 84,	85
,, ,, tuberculous		XXIV.	277
excision of, with sinus		XXIV.	304
jerk, absent in a case of hemiplegia . . .		XXVII.	47
swelling of left		XXIV.	286
Knee-joint, disease of		XXIV.	302
,, ,, with flexion of the leg . .		XXIV.	282
idiopathic osteomyelitis of femur invading .		XXIII.	223
Knight (*H. E.*), cases from Sir W. S. Church's wards .		XXVI.	289
report on influenza		XXVI.	223
Koch's tubercle bacillus		XXVI.	1, 2
Labour, complicated by disease of heart . .	XXV. 181 ;	XXVI.	311
induction of, in chorea gravidarum . . .		XXXIX.	7
premature, in dropsy		XXVI.	117
Labyrinth, extirpation of the, two cases of (*C. E. West*) .		XL.	93
Lachrymal gland, a case of tubercle of (*Jessop*) . . .		XXXV.	231
Lance (*H. W.*), with **Kanthack**, secondary infective lesions			
in lobar pneumonia		XXXII.	309
Landry's paralysis, a case of (*J. P.* and *J. L. Maxwell*) XXXVI. 173 ;		XL.	49
and rabies		XXVIII.	138
causation of		XXVIII.	138
electrical reactions in		XXVIII.	137
illustrations of		XXVIII.	137
microscopical examination of nerves in . . .		XXVIII.	148
post mortems in	XXVIII.	140, 143,	144
summary of cases		XXVIII.	149
Language, foulness of, in insane woman . . .		XXII.	4
Lankester (*A. O.*), on infantile diarrhœa . . .		XXI.	242
on punctured wounds		XXII.	364
,, re-fracture of the femur		XXI.	68
Laparotomies, cases of (*Harrison Cripps*) . . .		XXXV.	23
,, ,, (*D'Arcy Power*) . . .		XXXV.	40
,, ,, (*Willett* and *Cholmeley*) . .		XXXV.	205
Laparotomy, for impacted gall-stone . . .		XXVIII.	118
,, intussusception of bowel .	XXVIII. 101, 102,	114,	115
Laryngeal and palatal anæsthesia, in disseminated			
sclerosis (*W. J. Horne* and *F. Batten*) . . .		XXXII.	173
Laryngismus stridulus in typhoid fever . . .		XXV.	138
Larynx, abscess in, in malignant disease of . . .		XXIII.	153
congenital stricture of		XXV.	225
department for diseases of the . . .		XXI.	145

	VOL.	PAGE
Larynx, epithelioma of the	XXXIX.	221
necrosis of, in typhoid fever	XXV.	133
position of syphilitic ulcers in	XXV.	223
simple stricture of	XXV.	223
tuberculous tumours of	XXI.	37
ulceration of, in typhoid fever	XXXI.	113
web in	XXV.	224
Latham (*Peter Mere*), as a clinical teacher	XXIV.	321
statistics of acute rheumatism	XXIII.	280
Lawrence (*L. A.*), some functions of the middle ear	XXXV.	113
Lead-poisoning, with bosses on the metacarpal bones	XXI.	169
Leaking gastric ulcer, case of, treated by operation (*D'Arcy Power*)	XXXVIII.	6
typhoidal ulcer, case of (*D'Arcy Power*)	XXXVIII.	21
Lectures and Demonstrations, list of	XXXIX.	303
Lee (*W. E.*), some points of interest in the Maidstone epidemic	XXXIII.	93
Leeches, consumption of	XXII.	47
Leg, cases of fracture of (*Mayo, Willett*, and *Hawes*)	XXXVII.	270
elephantiasis of one, in a boy	XXXII.	181
epitheliomatous ulcer of	XXIV.	285
flexion of, with disease of knee-joint	XXIV.	282
rickets of	XXII.	240
traumatic gangrene of	XXXII.	192
Legg (*W.*), introductory address to the Abernethian Society	XLI.	237
Legs, hereditary progressive muscular atrophy commencing in	XXV.	141–145
Leiter's tubes, their use in Graves' disease	XXVIII.	25
Lens, removal of, in high myopia	XXXV.	242
spontaneous dislocation of	XXIX.	304
Leprosy in West Africa	XXXIX.	177
Lesion of fifth nerve-trunk	XXIX.	215
,, ,, ,, microscopical appearances in	XXIX.	217
Lesions, infective, in lobar pneumonia	XXXII.	309
Letter-writing, in insanity	XXIX.	123
Leucocytosis in scarlet fever	XXXII.	225
Leukæmia, splenic, treated by injections of defibrinated bullock's blood	XXII.	245
Leucoma of lip and tongue	XXV.	112
Levison (*H. A.*), albuminuria in the apparently healthy	XXXV.	169
Lid-symptoms in Graves' disease	XXVII.	133
Liebault, on hypnotism	XXV.	120
Life and works of Percivall Pott	XXX.	163
duration of (*Hamer*)	XXVI.	307
the tripod of (*Gee*)	XXXIII.	1
Ligature of external iliac for secondary hæmorrhage (*Harmer*)	XXXV.	269
of femoral (*D'Arcy Power*)	XXXV.	43
,, ,, deep	XXX.	224
,, ,, superficial	XXX.	224
,, internal carotid artery	XXVII.	56
,, popliteal artery	XXX.	224
,, veins (*see* Veins).		
Ligatures, preparation of	XXIX.	91
Light, electric, effect of on eye (*Jessop*)	XXXVII.	311
its effect on bacteria	XXVI.	10, 11
necessity for, in dwelling-houses	XXVI.	10
Limbs, disuse of, after severe disease	XXV.	201
pseudo-paralysis of	XXV.	201
Limbus corneæ, growths at (*Jessop*)	XXXVI.	258
Linea albicantes, formation of (*Weber*)	XXXIV.	303

	VOL.	PAGE
Lingual hemiatrophy, a case of (*Weber*)	XXXIV.	307
Linseed meal, consumption of	XXII.	44
Lint, report on	XXIX.	101
Lip, leukoma of, and tongue	XXV.	112
Lithotomy following lithotrity	XXII.	243
suprapubic, case of	XXXVI.	48
,, for encysted calculus	XXVII.	124, 128
Lithotrity, cases of	XXV.	232, 233
followed by lithotomy	XXII.	243
Liver, abscess of, with parametritis	XXI.	173
acute atrophy of	XXXII.	425
carcinoma, primary, of	XXXI.	106
carcinoma of, simulating abscess	XXIII.	148
cirrhosis of, in a child of eleven	XXVIII.	167
,, its connection with gout	XXIII.	293, 295
,, with obscure and fatal symptoms	XXVI.	57
condition of, in diabetes mellitus	XXV.	8
,, gout	XXV.	9
cystic disease of, and kidneys (*J. G. Forbes*)	XXXIII.	181
gummata in, and in kidneys	XXIX.	216, 217
hydatid, a case of (*D'Arcy Power*)	XXVII. 43 ; XXXVII.	43
,, of, and kidney	XXVII.	183, 240, 165
,, rupturing into bile-ducts	XL.	5
hydatids of	XXIX.	336, 338
,, post-mortem appearances in	XXIX.	337
primary malignant disease of (*Kanthack* and *Lloyd*)	XXXI.	105
pylephlebitis, essay on (*Langdon Brown*)	XXXVIII.	53
rupture of (*D'Arcy Power*)	XXXVII.	28
sarcoma of	XXXI	109
some remarks on the surgery of the gall-bladder and bile-ducts (*Walsham*)	XXXVII.	321
syphilitic disease of	XXIX.	67
Lobar pneumonia, secondary infective lesions in	XXXI.	309
Lockwood (*C. B.*), cases of syphilis	XXXI.	225
In Memoriam, Sir George Murray Humphry	XXXII.	xxxi
on hernia	XXVI.	312
,, syphilis	XXI.	240
Locomotor ataxy, in children (*Moore*)	XXIX.	261
syphilitic (*Forbes*)	XXXVIII.	81
Lowe (*G.*), surgical cases of interest	XXVII.	49
Lower jaw, arrest of development in	XXXII.	403
Lumbar muscles, equilibrium maintained by	XXIV.	242
Lumbrici, passage of many, in typhoid fever	XXI.	109
Lumbricus teres, santonin in	XXIV.	239
Lunacy Act, effect of new	XXIX.	116
Lunacy, the difference of mind in the two sexes	XXIV.	1
Lung, calcareous masses from (*West*)	XXXI.	353
carcinoma of	XXVIII.	80, 84
carnification of, secondary to effusion	XXVIII.	1
,, physical signs of	XXVIII.	2
cirrhosis of	XXVIII.	2
,, due to tubercle	XXVIII.	4
chronic solidification of base of (*Gee*)	XXVIII.	1
consolidation of, and intra-thoracic growths	XXVIII.	95
drainage of	XXVIII.	5
gangrene of, after typhoid fever	XXIII.	109, 113
,, treated by operation	XXV.	253
its manner of contraction in pleural effusion	XXVIII.	131
medullary carcinoma of	XXVIII.	88

	VOL.	PAGE
Lung, phthisis of left apex of, occurrence of vomiting (*Habershon*)	XXIV.	131
rupture of aneurysm into	XXVII.	42
sarcoma of	XXVIII.	77, 85, 87, 88
tissue, injections direct of	XXV.	67
and pleura, new growths of (*West*)	XXXIII.	109
disease, desirability of expectoration in certain forms of	XXI.	120
„ old specimens of, containing tubercle bacilli (*Harris*)	XXI.	45
Lungs, affections of, in acute rheumatism	XXIII.	280
condition of, in pulmonary stenosis	XXIII.	240
lympho-sarcoma of	XXIII.	231
syphilitic affection of (*Weber*)	XXXIV.	305
trophic nerves of	XXIII.	113
Lupus lymphaticus, case of	XXX.	11
Lymphadenoma	XXIV.	280
cases of purpura in (*Herringham*)	XXXVIII.	117
of mediastinal glands	XXII.	101
Lymphangioma of skin	XXX.	111
of tongue	XXIX.	143, 151
„ „ microscopical examination of	XXIX.	147
„ „ minute anatomy of	XXIX.	144, 147
„ „ operation for	XXIX.	144
„ „ treatment of	XXIX.	144
Lymphatic glands (*see* Glands).		
system in insanity	XXVIII.	63
Lyndon (*A.*), notes of a case of malignant pustule	XXIV.	315
on erysipelas	XXIV.	321
Macan (*J. J.*), history of diphtheritic paralysis	XXX.	129
Mackrell (*A. S.*), memoir of	XXVII.	xliii
Macroglossia, some remarks on (*Francis*)	XXIX.	143, 147
Macula, hæmorrhage into (*Jessop*)	XXXV.	241
Madura foot in West Africa	XXXIX.	178
Magnesia, sulphate of, consumption of	XXII.	45
Magnet, its use for foreign bodies in the vitreous	XXII.	311
Magnetism, *Puysegur,* his practice of	XXV.	117
„ *Faria, Abbé,* his practice of	XXV.	117
Maidstone epidemic (typhoid), some points of interest in (*W. E. Lee*)	XXXIII.	93
Malaria, a cause of paroxysmal hæmaturia	XXII.	139
Malay midwifery (*Myers*)	XXXV.	101
Mal des montagnes (*Hepburn*)	XXXI.	191
Malformation of iris	XXIX.	297
Malformations, cardiac, association of, with other congenital defects	XXX.	53
Malignant diphtheria, hæmorrhage in	XXIII.	17
disease, cases of, from the Department for Diseases of the Throat and Nose (*D'Arcy Power* and *W. J. Horne*)	XXXIX.	219
„ coincident with tuberculosis (*Forbes*)	XXXV.	183
„ with suppuration (*Marsh*)	XXIII.	147
„ of cervical glands	XXIII.	153
„ „ larynx	XXIII.	153
„ „ liver, primary (*Kanthack* and *Lloyd*)	XXXI.	105
„ „ testis, abscess with	XXIII.	152
endocarditis	XXVII.	41
„ (streptococci)	XXXII.	1
growth developed in floor of ulcer of breast	XXIII.	159
pustule (*Lyndon*), notes of a case of	XXIV.	297, 315

	VOL.	PAGE
Malleolus, external, ganglionic swelling over	XXI.	187
Malt extract, use of, in typhoid fever	XXI.	117
Mammary gland (*see* Breast).		
analysis of tumours of, removal during the year 1900 (*Morley Fletcher* and *E. H. Shaw*)	XXXVII.	295
carcinomata of, removed during the year 1900 (*Morley Fletcher* and *E. H. Shaw*)	XXXVII.	300
chronic mastitis of	XXXVII.	307
colloid carcinoma of	XXXVII.	302
multiple tumours of	XXXVII.	308
Mania, after injury to the hand	XXI.	166
suddenness of the attack	XXIII.	21
Marsh (*Howard*), abscess, acute, diagnosis of	XXXIV.	241
abscess and new growth, diagnosis between	XXXIV.	251
,, in connection with ribs	XXXIV.	242
,, points of interest in	XXXIV.	241
carcinoma of sigmoid flexure of colon, simulating an iliac abscess	XXXIV.	253
cheek, abscess of	XXXIV.	254
decayed wisdom tooth, leading to sinus of cheek	XXXIV.	254
diagnosis between new growths and inflammatory enlargements of bones	XXVIII.	7
,, of acute abscess	XXXIV.	241
iliac abscess imitated by carcinoma	XXXIV.	253
memoir of Sir James Paget, Bart.	XXXV.	i
,, ,, Sir William Savory, Bart.	XXXI.	i
new growths and inflammatory enlargements of bones, diagnosis between	XXVIII.	7
ossification of displaced periosteum	XXXIV.	251
Paget, Sir James, Bart., memoir of	XXXV.	i
pelvic abscess from injury	XXXIV.	255
periosteal abscess	XXXIV.	250
post-mammary abscess	XXXIV.	249
ribs, abscess in connection with	XXXIV.	242
Savory, Sir William, Bart., memoir of	XXXI.	i
" shirt-stud " abscess of the abdominal wall	XXXIV.	244
sinus in cheek from decayed wisdom tooth	XXXIV.	254
sub-gluteal abscess	XXXIV.	246
sub-pectoral abscess	XXXIV.	246
sub-periosteal abscess	XXXIV.	250
suppuration, the association of with malignant disease	XXIII.	147
Marshall (*C. F.*), multiple gangrenous dermatitis and purpura in enteric fever	XXVII.	189
Martha Ward (*see* Women's Ward).		
ovariotomy and hysterectomy in (*Harrison Cripps*)	XXXIX.	143
table of cases of abdominal section admitted into during 1898 (*Harrison Cripps*)	XXXV.	23
Martin (*P.*), notes of a case of aneurysm of the aorta, treated after Tufnell's plan	XXIII.	83
Martin (*Robert*), memoir of	XXVII. xxxiii	
Mason (*J.*), a case of strangulated obturator hernia, recovery	XXVII.	65
Masterman (*E. W. G.*), on rodent ulcer	XXVIII. 305 ; XXIX. 189	
some unusual forms of carcinoma of the breast, considered chiefly from the point of view of microscopic pathology	XXVII.	193
two cases of spreading gangrene around the mouth, occurring in adults	XXVII.	205
Mastitis, chronic, of mammary gland	XXXVII.	307
Mastoid disease, treatment of (*De Santi*)	XXXV.	103
suppuration	XXIX.	343

		VOL.	PAGE
Matron, St. Bartholomew's Hospital, duties of . . .		XXII.	41
,, ,, report of influenza .		XXVI.	235
Maturity, puberty, and infancy, diseases of		XXII.	353
Maude (*A.*), case of melanotic sarcoma of hard palate . .		XXVI.	169
Graves' disease, note on the use of Leiter's tubes to the præcordium		XXVIII.	25
nine cases of Graves' disease; ophthalmoplegia; remarks on the lid symptoms .		XXVII.	133
some rare clinical points in Graves' disease . . .		XXIX.	181
Maxilla, superior (*see* Upper Jaw).			
superior, gummatous mass of face with necrosis of bone		XXVI.	85
,, tumour of		XXIV.	291
Maxwell (*J. L.*), a case of Landry's paralysis . . .		XL.	49
Maxwell (*J. Preston*), a case of intracapsular fracture-dislocation of the head of the humerus, operation .		XXXVIII.	33
a case of Landry's paralysis		XXXVI.	173
and **Butlin** (*H. T.*), on the results of operations for cancer of the breast		XXIV.	49
May (*J. H.*), with **Kanthack**, prognosis and causes of death in diphtheria treated by antitoxin		XXXII.	335
Mayo (*J. A.*), surgical emergencies		XXXVII.	269
Meaning of the word "delirium" (*S. Gee*) . . .		XXXIII.	3
Measles, followed by albuminuria		XXVI.	26
Meckel's diverticulum, intussusception of . . .		XXVII.	171
Mediastinal glands, lymphadenoma of		XXII.	101
posterior, primary lympho-sarcoma of . . .		XXIII.	231
Mediastinum, abscess of		XXVIII.	94
anterior, sarcoma of		XXVIII.	78, 79, 82
tumour of, presenting difficulties in diagnosis .		XXXIII.	7
Medical diagnosis, value of ophthalmoscope in (*Napier*)		XXIV.	337
Medicine, clinical contributions to practical (*Duckworth*) .		XXI.	105
its relation to diet		XXVI.	313
on the study of biology in		XXIV.	65
the future of (*Spicer*)		XXV.	279
Medico-legal aspects of coal-gas poisoning . . .		XXI.	77
importance of determining the duration of pregnancy, difficulty by means of menstruation (*C. Godson*) .		XXIV.	167
Medulla, antero-lateral nucleus of, and its relation to the vaso-motor centre		XXV.	37
Medullary carcinoma of lung		XXVIII.	88
Melancholia, suicide and homicide in		XXI,	7
Melanotic sarcoma of intestine		XL.	131
of palate (*Maude*)		XXVI.	169
Melanuria, the diagnostic value of (*Garrod*) . . .		XXXVIII.	25
Membrane, from fauces in diphtheria, examined bacteriologically		XXX.	142
,, tracheotomy wound, examined bacteriologically		XXX.	140
Memoir of Dr. James Andrew (*Sir William S. Church*) . .		XXXIII.	xxix
W. Morrant Baker (*Alfred Willett*) . .		XXXII.	xxxix
Sir George Burrows, Bart. (*Sir James Paget*) . .		XXIII.	xxxiii
Alfred Coleman (*W. B. Paterson*) . . .		XXXVIII.	xxxiii
Dr. J. Matthews Duncan (*Sir William Turner*) .		XXVI.	xxxiii
Dr. Frederic J. Farre (*Sir William S. Church*) .		XXII.	xxxiii
Dr. Francis Harris (*S. Gee*) . . .		XXI.	xxxi
Sir George Humphrey (*C. B. Lockwood*) . .		XXXII.	xxxi
Dr. A. A. Kanthack (*A. A. Bowlby*) . . .		XXXV.	5
A. S. Mackrell		XXVII.	xliii
Dr. Robert Martin		XXVII.	xxxiii
Mark Morris, the Steward		XXXI.	19
Sir James Paget, Bart. (*Howard Marsh*) . .		XXXVI.	1

	VOL.	PAGE
Memoir of Henry G. Read (*W. B. Paterson*)	XXXVIII.	XXXV
Sir William Savory, Bart. (*Howard Marsh*)	XXXI.	1
Dr. Reginald Southey (*Henry Power*)	XXXV.	1
Sir Richard Thorne Thorne, K.C.B.	XXXVI.	27
Bowater J. Vernon (*Henry Power*)	XXXVII.	1
William J. Walsham (*D'Arcy Power*)	XXXIX.	xxxiii
Meningeal artery, exposure of (*D'Arcy Power*)	XXXV.	43
hæmorrhage	XXVIII.	156
Meninges, congenital and traumatic cysts of	XL.	75
Meningitis, case of, after removal of nasal polypus	XXXVI.	53
chronic, with optic neuritis	XXI.	223, 225, 228
posterior basic, local paralysis in	XL.	37
purulent, with indefinite symptoms	XL.	12
symptoms of, produced by teething	XXII.	224
tubercular, simulated in spastic paralysis	XXVIII.	263
Menorrhagia in influenza	XXVI.	200
Menstrual colic	XXII.	95
fever	XXII.	93
Menstruation in pregnancy	XXIV.	172, 173
in Raynaud's disease	XXVIII.	38
Mental disturbance, a case of, after operation (*Herringham*)	XXI.	165
Microbe of suppurative parametritis	XXIV.	39
Micro-organisms in acute infective osteo-periostitis	XXIX.	267
Microscopic pathology of carcinoma of breast (*Masterman*)	XXVII.	193
Microscopical appearances in lesion of fifth nerve-trunk	XXIX.	217
examination of lymphangioma	XXIX.	147
,, ,, nerves in Landry's paralysis	XXVIII.	148
Microzymes, their relation to disease	XXIV.	79
Middle ear, some functions of (*Lawrence*)	XXXV.	113
,, disease, and mastoid suppuration	XXIX.	343
,, ,, cases of (*Mayo, Willett,* and *Hawes*)	XXXVIII.	280
Middlesbrough, pneumonia at	XXVIII.	74
Midwifery, antiseptic measures in	XXIII.	45
experiences of an assistant of	XXII.	357
Malay (*Myers*)	XXXV.	101
native, in West Africa	XXXIX.	204
Midwives, education of	XXIII.	56
Miller (*J. T.*), and Tylden (*H. J.*), recent research in diabetes, with a note on the pathology of the pancreas	XXVII.	71
Miscellanies (*Gee*)	XXII.	89
Mitchell, enteritis and colic simulating intestinal obstruction	XXXII.	61
Mitral, cases of morbus cordis	XXII.	128
and aortic orifices confluent	XXIII.	162
stenosis with phthisis	XXIII.	249
Moore (*E. J.*), report on influenza	XXVI.	224
Moore (*Norman*), abscess of gall-bladder, two cases of	XXVIII.	123
anatomy, morbid, of gout, some observations on	XXIII.	289
ataxy, locomotor, in children	XXIX.	261
cardiac murmurs audible without touching the chest	XXVI.	165
children, locomotor ataxy in	XXIX.	261
fever, enteric, pericarditis in	XL.	19
gall-bladder, abscess of	XXVIII.	123
gout, some observations on the morbid anatomy of	XXIII.	289
hæmaturia, parasitic, two cases of	XXI.	89
jaundice, protracted, case of	XXVIII.	123
locomotor ataxy in children	XXIX.	261
murmurs, cardiac, audible without touching the chest	XXVI.	165
paraplegia, partial, in children	XXIX.	261
pericarditis in enteric fever	XL.	19
peritonitis, three cases of	XXIV.	149
The Book of the Foundation of St. Bartholomew's	XXI.	xxxix

		VOL.	PAGE
Morbid anatomy of gout	. . . . . .	XXIII.	291
proclivities, and physical characters	. . .	XXXIX.	63
Morbus Addisoni, case of	. . . .	XXIV.	253
effect of nitrite of amyl on the pulse	. . .	XXIV. 254, 256	
nitro-glycerine in	. . . . . .	XXIV. 255, 258	
treatment of	. . . . . .	XXIV.	258
Morbus cordis, congenital	. . . . .	XXVIII.	151
mitral, cases of	. . . . . .	XXII. 128, 129	
„ and aortic, cases of	. . . .	XXII. 119, 125, 127	
Morbus coxæ, its natural course	. . . .	XXIV.	324
mortality from	. . . . .	XXIV.	334
treatment	. . . . . .	XXIV.	323
Morphia, consumption of	. . . . .	XXII.	52
Morrant Baker, obituary notice of	. . .	XXXII. xxxix	
Morrice (*G. G.*), suppression of urine in diphtheria	.	XXVIII.	193
two illustrations of nervous diseases	. . .	XXXIX.	167
Morris (*Mark*), the steward, obituary notice of	. .	XXXI.	19
Mortality, after abdominal section	. . .	XXIX.	22
„ after removal of goître	. . .	XXV.	104
geographical distribution of, in the British Isles	.	XXXIX.	95
influenza	. . . . .	XXVI. 207, 208	
in intussusception of the bowel	. . .	XXVIII.	98
Morton (*C. A.*), notes of three cases of coal-gas poisoning, with remarks on the symptoms, as illustrated by these and other cases	. . . .	XXI.	73
the surgical treatment of increased intracranial pressure	XXXIII.	63	
Mountain sickness (*Hepburn*)	. . . .	XXXI.	191
Mouth, epithelioma of, associated with abscess	.	XXIII.	151
state of, during sleep, in cases of nasal obstruction	.	XXIX.	237
spreading gangrene of	. . . .	XXVII.	205
treatment of	. . . . .	XXVII.	210
Multiple mucous polypi of the bladder	. . .	XXIII.	236
polypi of rectum	. . . .	XXXII. 19, 21	
„ „ the lower bowel occurring thrice in one family	XXXIII.	225	
Mundy (*H.*), a peculiar case of spinal deformity	. .	XXXVI.	55
Munk (*W.*), Notæ Harveianæ	. . .	XXIII.	1
Murmurs, cardiac, audible, without touching the chest	.	XXVI.	165
„ the common hæmic	. . .	XXVII.	33
„ hæmic, area of	. . .	XXVII.	34
„ „ audible behind	. . .	XXVII.	34
„ „ dilatation of heart in	. .	XXVII.	39
„ „ effect of exertion on	. .	XXVII.	36
„ „ „ „ position on	. .	XXVII.	35
„ „ „ „ respiration on	. .	XXVII.	37
„ „ in anæmia	. . .	XXVII.	37
„ „ „ children	. . .	XXVII.	37
„ „ point of maximum intensity of	.	XXVII.	33
„ „ tension of pulse in	. .	XXVII.	40
mitral diastolic, their causation	. . .	XXIV.	197
Murray, on tumours of the cerebro-spinal system	.	XXIII.	350
„ „ spleen	. . .	XXIII.	356
Murrell (*G. F.*), on skin-grafting	. . .	XXIX.	353
report of a case of sporadic criticism treated by thyroid juice	. . . .	XXIX.	101
Muscarin, nitrate of, its effect in paralysis of the sympathetic nerve	. . . .	XXIX.	104
Muscles, atrophy of	. . . . .	XXIII.	89
electrical condition of, in sclerosis	. . .	XXI. 95, 96	
lumbar, equilibrium maintained by	. . .	XXIII.	69
of neck, cramp in	. . . .	XXII.	218

	VOL.	PAGE
Muscles, operations on	XXXIV.	294
papillary, their action	XXIII.	167
pectoral, congenital absence of	XXX.	125
the lumbar, their function	XXIV.	242
Museum, additions to	XXXI.	273
„ „ during 1897	XXXIII.	233
descriptive list of specimens added to during 1896 (*Kanthack*)	XXXII.	451
„ „ histological records	XXXII.	513
„ additions to (*Andrewes* and *Morley Fletcher*)	XXXIV.	331
„ „ specimens added to the Museum (*Fletcher*)	XXXVI.	275
list of specimens added to XXXVII. 363; XXXVIII. 187; XXXIX. 243		
of Hospital	XXII.	32
specimens of interest added to	XXVII.	169
Myasthenia gravis, a case of, with autopsy (*Batten* and *Morley Fletcher*)	XXXVI.	213
Mycosis fungoides, a case of (*J. A. Ormerod*)	XXXVII.	257
Myeloid sarcoma of tibia, a case of (*D'Arcy Power*)	XXXV.	49
Myers (*C. S.*), Malay midwifery	XXXV.	101
the conditions of life on a Torres Strait island	XXXV.	91
Myoma, multinodular, of uterus	XXIX. 39, 40	
of uterus, hysterectomy for	XXIX. 39, 40	
Myopathies, brief sketch of the	XXV. 141, 144	
Myopia, removal of lens in (*Jessop*)	XXXV.	242
Myxœdema and Graves' disease	XXIX.	182
„ „ thyroid extract in	XXIX.	182
Nævus, treatment of, by electricity	XXVIII.	725
„ „ electrolysis (*Lewis Jones*)	XXX.	205
Napier, on tumours of the orbit	XXV.	278
the value of the ophthalmoscope in medical diagnosis	XXIV.	337
Nares, sarcomatous polypi of	XXI.	148
Nasal chambers, examination of the, for obstruction	XXIII.	120
forceps	XXIII.	123
growths, effects of post-	XXIX.	236
obstruction	XXV.	274
„ and asthenia	XXIX.	250
„ „ epilepsy	XXIX.	250
„ breathing in	XXIX.	235
„ condition of triangles of the neck in	XXIX.	237
„ defective aëration of blood in	XXIX.	243
„ deformities of the chest in	XXIX.	247
„ its causation and treatment	XXVII.	15
„ mode of respiration in	XXIX.	237
„ restlessness at night in	XXIX.	243
„ snoring in	XXIX. 237, 245	
„ state of mouth during sleep	XXIX.	237
„ symptoms and consequences of	XXIX.	243
„ treatment of	XXIII.	119
polypi, a cause of obstruction	XXIII.	133
polypus, case of meningitis after removal of	XXXVI.	53
saw	XXIII.	127
septum, dislocation of from the superior maxillary crest	XXIII.	124
„ hypertrophy and œdema of	XXVII.	25
„ „ of	XXIII.	127
sinuses, accessory, chronic purulent catarrh of	XXX.	237
stenosis	XXVII.	285

	VOL.	PAGE
Nash (*W. G.*), on torsion of the spermatic cord causing strangulation of the testis and epididymis	XXIX.	163
Naso-pharyngeal examination	XXIII.	121
obstruction	XXIII.	134
polypi	XXIII.	136
polypus	XXIV.	309
Naso-pharynx, adenoid vegetations in	XXI.	152
Native methods of treatment in West Africa (*J. G. Forbes*)	XXXIX.	189
Neck, blow on, leading to caries and paraplegia	XXVII.	242, 245
congenital cystic hygroma of	XXIV.	277
cramp in muscles of	XXII.	218
fibromatous outgrowth in the skin of	XXVI.	147
spasm of muscles of	XXIV.	249
Necrosis of arytænoid cartilage in typhoid fever	XXV.	133
of bone, in fractures of femur	XXVIII.	11
,, inferior turbinated bone	XXIII.	133
,, lower jaw	XXVII.	179
,, olecranon from syphilis	XXVI.	86
,, palate	XXVII.	205
,, upper jaw	XXVI. 85 , XXVII.	205
Nephrectomy, case of (*Harrison Cripps*)	XXXV.	35
for calculous pyelitis	XXI.	121
Nephrorrhaphy, cases of (*D'Arcy Power*)	XXXV.	47
Nephritis, acute, in children	XXVI.	27
chronic interstitial, and urate of soda	XXIII.	293, 294
parenchymatous, and urate of soda	XXIII.	293, 294
and peritonitis	XXIX.	67
Nephritis of pregnancy	XXVI.	117
Nephro-lithotomy in calculous pyelitis	XXI.	121
Nerve, ascending root of fifth	XXIX.	215
,, ,, destructive lesion of	XXIX.	215
effects of nicotine in paralysis of right sympathetic	XXIX.	104
optic, atrophy of in insular sclerosis	XXII.	308
paralysis of right sympathetic	XXIX.	103
recurrent laryngeal, danger of wounding in operation for goitre	XXV.	103
right sympathetic, paralysis of	XXIX.	103
third, paralysis of superior division of	XXII.	313
ulnar, divided	XXIV.	281
Nerve-disease, peripheral, illustrations of	XXII.	169
Nerve-injury at birth	XXXII.	404
Nerve-lesion, destructive	XXIX.	215
Nerve-physiology in relation to disease	XXV.	27
Nerve-trunk, lesion of fifth	XXIX.	215
Nerves, examination of peripheral, in Landry's paralysis	XXVIII.	148
injury of, treated by electricity	XXVIII.	254
trophic of lungs	XXIII.	113
Nervous affections after typhoid fever	XXIII.	115, 116
Nervous diseases, two illustrations of (*G. G. Morrice*)	XXXIX.	167
Nervous disorder, five cases of	XXI.	59
Neuralgia, chronic case of	XXXVI.	54
in influenza	XXVI.	198
treated by electricity	XXVIII.	255
Neurasthenia and insanity	XXIX.	118
Neuritis, alcoholic	XXII.	182, 253
,, in women, three cases of multiple peripheral	XXII.	253
of anterior tibial nerve	XXII.	169
,, right peroneal nerve	XXII.	171
optic, cases of	XXI.	223, 238

	VOL.	PAGE
Neuritis, optic, followed by total blindness	XXI.	225, 228
,, intra-cranial disease	XXI.	223
,, with cerebral abscess	XXI.	228
,, ,, chronic meningitis	XXI, 223, 225,	228
peripheral, cases of	XXII, 179,	253
,, ,, from cold	XXII.	179
Neuroses of children (*F. H. Bainbridge*)	XXXVII.	343
Neurosis, removal of uterine appendages for	XXIX.	48
Newbolt (*G. P.*), on osteotomy	XXIII.	349
New growth and abscess, diagnosis between (*Marsh*)	XXXIV.	251
growths of lung and pleura (*S. West*)	XXXIII.	109
Nias (*J. B.*), some facts about Sydenham	XXVI.	189
Nicotine, effects of, in paralysis of right sympathetic nerve	XXIX.	104
Nitrite of amyl in morbus Addisoni	XXIV. 254, 255, 256,	258
Nitro-glycerine in morbus Addisoni	XXIV. 255,	258
Nitro-hydrochloric acid, in treating uric acid headache	XXIII.	201
Nodules in rheumatism	XXII. 213,	215
on finger-joints, an unusual form of (*Garrod*),	XXIX.	157
subcutaneous, fibroid, notes on the occurrence of, in		
gouty persons (*Sir Dyce Duckworth*)	XL.	15
Noma, in typhoid fever	XXV.	133
Non-restraint, its bad effect in certain cases of insanity	XXIV.	14
Noon (*L.*), cases from Mr. Bruce Clarke's wards	XL.	125
Normal physiological functions of the great omentum	XXX.	88
Nose Department, cases of malignant disease from	XXXIX.	219
epithelioma of, ala of	XXI.	151
feeding through, in tracheotomy	XXI.	81
foreign body in	XXVI.	271
operations for deflected septum	XXXIV.	270
papilloma of septum of	XXI.	150
sarcoma of the	XXXIX.	219
Nostril, foreign body in	XXVII.	57
osseous outgrowth of	XXI.	147
Notæ Harveianæ (*Munk*)	XXIII.	1
Nurses, age and experience of	XXVII.	273
number affected by diphtheria	XXVII.	264
Obituary notices (*see* Memoirs).		
Objects of the operation of symphysiotomy	XXX.	45
Obliteration of retinal artery (*Jessop*)	XXXVII.	314
Observations on osteo-arthritis, &c. (*Sir Dyce Duckworth*)	XXXV.	13
upon osteo-arthritis (*Derwent Parker*)	XXXVI.	177
Obstruction, intestinal, a case of	XXV.	169
,, cases of	XXXVII.	275
,, diagnosis of	XXV.	172
,, doubtful cause	XXVIII.	121
,, enteritis and colic simulating	XXXII.	61
,, from cancerous stricture	XXVIII. 113, 116,	117
,, ,, impacted gall-stone	XXVIII.	113
,, ,, intussusception	XXVIII. 97,	113
,, in hysteria	XXXIV.	314
,, nine cases of	XXVIII.	113
,, operation for	XXV.	171
,, right iliac colotomy in	XXX.	215
,, treatment after	XXV.	174
,, ,, of	XXIV.	320
in vena cava superior with hepatic cirrhosis	XXXII.	71
nasal, and epilepsy	XXIX.	250
,, ,, its treatment	XXIII.	119
,, cocaine in	XXIII.	120

	VOL.	PAGE
Obstruction, nasal, examination of the nasal chambers for	XXIII.	120
,, intra-nasal	XXII.	122
,, state of mouth during sleep	XXIX.	237
naso-pharyngeal	XXIII.	134
of sublingual duct with abscess	XXXIII.	105
,, submaxillary duct	XXXIII.	105
,, uterus in sarcoma of bladder	XXIV.	213
Obstructions of nose, due to changes in middle ear	XXVII.	15
,, ,, extra-nasal	XXVII.	25
,, ,, from septal causes	XXVII.	21
,, ,, intra-nasal	XXVII.	16
,, ,, its causation and treatment	XXVII.	15
,, ,, mental distress in	XXVII.	16
,, ,, symptoms of	XXVII.	16
Obturator hernia, symptoms of strangulated (*Mason*)	XXVII.	65
Œdema, a rare form of, in Graves' disease	XXIX.	187
fugitive case of, obscure origin, ending fatally	XXX.	195
in hypertrophy of heart, and renal disease	XXXII.	261
of arm	XXVII.	61
Œsophagotomy	XXIX.	97
Œsophagus, carcinoma of	XXVIII. 79 ; XXXIX.	223
,, ,, in connection with tuberculosis	XXXV.	183
remarks on carcinoma of	XXXV.	195
Ogle (*J.*), report on influenza	XXVI.	217
and Willoughby (*W. G.*), notes of twenty-two cases of diphtheria under the care of Sir Dyce Duckworth, in which tracheotomy was performed	XXVI.	173
Oil of cloves, its action on the absorption of gas by the intestine	XXII.	292
Olecranon, necrosis of, from syphilis	XXVI.	86
Omental cancers	XXIII.	357
Omentum, cancer of	XXIII. 357 ; XXVIII.	120
hydatids of	XXVII.	241
the great, diseases of	XXX.	105
,, ,, displacement of	XXX.	93
,, ,, injuries of the	XXX.	91
,, ,, its development, anatomy, physiology, and pathology (*McAdam Eccles*)	XXX.	81
,, ,, normal physiological functions of	XXX.	88
Operation, cases of gastric ulcer, treated by (*D'Arcy Power*)	XXXVIII.	5
case of leaking gastric ulcer, treated by (*D'Arcy Power*)	XXXVIII.	6
cases, report of (*S. P. Huggins, Walsham, and Smith*)	XXXIV.	253
for gall-bladder	XXVIII.	124, 126
,, hydatids	XXVIII.	241
,, intestinal obstruction	XXV.	171
,, lymphangioma of tongue	XXIX.	146
,, removal of goître, steps in the	XXV.	102
radical, for hernia	XXXIV.	282
,, ,, hydrocele (*Walsham*)	XXXIV.	285
Operations for hernia (*D'Arcy Power*)	XXXV.	45
,, hydrocele ,, ,,	XXXV.	47
mental disturbance after	XXI.	165
of sixteen months, and their lessons (*D'Arcy Power*)	XXXV.	37
on fasciæ (*Walsham*)	XXXIV.	294
,, gall-bladder	XXXVI.	43
,, harelip and cleft palate (*Walsham*)	XXXIV.	271
,, joints (*D'Arcy Power*)	XXXIV. 286 ; XXXV.	45
,, kidney	XXXV.	47
,, muscles (*Walsham*)	XXXIV.	294
,, nose, deflected septum	XXXIV.	270

	VOL.	PAGE
Operations, preparation of instruments for	XXIX.	91
„ „ the patient for	XXIX.	90
results of Halsted's, for cancer of breast (*Butlin*)	XXXVII.	264
„ „ in cancer of breast (*Butlin* and *Maxwell*)	XXXIV.	49
„ „ „ 1890	XXVII.	271
„ „ Mr. Butlin's	XXIX.	96, 97
Ophthalmic cases at the hospital	XXII.	33
„ and notes (*Jessop*)	XXXV. 231; XXXVII.	309
notes and cases	XXII. 305; XXXVI.	253
practice, use of cocaine in	XXII.	305
Ophthalmoplegia	XXVII.	133, 138
in Graves' disease	XXVII.	138, 147
interna and externa, probably syphilitic	XXII.	211
Ophthalmoscope in medical diagnosis (*Napier*)	XXIV.	337
Opisthotonos, remarks on the causation of (*Herringham*)	XXXVI.	31
Opium, in diabetes mellitus	XXV.	7
remarks on the administration of, for the relief of pain	XXXIX.	231
Optic, atrophy in diabetes insipidus, cases of (*Stanley Bousfield*)	XXXVI.	235
nerve, atrophy of, in insular sclerosis	XXII.	308
„ physiological effects of section (*Jessop*)	XXXVII.	309
neuritis (*see* Neuritis).		
Orang-outan, structure of brain of	XXVII.	227
Orbit, gunshot wounds of (*Jessop*)	XXXVII.	312
perforating wounds of	XXIV.	179
tumours of the (*Napier*)	XXV.	278
Orchidopexy, operation of (*D'Arcy Power*)	XXXV.	48
Orchitis in influenza	XXVI.	203
Organism, the reserve forces of the animal (*Harry Campbell*)	XXXVIII.	143
Ormerod (*J. A.*), cirrhosis of the liver in a boy	XXVI.	57
degeneration, subacute, of spinal cord	XL.	23
disseminated sclerosis	XXIV.	155
endocarditis, with cerebral embolism	XXVII.	41
general paralysis of the insane, cases resembling	XXI.	23
Landry's paralysis, illustrations of	XXVIII.	137
muscular atrophy, varieties of	XXIII.	89
mycosis fungoides, a case of	XXXVII.	257
paralysis of certain muscles of hip and thigh	XXXI.	45
peripheral nerve disease, illustrations of	XXII.	169
postero-lateral sclerosis, a case of	XXIX.	203
quiescent phthisis, cases of	XXII.	159
tabes dorsalis in husband and wife	XXV.	87
Orthopædic Department, notes from the	XXVIII.	199
Osseous outgrowths of the nostril	XXI.	147
Ossification of displaced periosteum	XXXIV.	251
of retina	XXIX.	302
Osteitis deformans, a case of (*Weber*)	XXXIV.	305
„ beginning in early life	XXXII.	403
of the femur following typhoid fever	XXIII.	220
„ „ „ lower end	XXIV.	306
Osteo-arthritis, in the joint-disease of bleeders	XXVI.	80
observations on (*Sir Dyce Duckworth*)	XXXV.	13
„ „ (*Derwent Parker*)	XXXVI.	177
Osteoclasia	XXVII. 217; XXXIV.	291
by Grattan's instrument	XXVII.	220
„ „ and Thomas's instrument	XXVII.	221
instrumental	XXVII.	218
manual	XXVII.	217
paralysis following	XXVII.	219
Osteoma of palate	XXII.	323

			VOL.	PAGE
Osteo-myelitis, diffuse idiopathic of femur, invading knee-joint			XXIII.	223
Osteo-periostitis, acute infective			XXIX.	265
,,	,,	amputations in	XXIX.	273
,,	,,	bones affected in	XXIX.	267
,,	,,	cases of	XXIX.	273
,,	,,	complications and sequelæ	XXIX.	271
,,	,,	diagnosis of	XXIX.	270
,,	,,	different names for	XXIX.	265
,,	,,	etiology of	XXIX.	265
,,	,,	frequency of, in the two sexes	XXIX.	265
,,	,,	involvement of joints in	XXIX.	272
,,	,,	micro-organisms in	XXIX.	267
,,	,,	pathology of	XXIX.	266
,,	,,	periosteum in	XXIX.	272
,,	,,	pneumonia in	XXIX.	272
,,	,,	prognosis in	XXIX.	273
,,	,,	pyæmic abscesses in	XXIX.	271
,,	,,	septicæmia in	XXIX.	272
,,	,,	symptomatology	XXIX.	268
,,	,,	treatment of	XXIX.	270
Osteotomy, for mal-union of the femur			XXI.	65
,, rickety curvature			XXII.	240
on (*Newbolt*)			XXIII.	349
Ostitis, following gonorrhœa			XXII.	263
Otitis media, cases of (*Mayo, Willett*, and *Hawes*)			XXXVII.	280
indications for treatment of the chronic suppurative form (*De Santi*)			XXXV.	103
intra-cranial complications of (*Bailey*)			XXXVII.	287
the complications of (*Bowes*)			XXXIV.	127
with cerebellar abscess			XXXIX.	37
Outgrowth from the Eustachian tube			XXIII.	136
Outgrowths, osseous, of the nostril			XXI.	147
Out-patients' rooms, foundation-stone laid			XXII.	43
Ovarian cyst, dermoid			XXIX.	28
multilocular		XXIX. 25, 26, 29, 30, 31, 32, 33, 36		
,, with dermoid			XXIX.	34
suppurating			XXIX. 32, 36, 37	
unilocular		XXIX. 24, 25, 28, 36, 37		
with double pedicle			XXIX.	35
,, twisted pedicle			XXIX. 24, 33	
Ovaries, cystic disease of both			XXIX.	24
and tubes, diseases of			XXIX.	50
,, ,, effects of			XXIX.	54
,, ,, prolapsed and fixed			XXIX.	49
,, ,, removal of			XXIX.	50
,, ,, "unsexing" after removal			XXIX.	55
Ovariotomy			XXVII. 61 ; XXXIV. 231	
adhesions in			XXIX.	13
case of double			XXXVI.	44
cases of			XXII. 229 ; XXXV. 23	
effect of, on an insane woman			XXII.	106
incision for			XXIX.	8
operating table for			XXIX.	2
operation of			XXIX.	7
the pedicle in			XXIX.	10
treatment of the peritoneum			XXIX.	16
use of drainage tube in			XXII.	235
Ovariotomy and hysterectomy in Martha Ward			XXXIX.	143

	VOL.	PAGE
Ovary, one cystic, the other papillomatous	XXIX.	25
presence of a third	XXIX.	47
suppurating	XXIX.	34
Overgrowth resembling acromegaly	XXXII.	405
Oxygen, action of in pneumonia (*P. E. Turner*)	XXXIV.	87
inhalation, coal-gas poisoning	XXI.	74, 78
inhalations in anæmia	XXXII.	321
Paget (*Sir James, Bart.*), memoir of	XXXVI.	1
(*Stephen*), on abdominal abscesses	XXI.	242
„ medical treatment of surgical diseases	XXIII.	354
„ tumours of the palate	XXII.	315
Paget's disease of bone (*Weber*)	XXXIV.	305
Pain in intra-thoracic growths	XXVIII.	91
„ right lumbar region	XXIV.	293
relief of, in cancer of tongue	XXIX.	85
Palatal and laryngeal anæsthesia, in disseminated sclerosis (*Horne* and *Batten*)	XXXII.	173
Palate, adenomata of	XXII.	330
calcareous deposits in	XXII.	323
carcinoma of	XXII.	351
cartilaginous and bony growths of	XXII.	323
cleft, and harelip, operations on	XXXIV.	271
hard, melanotic sarcoma of	XXVI.	169
necrosis of	XXVII.	205
papilloma	XXII.	325
paralysis of the, in posterior basic meningitis	XL.	38
polypoid and warty growths on	XXII.	324
sarcoma of	XXII.	345
tumours of	XXII.	315
vascular growths of	XXII.	320
Pallor, in chloroform anæsthesia	XXX.	27
Palmar fascia, contraction of, in relation to gout and rheumatism	XXXII.	119
Pancreas, acid spirit or glycerine extract of	XXIX.	134
brine extract of	XXIX.	132
„ „ diastasic power of	XXIX.	133
„ „ tryptic power of	XXIX.	134
cancer of	XXX. 5 ; XXXVII.	337
experiments with fresh pulp of	XXIX.	126
glycerine extract of, diastasic power	XXIX.	134
„ „ lipolytic action of	XXIX.	126, 128
„ „ tryptic action of	XXIX.	134
sarcoma of	XXVIII.	85
tumour of	XXXV.	34
Pancreatic ferment, diastasic action of	XXIX.	128
lipolytic action of	XXIX.	128
procedure with	XXIX.	126
proteolytic action of	XXIX.	128
rennet action of	XXIX.	128
tryptic value of	XXIX.	127
Pancreatic ferments, in brain disease	XXIX.	130, 136
in diabetes	XXIX.	132, 137
„ disease	XXIX.	125
„ „ conclusions from experiments	XXIX.	141
„ fevers	XXIX.	131, 136
„ heart disease	XXIX.	130, 135
„ phthisis	XXIX.	132, 137
„ pneumonia	XXIX.	129, 131
„ „ and heart disease	XXIX.	129, 135

	VOL.	PAGE
Pancreatic ferments in renal disease	XXIX.	132, 137
in suppurative or malignant disease . . .	XXIX.	131, 136
the, iodine, standard solution of, for . . .	XXIX.	127
Papillary muscles, action of	XXIII.	167
Papillitis, case of double, with recovery (*Jessop*) . .	XXXVI.	263
Papilloma of ovary	XXIX.	25
of palate	XXII.	325
,, septum of nose	XXI.	150
,, trachea	XXI.	147
Paracentesis thoracis, followed by albuminous expectoration	XXII.	99
Paralysis, after diphtheria	XXVII.	263, 287
alcoholic, pathology of	XXXII.	407
agitans, tremors of legs and arms resembling . .	XXV.	276
atrophic	XXIII.	89
,, of deltoid	XXIII.	90
,, of flexors of forearm . . .	XXIII.	90, 95
,, of legs	XXIII.	101
,, of spinati	XXIII.	90
Bell's, associated with herpes zoster . . .	XXXIX.	167
bulbar, progressive	XXIII.	93
,, without anatomical change . .	XXXVI.	213
brass founders'	XXV.	78
cases resembling general paralysis of the insane .	XXI.	23
connected with alcoholism	XXII.	171, 253
diphtheritic	XXVII.	287
facial, cases of	XXII.	172
,, in Graves' disease	XXVII.	138
following antitoxin	XXXI.	101
,, blow on neck	XXVII.	242
,, osteoclasia	XXVII.	219
from pressure on cord	XXVII.	245
general, of adolescence (*Weber*) . . .	XXXIV.	312
,, ,, the insane, on (*Farrar*) . .	XXIV.	317
,, pressure on the brain in . .	XXVIII.	55
,, syphilis a cause of (*Forbes*) . .	XXXVIII.	68
,, trephining the skull in . . .	XXVIII.	55
,, uncertainty of diagnosis in . .	XXVIII.	57
infantile, treatment by electricity . . .	XXVIII.	253
Landry's, a case of (*J. L. Maxwell*) . . .	XL.	49
,, ,, (*J. P. Maxwell*) . .	XXXVI.	173
,, ,, illustrations of (*Ormerod*) .	XXVIII.	137
local, in posterior basic meningitis (*Langdon Brown*)	XL.	37
muscular, in typhoid fever	XXV.	138
of abductors of the vocal cords (*Garrod*) . .	XXII.	209
,, certain muscles of hip and thigh (*Ormerod*) .	XXXI.	45
,, extensors of knees	XXII.	181
,, palate, in posterior basic meningitis . .	XL.	38
,, right sympathetic nerve	XXIX.	103
,, ,, ,, ,, action of reagents in a case of	XXIX.	103
,, ,, effect of exercise on . .	XXIX.	104
,, ,, ,, heat in . . .	XXIX.	104
,, ,, ,, nicotine in . .	XXIX.	104
,, ,, ,, nitrate of muscarin in . . .	XXIX.	104
,, ,, ,, nitrate of pilocarpine in . .	XXIX.	104
,, ,, ,, ,, ,, nitrite of amyl in .	XXIX.	104
,, third nerve, superior division . . .	XXII.	31

		VOL.	PAGE
Paralysis, progressive, bulbar	. . . .	XXIII.	93
pseudo-hypertrophic in an adult (*Fletcher*)	. .	XXIX.	327
,, ,, and progressive muscular atrophy	. . . .	XXIX.	329
spastic, absence of bed-sores in	. . .	XXVIII. 269, 279	
,, articulation in	. . . .	XXVIII.	277
,, condition of limbs in	. . .	XXVIII. 264, 273	
,, convulsions in	. . . .	XXVIII.	271
,, delusions in	. . . .	XXVIII.	275
,, dysphagia in	. . . .	XXVIII.	265
,, electrical reaction of muscles in	. .	XXVIII. 267, 278	
,, emaciation in	. . . .	XXVIII. 263, 279	
,, emotional condition in	. . .	XXVIII.	263
,, examination of larynx in	. . .	XXVIII.	268
,, inspiratory laugh in	. . .	XXVIII.	279
,, loss of control of sphincters in	. .	XXVIII.	263
,, mental condition in	. . . .	XXVIII.	272
,, nervous system in	. . .	XXVIII.	272
,, of all the muscles	. . .	XXVIII.	263
,, reflexes in	. . . .	XXVIII. 263, 272, 275	
,, resembling trismus	. . .	XXVIII.	279
,, sensation in	. . . .	XXVIII.	275
,, sweating in	. . . .	XXVIII. 265, 274	
,, temperature in	. . .	XXVIII. 266, 273	
syphilitic, a case of (*Weber*)	. . .	XXXIV.	308
Parametritis, progressive suppurative	. . .	XXIV.	39
,, ,, microbe of	. .	XXIV.	39
with abscess of the liver	. . .	XXI.	173
Paranæsthesia and paraplegia	. . .	XXI.	140
Paraplegia, alcoholic	. . . .	XXII.	253
from blow on neck	. . . .	XXVII. 242, 245	
hereditary, spastic	. . . .	XXVII.	7
infantile	. . . .	XXIX.	263
partial, in children	. . . .	XXIX. 261, 262	
sacral decubitus in	. . . .	XXI.	140
spastic, infantile, hereditary (*Gee*)	. .	XXV.	81
,, and lateral sclerosis	. . .	XXVII.	14
syphilitic	. . . .	XXII. 251 ; XXXVIII. 78	
with jumping movements after shock	. .	XXI.	62
and paranæsthesia	. . .	XXI.	140
Paresis, in spastic paralysis	. . .	XXVIII.	271
right sided	. . . .	XXVIII.	263
Parietal bone, fracture of	. . . .	XXVII.	183
Parotid abscess	. . . .	XXI.	114
bubo, in typhoid fever	. . .	XXI.	112
gland, inflammation of, in punctured wound of intestine		XXVII.	177
region, growth in	. . . .	XXIV.	279
,, swelling in	. . . .	XXIV.	283
Paroxysmal hæmaturia (*Herringham*)	. .	XXII.	133
Patella, refracture of	. . .	XXI. 68 ; XXX. 230	
starred fracture of	. . . .	XXVII.	211
Patellar ligament, swelling over its outer side	. .	XXIV.	298
reflex, value of, in diphtheria	. . .	XXX.	151
Paterson (*H. J.*) on Thiersch's skin-grafting	. .	XXXII.	161
on value of Ehrlich's section	. . .	XXXII.	217
Pathology, microscopic, of carcinoma of breast (*Masterman*)		XXVII.	193
of alcoholic paralysis	. . .	XXXII.	410
of the great omentum (*McAdam Eccles*)	. .	XXX.	81
,, hæmoptysis	. . . .	XXI.	51
,, horns, warts, and epitheliomata (*Foulerton*)	.	XXV.	105

	VOL.	PAGE
Pathology of insanity	xxvIII.	58
„ intra-thoracic growths	xxvIII.	89
„ pancreas (*Miller* and *Tylden*)	xxvII.	71
„ Raynaud's disease (*Huig*)	xxvIII.	29
and prognosis of glioma of the retina, some points in the (*Jessop*)	xxxvIII.	159
„ therapeutics, action and reaction in (*Weber*)	xxxIX.	139
Patients, preparation of, for operation	xxIX.	6
the numbers of, since 1836	xxII.	55
Paton (*E. Percy*), pericæcal suppuration with cerebral symptoms	xxx.	63
Pectoral muscles, absence of	xxx.	125
Pedicle, double, to ovarian cyst	xxIX.	35
in ovariotomy, treatment of	xxIX.	10
„ „ slipping of ligature of	xxIX.	30
twisted, of ovarian tumour	xxIX.	24, 33
Pediculi, a cause of high temperature	xxIX.	332
„ „ „ taches bleuâtres	xxIX.	332
Peliosis in rheumatism	xxvII.	3
Pelvic abscess from injury (*Marsh*)	xxxIV.	255
glands, abscess complicating cancer of	xxIII.	152
Pelvis, fracture of, with ruptured bladder	xxxII.	199
hydatid, a case of	xxxVI.	45
of boy with extroversion of bladder	xxvII.	170
Pemphigus, acute	xxII.	227
„ case of (*Herringham*)	XL.	33
Penis, epithelioma of	xxIV.	302
glans, horns on	xxv.	107
Perforated duodenal ulcer, cases of (*D'Arcy Power*)	xxxVII.	46
„ „ treated by operation (*Power*)	xxxVIII.	14
gastric ulcer, cases of (*D'Arcy Power*)	xxxVII.	50
„ „ treated by operation (*D'Arcy Power*)	xxxVIII.	10
Pericardial effusion, and intra-thoracic growths	xxvIII.	94
Pericarditis, cases of	xxII.	213
in enteric fever (*Norman Moore*)	XL.	19
rheumatic, age in	xxIII.	278
„ frequency of	xxIII. 269, 278	
„ „ „ in men	xxIII.	278
„ „ mortality in	xxIII.	281
Pericardium, diseases of	xxxII.	37
effusion in, distinguished from tumour	xxvIII.	94
Perimetritis	xxIX.	52
Perinæum, drainage of bladder through	xxvII.	120
Periostitis after gonorrhœa	xxII.	263
„ typhoid fever	xxI.	107
Peripheral nerve-diseases, illustrations of	xxII.	169
neuritis, cases of	xxII. 179, 253	
„ „ „ from cold	xxII.	179
Peritoneum, acute effusion into, caused by tapping	xxIV.	151
chronic adhesions in	xxvII.	247
fæcal extravasation into	xxvIII.	117
opening of, for relief of pain	xxIV.	149
Peritonitis, a case of acute septic (*D'Arcy Power*)	xxxVIII.	22
cases of (*D'Arcy Power*)	xxxVII.	38
„ „ (*Mayo, Willett,* and *Hawes*)	xxxVII.	277
in a case of distended gall-bladder	xxv.	252
tuberculous (*Harrison Cripps*)	xxxV.	33
„ case of (*D'Arcy Power*)	xxxV.	40
Peroneal nerve, neuritis of right	xxII.	171
Phagedæna, distinguished from gangrene	xxv.	76

	VOL.	PAGE
Phalanx, distal, its condition in whitlow	xxv.	189
Pharmacopœias of the Hospital	xxii.	1
Pharyngeal tonsil, hypertrophy of	xxiii.	135
Pharynx, irritable	xxv.	211
,,　　　treatment of	xxv.	212
Philanthropos Theophilus, his six gifts . . .	xxi.	231
Phillips (*Ll. C. P.*), a case of xerodermia pigmentosa .	xxxi.	221
Phrenology and physiognomy : what are they worth ?	xxi.	244
Phthisis, antiseptic treatment of	xxv.	49
bacillary, after typhoid fever	xxi.	115
blood casts in	xxx.	253
cases of hæmoptysis in	xxii.	200
,, ,, quiescent	xxii.	159
coagulability of the blood in	xxvii.	92
conditions tending to the promotion of, in dwelling-house	xxvi.	13
deaths from, in Leicester and Chelmsford . .	xxvi.	3
effects of drainage on death-rate . . .	xxvi.	8
heredity of	xxvi.	263
how affected by influenza	xxvi. 209, 260	
in pulmonary stenosis	xxiii.	240
,, the Hebrides	xxv.	51
injections of sulphuretted hydrogen gas in . .	xxv.	66
mortality from, in England and Wales . .	xxvi.	1, 2
of	xxxii.	31
statistics of vomiting in	xxiv. 138, 139.	
subcutaneous injection of balsam of Peru in . .	xxvi.	89
tendency to, in congenital heart-disease . .	xxiii.	240
treatment of	xxvi.	88
,,　　,,　by antiseptics . . .	xxvi.	87
,,　　,,　,, benzosol . . .	xxvi.	102
,,　　,,　,, curative medicines . .	xxvi.	91
,,　　,,　,, inhalation of hot air . .	xxvi.	91
,,　　,,　,, instillation . . .	xxvi.	92
,,　　,,　,, rectum . . .	xxvi.	91
,,　　,,　with corrosive sublimate . .	xxvi.	100
,,　　,,　,, helenine . . .	xxvi.	100
,,　　,,　,, periodate crystals .	xxvi.	101
,,　　,,　,, tar . . .	xxvi.	100
with aortic incompetence	xxiii.	248
,, mitral stenosis	xxiii.	249
vomiting in left apex disease . . .	xxiv.	131
Physical characters and morbid proclivities . .	xxxix.	63
Physics, arrangement for the teaching of . . .	xxii.	155
Physiology, forensic (*Atkinson*)	xxxix.	127
in relation to disease	xxv.	27
of great omentum (*McAdam Eccles*) . . .	xxx.	81
,, brain and spinal cord	xxv.	28
Pigeons, action of aconite on	xxii. 275, 277, 279	
Pilocarpine, nitrate of, effect in paralysis of right sympathetic nerve	xxix.	104
Pineal gland, its origin	xxv.	40
Plague, a short account of the second epidemic at Bhiwudi (*Dalàl*)	xxxv.	119
points of interest in connection with (*Sandilands*) .	xxxvi.	61
Plants and animals, their relationship . . .	xxiv.	65
dietetic values of food-stuffs prepared by . .	xxx.	113
Pleura and lungs, new growths of	xxxiii.	109
syphilitic affection of (*Weber*) . . .	xxxiv.	305
Pleural effusions (*Gow*)	xxiii.	357
contraction of lung in	xxviii.	181

	VOL.	PAGE
Pleurisy in influenza	XXVI.	202
with effusion, the etiology of (*Hedges*)	XXXVI.	75
„ empyema	XXXII.	35
Pleuritic effusion, and intra-thoracic growths . . .	XXVIII.	95
distinguished from pericardial	XXVIII.	95
its mode of action on the lung	XXVIII.	131
leading to carnification of lung	XXVIII.	1
serous, discharged through lung	XXIII.	36
Pneumococcus, action of oxygen on (*P. E. Turner*). . .	XXXIV.	87
Pneumonia, a cause of cirrhosis of lung	XXVIII.	2
acute lobar, in children	XXVI.	289
„ „ abdominal symptoms in . . .	XXVI.	289
and the pneumococcus in reference to the action of		
oxygen (*P. E. Turner*)	XXXIV.	87
at Middlesborough	XXVIII.	174
bacillus of (*Klein*)	XXVIII.	176
bacteriology of	XXVIII.	177
cases of, injected with strychnia	XXII. 121, 122	
causes of	XXVI.	305
croupous, bacteriology of	XXVIII.	173
„ etiology of	XXVIII.	173
„ pulse and respiration in . . .	XXVIII.	231
deglutition, after tracheotomy	XXI.	80
embolism of right coronary artery	XXXII.	7
lobar, secondary infective lesions in . . .	XXXII.	309
local, in tracheotomy	XXI.	80
with endocarditis	XXII.	5
Pneumoniæ, diplococcus	XXVIII.	174
Pneumothorax, cases of spontaneous (*Harris*) . . .	XXIII.	33
due to gangrene of lung	XXIII.	113
recurrent	XXVI.	294
value of the bell-sound in	XXIII.	44
Points of interest in the Maidstone epidemic (typhoid) . .	XXXIII.	95
Poisoning, and insanity	XXIX.	122
by coal-gas, three cases of	XXI.	73
„ lead, case of, with bosses on the metacarpal		
bones	XXI.	169
„ sulphuretted hydrogen	XXII.	301
Poliomyelitis, anterior, acute	XXIII.	90
„ chronic	XXIII.	91
„ subacute	XXIII.	91
syphilitic, a case of	XXII.	250
Polyneuritis, a case of puerperal (*Weber*) . . .	XXXIV.	305
Polypi, fibrous, of naso-pharynx	XXVIII.	71
„ „ removal of	XXVIII.	71
„ „ treatment of	XXVIII.	72
gelatinous, „	XXVIII.	70
„ „ treatment of . . .	XXVIII.	72
multiple, of the bladder	XXIII.	236
„ „ „ lower bowel	XXIII.	225
„ „ „ rectum	XXXII. 19, 21	
nasal	XXVII.	19
„ a cause of obstruction	XXIII.	133
„ fibrous	XXVII.	30
„ gelatinous	XXVII.	30
„ symptoms of	XXVII.	20
naso-pharyngeal	XXIII.	136
„ „ cases of	XXVIII.	69
„ „ removal of	XXVIII.	69

	VOL.	PAGE
Polypi of the rectum in a mother and child	XXVI.	299
sarcomatous, of nose	XXI.	148
Polypoid growth of palate	XXII.	324
Polypus, malignant, of antrum	XXVII.	31
nasal, meningitis following removal of . . .	XXXVI.	53
naso-pharyngeal	XXIV.	309
Popliteal artery, ligature of (*Walsham*)	XXXIV.	301
superficial femoral, and deep femoral arteries, with their corresponding veins, ligature of . . .	XXX.	224
Portal vein, changes in calibre of	XXXVII.	75
,, ,, composition of the blood in . .	XXXVII.	75
diseases of	XXXVII.	70
inflammatory condition of	XXXVII.	53
morbid anatomy of	XXXVII.	76
Position of incision in whitlow	XXV.	191
,, ,, through the skin, in removal of goitre .	XXV.	102
,, jugular vein, and carotid artery, in removal of goitre	XXV.	102
Posterior rhinoscopy in nasal obstruction	XXIII.	121
Post-mammary abscess (*Marsh*)	XXXIV.	249
Post-nasal vegetations	XXIII.	134
Potassium, bromide, consumption of	XXII.	48
iodide ,, ,, ...	XXII.	48
its possible use in the animal economy . . .	XXIV.	74
,, ,, ,, ,, plants	XXIV.	74
Post mortem appearances in hydatids of liver . . .	XXIX.	337
examinations in chorea	XXIV. 56, 57,	59
Post mortems, at the Hospital	XXII.	37
in Landry's paralysis	XXVIII. 140, 143,	145
Pott (*Percivall*), life and works of	XXX.	163
life of	XXX.	165
as writer	XXX.	179
synopsis of works	XXX.	182
Pott's fracture, cases of (*Mayo, Willett,* and *Hawes*) . .	XXXVII.	271
,, old standing	XXIV.	295
Powell (*H. A.*), a report of four cases of severe head injury .	XXVII.	183
Power (*D'Arcy*), a case of absence of kidney . . .	XXXV.	48
,, ,, acute septic peritonitis . .	XXXVIII.	22
,, ,, dermoid cyst, presacral . .	XXXVII.	42
,, ,, endothelioma . . .	XXXVII.	44
,, ,, hytadid of liver . . .	XXXVII.	43
,, ,, rupture of first part of duodenum .	XXXV.	41
,, ,, ,, ,, kidney . . .	XXXVII.	29
,, ,, ,, ,, liver . . .	XXXVII.	28
,, ,, tuberculous peritonitis . .	XXXVII.	40
a year's abdominal operations . . .	XXXVII.	27
cases of intussusception . . .	XXXVII.	32
,, laparotomies	XXXV.	40
,, nephrorrhaphy	XXXV.	47
,, perforated duodenal ulcer .	XXXVII.	46
.. ,, gastric ulcer . .	XXXVII.	50
,, peritonitis	XXXVII.	38
,, polyorromenitis . . .	XXXVII.	38
,, pyonephrosis	XXXV.	47
exposure of meningeal artery	XXXV.	43
injuries of abdomen	XXXVII.	28
ligature of femoral artery	XXXV.	43
myeloid sarcoma of tibia	XXXV.	49
notes of an experiment on the induction of false albuminuria . , , ...	XXIII.	173

		VOL.	PAGE
Power (*D'Arcy*), on the cure of king's evil	. . . .	XXVII.	282
operations for hernia	. . . . .	XXXV.	45
,, ,, hydrocele	. . . . .	XXXV.	47
,, on joints	. . . . .	XXXV,	45
,, ,, kidney	. . . . .	XXXV.	47
perforated duodenal ulcer treated by operation	. .	XXXVIII.	14
,, gastric ulcer treated by operation	. .	XXXVIII.	10
primary sarcoma of vagina in children	. . .	XXXI.	121
some cases of gastric and intestinal perforation, and the lessons they teach	. .	XXXVIII.	5
,, ,, gastric surgery	. . . .	XXXIX.	19
surgical discussion on strumous arthritis	. . .	XXV.	271
the operations of sixteen months, and their lessons	.	XXXV.	37
treatment of ganglion	. . . . . .	XXXV.	50
and **Horne** (*W. Jobson*), on some cases of malignant disease from the Department for Diseases of the Throat and Nose	.	XXXIX.	219
Power (*Henry*), on medicine in the Middle Ages	. .	XXIII. '	345
secondary cataract	. . . .	XXXIV.	5
Pregnancy, complicated with heart-disease	. . . .	XXV.	181
dropsy in	. . . .	XXVI.	115
duration of, difficulty of determining its medico-legal importance (*C. Godson*)	. . .	XXIV. 167,	169
,, ,, (*Graham*)	. . . . .	XXV.	177
eclampsia of	. . . . . .	XXVI.	115
in influenza	. . . .	XXVI.	203
,, nephritis	. . . . . .	XXVI.	117
,, Raynaud's disease	. . . .	XXVIII.	38
,, renal affections (*Griffith*)	. . .	XXVI.	115
menstruation occurring during	. . .	XXIV. 172,	173
Premature labour in dropsy	. . . . .	XXVI.	117
Preparation of instruments	. . . . .	XXIX.	91
of patients before operation	. . . . .	XXIX.	6
Prescribing at the Hospital	. . . . . .	XXII.	38
Present position of symphysiotomy	. . . .	XXX.	27
Priapism, painful, persistent (*H. V. Pryce*)	. . .	XXXVIII.	99
Prize (*Horton-Smith*)	. . . .	XXXVII.	53
,, (*Stephen Scott*)	. . . .	XXXV.	131
Procidentia uteri	. . . .	XXVII.	59
Production of gout by drugs	. . . . . .	XXIV.	225
Prognosis, after operation, in glioma of the retina (*Jessop*)	.	XXXIX.	213
in albuminuria (*Lewis Jones*)	. . . .	XXVI.	307
,, cases of diphtheria, treated by antitoxin (*Kanthack* an'd *May*)	. .	XXXII.	335
of simple gastric ulcer (*Habershon*)	. . .	XXVII. 149,	159
,, tetanus (*Worthington*)	. . . .	XXXI.	137
Prostate, enlargement of	. . . . . .	XXVII.	249
,, ,, with hæmorrhage	. . .	XXV.	232
hæmaturia from	. . . . . .	XXV.	229
incision of	. . . .	XXVII.	122
Prostatic atrophy, relation of testes to (*Bruce Clarke*)	.	XXXV.	249
Pruen (*S. T.*), on alcohol	. . . . . .	XXII.	360
Pruritus, boro-glyceride in	. . . . .	XXI.	119
Pryce (*H. Vaughan*), painful persistent priapism	.	XXXVIII.	99
Puberty, infancy, and maturity, diseases of	. .	XXII.	353
Puerperal eclampsia	. . . . . .	XXII.	358
fever (*see* Fever, Puerperal).			
polyneuritis, a case of (*Weber*)	. . . .	XXXIV.	305
women, immunity of, from diphtheria infection	.	XXX.	151
Pullen (*R. S.*), case of foreign body in the nose	. .	XXVI.	271

	VOL.	PAGE
Pulmonary circulation, conditions of (*Michael Foster*) . .	XXVIII.	257
hæmorrhage	XXVII.	83
tuberculosis, associated with congenital cardiac disease	XXIII.	239
vessels, hæmoptysis due to ulceration of the walls of .	XXI.	53
Pulsation, arrested, in arteries	XXV.	258
Pulse, cause of slowness of, in diphtheria	XXVIII.	193
effect of amyl-nitrite on the, in morbus Addisonii .	XXIV. 254,	258
frequency of, in pneumonia	XXVIII.	231
irregularity of, in intra-thoracic growths . . .	XXVII.	92
tension of, in hæmic murmurs	XXVII.	40
Pulse-respiration ratio, in croupous pneumonia . .	XXVIII.	231
Pulsus paradoxus	XXI.	87
Punctured wounds (*see* Wound).		
Pupil, in chloroform anæsthesia	XXX.	20
value of the, as an aid to diagnosis . . .	XXV.	38
Pupils, in coal-gas poisoning	XXXI.	77
inequality of, in intra-thoracic growths . . .	XXVIII.	92
Purkinje's cells in cerebellar disease . . .	XXIV.	246
Purpura, as it occurs in sarcoma, lymphadenoma, and		
tubercle	XXXVIII.	117
in enteric fever	XXVII. 189,	191
„ influenza	XXVI.	201
„ paroxysmal hæmaturia	XXIII.	137
notes of two cases of	XXV.	165
treatment of	XXV.	166
use of turpentine in	XXV. 166 ; XXVII.	95
Purulent catarrh, chronic, of the accessory nasal sinuses .	XXX.	237
„ „ frontal sinuses . .	XXX.	244
Pus, foul-smelling, in tympanum	XXIX.	345
Pustule, malignant, notes of a case of (*Lyndon*) . .	XXIV. 297,	315
Putrefactive bacilli, inhalations of	XXV.	66
Pyæmia, aural	XXX.	247
case of, due to streptococcus pyogenes, in which the		
serum treatment failed (*Horder*) . . .	XXXIII.	89
from middle-ear disease	XXIX.	344
and septicæmia	XXIII.	46
Pyelitis, calculous, nephrectomy for	XXI.	121
„ nephro-lithotomy in a case of . .	XXI.	125
Pylephlebitis (*Langdon Brown*)	XXXVII.	53
bibliography of	XXXVII.	178
record of the cases in St. Bartholomew's Hospital . .	XXXVII.	155
suppurative	XXXVII.	95
„ diagnosis of	XXXVII.	125
„ prognosis of	XXXVII.	127
table of	XXXVII.	136
Pylethrombosis (*Langdon Brown*)	XXXVII.	60
causes of	XXXVII.	71
diagnosis of	XXXVII.	89
etiology and pathology of	XXXVII.	60
prognosis of	XXXVII.	90
septic causes of	XXXVII.	71
signs and symptoms of	XXXVII.	80
treatment of	XXXVII.	92
Pylorectomy, for carcinoma	XL.	133
Pyonephrosis, cases of (*D'Arcy Power*) . . .	XXXV.	47
Pyosalpinx	XXIX.	52
case of (*Harrison Cripps*)	XXXV.	32
Pyrexia, in spastic paralysis	XXVIII.	266
slightness of, in malignant diphtheria . . .	XXIII.	17

	VOL.	PAGE
Quacks and quackery	XXI.	248
Quadriceps tendon, case of rupture of (*Mayo, Willett*, and Hawes)	XXXVII.	273
Quassia, introduction and consumption of . . .	XXII.	45
Quinine, consumption of	XXII.	47
in paroxysmal hæmaturia	XXII.	140
Rabies and Landry's paralysis	XXVIII.	138
Race, geographical distribution of, in the British Isles .	XXXIX.	94
Radical cure of right inguinal hernia, operation for, followed by gangrenous appendicitis (*J. Findlay Alexander*)	XL.	153
operation for hydrocele (*Walsham*). . . .	XXXIV.	285
Radius, congenital absence of	XXXII.	400
swelling in or about head of	XXIV.	310
Ranking (*J. E.*), three medical cases	XXII.	245
Rash, ether	XXXII.	79
in influenza	XXVI.	201
Raven (*Thomas F.*), some aspects of infectious diseases, and shock in their etiology	XXXVII.	205
Rawling (*L. B.*), on congenital and traumatic cysts of the brain and meninges	XL.	75
Raynaud's disease, a case of (*Haig*) . . .	XXVIII.	29
changes in the blood in	XXVIII.	37
enlargement of the spleen in	XXVIII.	37
etiology of	XXVIII.	33
in paroxysmal hæmaturia	XXII.	138
menstruation and pregnancy in . . .	XXVIII.	38
pathology of	XXVIII.	29
Read (*H. G.*), memoir of	XXXVIII.	xxxv
Rebuilding of the Hospital	XXII.	22, 32
Recession of triangles of the neck, in cases of nasal obstruction	XXIX.	237
Rectal hernia	XXVII.	61
injection of sulphuretted hydrogen gas . .	XXV.	66
Rectum, communicating with broad ligament cyst .	XXIX.	34
dilatation of	XXIV.	260
fissure of (*Goodsall*)	XXVIII.	205
foreign body in	XXVII.	57
growth in	XXXII.	21
impacted fæces in	XXVII.	250
multiple polypi in	XXIII.	225
„ „ of	XXXII.	19, 21
operations on (*Walsham*)	XXXIV.	293
polypi in	XXVI.	229
polypoid growths with fissure of . . .	XXVIII.	207
procidentia of	XXVII.	59
retention of fæcal mass in	XXVII.	58
twenty cases of foreign bodies in (*Goodsall*) . .	XXIII.	71
Recurrent carcinoma, in breast	XXIV.	286
epithelioma beneath jaw	XXIV.	287
sarcoma of humerus	XXIV.	205
„ „ scapula	XXIV.	302
scirrhus of breast	XXIV.	309
Reece (*R. J.*), a case of a piece of glass in the eyeball for seven years and ninety-four days . . .	XXIV.	201
on compound fractures	XXIII.	347
„ the medical organisation of the volunteer force	XXIV.	319
Reflexes in spastic paralysis	XXVIII.	265, 273
Refracture of the femur	XXI.	68
Relapses, in acute rheumatism	XXIII.	281
in influenza	XXVI.	199

	VOL.	PAGE
Relation of gout and rheumatism to Dupuytren's contraction (*Hedges*)	XXXII.	119
Removal of a large goitre, method of operation	XXV.	97
of goitre, cases of	XXXVI.	49
„ „ danger of carbolic acid dressings in	XXV.	103
„ „ methods of applying bandages after	XXV.	103
„ „ mortality of	XXV.	104
„ „ position of incision through the skin in	XXV.	102
„ „ „ „ jugular vein, and carotid artery in	XXV.	102
„ „ steps in the operation for	XXV.	102
„ „ successful (*Jessop* and *Berry*)	XXV.	97
„ „ suture used in	XXV.	103
„ half of lower jaw	XXIII.	238
„ kidney	XXI.	121
„ lens in high myopia (*Jessop*)	XXXV.	242
„ nasal polypus, case of meningitis after	XXXVI.	53
„ turbinate bones in Graves' disease	XXVIII.	28
„ uterine appendages for hystero-epilepsy	XXIX.	48
„ „ „ „ threatened insanity	XXIX.	48
Renal affection of pregnancy and parturition, note on the	XXVI.	115
albuminuria in children (*Herringham*)	XXVI.	25
contusion, a case of (*Mayo, Willett,* and *Hawes*)	XXXVIII.	271
disease, hypertrophy of heart, and œdema	XXXII.	261
dropsy, sudden disappearance of (*Weber*)	XXXIV.	303
hæmaturia	XXV.	230
surgery, two contributions to	XXI.	121
Rendel (*A. B.*), on cerebral hæmorrhage	XXVII.	285
Report from Electrical Department	XXII.	57
of operation cases (*Huggins, Walsham,* and *Smith*)	XXXIV.	263
„ special committee, on Apothecaries Shop	XXII.	30
Medical, of the Anglo-French Commission on the western frontier of the Gold Coast Colony (1902–1903) (*J. G. Forbes*)	XXXIX.	171
of year's work in Electrical Department (*H. Lewis Jones*)	XXXIII.	169
on influenza (*Habershon*)	XXVI.	239
„ „ (*Knight*)	XXVI.	223
„ „ (*E. T. Moore*)	XXVI.	224
„ „ Matron, St. Bartholomew's Hospital	XXVI.	235
„ „ Resident Officer, Royal Free Hospital	XXVI.	247
„ „ „ Officers, St. Bartholomew's Hospital	XXVI.	210
„ lint	XXIX.	101
„ sporadic cretinism and thyroid juice (*Murrell*)	XXIX.	101
Resection, intestinal (*R. C. Bailey*)	XXXIII.	55
of ribs for gangrene of lung	XXV.	254
„ „ in actinomycosis	XXXI.	25
Reserve force of the heart (*Harry Campbell*)	XXXVIII.	144
Respiration, frequency of in pneumonia	XXVIII.	231
nature of in nasal obstruction	XXIX.	237
Respirator, Cargill's, in nasal disease	XXIII.	128
Respirators, their use	XXV.	54
Respiratory sounds, the theories of	XXVI.	103
Results of embolism	XXVIII.	229
„ Halsted's operations for cancer of breast (*Butlin*)	XXXVII.	264
„ removal of glands	XXIX.	95
„ opening of joints	XXIX.	93
Retention and retraction of drainage tube	XXII.	236
of urine, cases of (*Mayo, Willett,* and *Hawes*)	XXXVII.	282
„ „ in women (*McAdam Eccles*)	XXIX.	350
Retina, atrophy of optic disc in diabetes insipidus (*Bousfield*)	XXXVI.	235
glioma of (*Jessop*)	XXXVI.	253

		VOL.	PAGE
Retina, hæmorrhage into (*Jessop*)	. . . . .	xxxv.	247
,, ,, macula of (*Jessop*)	. . .	xxxv.	241
ossification of (*Bullar*)	. . . . .	xxix.	302
papillitis, with recovery (*Jessop*)	. . .	xxxvi.	263
prognosis, after operation, in glioma of the (*Jessop*)	.	xxxix.	213
some points in the pathology of glioma of the (*Jessop*)	.	xxxviii.	159
Retinal artery, obliteration of (*Jessop*)	. . . . .	xxxvii.	314
Retraction of head, in typhoid fever	. . . . .	xxii.	224
Rheumatic fever (*see* Rheumatism, Acute).			
hyperpyrexia	. . . . .	xxvii.	286
fever without arthritis	. . . . .	xxiv.	21
Rheumatism, acute, affection of lungs in	. .	xxiii.	280
,, concurrent diseases in	. . .	xxiii.	286
,, definition of	. . .	xxiii.	270
,, duration of	. . .	xxiii.	286
,, examination of nearly seven hundred			
cases (*Sir W. S. Church*).	.	xxiii.	269
,, frequency of endocarditis in	.	xxiii. 269, 273, 275	
,, ,, ,, pericarditis in	.	. xxiii. 269, 278	
,, hyperpyrexia in	. . . .	xxiii.	285
,, mistaken for variola	. . .	xxi.	136
,, mortality	. . . .	xxiii.	280
,, relapses in	. . . .	xxiii.	281
,, statistics in (*Latham*)	. . .	xxiii.	280
,, temperature in	. . .	xxiii.	283
,, treatment of	. . . .	xxiii.	285
aconite in	. . . . .	xxiv.	23
and the erythemata	. . . . .	xxiv.	53
discussion on	. . . . .	xxiv.	322
erythema multiforme in	. . . . .	xxvii.	5
fatal case of, with hæmorrhagic erythema (*Sir Dyce*			
Duckworth)	. . . .	xxvii.	1
gonorrhœal	. . . . . .	xxii.	261
its relation to chorea	. . . . .	xxvi.	265
nodules in	. . . . . .	xxii. 213, 215	
occurrence of erythema multiforme and nodosum (*Garrod*)	xxiv.	43	
peliosis in	. . . . . .	xxvii.	3
relation of chorea gravidarum to	. . .	xxxix.	4
urticaria in	. . . . . .	xxvii.	5
with purpura (*Sir Dyce Duckworth*)	. . .	xxvii.	1
Rheumatoid arthritis, observations on (*Sir Dyce Duckworth*)	xxxv.	13	
observations upon (*Derwent Parker*)	. . .	xxxvi.	177
Rhinitis, or nasal catarrh	. . . . .	xxvii.	17
Rhinoscopy, posterior, in nasal obstruction	. .	xxiii.	121
Rhythmical jerking in Graves' disease	. . .	xxix.	185
Rib, fracture of, followed by sarcoma	. . .	xxii.	247
Ribs, abscess in connection with (*Marsh*)	. . .	xxxiv.	242
cases of fracture of (*Mayo, Willett,* and *Hawes*)	.	xxxvii.	271
fractures of, in the insane	. . .	xxvi. 15 ; xxvii. 50	
resection of, for gangrene of lung	. . .	xxv.	254
sarcoma following fracture of	. . .	xxii.	247
Rickets, extreme, of legs, treated by osteotomy	. .	xxii.	240
Right iliac colotomy for intestinal obstruction	. .	xxx.	215
Rigidity, and jactitation of limbs in typhoid fever	.	xxv. 134, 136, 137	
spastic, electrical reactions of muscles in (*Sir Dyce*			
Duckworth and *Tooth*)	. . . .	xxviii.	263
,, two cases of	. . . .	xxviii.	263
Rigor and collapse in typhoid fever	. . . .	xxxii.	107
Rivers (*W. H. R.*), a case of spasm of the muscles of the			
neck causing protrusion of the head	. .	xxiv.	249

	VOL.	PAGE
Rivers (*W. H. R.*), delirium, and its allied conditions . .	XXV.	279
on hysteria	XXVII.	285
„ neurasthenia	XXIX.	350
Roberts (*Hubert*), history and present position of symphysistomy	XXX.	27
on puerperal eclampsia	XXIX.	351
Rodent ulcer	XXIX.	189
age of occurrence	XXIX.	197
clinical appearance of	XXIX.	187
condition of lymphatics in	XXIX.	191
diagnosis of	XXIX.	199
duration of	XXIX.	198
early stages of	XXIX.	191
etiology of	XXIX.	196
frequency of	XXIX.	189
growth of	XXIX.	190, 198
its nature and origin (*Ferguson*)	XXI.	101
malignancy of	XXIX.	196
on (*Masterman*)	XXVIII. 305; XXIX.	189
microscopical characters of	XXI.	102
microscopy of	XXIX.	193
of face	XXIV.	301
„ „ and tumour of the antrum . . .	XXIV.	284
original growth	XXIX.	195
pathology of	XXIX.	192
sex in	XXIX.	198
situation of	XXIX.	191
treatment of	XXIX.	200
Rolleston (*H. D.*), the causation of mitral diastolic murmurs	XXIV.	197
treatment by hypnotic suggestion . . .	XXV.	115
and **Crouch** (*C. P.*), a case of intestinal obstruction	XXV.	169
Roughton (*E. W.*), experiences of a midwifery assistant	XXII.	357
on coma	XXI.	249
„ nasal obstruction	XXV.	274
„ parametritis and abscess of the liver . .	XXI.	173
Rules for the patients	XXII.	40
Rundle (*Henry*), varicocele in relation to admission to the Services	XXXV.	51
Rupture of aneurysm into lung	XXVII.	42
„ bowel	XXVIII.	117
„ eyeball	XXII.	310
„ first part of duodenum, case of (*D'Arcy Power*) .	XXXV.	41
„ gall-bladder, a case of (*Walsham*) . .	XXXVII.	341
„ hydatid of liver into bile-ducts . . .	XL.	5
„ kidney (*D'Arcy Power*)	XXXVII.	29
„ liver (*D'Arcy Power*)	XXXVII.	28
„ small intestine, case of	XXXVI.	41
„ spleen, cases of	XXXVI.	42
Ruptured kidney	XXXII.	196
Sacro-iliac disease following acute periostitis of tibia .	XXIII.	261
Sacrum and coccynx, sinuses over (*Goodsall*) . .	XXIV.	229
Salicylate of soda, introduction and consumption of .	XXII.	54
Salpingitis, tubercular	XXIX.	51
Salt in hæmoptysis	XXVII.	96
Sandilands (*J. E.*), points of interest in connection with plague, illustrated by the Aden epidemic of 1900 .	XXXVI.	61
Santi (*P. R. W. de*), on malignant disease of the rectum	XXIV.	338
the indications for opening the mastoid in chronic suppurative otitis media	XXXV.	103

		VOL.	PAGE
Santonin, its uses in cases of bilharzia		XXI.	92
,, ,, lumbricus teres		XXXIV.	239
Sapræmia		XXIII.	47
Sarcoma between bladder and rectum, a case of		XXIV.	213
cases of purpura in (*Herringham*)		XXXVIII.	117
melanotic, of intestine		XL.	131
,, ,, palate (*Marsh*)		XXVI.	169
myeloid of tibia, a case of (*D'Arcy Power*)		XXXV.	49
of bones of thigh and leg (*Butlin* and *Colby*)		XXXI.	31
,, brain		XXVI.	112
,, choroid, cases of (*Jessop*)		XXXV.	239
,, femur		XXIV.	305
,, humerus		XXIV.	205, 207
,, jaw, upper		XXIV.	310
,, ,, and nose		XXXIX.	219
,, knee-joint		XXXII.	184
,, liver		XXXI.	109
,, lung		XXVIII.	77, 85, 87, 88
,, mediastinum		XXVIII.	78
,, ,, and rib		XXII.	247
,, nose, and upper jaw		XXXIX.	219
,, palate		XXII.	345
,, ,, treatment of		XXII.	350
,, pancreas		XXVIII.	85
,, rib		XXII.	247
,, scapula, recurrent		XXIV.	302
,, spinal cord		XXIII.	142
primary, of liver		XXXI.	109
,, ,, mediastinal glands		XXIII.	231
,, ,, vagina (*Gow*)		XXVII.	97
,, ,, ,, in children (*D'Arcy Power*)		XXXI.	121
,, ,, ,, age of occurrence		XXVII.	106
,, ,, ,, diagnosis of		XXVII.	107
,, ,, ,, duration of		XXVII.	107
,, ,, ,, recurrence of		XXVII.	107
,, ,, ,, symptoms of		XXVII.	106
simulating abscess		XXIII.	147, 148
tables of central, of bone		XXXI.	43
,, ,, sub-periosteal		XXXI.	41
unusual form of		XL.	125
Sarcomatous polypi of nares		XXI.	148
Saunders (*Sir Edwin*), report on condition of the Hospital		XXVII.	269
Savory (*Sir William, Bart.*), cases from his wards		XXIII.	213
memoir of		XXXI.	1
Saw, nasal		XXIII.	127
Scalds, cases of (*Mayo, Willett,* and *Hawes*)		XXXVII.	279
Scapula, a case of excision of		XXIV.	205, 207
displacement of angle of		XXXIV.	235
Scarlatina, a source of puerperal fever		XXIII.	51
Scarlet fever, in Sitwell Ward		XXVII.	272
leucocytosis in		XXXII.	25
on (*Humphreys*)		XXVII.	281
,, (*Scholefield*)		XXIX.	353
Scholefield (*R. E.*), on scarlet fever		XXIX.	353
Sciatica treated by electricity		XXVIII.	255
Science, teaching of, preliminary, at St. Bartholomew's		XXII.	149
Sclerosing tuberculosis simulating scirrhous carcinoma		XL.	107
Sclerosis, amyotrophic lateral		XXII.	94, 95, 97
disseminated, a case of		XXIV.	155

			VOL.	PAGE
Sclerosis, disseminated, microscopic appearance of	. .	.	XXIV.	158
„	post-mortem appearance of cord in	.	XXIV.	157
„	syphilitic in origin (*Forbes*)	. .	XXXVIII.	83
„	with palatal and laryngeal anæsthesia			
	(*W. J. Horne*, with *F. Batten*)	.	XXXII.	173
insular, commencing with diplopia and optic nerve				
atrophy	. . . .	.	XXII.	308
of spinal cord, some cases of (*Garrod*)	. .	.	XXI.	93
„ „ „ electrical condition of muscles in	.	XXI.	95
„ „ „ with unilateral tremors	. .	.	XXI.	94
postero-lateral, of cord	. . . .	.	XXIX.	203
„ „ „ bibliography of	. .	.	XXIX.	212
„ „ changes in	. .	.	XXIX.	208
„ „ „ microscopical character	.	XXIX.	209
„ „ „ various names of	.	XXIX.	210
Sclerotic, rupture of, stitched up, with recovery	. .	.	XXII.	310
Scott (*S. K.*), perforation of intestine in typhoid fever	.	XXXIX.	133
tuberculosis of the female breast	. . .	.	XL.	97
and **Gardner** (*H. W.*), a case of erythema iris	.	XXXVIII.	135
Scott (*Stephen*), Prize Essay on Hypopyon (*Turner*)	. .	.	XXXV.	131
Scrotum, malignant disease of	. . . .	.	XXV.	193
„ „ „ condition of glands in	.	XXV.	197
„ „ cures by operation	. .	.	XXV.	195
„ „ mortality of operations for	.	XXV.	194
„ „ „ repeated operations for	.	XXV.	197
„ „ „ operative surgery of	.	XXV.	193
Scurvy, infantile	. . . . . .	.	XXV.	86
Second year's surgery at St. Bartholomew's Hospital	.	XXX.	227
Secondary cataract (*H. Power*)	. . . .	.	XXXIV.	5
hæmorrhage from femoral artery, a case of ligature of				
external iliac artery (*Harmer*)	. . .	.	XXXV.	269
Senile gangrene	. . . . . .	.	XXX.	69
in a man aged forty-five (*E. E. Young*)	. .	.	XXXIX.	235
Sepsis in parturient women	. . . .	.	XXIII.	48, 50
Septicæmia and pyæmia	. . . .	.	XXIII.	46
in puerperal fever	. . . .	.	XXIII.	46
treated with antistreptococcic serum	. .	.	XXXII.	23
Septum auriculorum, imperfect	. . .	.	XXVIII.	152
narium, blood tumours in	. .	.	XXVII.	21
„ conditions causing nasal obstruction	.	XXVII.	20
„ deviations of	. . .	.	XXVII.	22
„ „ accompanied by spurs	.	XXVII.	24
„ dislocations of	. . .	.	XXVII.	24
„ gummata of	. . .	.	XXVII.	21
„ hypertrophy and œdema of	.	XXVII.	25
„ spurs on	. . . .	.	XXVII.	23
nasal, deflected, operations for (*Walsham*)	.	XXXIV.	270
„ enchondrosis of	. . .	.	XXIII.	126
„ exostosis of	. . . .	.	XXIII.	126
„ gummata of the	. . .	.	XXIII.	128
„ hæmatoma of the	. . .	.	XXIII.	128
„ hypertrophy of the	. . .	.	XXIII.	127
„ periostitis of the	. . .	.	XXIII.	128
„ spontaneous deviation of the	.	XXIII.	123
ventriculorum, imperfect	. . .	.	XXVIII.	152
Serum albumen, its action injected subcutaneously	.	XXIII.	173
antistreptococcic	. . . . .	.	XXXII.	23
of the blood, its condition in cyanosis	. .	.	XXII.	144
reaction in typhoid fever (*Churchill*)	. .	.	XXXIV.	205

	VOL.	PAGE
Serum treatment, failure of, in a case of chronic strepto-coccus pyæmia (*Horder*)	XXXIII.	89
Sequelæ, early, of severe faucial diphtheria	XL.	41
of gonorrhœa, rarer	XXII.	261
,, influenza	XXVI. 253, 262	
Sex in intra-thoracic growths	XXVIII.	75
,, intussusception of bowel	XXVIII.	97
Sexes, the difference in mind in lunacy	XXIV.	1
Sexual complications in insanity	XXII.	103
element in women, in insanity	XXIV.	10
Shaw (*T. Claye*), (*see* Claye-Shaw (*T.*)).		
fractured ribs in the insane	XXVI.	15
on insanity with sexual complications	XXII.	103
,, the commencement and end of insanity	XXIII.	19
,, ,, earlier stages of insanity	XXIX.	109
,, ,, expression of emotion	XXXVI.	243
,, ,, forecast of destructive impulses in the insane	XXI.	1
surgery and insanity	XXVIII.	55
(*E. H.*) and **Fletcher** (*Morley*), analysis of tumours of breast removed during the year 1900	XXXVII.	295
(*E. H.*) and **Fletcher** (*Morley*), carcinomata of mammary gland removed during 1900	XXXVII.	300
Shock, followed by paraplegia and jumping movements	XXI.	62
some aspects of its etiology (*T. F. Raven*)	XXXVII.	205
Shore (*T. W.*), on a case of muscular atrophy and gangrene of the lung after typhoid fever	XXIII.	109
on coagulation of the blood	XXIII.	353
,, hemiplegia	XXI.	238
,, some recent advances in nerve-physiology considered in relation to disease	XXV.	27
,, the study of biology in relation to medicine	XXIV.	65
and **Womack** (*F.*), preliminary scientific teaching at St. Bartholomew's Hospital	XXII.	149
Shoulder, case of intracapsular fracture-dislocation at (*Maxwell*)	XXXVIII.	33
dislocation of, without rupture of the capsule (*Evill*)	XXIV.	163
swelling of the left	XXIV.	297
Shoulder-joint, amputation at XXI. 183; XXIV. 205; XXXIV. 247; XXXVII. 283		
Shrubsall (*F. C.*), physical characters and morbid proclivities	XXXIX.	63
Sidebotham (*E. J.*), on the treatment of intestinal obstruction	XXIV.	320
notes on two cases of cerebral hæmorrhage, and a case of jaundice with delirium	XXIII.	179
Sigmoid flexure, carcinoma of, simulating an iliac abscess	XXXIV.	253
idiopathic dilatation of (*Herringham* and *Bruce Clarke*)	XXXI.	57
five cases of volvulus of (*Bird*)	XXXVI.	199
Silk-worm gut for sutures	XXVIII.	21
in abdominal section	XXIX.	18
Sinus, longitudinal, thrombosis of	XXVIII.	151
of knee, with excision	XXIV.	304
the lateral, exposure of	XXIX. 345, 346	
,, removal of clot from	XXIX.	346
Sinuses, ethmoidal, purulent catarrh of	XXX.	243
frontal ,, ,, ,,	XXX.	244
nasal ,, ,, ,,	XXX.	237
over the sacrum and coccyx (*Goodsall*)	XXIV.	229
Sitwell Ward, case of scarlet fever after operation in	XXVII.	272
Skiagraphy in diseases of the chest (*H. Walsham*)	XXXIV.	29
Skin affections in kidney disease	XXII.	226
cleavage, lines of (*Weber*)	XXXIV.	303

	VOL.	PAGE
Skin Department, cases from (*West*)	XXXI.	263
disease, a case of erythema iris (*Gardner* and *Scott*)	XXXVIII.	135
,, ,, ,, mycosis fungoides (*Ormerod*)	XXXVII.	257
,, two cases of tinea favosa capitis (*Sir Dyce Duckworth*)	XXXVIII.	155
gangrene of, in typhoid fever	XXVII.	189
lymphangioma of	XXX.	111
unusual pigmentation of	XXVII.	109
Skin-grafting, on	XXIX.	253
by Thiersch's method	XXXII.	161
Skinner (*James*), notes of surgical cases in the Edinburgh Infirmary	XXXVII.	215
Skull, cases of fracture of (*Mayo, Willett,* and *Hawes*)	XXXVII.	271
,, trephining (*Walsham*)	XXXIV.	266
compound depressed fracture of	XXIX.	227
fracture of base of	XXV. 241 ; XXIX.	226
,, ,, ,, , insanity following	XXVII.	185
fractured base of, with remarkable eye symptoms (*Willett* and *Wood-Hill*)	XXXIV.	257
in insanity, effect of operation on the	XXVIII.	68
trephining of, in insanity	XXVIII.	55
Sleep, condition of brain in	XXV.	151
distressed, in nasal obstruction	XXIX.	236
respiration during	XXIX.	236
Sleeping-sickness in West Africa	XXXIX.	178
Small intestine, strangulation of, in fossa intersigmoidea (*McAdam Eccles*)	XXXI.	177
Smallpox, arrangements for	XXII.	37
Bishop of Worcester on	XXII.	37
Hospitals, sites for	XXIV.	27
Smashes, cases of surgical (*Mayo, Willett,* and *Hawes*)	XXXVII.	282
Smell, the sense of in Graves' disease	XXIX. 181,	185
Smith (*G.*), **Walsham** (*W. J.*), and **Huggins** (*S. P.*), report of operation cases	XXXIV.	263
Smith (*Sir Thomas*), a case of abdominal cyst	XXXIV.	1
a report of two cases of aneurysm treated by the injection of coagulating fluid into the sac	XXVII.	253
cases from his wards (*Jowers*)	XXIII.	231
cases from wards	XXXII.	19
three cases of multiple polypi of the lower bowel in one family	XXIII.	225
and **Willett**, (*Edgar*), fibromatous growths in the skin of the neck, with disseminated tubercles	XXVI.	147
(*T. R.*), with **Cozens** (*C.*), two cases of impaction of vegetable foreign body, one in the submaxillary, the other in sublingual salivary duct, leading to obstruction of the duct, and formation of an abscess in the gland	XXXIII.	105
Snake-bites, native treatment of, in West Africa	XXXIX.	199
Snoring, in nasal obstruction	XXIX. 237,	245
Sodium phosphate, impurity	XXIV.	223
,, its action in gout	XXIV.	221
salicylate, in acute rheumatism	XXIII.	285
,, in diabetes mellitus	XXV.	7, 12
,, its action in gout	XXIV. 221,	224
urate, and degeneration of aortic valves	XXIII.	292
,, in joints	XXIII.	291
,, presence of, in gout	XXIII.	291
,, ,, parenchymatous nephritis	XXIII. 293,	294
Soft palate and tongue, a case of deviation of (*Weber*)	XXXIV.	307

	VOL.	PAGE
Soils for building sites	XXVI.	3
Solvents of diphtheritic membrane	XXX.	149
Somnambulism following fright	XXI.	63
Sore-throats among nurses, diphtheria bacillus, in series of	XXXII.	145
Sounds, respiratory, the place of their origin	XXI.	192
Southey's tubes, use of	XXVII.	247
Space around houses, necessity for	XXVI.	7
Spasm of the muscles of the neck	XXIV.	249
Spasmodic dysmenorrhœa (*C. Godson*)	XXIV.	167
Spasms, chronic, in Graves' disease	XXIX.	185
of muscles of the thumb and forearm	XXII.	217
Spastic condition of muscles after amputation of the finger	XXIV.	294
paralysis (*see* Paralysis).		
rigidity of left arm after wound of finger	XXIV.	302
talipes (*Kent Hughes*)	XXXV.	181
Spaying	XXIX.	56
Specific gravity of the blood in health and disease, on the (*Lloyd Jones*)	XXIV.	314
Specimens added to Museum, list of	XXXII.	451
,, ,, in 1897	XXXIII.	233
Speech, affection of in the insane	XXIII.	31
loss of, in typhoid fever	XXI.	106
Spencer (*W. G.*), on the dressing of wounds	XXIII.	352
varicocele, its origin in persistence of fœtal veins	XXIII.	137
Spermatic cord, chronic inflammation of	XXIX.	176
torsion of, its cause	XXIX.	177
,, ,, diagnosis of	XXIX.	177
,, ,, reduction of	XXIX.	170
,, ,, seat of	XXIX.	177
,, ,, side on which it occurs	XXIX.	177
,, ,, symptoms of	XXIX.	177
,, ,, treatment of	XXIX.	178
,, ,, twists in	XXIX.	177
,, ,, with strangulation of epididymis and testis (*Nash*)	XXIX. 163, 165, 168, 169	
Sphenoidal sinuses, purulent catarrh of	XXX.	243
Sphincters, condition of, in spastic paralysis	XXVIII. 265, 277	
Spicer (*Holmes*), on future of medicine	XXV.	279
on hereditary influences	XXII.	361
osteotomy of the femur	XXI.	65
Spinæ, erectores, their function	XXIII.	69
Spinal caries, on (*Gardner*)	XXIII.	357
column, injury and disease of	XXI.	258
Spinal cord, ascending antero-lateral tract of	XXIII.	141
cases of sclerosis of	XXI.	93
changes in postero-lateral sclerosis	XXIX.	208
crushing of	XXI.	140
curvature, with loss of sensation to heat and cold	XXVIII.	213
dilatation of canal of	XXVIII.	219
hæmorrhage into	XXI.	140
homology of its central canal	XXV.	43
method of microscopical examination of	XXI.	141
microscopic examination of	XXIII.	111
mixed tract of	XXI.	138
sarcoma of	XXIII.	142
symptoms in typhoid fever	XXI.	111
syphilitic disease of	XXVIII.	78
topographical anatomy of	XXI.	137
Spinal deformity, cases of, associated with myopathy of the spinal muscles (*Mundy*)	XXXVI.	55

	VOL.	PAGE
Spine, concussion of	XXI.	259
fracture of	XXI.	259
„ with dislocation	XXI.	140
Spleen, condition of, in malignant diphtheria	XXIII.	17
dislocated, operation for	XXVI.	144
dislocation of, cause of	XXVI.	142
effect of removal (*D'Arcy Power*)	XXXVII.	42
enlarged and dislocated	XXVI.	131
enlargement of, with tenderness	XXVII.	227
infarcts in	XXVII.	42, 46
retention of uric acid by	XXV.	9
rupture of (*D'Arcy Power*)	XXVII.	31
ruptured, cases of	XXXVI.	42
suppuration of	XXXVII.	109
tumours of the (*Murray*)	XXIII.	356
Splenectomy	XXVI.	139
Splenic leukæmia, treated by injections of defibrinated bullock's blood	XXII.	245
Splints, Bavarian and similar	XXII.	369
Sponges, for abdominal section	XXIX.	5
Sputum, in intra-thoracic growths	XXVIII.	91
Staff, Hospital, directions to the	XXII.	34
medical and surgical	XXXIX.	302
nursing, effect of influenza on	XXVII.	261
Staggering, cerebellar	XXIII.	65, 67
in cats (*Herringham* and *Andrewes*)	XXIV.	241
cerebellar disease (*Herringham* and *Andrewes*)	XXIV.	241
Standage (*R. F.*), two cases of tetanus	XXVII.	211
Stanley's case of patent urachus described (*Doran*)	XXXIV.	33
Staphylococcic infection, on a case of (*Sir Lauder Brunton*)	XXXIX.	227
Starch, how formed	XXIV.	71
standard solution of, for pancreatic ferments	XXIX.	127
Statistics of acute rheumatism (*Latham*)	XXIII.	280
intra-thoracic growths	XXVIII.	76
Steavenson (*W. E.*), report from the Electrical Department	XXII.	57
thirty cases of fibro-myomata of the uterus, treated by electricity	XXIV.	89
Steedman, (*J. F.*), accidents in the cricket-field	XXXVI.	221
Stenosis, mitral, its connection with phthisis	XXIII.	249
pulmonary „ „	XXIII.	240
nasal	XXVII.	285
of air-passages	XXV.	223
Sterilization in Cæsarian section	XXIX.	50
removal of uterine appendages for	XXIX.	49
Sterilizers	XXIX.	4
Sterility, cured by dilatation with metallic bougies	XXIV.	170
Sterno-mastoid, division of, in wryneck	XXIV.	251
Stevens (*C. R.*), on the environment of medicine and surgery	XXIX.	352
Steward, The, St. Bartholomew's Hospital, obituary notice	XXXI.	19
Stomach, carcinoma of	XXVIII.	80
dilatation of, in gastric ulcer	XXVII.	155
diphtheritic membrane in	XXV.	69
perforated ulcers of, cases of	XXXVII.	50, 277
perforating ulcer of, treated by operation (*D'Arcy Power*)	XXXVIII.	10
„ ulcers of, the surgical treatment of	XXXIX.	19
ulcer of (*see* Ulcer, Gastric).		
Stomachic phenomena during chloroform anæsthesia (*Gill*)	XXXIV.	107
Stone, in bladder (*see* Calculus Vesical).		
„ kidney	XXI. 122 ; XXV. 231	
„ gall-bladder, distended	XXV.	252
removal of, from kidney	XXI.	126

		VOL.	PAGE
Stools, green		XXI. 110 ; XXXIII.	13
Strabismus, external, with hysterical stupor		XXI.	59
Strangulation of epididymis		XXIX.	163
,, intestine		XXIV.	152
,, small intestine in fossa intersigmoidea (*McAdam Eccles*)		XXXI.	177
Streptococci, in pneumonia		XXVIII.	176
Streptococcus pyæmia, case of, in which the serum treatment failed (*Horder*)		XXXIII.	89
Streptomycosis or **septicæmia**, treated with antistreptococcic serum		XXXII.	23
Stricture, cancerous, of bowel		XXVIII. 113, 116,	117
cicatricial, of air-tubes		XXV.	223
of trachea and bronchi		XXV.	225
simple, of larynx		XXV.	223
tuberculous, of ileo-cæcal valve		XL.	128
Strictures treated by electricity		XXVIII.	256
Strychnia, hypodermic injection of, in cases of cardiac failure (*Habershon*)		XXII.	115
introduction and consumption of		XXII.	52
solution for hypodermic injection		XXII.	119
use of, in the uric acid headache		XXIII.	206
Stupor, hysterical, with external strabismus		XXI.	59
Styan (*T. G.*), cases from Sir William Church's wards		XXI.	211
Styptics and styptic sprays in hæmoptysis		XXVII.	95
Subarachnoid hæmorrhage		XXVIII. 152, 153,	155
Subgluteal abscess (*Marsh*)		XXXIV.	246
Sublingual duct, obstruction of, by foreign body		XXXIII.	105
Submaxillary duct, ,, ,, ,, ,,		XXXIII.	105
,, gland, inflammation of, in punctured wound of intestine		XXVII.	177
Subpectoral abscess (*Marsh*)		XXXIV.	246
Subperiosteal abscess (*Marsh*)		XXXIV.	250
Subsoil water, in its importance to health		XXVI.	5
Sudden death, in infants (*Thursfield*)		XXXVIII.	129
remarks upon (*Horder*)		XXXV.	154
Sugar, its mode of production		XXIV.	72
Suggestion, hypnotic, treatment by		XXV. 115,	118
verbal, in treatment of disease		XXV.	122
Suicide, among epileptics		XXI.	3, 7
and insanity		XXIX.	118
in imbeciles		XXI.	4
,, melancholia		XXI.	7
,, the insane		XXI. 2 ; XXIII.	29
Sulphuretted hydrogen, effects of absorption of		XXII.	302
gas, rectal injections of		XXV.	66
Superficial femoral, deep femoral, and popliteal arteries, with their corresponding veins, ligature of		XXX.	223
Supernumerary auricle		XXIV.	284
Suppression of urine, case of (*D'Arcy Power*)		XXXV.	48
,, ,, in diphtheria (*Morrice*)		XXVIII.	193
Suppuration, acute, of joints, connected with gonorrhœa		XXII.	263
long standing, treated by continuous warm baths		XXIII.	255
,, ,, followed by malignant disease		XXIII.	157
of gall-bladder		XXVIII.	51
,, kidney		XXIII.	345
,, mastoid		XXIX.	343
pericæcal, with cerebral symptoms		XXX.	63
Suppurative pylephlebitis		XXXVII.	95
treatment of		XXXVII.	129

	VOL.	PAGE
Supra-pubic lithotomy, case of	xxxvi.	48
Supra-renal capsules, cases of hæmorrhage into (*Talbot*)	xxxvi.	207
Supra-renals, deposit in	xxvii.	109
Surgery, a year's (*Butlin*)	xxix.	89
a second year's, at St. Bartholomew's Hospital (*Butlin*)	xxx.	227
and insanity	xxviii.	55
aseptic and antiseptic methods in	xxix.	89
gastric, some cases of (*D'Arcy Power*)	xxxix.	19
hæmorrhage in	xxii.	355
renal, two contributions to	xxi.	121
of the gall-bladder and bile-ducts, some remarks on (*W. J. Walsham*)	xxxvii.	321
Surgical cases of interest (*Lowe*)	xxvi.	49
consultations	xxiv.	273
emergencies (*Mayo, Willett,* and *Hawes*)	xxxvii.	269
emphysema	xxvii.	212
experience, the lessons of a year's (*D'Arcy Power*)	xxxvi.	37
smashes, cases of (*Mayo, Willett,* and *Hawes*)	xxxvii.	282
treatment of hydatids	xxviii.	235
Suture used in removal of goître	xxv.	103
Sutures in abdominal section	xxviii.	21
silver, inserted and left in the tibiæ	xxii.	242
Sweating in spastic paralysis	xxviii.	265
„ typhoid fever	xxv.	139
Syrinogomyelia, a case of (*Weber*)	xxxiv.	313
Sydenham, some facts about (*Nias*)	xxvi.	189
Sylvius, glioma of the aqueduct of, a case of (*Herringham*)	xxxvi.	31
Symonds (*H.*), two cases of abdominal tumour and a case of gangrene of lung treated by operation	xxv.	249
Sympathetic iritis	xxix.	302
nerve, right, effects of nicotine in paralysis of	xxix.	104
„ „ paralysis of	xxix.	103
Sympson (*E. M.*), notes on two cases of intra-cranial tumour	xxiii.	186
on omental cancers	xxiii.	357
Symphysiotomy, history and present position of	xxx.	27
indications for	xxx.	42, 48
cases of (*Pinard*)	xxx.	31
Symptoms, misleading or seemingly unimportant, in certain diseases	xl.	1
of intra-thoracic growths	xxviii.	91
„ intussusception of bowel	xxviii.	98
„ nasal obstruction	xxiii. 119; xxix.	243
„ obstruction of nose	xxvii.	15
Synchondrosis, separation of sacro-iliac	xxvii.	51
Synopsis of works of Pott	xxx.	182
Synovial cysts in connection with joints	xxi.	117
Syphilis, a cause of general paralysis (*Forbes*)	xxxviii.	68
„ „ spinal disease (*Forbes*)	xxxviii.	78
affecting the joints	xxvi.	83
cases of (*Lockwood*)	xxxi.	225
connection with hæmaturia	xxii.	141
fibrosis of heart wall, as result of	xxxix.	11
heredity in relation to the nervous system (*Forbes*)	xxxviii.	37
on (*Lockwood*)	xxi.	240
native treatment of, in West Africa	xxxix.	197
necrosis of olecranon from	xxvi.	86
„ „ upper jaw from	xxvi.	85
of the heart (*Herringham*)	xxxix.	9
Syphilitic affection of the lungs and pleuræ (*Weber*)	xxxiv.	305
disease of joints	xxvi.	83

		VOL.	PAGE
Syphilitic disease of knee		XXVI.	83, 84, 85
,, ,, liver		XXIX.	67
disseminated sclerosis (*Forbes*)		XXXVIII.	83
fissure of anus, symptoms of (*Goodsall*)		XXVIII.	205
gummata of face		XXVI.	85
locomotor ataxy (*Forbes*)		XXXVIII.	81
paralysis, a case of (*Weber*)		XXXIV.	308
ulcers, position of, in larynx		XXV.	222
Tabes dorsalis in husband and wife		XXV.	87
post-mortem appearances in		XXV.	93
syphilitic		XXXVIII.	81
Table for operations		XXIX.	2
Tables, for dressings and instruments		XXIX.	3
Tables, Statistical, or others—			
abdominal section, appendix of cases for ovariotomy, &c., in the Women's Ward at St. Bartholomew's Hospital (*Harrison Cripps*)		XXIX.	24
,, ,, table of cases of, in Martha Ward during 1898 (*Harrison Cripps*)		XXXV.	27-35
a year's abdominal operations, tabulated (*D'Arcy Power*)		XXXVII.	27
,, surgery at St. Bartholomew's Hospital		XXIX.	93
a second year's surgery, list of cases (*H. T. Butlin*)		XXX.	227
Addison's disease, tables of temperature in (*A. Wallace*)		XXIV.	256
albuminuria in the apparently healthy, summary of cases in tabular form (*H. A. Levison*)		XXXV.	174
alcoholic cirrhosis, statistical results of an examination of 131 cases (*R. A. Yeld*)		XXXIV.	216
anæmia, charts of the changes produced by oxygen inhalations (*F. M. Burnett*)		XXXII.	322
analysis of English and Indian wheats		XXX.	117
,, ,, forty cases of intussusception, with tables (*W. McAdam Eccles*)		XXXIII.	146
,, ,, the tumours of the breast removed at St. Bartholomew's Hospital during the year 1900, tabular statement of (*Morley Fletcher* and *E. H. Shaw*)		XXXVII.	295
aneurysm, aortic, table of diet in		XXIII.	85
antiseptic measures in midwifery, table showing mortality among patients admitted to the lying-in wards of the General Lying-in Hospital during successive periods of four months each, from 18th Sept. 1883 to 31st Dec. 1884		XXIII.	54
,, treatment of phthisis, table of first hundred in-patients treated with instillations (*Vincent D. Harris*), Part I.		XXV.	57
,, ,, phthisis, table of cases treated (*Vincent D. Harris*), Part II.		XXVI.	93
appendicitis, cases of, in Mr. Willett's wards, tables laparotomy		XXXV.	213
,, ,, under the care of Mr. Butlin during the two years from Oct. 1896 to 30th Sept. 1898 inclusive, classification of		XXXIV.	71
Aronson's antitoxin, cases of diphtheria treated by, tables of (*H. J. May* and *A. A. Kanthack*)		XXXVI.	369

		VOL.	PAGE

Tables, Statistical, or others (*continued*)—

arteritis, in relation to enteric fever, tables of (*G. A. Auden*) . . . . **xxxv.** 74

bacillus recognised in membrane from tracheotomy cases, table . . . . **xxx.** 140–146

bacteriology of acute broncho-pneumonia, summary of conclusions (*P. Horton-Smith*) , ... **xxxiii.** 51

Bertoni's ether, tables of formulæ of the amyl alcohols . **xxviii.** 282

blood-corpuscles in diabetic patients, table showing the number of red and white in diabetes (*S. H. Habershon*) . . . . **xxvi.** 159

brain, abscess of, tables . . . . **xxxiv.** 127

„ and meninges, tables of congenital and traumatic cysts (*L. B. Rawling*) . . . . . **xl.** 81

breads, percentage composition of various (*Sir Lauder Brunton* and *T. W. Tunnicliffe*) . . . **xxxiii.** 159

„ relative digestibility of white and brown, conclusions formulated (*Sir Lauder Brunton* and *T. W. Tunnicliffe*) . . . . . **xxxii.** 167

Bright's disease, chronic, tables showing kidney disease to be a frequent cause of sudden death (*T. J. Horder*) . . . . **xxxv.** 157

broncho-pneumonia, bacteriological analysis of results obtained (*P. Horton-Smith*) . . . . . **xxxiii.** 41

cancer of the breast, the results of operations by Mr. Butlin, between the years 1880 and 1895 inclusive, on 129 patients (*H. T. Butlin* and *J. P. Maxwell*) . . . . **xxxiv.** 53

„ primary, of the lung, table of ages in (*S. West*) . **xxxii.** 121

cardiac hypertrophy and œdema, relationship of, to chronic renal disease, tables . . . **xxxii.** 269–307

carminatives, their action upon the absorption of gas by the intestines, synopsis of experiments (*Sir Lauder Brunton* and *J. T. Cash*) . . . . **xxii.** 296

chorea, curves of Charts I. and II. . . . . . **xxxii.** 388

„ etiology of, tables of . . . . . **xxxii.** 384

„ history of rheumatism in 85 per cent. of cases during 13 years, from 1883 to 1897 (*Sir Dyce Duckworth*) . . . . **xxxvii.** 20

cirrhosis of liver in a boy aged ten, table of temperature in . . . . **xxvi.** 67

congenital and traumatic cysts of the brain and meninges, tables of . . . . . . **xl.** 84

croup and tracheotomy, results of early tracheotomy . **xxiv.** 143

cystic disease of kidneys and liver, summary of cases from St. Bartholomew's Hospital (*J. Forbes*) . . . . **xxxii.** 218

„ „ „ the kidneys, statistics of cases (*J. Forbes*) . . . . . . **xxxiii.** 185

death, sudden, tables showing the frequency of kidney disease in (*T. J. Horder*) . . . . . **xxxv.** 157

diabetes insipidus, chart of the visual fields . . . **xxxvi.** 240

„ mellitus, salicylate of soda in, tabulated examination of urine (*A. Haig*) . . . . **xxv.** 19

diphtheria and throat disease in St. Bartholomew's Hospital during 1890, tables of (*Sir W. Church*) . . . . **xxvii.** 264–271

„ bacteriological investigations in . . **xxxi.** 96

„ cases treated by antitoxin in which an autopsy was performed . . . **xxxii.** 337

		VOL.	PAGE
Tables, Statistical, or others (*continued*)—			
diphtheria, cases treated by antitoxin in which no autopsy (*May* and *Kanthack*)	. .	XXXII.	340
,, examination, bacteriological, of membrane on the fauces		XXX.	142
,, non-tracheotomy cases under antitoxin treatment (St. Bartholomew's Hospital)		XXXII.	355
,, pulse-rate in suppression of urine in	.	XXVIII.	195–197
,, tracheotomy cases under antitoxin treatment (St. Bartholomew's Hospital)	. .	XXXII.	354
Depuytren's contraction of palmar fasciæ, tables of the relation of gout and rheumatism to (*C. E. Hedges*)		XXXII.	138
Electrical Department, list of cases under treatment in 1897 (*H. Lewis Jones*) .	.	XXX.	170
,, ,, table of In-Patients (*W. E. Steavenson*) . . .		XXII.	58 84
electrical reactions in peripheral nerve disease, tables of		XXII.	177
elephantiasis of one leg in a boy, measurements in inches		XXXII.	183
endocarditis, malignant, charts giving results of bacteriological examination in 24 cases, with nature of organism present (*A. M. Ware*) . . .		XXXV.	257
enteritis and colic simulating intestinal obstruction, chief points in four cases for comparison (*Smith, Willett, Marsh,* and *Butlin*) . . ; . .		XXXII.	66
etiology of enteric fever, tables of . . .		XXXV.	61
,, ,, pylephlebitis, suppurative, tables of	.	XXXVII.	95
,, ,, pylethrombosis, tables of (*Langdon Brown*) .		XXXVII.	140
fibro-myomata of uterus treated by electricity, measurements taken by Dr. Gordon		XXIV.	94
filariasis		XXXIX.	185
fractured ribs in the insane, table showing the weight required to cause fracture of the rib, and the seat of the fracture (*T. Claye Shaw*) . .		XXVI.	21
gastric surgery, cases of, tabulated (*D'Arcy Power*)		XXXIX.	20
glands, mesenteric, remaining caseous, rendering children liable to general acute tuberculosis, tables (*W. P. Herringham*)		XXIX.	64
glioma of retina, analysis of 83 cases (*W. H. Jessop*)	.	XXXIX.	216
gout, excretion of uric acid, charts of diet and treatment (*A. Haig*)		XXIV.	218
,, morbid, anatomy of, tables of (*N. Moore*)	.	XXIII.	291
growths, sprouting, endocardial, table . .		XXVIII.	224
hæmic cardiac murmur, tabulated notes on the common (*A. E. Garrod*)		XXVII.	35
human pancreatic ferments in disease, tables of results with (*V. Harris* and *Crace-Calvert*) . . .		XXIX.	129
hydatids, discharge of 300 from suppurating thoracic cyst, measurements of chest in, recovery		XXV.	216
,, table of constituents of normal hydatid fluid		XXVIII.	236
hypopyon, table of statistics of 189 cases (*P. E. Turner*)		XXXV.	133
hysterectomy and ovariotomy in Martha Ward, record of cases from June 1897 to July 1903, tables (*Harrison Cripps*)		XXXIX.	154
infectious diseases, list requiring the compulsory notification of (*R. Thorne Thorne*)		XXIV.	56
Influenza epidemic, mortality chart of the Cholera of 1848 and of the Influenza of 1847–48 . .	.	XXVI.	207

	VOL.	PAGE
Tables, Statistical, or others (*continued*)—		
Influenza epidemic, returns of the Registrar-General for the five weeks during which the epidemic was at its height	XXVI.	208
,, table of cases admitted into and arising in the wards	XXVI.	206
,, table of temperature in cases	XXVI.	200
,, table showing the weekly averages of patients attending in the Casualty Department in corresponding weeks of different years	XXVI.	195
intussusception, analysis of forty cases of, with tables (*W. McAdam Eccles*)	XXXIII.	146
,, summary of 96 cases of (*W. McAdam Eccles*)	XXXVII.	194
Klein's antitoxin, tables of cases of diphtheria treated by (*H. J. May* and *A. A. Kanthack*).	XXXII.	368
Landry's paralysis, brief summary of cases (*J. A. Ormerod*).	XXVIII.	137
lessons of a year's surgical experience, operations tabulated (*D'Arcy Power*)	XXXVI.	40
leucocytosis of scarlet fever, appendix of cases	XXXII.	241
mammary gland, relative frequency of tuberculosis in, compared with other diseases, cases of, and tables (*S. R. Scott*)	XL.	99–118
mixed nephritis, tabulated cases of	XXXII.	305
muscular atrophy, tables showing reactions to faradisation and galvanism in varieties of (*J. A. Ormerod*).	XXIII.	91
nasal breathing in nasal obstruction, table of cases in	XXIX.	238
neoplasm of the bladder, table showing all the cases admitted into St. Bartholomew's Hospital during the six years 1889–1894 inclusive (*T. J. Horder*)	XXXII.	211
new growths of the lung and pleura (*S. West*)	XXXIII.	121
,, ,, tabular arrangement of operations for removal of	XXXII.	212
œsophagus, summary of sixty-one cases of carcinoma of (*J. G. Forbes*)	XXXV.	194
operations of sixteen months and their lessons, list of (*D'Arcy Power*)	XXXV.	39
otorrhœa, chronic purulent, results of twenty-six operations for (*P. R. W. De Santi*)	XXXV.	109
oxygen inhalations, treatment of anæmia by, chart of	XXXII.	323
palate, tumours of the, tables of (*S. Paget*)	XXII.	326
pemphigus, case of acute, table of temperature in (*W. P. Herringham*).	XL.	34
peritonitis, chronic, tables of tubercular (*W. P. Herringham*)	XXIX.	70
phthisis, tables of antiseptic treatment of (*V. D. Harris*)	XXV. 57; XXVI. 93	
physical types, and certain diseases, tables of (*F. C. Shrubsall*).	XXXIX.	111
pleurisy, primary, with serous effusion, table of statistics (*C. E. Hedges*)	XXXVI. 83–145	
pneumonia, and the pneumococcus, tables of pneumonia, croupous, pulse, and respiration ratio in tables I.	XXVIII. 232, 233	
,, effect of oxygen on (*P. E. Turner*)	XXXIV. 100–104	
,, lobar, secondary infective lesions in, tables	XXXII. 316–319	

		VOL.	PAGE

Tables, Statistical, or others (*continued*)—

pregnancy, duration of, analysis of a series of 236 cases
(*A. R. Graham*) . . . . xxv. 178

prognosis after operation in glioma of retina, tabulated
analysis of 83 cases (*W. H. Jessop*) . . xxxix. 213

„ and causes of death in cases of diphtheria
treated by antitoxin, tables of . . . xxxii. 337

pulse-rate in suppression of urine in diphtheria, tables
of . . . . xxviii. 195-197

pylephlebitis, suppurative, tables of (*W. Langdon Brown*) xxxvii. 142

pylethrombosis, tables of (*W. Langdon Brown*) . . xxxvii. 140

renal surgery, urine charts in two cases (*W. J. Walsham*) xxi. 124, 127

report, medical, of the Anglo-French Boundary Commission, tables of results of blood examination for
filariasis, &c. (*J. Graham Forbes*) . . . xxxix. 185

results of operations for primary cancer of the breast,
performed during the years 1895, 1896, 1897, tables
of the (*H. T. Butlin*) . . . . . . xxxvii. 263

rheumatism and cardiac affections, examination of
nearly 700 cases, tables of (*Sir W. S. Church*) . xxiii. 272

rheumatic curves, Chart III. . . . . . xxxii. 388

ribs fractured in the insane, table showing the weight
required to cause fracture of the rib, and the seat
of the fracture (*T. Claye Shaw*) . . . . xxvi. 21

rodent ulcer, cases tabulated (*E. W. G. Masterman*) . xxix. 189

sarcoma, primary, of vagina, table of cases of (*W. J. Gow*) xxvii. 104

scarlet fever, tables and charts (*Humphreys*) . . xxvii. 281

„ „ the leucocytosis, appendix of cases . xxxii. 241

scrotum, malignant disease of, tabulated results of
operations (*H. T. Butlin*) . . . . . xxv. 196

skin-grafting, table of cases treated by Thiersch's
method of (*H. J. Paterson*) . . . . xxxii. 171

staphylococcic infection, case of, table of temperature
in (*Sir Lauder Brunton*) . . . . . . xxxix. 229

suppuration of long standing, treatment by continuous
warm baths, chart showing range of temperature
during twelve hours . . . . . . xxiii. 266

suppurative otitis media, statistical tables on its complications (*T. A. Bowes*) . . . . xxxiv. 188-191

syphilis, hereditary, its influence on the nervous system,
analysis of cases (*J. Graham Forbes*) . . . xxxviii. 39

tabes dorsalis, tabular report of sensory power in lower
limbs (*J. A. Ormerod*) . . . . . xxv. 88, 91

temperature in Addison's disease, tables of (*A. Wallace*) xxiv. 256

„ „ cirrhosis of liver in a boy aged ten, table
of . . . . xxvi. 67

„ „ head, injuries of, table of (*McAdam
Eccles*). . . . . xxix. 227, 228, 230

„ „ septicæmia, charts of . . . . xxxiv. 127

„ „ staphylococcic infection, table of (*Sir
Lauder Brunton*) . . . . . xxxix. 229

„ „ suppuration of long standing, range of . xxiii. 266

„ „ typhoid fever, tables of . . . . xxxii. 15

throat-disease and diphtheria, prevalence of, in St. Bartholomew's Hospital during 1890 (*Sir W. S. Church*) xxvii. 264, 271

thyroid juice in sporadic cretinism, table, heights and
weights of patients . . . . xxix. 102

tracheotomy and croup, results of early . . . xxiv. 143

„ tables of thirty cases requiring (*G. H.
Holden*) . . . . . . xxviii. 162

	VOL.	PAGE
Tables, Statistical, or others (*continued*)—		
trephining the skull in forms of insanity, results of (*T. Claye Shaw*)	XXVIII.	55
tuberculosis and malignant disease, tables	XXXV.	190
„ of female breast, tables (*S. R. Scott*)	XL.	118
tuberculous infection in children, tables from the post-mortem records of St. Bartholomew's Hospital, for 1893, 1894 (*G. A. Auden*)	XXXV.	79
„ infection of the lymphatic glands in children, tables taken from the post-mortem records of the Children's Hospital, Great Ormond Street (*F. E. Batten*)	XXXI.	183
tumours of the palate, tables of (*S. Paget*)	XXII.	326
typhoid fever, etiology of, tables	XXXV.	61
ulcer, duodenal, perforated, table of food given by month	XXXVIII.	15
„ gastric, simple, table of cases on the prognosis of (*S. H. Habershon*)	XXVII.	150–158
„ rodent, tabulated analysis of cases (*E. W. G. Masterman*)	XXIX.	191
uric acid headache, tables (*A. Haig*)	XXIII.	221
urine in diphtheria, tables of pulse-rate in suppression of	XXVIII.	195–197
vagina, primary sarcoma of, table of cases (*W. J. Gow*)	XXVII.	104
variation in number of white blood-corpuscles in diabetic patients, tables (*S. H. Habershon*)	XXVI.	159
varicocele in the Navy, table with rejections for (*H. Rundle*)	XXXV.	52
vomiting in phthisis, tables respecting (*S. H. Habershon*)	XXIV.	139
Tache cérébrale in typhoid fever	XXV.	139
Taches bleuâtres, from pediculi	XXIX.	332
in empyema	XXIX.	333
note on (*Sir Dyce Duckworth*)	XXIX.	331
Tachycardia, cases of	XXIX.	291
Talbot (*Eustace*), cases of hæmorrhage into the supra-renal capsules	XXXVI.	207
Talipes equinus, a new kind of (*Kent Hughes*)	XXXV.	181
causes of	XXVIII.	200
treatment at birth	XXVIII.	200
severe	XXIV.	279
Tannin, solution of, injected into aneurysmal sac	XXVII.	257
Tarsectomy, operation of	XXVIII.	203
Taylor (*Everley*), on jottings from general practice	XXIV.	321
Teeth, removal of, in cancer of tongue	XXIX.	86
Teething, causing symptoms resembling meningitis	XXII.	224
Temperature, in acute rheumatism	XXIII.	283
in a case of morbus Addisoni	XXIV.	256
„ influenza	XXVI.	200
„ intra-thoracic growths	XXVIII.	93
„ relation to injuries of the head (*McAdam Eccles*)	XXIX.	225
„ in spastic paralysis	XXVIII.	266, 273
modifications in the action of aconite produced by	XXII.	271
of a case of cirrhosis of liver	XXVI.	69
Tendon, case of rupture of quadriceps (*Mayo, Willett,* and *Hawes*)	XXXVII.	273
peroneus longus, shortening of for dislocation	XXXIV.	295
Tendons, flexor, their range of movement in whitlow	XXV.	192
operations on (*Walsham*)	XXXIV.	294
Testes, operations on (*D'Arcy Power*)	XXXV.	48
relation of, to prostatic atrophy (*Bruce Clarke*)	XXXV.	249

	VOL.	PAGE
Testis, abscess of, with malignant disease	XXIII.	152
axial rotation of	XXIX.	166
ectopic	XXIX.	166
fungus of	XXVII.	52
gangrene of	XXIX.	172
incompletely descended, in torsion of cord	XXIX. 163, 165, 168, 169	
sarcoma of, simulating abscess	XXIII.	148
strangulation of (*Nash*)	XXIX. 163, 165, 166, 168, 169, 170	
tumour of	XXIV. 295, 308	
undescended	XXIV. 290 ; XXIX. 173	
Tetanus, chloroform in	XXVII. 212, 214	
difficulty of feeding in	XXVII. 212, 214, 215	
following punctured wound of hand	XXVII.	213
„ nephro-lithotomy	XXI.	125
neonatorum, a case of (*Ware*)	XXXVI.	195
prognosis of (*Worthington*)	XXXI.	137
subacute, treated by chloral hydrate and bromide of potassium	XXIII.	234
two cases of	XXVII.	211
Tetany, symptoms intermediate between it and chorea	XXVI.	65
Theatre, for abdominal section	XXIX.	1
„ „ „ mode of preparing	XXIX.	6
Theophilus Philanthropos, his Six Gifts	XXI.	231
Theory of the respiratory sounds	XXI.	196
Therapeutics and **pathology**, action and reaction in	XXXIX.	139
Thiersch's method of skin-grafting	XXXII.	161
Thigh, swelling, deep-seated on upper third	XXIV.	278
Third nerve, paralysis of superior division of	XXII.	313
Thoracic hydatids	XXVIII.	238
Thorax, compression of, causing sub-conjunctival hæmorrhage	XXXVIII.	179
conditions of, during inspiration	XXVIII.	259
hydatid cysts in	XXVIII.	239
suppurating hydatid in	XXV.	214
the artificial	XXI. 191, 207	
Thorne (*Sir Richard T.*), cleanliness in its relation to health	XXIV.	313
memoir of	XXXVI.	27
some medical points relating to the provision of isolation hospitals	XXIV.	25
the dwelling-house in relation to tubercular consumption	XXVI.	1
Throat department, cases of malignant disease from the (*D'Arcy Power* and *W. J. Horne*)	XXXIX.	219
disease within the Hospital, during the year 1890	XXVII.	261
Thrombosis of longitudinal sinus	XXVIII.	151
Thursfield (*Hugh*), sudden death in infants, associated with enlargement of the thymus gland	XXXVIII.	129
Thymus gland, enlargement of, associated with sudden death in infants (*Thursfield*)	XXXVIII.	129
Thyroidectomy in Graves' disease	XXVIII.	27
Thyroid extract, in Graves' disease	XXIX.	182
„ „ myxœdema	XXIX.	182
„ its use in sporadic cretinism (*Murrell*)	XXIX.	102
gland, carcinoma of	XXVIII.	79
„ case of partial removal of	XXXVI.	49
cyst, removal of, followed by ulceration opening into trachea	XXIII.	218
Tibia, acute periostitis of	XXIII.	259
cases of compound fracture of (*Mayo, Willett,* and *Hawes*)	XXXVII.	270
myeloid sarcoma of (*D'Arcy Power*)	XXXV.	49
swelling of lower end of	XXIV.	281

	VOL.	PAGE
Tibia, swelling of upper third of right	XXIV.	283
„ over right	XXIV.	278
ununited fracture of	XXIV.	288
Tibiæ, osteotomy of, for rickets	XXII.	240
silver sutures inserted and left in	XXII.	242
Tibial nerve, anterior, neuritis of	XXII.	169
Tinea favosa capitis, two cases of, recovery under treatment with izal (*Sir Dyce Duckworth*)	XXXVIII.	155
Tinnitus aurium, treated by electricity	XXVIII.	254
in Graves' disease	XXVII.	138
Toes, gangrene of	XXIV.	280
Tongue, acute abscess of	XXV.	257
and soft palate, a case of deviation of (*Weber*)	XXXIV.	307
cancer of	XXIX.	85
congenital overgrowth of	XXIX.	156
dryness of	XXIV.	289
epithelioma of	XXIV.	288
hæmangioma of	XXIX.	149
hæmato-lymphangioma of	XXIX.	149
hypertrophy of	XXIX.	154
„ „ associated with epilepsy	XXIX.	155
„ „ „ „ irritation	XXIX.	155
infective granulomata of (*Francis*)	XXIX.	156
leukoma of, and lip	XXV.	112
lymphangioma of, microscopical examination of	XXIX.	147
„ „ operation for	XXIX.	146
„ „ treatment of	XXIX.	144
removal of, for cancer	XXIX.	87
ulcers of the	XXIV.	83
„ on the	XXIV.	287
wasting of	XXIII.	93, 95
Tonsil, pharyngeal, hypertrophy of	XXIII.	135
Tonsils, enlarged, and adenoid vegetations	XXVII.	25
operations on (*Walsham*)	XXXIV.	271
Tonsillitis in rheumatism	XXIV.	46
Tooth, decayed wisdom, leading to sinus of cheek (*Marsh*)	XXXIV.	254
extraction of, causing angina Ludovici	XXVII.	178
Tooth (*Howard*), a contribution to the topographical anatomy of the spinal cord	XXI.	137
destructive lesion of the fifth nerve-trunk, an anatomical study	XXIX.	215
hereditary spastic paraplegia	XXVII.	7
note on the ascending antero-lateral tract	XXIII.	141
observations on epilepsy	XXXI.	63
on hereditary progressive muscular atrophy, commencing in the lower extremities	XXV.	141
pathology of alcoholic paralysis	XXXII.	407
and **Duckworth** (*Sir Dyce*), two cases of general spastic rigidity	XXVIII.	263
Torres Straits Island, the conditions of life on a (*Myers*)	XXXV.	91
Torsion of spermatic cord (*Nash*)	XXIX.	163, 165, 168, 169, 170
„ „ „ age of occurrence	XXIX.	176
Trachea, and bronchi, simple stricture in	XXV.	225
foreign body passing down, exit through abscess in axilla (*Good*)	XXVII.	251
method of removing membrane or mucus from	XXI.	84
obstruction of	XXIX.	324
papilloma of	XXI.	147
stenosis of, its effects	XXIX.	325
ulceration of thyroid cyst into	XXIII.	218

		VOL.	PAGE
Tracheal obstruction, causing expiratory dyspnœa and emphysema		XXIX.	323
Tracheotomy, after-treatment of		XXVIII.	160
cases illustrating the after-treatment of (*Habershon*)		XXI.	61–87
cause of local pneumonia in		XXI.	80
feeding through the nose in		XXI.	81
for tuberculous laryngitis		XXVII.	89
in croup (*Hamer*)		XXIV.	141
„ diphtheria		XXVI.	173
„ Graves' disease		XXVIII.	28
instruments required		XXVIII.	157
membrane from, examined bacteriologically .		XXX.	140
on (*Drage*)		XXII.	354
on (*Holden*)		XXVIII.	157
percentages of recovery from		XXIV.	147
the after-treatment of (*Habershon*) . . .		XXI.	79
use of sprays in		XXVIII.	100
when to be done		XXIV.	145, 146
Training, effect of, on the urine		XXIV.	6
Trance, condition of, after an operation for hernia		XXI.	166
Traumatic cysts of the brain and meninges . .		XL.	75
gangrene of leg		XXXII.	192
hernia		XXVII.	51
Treatment, by hypnotic suggestion . . .		XXV.	118
of alcoholism by hypnotism		XXV.	126
„ chronic ulcers of the tongue by excision .		XXIV.	83
„ disuse of limbs after severe disease .		XXV.	210
„ early sequelæ of severe faucial diphtheria .		XL.	41
„ fistulous opening into bladder . . .		XXIV.	259
„ ganglion		XXXV.	50
„ gout		XXVI.	270
„ hæmoptysis	XXVII.		81, 85, 93
„ harelip		XXXIV.	271
„ hydatid cyst in liver		XXVII.	164
„ influenza		XXVI.	209
„ insomnia		XXV.	151
„ intussusception of bowel . . .		XXVIII.	99
„ lymphangioma of tongue . . .		XXIX.	144
„ Morbus Addisonii		XXIV.	258
„ nævus by electrolysis		XXX.	205
„ obstructions of nose		XXVII.	15
surgical, of increased intra-cranial pressure .		XXXIII.	63
Trembling in Graves' disease		XXVII.	142
Tremors, hysterical		XXI.	61
of the legs and arms, resembling paralysis agitans		XXI.	61
unilateral, in sclerosis		XXI.	94
Trephining, cases of		XXXVI.	52
in traumatic epileptiform convulsions . .		XXVI.	69
the skull, cases of		XXXIV.	266
„ „ for cerebral abscess . .		XXXIV.	266
„ „ „ chronic hydrocephalus . .		XXXIV.	269
„ „ „ compound depressed fracture of .		XXXIV.	268
„ „ „ fissured fracture of . . .		XXXIV.	269
„ „ „ general paralysis . . .		XXVIII.	58
„ „ „ insanity		XXVIII.	55
„ „ „ necrosis of		XXXIV.	269
„ „ „ paralysis of face and arm . . .		XXXIV.	269
„ „ „ sepsis, after injury . . .		XXIX.	97
„ „ „ traumatic epileptiform convulsions .		XXVI.	69
Tripod of life (*Gee*)		XXXIII.	1

	VOL.	PAGE
Trismus, after nephro-lithotomy	XXI.	125
Trophic nerves of lungs	XXIII.	113
Tubal disease, and perimetritis	XXIX.	52, 53
„ frequency of	XXIX.	53
gestation	XXIX.	42
„ case of (*Harrison Cripps*)	XXXV.	28
Tube, Eustachian, outgrowths from	XXIII.	136
Tubes, Fallopian, distension of	XXIX.	51
Leiter's in Graves' disease (*Maude*)	XXVIII.	25
Tubercle bacillus (*Koch's*)	XXVI.	1, 2
caseating, in cerebellum	XXIII.	188
cases of purpura in (*Herringham*)	XXXVIII.	117
cirrhosis of lung due to	XXVIII.	4
in chronic peritonitis	XXIX.	63
inoculation of	XXV.	52
in other parts of the body, and disease of knee	XXIV.	308
of lachrymal gland, a case of (*Jessop*)	XXXV.	231
Tubercles, disseminated about body	XXVI.	147
Tubercular consumption, relation to dwelling-house	XXVI.	1
disease of urinary tract	XXXII.	200
meningitis, producing localising symptoms in a case of cerebral tuberculosis (*G. C. Garratt*)	XXX.	211
„ simulated in spastic paralysis	XXVIII.	263
peritonitis, treatment	XXIX.	81
tumour of cerebellum	XXIII.	186
Tuberculosis, pulmonary, its association with heart-disease	XXIII.	239
„ with aneurysm	XXIII.	246
„ „ pigmentation of skin	XXVII.	109
coincident with malignant disease	XXXV.	183
infection of lymphatic glands in children	XXXI.	183
of the female breast	XL.	96
Tuberculous disease of knee and ankle	XXIV.	276
infection in children, the focus of (*Auden*)	XXXV.	79
meningitis, draining of ventricles in	XXXIII.	82
stricture of the ileo-cæcal valve	XL.	128
tumours of the larynx (*Kidd*)	XXI.	37
Tufnell's treatment of aneurysm	XXI. 220; XXIII. 84; XXVII.	254
Tumour, abdominal, distended gall-bladder	XXV.	252
„ two cases of	XXV.	249
at base of brain	XXVI.	107
cerebral, a case with hæmorrhage	XXIII.	179
„ microscopical examination of	XXIII.	180
congenital, in an infant	XXIV.	276
fibrous, of dura mater	XXVII.	171
in left loin	XXIV.	282
mediastinal	XXVIII.	73, 80, 81
„ presenting difficulties in diagnosis, a case of (*Sir Dyce Duckworth*)	XXXIII.	7
„ (*see* Intra-thoracic growths).		
of antrum	XXIV.	284
„ bladder	XXIV.	292
„ breast	XXIV. 293, 298, 299, 308; XXVII.	201
„ cerebellum	XXIII.	65
„ groin	XXXII.	194
„ left breast, the other having been previously removed	XXIV.	286, 304
„ „ epigastric region	XXIV.	289
„ „ hypochondrium	XXIV.	298
„ mediastinum, presenting difficulties in diagnosis	XXXIII.	77
„ neck	XXIV.	299

	VOL.	PAGE
Tumour of scalp	XXIV.	292, 299
,, superior maxilla	XXIV.	291
,, testis	XXIV.	295, 308
tubercular, of cerebellum	XXIII.	186
Tumours, cystic, of lower jaw	XXII.	238
,, ,, palate	XXII.	319
fibrous and fibroid, of pelvic platysma . . .	XXIX.	50
hepatic, on (*Haviland*)	XXIII.	356
implicating right sympathetic nerve . . .	XXIX.	103
medical discussion on (*Habershon*)	XXV.	279
of the bladder, on (*Heaton*)	XXV.	280
,, ,, ,, villous	XXV.	230, 233
,, ,, cerebro-spinal system (*Murray*) . . .	XXIII.	350
,, ,, Fallopian tubes	XXIX.	50
,, ,, mammary gland, removed during 1900, analysis of (*Morley Fletcher* and *E. II. Shaw*) . . .	XXXVII.	295
,, ,, ,, ,, multiple . . .	XXXVII.	308
,, ,, orbit (*Napier*)	XXV.	278
,, ,, palate	XXII.	315
,, ,, spleen (*Murray*)	XXIII.	356
operations for removal of (*D'Arcy Power*) . .	XXXV.	49
removal of, results	XXIX.	94
sarcomatous, of fractured ribs	XXII.	247
tuberculous, of the larynx (*Kidd*)	XXI.	37
Tunnicliffe (*F. W.*), nine cases of intestinal obstruction due to various causes, with some remarks by Mr. Bruce Clarke	XXVIII.	113
two cases of hydatid tumours ; one of the liver ; one of the kidney	XXVII.	163
and **Sir Lauder Brunton**, on the relative digestibility of white and brown bread	XXXIII.	157
,, ,, ,, acute atrophy of liver .	XXXII.	425
Turbinal bodies, erection of galvano-cautery in . .	XXVII.	17
hypertrophy and œdema of, galvano-cautery in . .	XXVII.	16, 17
morbid conditions of, causing obstruction . .	XXVII.	16
Turbinal bones, hypertrophy of	XXVII.	18
removal of, in Graves' disease	XXVIII.	28
Turnbull (*G. L.*), on hypnotics	XXV.	280
Turner (*P. E.*), on hypopyon	XXXV.	131
on pneumonia and the pneumococcus . . .	XXXIV.	87
Turpentine in purpura	XXV. 166 ;	XXVII. 95
Tylden (*H. J.*), notes from the Casualty Department .	XXVI.	263
memoir of	XXVIII.	299
on coma	XXIV.	318
,, diabetes	XXVII.	283
,, typhoid fever	XXVIII.	289
and **Miller** (*J. T.*), recent researches in diabetes, with a note on the pathology of the pancreas . .	XXVII.	71
Tympanum, foul-smelling pus in	XXIX.	345, 346
Typhoid fever (*see* Fever, Typhoid).		
Ulcer, duodenal, gastro-enterostomy for . . .	XL.	71
,, perforated, cases of (*D'Arcy Power*) . .	XXXVII.	46
,, perforating, treated by operation (*D'Arcy Power*)	XXXVIII.	14
gastric, age occurrence of	XXVII.	150
,, cases of perforated, XXXVII. 50, 277 ; XXXVIII. 8, 9, 10, 12 ; XXXIX. 20, 23 ; XL. 69.		

	VOL.	PAGE
Ulcer, gastric, causes of relapse of	XXVII.	156
,, dilatation of stomach in	XXVII.	155
,, duration of	XXVII.	151
,, influence of age on prognosis	XXVII.	159
,, leaking, case of, treated by operation (*D'Arcy Power*)	XXXVIII.	6
,, perforated, bacteriology of	XXXVII.	52
,, ,, (*D'Arcy Power*)	XXXVII.	50
,, ,, (*Mayo, Willett,* and *Hawes*)	XXXVII.	277
,, prognosis of simple (*Habershon*)	XXVII.	149
of breast, malignant, growth developed in floor of	XXIII.	159
,, face, rodent, and tumour of antrum	XXIV.	284
,, leg, epitheliomatous	XXIV.	285
on tongue	XXIV.	287
,, ,, treated by excision	XXIV.	83
rodent (*Masterman*)	XXVII.	305
,, microscopal characters of	XXI.	102
,, nature and origin of (*Ferguson*)	XXI.	101
,, of antrum	XXIV.	284
,, ,, face	XXIV.	284
typhoidal, leaking, case of (*D'Arcy Power*)	XXXVIII.	21
Ulceration of the colon	XXIII.	213
,, ,, ,, and cæcum	XXIII.	215
,, ,, larynx in typhoid fever	XXXI.	113
,, ,, pulmonary vessels, hæmoptysis due to	XXI.	53, 58
Ulcerative endocarditis, a cause of aneurysm	XXII. 190 ; xxv.	273
Ulcers, syphilitic, position of in larynx	XXV.	223
Ulnar nerve, division of	XXIV.	281
Umbilical hernia of thirty years' standing	XXVIII.	119
two cases of	XXVIII. 113, 119,	120
Umbrella for clergyman at the Hospital	XX.	36
Undescended testis	XXIV.	290
Upper jaw (*see* Maxilla), epithelioma of	XXIV.	311
necrosis of, from syphilis	XXVI.	85
sarcoma of the	XXXIX.	219
Urachal cysts, observations on (*Doran*)	XXXIV.	33
Urachus, Stanley's case of patent, with observations on urachal cysts (*Doran*)	XXXIV.	33
Urate of soda (*see* Sodium, Urate).		
Urea, amount of, in gout	XXIV. 218, 220,	222
and uric acid	XXIV.	74
Urethra, calculus impacted in	XXXVI.	47
foreign body in (*Mayo, Willett,* and *Hawes*)	XXXVII.	282
hæmaturia from	XXV.	229
on rupture of	XXII.	362
operations on (*Walsham*)	XXXIV.	293
traumatic rupture of (*Mayo, Willett,* and *Hawes*)	XXXVII.	281
Urethral stricture, treatment by electricity	XXVIII.	206
Urethrotomy, case of impacted calculus	XXXVI.	47
Uric acid, absent from the blood in fevers	XXVI.	43
amount of in diabetic urine	XXV.	10
,, ,, gout	XXIV. 218, 220,	222
calculi	XXI.	89
excretion of, in a case of gout (*Haig*)	XXIV.	217
,, ,, influenced by some drugs	XXIV.	217
headache, effect of diet on	XXIII. 204,	206
,, its factors	XXXIII.	207
,, some clinical features of (*Haig*)	XXIII.	201
,, theory of its production	XXIII.	206
,, treated by nitro-hydrochloric acid	XXIII.	201

	VOL.	PAGE
Uric acid, headache, use of strychnine in	XXIII.	206
in the blood, effect of alkalies on	XXVI.	49
its relation to urea	XXVI.	35, 54
quantity in the blood and tissues (*Haig*)	XXVI.	33
,, ,, ,, in cases of morbus cordis	XXVI.	41
,, ,, ,, ,, pneumonia	XXVI.	40
retention of, in the spleen	XXV.	9
Urinary tract, tubercular disease of	XXXII.	200
Urine, a case of suppression of (*D'Arcy Power*)	XXXV.	48
bloody, a sign of infantile scurvy	XXV.	85
cases of extravasation of (*Mayo, Willett, and Hawes*),	XXXVII.	281
,, retention of (*Mayo, Willett, and Hawes*),	XXXVII.	282
charts of the, in calculous pyelitis	XXI.	124, 127
containing bloody coagula	XXVIII.	249
effect of training on	XXIV.	6
extravasation of	XXXVII.	281
fæces present in the	XXIV.	258
free fat in	XXI.	117
in a case of fistulous opening between bladder and intestine	XXIV.	259
,, pregnancy	XXVI.	116
retention of, cases of	XXXVII.	282
,, in typhoid fever	XXV.	139
,, ,, women (*McAdam Eccles*)	XXIX.	350
suppression of, a case of	XXXV.	48
,, ,, ,, (*Gow*)	XXV.	272
,, ,, in diphtheria (*Morrice*)	XXVIII.	193
typhoidal, Ehrlich's test for	XXVI.	290
Urticaria, caused by hydatid fluid	XXVIII.	236
in rheumatism	XXVII.	5
occurrence of, in paroxysmal hæmaturia	XXII.	137
Uterine appendages (*see* Appendages, Uterine).		
Uterus, dysmenorrhœa, cured by dilatation of the os	XXIV.	170
fibro-myomata of, treated by electricity	XXIV.	89
hysterectomy for fibroids of	XXIX.	38
multinodular myoma of	XXIX.	39, 40
ruptured, case of	XXXV.	33
Vaccinia, of lids and conjunctiva, cases of (*Jessop*)	XXXV.	237
Vagina, atresia of	XXXIV.	232
primary sarcoma of (*Gow*)	XXVII.	97
,, ,, in children (*D'Arcy Power*)	XXXI.	121
wounds of	XXXIV.	236
Value of Ehrlich's reaction in diagnosis of typhoid fever	XXXII.	217
,, ,, test for typhoidal urine	XXVI.	290
,, injection of boro-glyceride in cystitis	XXI.	120
,, post mortem examinations in hæmaturia	XXII.	144
,, the pupil, as an aid to diagnosis	XXV.	38
the diagnostic, of melanuria	XXXVIII.	25
Valve, ileo-cæcal, tuberculous stricture of	XL.	128
Valves of the heart (*see* Heart, Mitral, Tricuspid, and Pulmonary).		
cardiac, their action on intra-thoracic pressure	XXVIII.	260
and heart, abnormal foramina of	XXVI.	314
Valvular, congenital, defects (*Weber*)	XXXV.	147
Varicella, distinction of the rash from variola	XXI.	136
Varicocele, in relation to admission to the Services (*Rundle*)	XXXV.	51
its origin in persistence of fœtal veins	XXIII.	137
operation for (*D'Arcy Power*)	XXXV.	44
,, ,, results	XXIX.	95
radical operation for (*Walsham*	XXXIV.	285

	VOL.	PAGE
Varicose veins, operations for, results	XXIX.	95
„ on (*Walsham*)	XXXIV.	285
„ „ (*D'Arcy Power*)	XXXV.	44
Variola, as seen in the Casualty Department	XXI.	131
course and treatment of (*Innes*)	XXII.	356
diagnosis from acute rheumatism	XXI.	136
Vascular growths of palate	XXII.	32
Vaseline, introduction and consumption of	XXII.	55
Vasomotor centre	XXV.	37
Vegetations, adenoid, in vault of pharynx	XXIII.	134
„ of naso-pharynx	XXI.	152
Vein, femoral deep, ligature of	XXX.	224
„ superficial, ligature of	XXX.	224
jugular „	XXIX. 345,	346
popliteal „	XXX.	224
jugular, and artery, carotid, position of in removal of goitre	XXV.	102
enlarged in intra-thoracic growths	XXVIII.	92
fœtal, persistence of, a cause of varicocele	XXIII.	137
operations on (*D'Arcy Power*)	XXV.	44
prostatic, a rupture of	XXV.	229
Vena cava superior, occulsion of	XXXII.	74
Venesection, in hæmoptysis	XXVII.	87
Ventricle, left, mode of expansion of	XXIV.	200
„ suction-pump, action of	XXIV.	199
Ventricles, drainage of, in tuberculous meningitis	XXXIII.	82
Vermiform appendix, hernia of (*McAdam Eccles*)	XXXII.	93
hernia, femoral of	XXVII.	179
and cæcum in sac of left femoral hernia	XXVII.	180
removal of (*D'Arcy Power*)	XXXVII.	28
Vernon (*Bowater J.*), memoir of	XXXVII.	1
Vertebræ, dorsal, fracture and dislocation of	XXI.	140
eroded by aneurysm of aorta	XXI.	219
Victoria Park Hospital, notes on the influenza epidemic at	XXVI.	259
Vienna, medical school of (*Johnson*)	XXV.	275
paste, in cancer of the breast	XXIII.	57
Villous carcinoma of the breast	XXIV.	263
Viscera, innervation of	XXIII.	113
relation of nervous system to	XXV.	33
Vitreous, hæmorrhage, new vessels in (*Jessop*)	XXXV.	247
magnet, its use in foreign bodies in the	XXII.	311
Vocal cords, a case of paralysis of the abductors of the, with lesions of several cranial nerves	XXII.	209
observations on	XXIV.	261
position of, in speaking	XXIV.	261
Voice, character of, in adenoid vegetations	XXVII.	27
in intra-thoracic growths	XXVIII.	92
Volvulus, five cases of (*Robert Bird*)	XXXVI.	199
Vomiting, as an early sequel of severe faucial diphtheria	XL.	41
caused by compression of the pneumogastric	XXIV.	132
fæcal and enemata (*Weber*)	XXXIV.	314
from irritation of the pneumogastric	XXIV.	135
how caused	XXIV.	131
in phthisis of left apex (*Habershon*)	XXIV.	131
„ „ reflex	XXIV.	137
„ „ statistics of	XXIV. 138,	139
Wallace (*A.*), clinical notes and observations from the Essex and Colchester Hospital	XXIV. 253; XXV. 201; XXVII.	239
report on influenza at Colchester	XXVI.	251

		VOL.	PAGE
Wallis (*F. C.*), on injuries in and about joints		XXI.	251
the surgical treatment of hydatids		XXVIII.	235
Walsham (*Hugh*), the X-rays in diseases of the chest		XXXIV.	29
Walsham (*W. J.*), memoir of		XXXIX. xxxiii
nasal obstruction and its treatment		XXIII.	119
,, ,, its causation and treatment		XXVII. 15, 285
nose operations for deflected septum		XXXIV.	251
notes from the Orthopædic Department		XXVIII.	119
on chronic purulent catarrh of the accessory nasal sinuses		XXX.	237
operations on fascia		XXXIV.	294
,, ,, harelip, and cleft palate		XXXIV.	271
,, ,, joints		XXXIV.	286
,, ,, muscles		XXXIV.	294
,, ,, varicose veins		XXXIV.	285
osteoclasis		XXVII.	217
our surgical consultations		XXIV.	273
radical operation for hernia		XXXIV.	282
,, ,, ,, hydrocele		XXXIV.	285
removal of lymphatic glands		XXXIV.	298
rupture of gall-bladder		XXXVII.	341
some remarks on the surgery of the gall-bladder and bile-ducts		XXXVII.	321
surgical emergencies admitted into the wards of		XXXVII.	269
three cases of large naso-pharyngeal polypi, with remarks on the removal of such growths		XXVIII.	69
two cases of mastoid suppuration following middle-ear disease		XXIX.	343
two contributions to renal surgery		XXI.	121
Smith (*Gilbert*), and **Huggins** (*S. P.*), report of operation cases		XXXIV.	263
Ware (*A. M.*), a case of tetanus neonatorum		XXXVI.	195
the relation of bacteriology to the pathology and symptoms of malignant endocarditis		XXXV.	253
Waring (*H. J.*), a case of actinomycosis hominis		XXVII.	173
acute infective periostitis		XXIX.	265
report on dressings, water, and air of operating theatre		XXIX.	100
and **Eccles** (*McAdam*), cases from Mr. Langton's wards		XXVII.	177
Warm baths, use in long-standing suppuration		XXIII.	255
Warts and epitheliomata		XXV. 106, 107
,, pathology of		XXV.	105
Warty growths, of palate		XXII.	329
Water-closets at the Hospital		XXII.	43
Water of theatre, report on		XXIX.	100
Waters, alkaline, their use in diabetes mellitus		XXV.	11
mineral, of London		XXII.	18
,, their use in the Hospital		XXII.	14
Watts (*H.*), cases from Mr. Baker's wards		XXIV.	205
Webb (*H. S.*), annals in the life of a country doctor		XXXIV.	231
Weber (*F. Parkes*), a case of facial paralysis, of syphilitic origin		XXXIV.	308
,, lingual hemiatrophy		XXXIV.	307
a note on action and reaction in pathology and therapeutics		XXXIX.	139
cerebral hæmorrhage in a child		XXXIV.	311
congenital valvular defects on the left side of the heart		XXXV.	147
enemata in vomiting		XXXIV.	314
formation of lineæ albicantes		XXXIV.	303
general paralysis of adolescence		XXXIV.	312
hydrocephalus, primary and internal, in an adult		XXXIV.	307

	VOL.	PAGE
Weber (*F. Parkes*), hysterical intestinal obstruction . .	XXXIV.	314
lingual hemiatrophy, a case of	XXXIV.	307
notes on some cases at the German Hospital . .	XXXIV.	308
on abnormal foramina in the heart and its valves . .	XXVI.	314
on the significance of albuminuria in pulmonary phthisis	XXVIII.	303
syphilitic affection of lungs	XXXIV.	305
and **Arkwright** (*J. A.*), pseudo-bulbar paralysis following a lesion of the right side of the brain, pointing to the probable existence of defect on the left side, previously latent	XXIX.	253
Weights required to produce fractures of the ribs in the insane	XXVI.	21
Wells, on rupture of the urethra	XXII.	362
West (*C. E.*), two cases of extirpation of the labyrinth . .	XL.	93
,, ,, intra-cranial cases	XXXIX.	37
(*R.*), on carbuncle	XXIX.	354
(*Samuel*), a case of hæmorrhagic typhoid . .	XXXI.	259
blood-casts in phthisis	XXX.	253
case of profuse diarrhœa, causing death in man from tropics	XXXII.	87
cases from the Skin Department	XXXI.	263
clinical notes and observations	XXII.	213
fetid empyema	XXXII.	83
five cases of functional nervous disorder . . .	XXI.	59
new growths of lung and pleura · . . .	XXXIII.	109
observations upon the pulse-respiration ratio in croupous pneumonia	XXVIII.	231
on calcareous masses from lung	XXXI.	253
,, influenza	XXVI.	312
profuse non-fatal hæmoptysis	XXI.	51
simple cicatricial stricture of the air-tubes . .	XXV.	223
the influenza epidemic of 1890 as experienced at St. Bartholomew's Hospital, and the Royal Free Hospital, with reports from the resident officers .	XXVI.	193
three cases of dermatitis herpetiformis, with some instances of local bullous eruption following poisoned wounds, and remarks . . .	XXIX.	313
West Africa, ainhum, in'filariasis in	XXXIX.	182
Gold Coast (*see*).		
goundou in	XXXIX.	179
guinea-worm, native treatment of in . . .	XXXIX.	194
gynæcology, native, in	XXXIX.	204
leprosy in	XXXIX.	177
madura foot in	XXXIX.	178
midwifery, native, in	XXXIX.	204
native method of treatment in (*J. G. Forbes*) . .	XXXIX.	189
White (*C. Percival*), a case of cardiac disease complicating pregnancy and labour	XXV.	81
heart disease complicating labour	XXVI.	311
(*C. Powell*) bacteriological investigations in diphtheria .	XXXI.	87
Whitlow, diagnosis of implication of the sheath of the tendon in	XXV.	189, 190
importance of not incising sheath of tendons .	XXV.	187
incisions in, their position	XXV.	191
treatment of	XXV.	185
various degrees of	XXV.	185
Widal's serum reaction in typhoid fever, notes on . .	XXXIV.	205
Wigmore (*F. H.*), experiences of a house-surgeon . .	XXIII.	346
on certain diseases of infancy, puberty, and maturity .	XXII.	353

	VOL.	PAGE
Wilkie (*J.*), on physiology in brain-surgery	XXIII.	346
Willett (*Alfred*), cases from his wards	XXI.	65
memoir of W. Morrant Baker	XXXII.	xxxix
and **Cholmeley** (*M. A.*), cases of appendicitis	XXXV.	205
laparotomies	XXXV.	205
and **Wood-Hill** (*H. G.*), on a case of fractured base of the skull with remarkable eye-symptoms	XXXIV.	257
(*Edgar*), an account of some of the more interesting specimens recently added to the Museum	XXVII.	169
ether rash	XXXII.	79
lymphangioma of skin	XXX.	111
notes of surgical cases in the Edinburgh Infirmary, during 1804–6	XXXVII.	215
some operations on the stomach and intestines	XXIX.	351
and **Smith** (*T.*), fibromatous growths in the skin, with disseminated tubercles about the body	XXVI.	147
(*J. A.*), surgical emergencies	XXXVIII.	209
Mayo, and **Hawes**, a case of contusion of kidney	XXXVII.	282
cases of fractures	XXXVII.	269
,, ,, perforated gastric ulcer	XXXVII.	277
,, ,, disease of joints	XXXVII.	281
,, ,, hernia	XXXVII.	277
,, ,, injury to and disease of genito-urinary system	XXXVII.	281
,, ,, intestinal obstruction	XXXVII.	275
,, ,, middle ear disease	XXXVII.	280
,, ,, surgical emergencies	XXXVII.	269
,, ,, surgical smashes	XXXVII.	282
Williams (*H.*), report on influenza	XXVI.	229
Willoughby (*W. G.*), report on influenza	XXVI.	227
and **Ogle** (*J. G.*), notes of twenty-two cases of diphtheria under the care of Sir Dyce Duckworth, M.D., in which tracheotomy was performed	XXVI.	173
Wingfield (*H.*), on hypnotism	XXVII.	284
Wool, absorbent, report on	XXIX.	100
Womack (*F.*), on the rate of cooling of the body after death	XXI.	252
the rate of cooling of the body after death	XXIII.	193
and **Shore** (*T. W.*), preliminary scientific teaching at St. Bartholomew's Hospital	XXII.	149
Women, alcoholic neuritis in	XXII.	253
peripheral neuritis in	XXII.	253
retention of urine in (*McAdam Eccles*)	XXIX.	350
Wood-Hill (*H. G.*), and **Willett** (*Alfred*), fractured base of the skull with remarkable eye-symptoms	XXXIV.	257
Worcester (*Bishop of*), on smallpox at the Hospital	XXII.	37
Works of Percivall Pott	XXX.	182
Worry, a cause of insanity	XXVIII.	60
mental, in hæmaturia, effects of	XXII.	137
Worthington (*G. V.*), prognosis of tetanus	XXXI.	137
cases from Sir T. Smith's wards	XXXII.	19
Wound, gunshot, of the brain	XXIX.	228
poisoned, followed by bullous eruption	XXIX.	313
punctured, extending through ischio-rectal space into pelvis	XXXIV.	255
punctured, of hand	XXVII.	213
,, ,, intestine	XXVII.	177
lacerated, of chest and abdomen	XXVII.	50
,, ,, internal carotid artery	XXVII.	54
,, ,, knee and leg	XXVII.	53
,, ,, vagina, hæmorrhage from	XXXIV.	236

	VOL.	PAGE
Wounds, dressing of	XXIII.	352
gunshot, of orbit, effects on eye (*Jessop*) . . .	XXXVII.	312
perforating, of orbit	XXIV.	179
punctured (*Lankester*)	XXII.	364
treatment of	XXVI.	303
Wrist-drop	XXIV.	300
Wrist-joint, disease of	XXIV. 285,	309
Wryneck	XXIV.	249
Xerodermia pigmentosa (*Phillips*)	XXXI.	221
X-rays, in diseases of the chest (*H. Walsham*) . .	XXXIV.	29
Year's abdominal operations (*Power*)	XXXVII.	27
surgery (*Butlin*)	XXIX.	89
,, second (*Butlin*)	XXX.	227
work in the Electrical Department (*Lewis Jones*) .	XXXIII.	169
Yeld (*R. A.*), on alcoholic cirrhosis	XXXIV.	215
Young (*S. L. O.*), on abscess of the brain . . .	XL.	53

THE END

Printed by BALLANTYNE, HANSON & Co.
Edinburgh & London

STATISTICAL TABLES

OF THE

𝔓atients under 𝔗reatment

IN THE WARDS OF

ST. BARTHOLOMEW'S HOSPITAL

DURING 1904,

BY

THE MEDICAL REGISTRARS,

P. HORTON-SMITH HARTLEY, M.D. (CANTAB.), F.R.C.P.,
T. J. HORDER, M.D.,

AND

THE SURGICAL REGISTRAR,

G. E. GASK, F.R.C.S.

London:

PRINTED BY CHARLES SKIPPER AND EAST,

49, GREAT TOWER STREET, E.C.

1905.

ST. BARTHOLOMEW'S HOSPITAL.

1905.

The Medical and Surgical Staff.

Consulting Physicians.
Sir W. S. CHURCH, Bart., K.C.B.; Dr. HENSLEY.
Sir LAUDER BRUNTON, F.R.S.; Dr. GEE.

Consulting Surgeons.
Sir THOMAS SMITH, Bart., K.C.V.O.; Mr. WILLETT; Mr. BUTLIN;
Mr. MARSH; Mr. LANGTON.

Consulting Ophthalmic Surgeon.
Mr. HENRY POWER.

Physicians.
Sir DYCE DUCKWORTH; Dr. NORMAN MOORE; Dr. SAMUEL WEST;
Dr. ORMEROD; Dr. HERRINGHAM.

Surgeons.
Mr. HARRISON CRIPPS; Mr. BRUCE CLARKE;
Mr. ANTHONY BOWLBY, C.M.G.; Mr. LOCKWOOD; Mr. D'ARCY POWER.

Assistant-Physicians.
Dr. TOOTH, C.M.G.; Dr. GARROD; Dr. CALVERT;
Dr. MORLEY FLETCHER; Dr. DRYSDALE.

Assistant-Surgeons.
Mr. WARING; Mr. ECCLES; Mr. BAILEY; Mr. HARMER;
Mr. RAWLING.

Physician-Accoucheur.
Dr. CHAMPNEYS.

Assistant-Physician-Accoucheur.   Surgeon to Obstetric Wards.
Dr. W. S. A. GRIFFITH.   Mr. HARRISON CRIPPS.

Ophthalmic Surgeons.
Mr. JESSOP; Mr. HOLMES SPICER.

Aural Surgeon.
Mr. CUMBERBATCH.

Dental Surgeons.
Mr. PATERSON; Mr. ACKERY.

Assistant Dental Surgeons.
Mr. ACKLAND; Dr. AUSTEN.

Medical Officer in charge of Electrical Department.
Dr. LEWIS JONES.

Pathologist.
Dr. ANDREWES.

Administrators of Anæsthetics
Mr. GILL; Mr. EDGAR WILLETT.

Medical Registrars.   Surgical Registrar.
Dr. HORTON-SMITH HARTLEY; Dr. HORDER.   Mr. GASK.

Casualty Physicians.
Dr. TALBOT; Dr. BRANSON.

CONTENTS.

	PAGE.
Number of Beds	iv.
General Statement of the Patients under Treatment during the year	iv.
Patients brought in Dead	iv.
Occupations of the Male Patients	v.
Occupations of the Female Patients	viii.

MEDICAL REPORT—

Preface to the Medical Tables 11

TABLE I.—Showing the Total Number of Cases of each Disease under Treatment during the Year 1904, with the Results 12

Abstract of Table I. 37

Index to Medical Cases, showing Diseases and chief Symptoms 38

Index to Register of Medical Post-mortem Examinations 60

SURGICAL REPORT—

Preface to the Surgical Report... 72

TABLE I.—Showing the Total Number of Cases under Treatment during the Year 1904, with the comparative frequency and mortality of each Disease at different ages 73

Abstract of Table I. 117

TABLE II.—Showing the Surgical Operations performed 118

Statistics of Anæsthetics 154

Appendix 155

Sub-Table showing the number of Cases of Erysipelas, Pyæmia, &c. ... 190

Table of Statistics of Appendicitis 192

Index to Register of Surgical Post-mortem Examinations 194

ST. BARTHOLOMEW'S HOSPITAL.

1904.

Number of Beds in	Medical Wards	... ...	239
„ „	„ Wards for Diseases of Women	... ...	32
„ „	„ Surgical Wards	... ...	335
„ „	„ Ophthalmic Wards ...	... ...	25
„ „	„ General and Isolation	... ...	39
			670

GENERAL STATEMENT OF THE PATIENTS UNDER TREATMENT DURING THE YEAR 1904.

Patients remaining in, January 1st, 1904 :—

Medical 245
Surgical ... ... 314 } ... 559

Admitted during the year 1904 :—

Medical 2,594
Surgical ... ... 3,995 } ... 6,589

} ... 7,148

Discharged :—

Medical 2,256
Surgical ... ... 3,730 } ... 5,986

Died :—

Medical 343
Surgical ... ... 261 } ... 604

Remaining in, January 1st, 1905 :—

Medical 240
Surgical ... ... 318 } ... 558

} ... 7,148

Patients brought in Dead :—

Medical 13
Surgical ... ... 5 } ... 18

Dying in the Surgery or Surgery Ward :—

Medical 32
Surgical ... ... 9 } ... 41

} ... 59

Patients admitted to Surgery Ward during the year 1904 (not included in the above statistics) :—

Medical 169
Surgical ... ... 127 } ... 296

Average duration of stay of Patients ... ... 29·38 days.

OCCUPATIONS OF MALE PATIENTS.

Accountant	1	Cabmen	26	Detectives	3
Accoutrement maker	1	Call boy	1	Dispensers	3
Acrobat	1	Cane worker	1	Distillers	2
Actors	4	Canteen attendant	1	Diver	1
Agents	4	Capsule makers	2	Dock labourers	13
Apprentice	1	Caretakers	4	Domestic servants	3
Army pensioners	4	Carmen	143	Drapers	3
Army reservist	1	Carpenters	50	Drapers' assistants	9
Artist's model	1	Carpet planners	2	Draymen	5
Asphalte workers	3	Carriage cleaners	2	Drillers	2
Asylum attendants	4	Cashiers	3	Driver	1
		Cask maker	1	Druggists' assistants	2
		Cat's meat man	1	Dustmen	4
		Cattle drivers	2	Dyer	1
Bacon drier	1	Cellarmen	8		
Bag maker	1	Cement worker	1		
Bakers	18	Chaff cutters	2		
Bakers' assistants	2	Chairmakers	7	Electricians	17
Bank messengers	2	Chartered accountant	1	Electro-plater	1
Barbers	2	Chauffeurs	3	Engine cleaners	10
Barge builders	2	Checkers	3	Engine drivers	6
Barmen	8	Cheesemongers'		Engineers	42
Barrister	1	assistants	3	Engineers' labourers	9
Basket makers	4	Chef	1	Engineer's pattern	
Billiard markers	2	Chemists	3	cutter	1
Billposter	1	Chemists' assistants	3	Errand boys	28
Bird cage maker	1	Chimney sweeps	3	Excavator	1
Blacking maker	1	Cigar makers	2		
Blacksmiths	26	Civil engineers	3		
Boiler makers	3	Civil servant	1		
Bookbinders	15	Clergymen	5	Factory manager	1
Book-edge gilders	2	Clerks	151	Factory workers	2
Booking clerk	1	Clock maker	1	Farmers	14
Bookkeeper	1	Club attendant	1	Farmers' labourers	12
Book porters	3	Coach builders	4	Farriers	10
Booksellers	2	Coachmen	37	Firemen	8
Bookseller's assistant	1	Coal porters	11	Firewood cutter	1
Bootblack	1	Coffee stall keepers	2	Fisherman	1
Boot laster	1	Collar maker	1	Fish market porters	2
Boot makers	33	Collectors	7	Fishmongers	7
Bottle maker	1	Colonial sampler	1	Fitters	5
Bottle washers	2	Commercial travellers	10	Florists	3
Bow and arrow maker	1	Commissionaires	2	Footmen	5
Box makers	10	Compositors	8	Foremen	4
Brass burnishers	3	Confectioners	5	Foundry man	1
Brass finishers	9	Conjurer	1	French polishers	17
Brass moulders	2	Cooks	19	Fret-worker	1
Brewers' labourers	4	Coopers	4	Fruiterers	11
Bricklayers	32	Corn merchant	1	Furnisher	1
Bricklayers' labourers	7	Coroner's officer	1	Furniture maker	1
Brick maker	1	Corset makers	2	Furniture removers	2
Brush makers	7	Costermongers	11	Furriers	2
Builders	7	Cowmen	4		
Builder's clerk	1	Curriers	2		
Builders' labourers	6	Customs officers	2		
Butchers	33	Cycle makers	4	Galvanisers	2
Butlers	11			Gamekeepers	2
				Gardeners	42
		Dairymen	5	Gas fitters	15
Cabinet makers	28	Decorators	7	Gas-meter makers	2
Cable joiner, G.P.O.	1	Dentist's assistant	1	General dealers	9
				Gilders	2

Glass bevellers	... 5	Labourers ...	... 261	Organ grinder	... 1
Glass blowers	... 3	Lamp lighters	... 2	Ostler	... 1
Glass cutters ...	... 2	Laster ...	... 1	Overseer ...	... 1
Glass silverer...	... 1	Lathe workers	... 2		
Glaziers	... 6	Laundrymen ...	... 3		
Gold blockers	... 2	Lavatory attendants	2	Packers	42
Gold dredger ...	... 1	Law writers ...	... 3	Packing-case makers	7
Goldsmith ...	... 1	Lead workers...	... 6	Page boys	2
Golf caddies ..	... 1	Leather workers	... 4	Painters	55
Greengrocers ...	... 4	Letter carrier...	... 1	Pantryman ...	... 1
Grocers ...	... 6	Library assistants	... 2	Paper-bag maker	... 1
Grocers' assistants	... 12	Licensed victuallers ...	2	Paper hangers	... 4
Grooms ...	... 3	Lift attendants	... 8	Paper makers	... 4
Gum-boiler ...	... 1	Lightermen ...	... 8	Pastrycook ...	... 1
Gunners ...	... 1	Lithographers	... 9	Paviors	2
		Locksmiths ...	... 3	Pawnbrokers' assistants	2
		Lodging house keeper	1	Pencil packers	... 2
Hairdressers ...	... 7			Pensioners ...	... 4
Hair-sorters ...	... 2	Machinists ...	... 10	Photographers	... 7
Hallporter ...	... 1	Mail van driver	... 3	Physician ...	... 1
Hammermen ...	... 3	Malt worker ...	... 1	Pianist ...	... 1
Harness maker	... 1	Manager ...	... 1	Pianoforte makers ...	2
Hatters ...	... 2	Mantle cutters	... 4	Picture-frame makers	4
Hawkers ...	... 11	Marble cutter	... 1	Pipe makers ...	... 2
Hay-trusser ...	... 1	Marines ...	... 3	Plasterers ...	... 5
Helmet maker	... 1	Marine store dealer ...	1	Plateglass cutters	... 2
Horse dealer ...	... 1	Market gardener ...	1	Platelayers ...	... 8
Horsehair curler	... 1	Mason	1	Plumbers ...	... 15
Horsehair dealer	... 1	Mattress makers	... 2	Policemen ...	... 11
Horsekeepers ...	... 23	Mechanics ...	... 2	Polisher ...	... 1
Horse slaughterer	... 1	Medical practitioners	7	Porters ...	... 115
Hosier ...	... 1	Medical students	... 14	Postmen ...	... 7
Hosier's assistant	... 1	Merchant ...	... 1	Post office assistants	3
Hospital porter	... 1	Messengers ...	... 17	Post office sorters	... 3
Hotel porter ...	... 1	Metal workers	... 8	Potmen ...	... 9
House decorators	... 2	Mica worker ...	... 1	Poultry farmer	... 1
Housekeepers...	... 2	Militiaman ...	... 1	Press boy ...	... 1
House physicians	... 5	Milkmen ...	... 9	Priest	1
House surgeon	... 1	Miller	.. 1	Printers ...	... 57
Huntsman ...	... 1	Mineral-water bottler	1	Professional singer	... 1
		Miners ...	... 3	Provision dealers	... 2
Ice cream maker	... 1	Missionary ...	... 1	Publicans ...	... 5
Income-tax collector	1	Moulders ...	... 2		
India-rubber workers	4	Musical-instrument		Railway checker	... 1
Indigo planters	... 2	maker	... 1	Railway foreman	... 1
Innkeeper ...	... 1	Music copyist	... 1	Railway guards	... 2
Instrument makers ...	4	Musicians ...	... 2	Railway porters	... 19
Insurance agents	... 2			Railway signalman ...	1
Iron workers ...	... 9	Naval officer ...	... 1	Rate collector...	... 1
		Navvies ...	... 2	Reading boy ...	... 1
Jewellers ...	... 2	Newsvendors...	... 3	Reporter ...	... 1
Jockey ...	... 1	Night gatekeeper	... 1	Riding-school orderly	1
Joiners ...	... 6	Night watchmen	... 3	Rifle viewer ...	... 1
Journalists ...	... 4			Road sweepers	... 2
		Office boys ...	... 15	Rope makers ...	... 2
		Oilman ...	... 1		
Kitchen boys...	... 3	Omnibus conductors...	2		
Kitchen porters	... 4	Omnibus drivers ...	3	Sack maker ...	... 1
Knife grinder	... 1	Organ builder	... 1	Saddler ...	... 1

OCCUPATIONS OF MALE PATIENTS *(continued)*.

Sailors...	16	Solicitors	2	Tram conductors	5
Salesmen	4	Stablemen	5	Tram drivers...	3
Sanitary inspector	1	Stationers	2	Travellers	6
Sausage maker	1	Station foreman	1	Turners (wood)	2
Saw maker	1	Stevedores	7	Typists	4
Sawmill hand	1	Stewards	3		
Sawyers	5	Stickmaker	1	Umbrella makers	4
Scaffolders	3	Stockbrokers' clerks	2	Undertakers ...	2
Scavengers	6	Stokers	14	Upholsterers ...	8
Schoolboys	496	Stone cutter	1		
Schoolmasters	3	Stonemasons	9		
Secretary	1	Store keepers...	2	Valets ..	5
Sewing machine maker	1	Straw hat makers	2	Van boys	32
Shepherds	2	Students	4	Verger...	1
Ship engineers	2	Surgeons	2	Veterinary surgeon ...	1
Ship fireman ...	1	Surgical instrument		Violinist	1
Ship painter ...	1	makers	4	Vulcanite worker	1
Ship stewards	4	Surveyors	3		
Shipwrights ...	3			Waiters	16
Shoeblacks	2	Table maker ...	1	Walking stick makers	2
Shoeing smiths	2	Tailors	21	Warehousemen	60
Shoemakers ...	3	Tea warehousemen	3	Waste-paper sorter ...	1
Shop assistants	28	Telegraphists	4	Watchmakers	6
Shopkeeper	1	Telegraph linesman...	1	Watchmen	2
Shunters	4	Telegraph messengers	8	Waterside labourers ...	6
Signalmen	3	Telephone clerk	1	Wheelwrights	7
Sign writers ...	2	Telephone linesman...	1	Window cleaners	12
Silk spinner ...	1	Thermometer makers	4	Wine packers...	3
Silver polishers	4	Tie cutters	3	Wood workers	16
Silversmiths ...	2	Timber porter	1		
Skin dressers...	4	Timekeepers ...	3		
Slaters...	3	Tin workers ...	14	Infants	362
Soap maker ...	1	Tobacco sorters	3		
Soldiers	19	Toy makers ...	2	No occupation	52

OCCUPATIONS OF FEMALE PATIENTS.

Actress	... ...	1	Flower makers	...	8
Artificial flower makers		4	Flower sellers	...	1
Asylum nurse	... ...	1	Forewomen ...	...	3
			French polishers	...	10
			Fruit seller	... ...	1
Bag makers	... ...	2	Furriers	... ...	2
Barmaids	... ...	10	Fur sewers	... ...	4
Basket makers	... ...	2			
Billiard-shade makers		2			
Blouse maker	...	1	General dealers	...	4
Boarding-house keepers		4	Gold and silver polisher		2
Bookbinders ...	...	2	Governesses ...	...	15
Bookfolders ...	...	10	Greengrocers ...	...	2
Bookkeepers	...	7	Gum workers...	...	2
Boot workers...	...	4			
Bottle washers	...	2			
Box makers ...	...	23	Hawkers	... ...	4
Brace maker ...	...	1	Hosier	... ...	1
Brush makers	...	4	Housekeepers	...	23
Buttonhole makers	...	2	Housewives and house-		
			workers	...	1,281
Canvas stamper	...	1			
Capsule maker	...	1	Ironers	... ...	6
Cardboard workers	...	4			
Caretakers	... ...	2	Jewel polishers	...	2
Cashiers	... ...	3			
Chair caners ...	...	2	Lace makers ...	...	2
Chambermaids	...	2	Lacquerer	... ...	1
Charwomen ...	...	26	Lady's maids	...	18
Chocolate coverer	...	1	Laundresses ...	...	32
Chocolate makers	...	2	Lavatory attendant ...		1
Church keeper	...	1	Lead-pencil polisher		1
Cigarette makers	...	2	Leather workers	...	2
Cigar makers...	...	4			
Clerks ...	...	11			
Cloth worker	...	1	Machine ruler	...	1
Coffee shop assistants		2	Machinists ...	...	50
Collar ironers...	...	2	Mantle makers	...	4
Collar makers	...	2	Match-box maker	...	1
Collar turners	...	2	Mat maker ...	...	1
Companions ...	...	7	Matron	...	1
Confectioners...	...	7	Menthol moulder		1
Convent sister	...	1	Milliners	...	16
Cooks	...	57	Mothers' helps	...	8
Cutters	... ...	2	Music teachers	...	8
Dairy maids ...	...	2			
Domestic servants	...	171	Needleworkers	...	18
Drapers' assistants	...	6	Net maker ...	...	1
Dressmakers	...	41	Nursemaids ...	...	11
			Nurses (children's) ...		7
			„ (hospital)	...	48
Electric-wire worker		1	„ (monthly)	...	10
Embosser	... ...	1	„ (sick)	...	17
Embroidery makers ...		2			
Envelope folders	...	4	Office cleaners	...	10
			Ostrich-feather curlers		2
Factory workers	...	6			
Fancy-bottle-cap maker		1	Packers	... ...	7
Feather workers	...	3	Paper-bag makers	...	2

Parlourmaids...	...	9
Pattern mounters	...	3
Phonograph retoucher		1
Photo-frame makers...		3
Professional singer ...		1
Pupil teachers	...	2
Purse maker ...	...	1
Rubber worker	...	1
Saleswomen	...	4
School girls ...	...	340
School mistresses	...	8
Secretaries	...	2
Shirt ironer ...	...	2
Shirt maker ...	...	4
Shop assistants	...	21
Shopkeepers	...	5
Silver polisher	...	1
Stall keepers ...	...	2
Stamp gummer	...	1
Stewardess	...	1
Still-room maids	...	3
Tailoresses	...	18
Teachers	...	8
Tea weighers	...	2
Telegraphist ...	...	1
Theatre attendant ...		1
Tie makers ...	...	3
Tin workers ...	...	2
Tobacco workers	...	3
Tooth-brush makers...		2
Typists	... ...	4
Umbrella makers	...	7
Upholsteress ...	...	1
Waistcoat makers	...	2
Waitresses	...	15
Ward maids ...	...	13
Warehouse messenger		1
Washerwomen	...	9
Waterproof maker ...		1
Wire worker ...	...	1
Wood-bundle maker		1
Workhouse superin-		
tent		1
Infants	... ...	252
No occupation	...	35

MEDICAL REPORT.

PREFACE TO THE MEDICAL TABLES.

Indices of Medical Cases and of the Post-mortem Register for the year are appended to the Statistical Tables.

The system of classification introduced in 1895 has been continued. The Medical cases (with the exception of those in Radcliffe and Isolation Wards, which are bound together under the name of Radcliffe), are bound and indexed according to the Physician under whose care they were.

Thus of Male Patients : —

Those under Dr. Gee and Dr. Herringham are bound in
   Vol. I.
   „   „   Sir Dyce Duckworth are bound in Vol. II.
   „   „   Dr. Norman Moore   „   „   III.
   „   „   Dr. Samuel West   „   „   IV.
   „   „   Sir Lauder Brunton and Dr. Ormerod are
        bound in Vol. V.

The Female cases are similarly numbered, and those under Dr. Champneys are bound in Vol. VI.

Also following the plan introduced in 1895, Alphabetical Indices of Patients' names, and of their diseases and chief symptoms, have been embodied in special volumes, one for Male and one for Female cases. These volumes are kept with the notes of the year.

It may be mentioned that the Tables and Indices which follow are not strictly comparable with each other. In Table I. each case only occurs once under the chief disease or symptom, whereas in the Clinical Index prominent secondary symptoms and special methods of treatment are included. Again, the Post-mortem Index includes records of a number of Patients brought in dead or dying in the Surgery Ward, who, not having been admitted to the Hospital, appear neither in Table I. nor in the Clinical Index.

TABLE I.

DISEASE	Total	Discharged M.	Discharged F.	Died M.	Died F.
GENERAL DISEASES.					
A.					
Diphtheria	18	10	2	3	3
Erysipelas	3	1	2		
Fever	19	11	8		
Influenza	21	11	10		
Malaria	11	11			
Malta Fever	1		1		
Measles	16	11	5	1	1
Pertussis	10	5	4		
Pyæmia	1			1	
Scarlet Fever	8	1	7		
Tetanus	1	1		1	
Tuberculosis	15			9	6
Typhoid Fever	60	29	23	4	4
Varioloid	1		1		
Total	185	90	63	16	14

TABLE I. (continued).

DISEASE.	Total	Discharged M.	Discharged F.	Died M.	Died F.
GENERAL DISEASES. **B.**					
Addison's Disease ...	3	2	...	...	1
Alcoholism ...	4	2	1	1	...
Anæmia ...	25	6	19	...	1
" Pernicious ...	5	1	1	2	1
Arthritis (Gonorrhœal) ...	6	4	2	...	...
" (Multiple) ...	3	...	3	...	...
Catarrh, Universal...	1	...	1	...	...
Debility ...	3	...	3	...	...
Diabetes, Mellitus ...	18	7	9	2	...
" Insipidus...	4	1	3	...	...
Exophthalmic Goître ...	20	5	13	...	2
Glycosuria ...	2	...	2	...	...
Gout ...	11	10	1	...	...
Hæmoglobinuria, Paroxysmal ...	1	1	...	...	...
Hæmophilia ...	2	2	...	...	...
Leukæmia, Lymphatic ...	2	...	...	2	...
" Myelogenic ...	4	4	...	...	...
Lymphadenoma ...	6	3	1	2	...

TABLE I. (*continued*).

DISEASE	Total	Discharged M	Discharged F	Died M	Died F
GENERAL DISEASES, B (*continued*).					
Marasmus ...	6	3	...	2	1
Myxœdema ...	4	...	4	...	...
Osteo-arthritis ...	15	5	10	...	...
Purpura ...	1	1	1	...	...
Rheumatism, Acute ...	144	70	67	3	4
" Chronic ...	1	...	1	...	...
Rickets ...	10	2	7	1	1
Scurvy, Infantile ...	1	...	1	1	...
Syphilis ...	5	...	4	...	...
Typho-toxin Inoculation ...	3	2	1	...	...
Total ...	310	132	153	15	10

TABLE I. (continued).

DISEASE.	Total.	Discharged. M.	Discharged. F.	Died. M.	Died. F.	Under 5. Disch. M.	Under 5. Disch. F.	Under 5. Died M.	Under 5. Died F.	−10. Disch. M.	−10. Disch. F.	−10. Died M.	−10. Died F.	−15. Disch. M.	−15. Disch. F.	−15. Died M.	−15. Died F.	−20. Disch. M.	−20. Disch. F.	−20. Died M.	−20. Died F.	−30. Disch. M.	−30. Disch. F.	−30. Died M.	−30. Died F.	−40. Disch. M.	−40. Disch. F.	−40. Died M.	−40. Died F.	−50. Disch. M.	−50. Disch. F.	−50. Died M.	−50. Died F.	−60. Disch. M.	−60. Disch. F.	−60. Died M.	−60. Died F.	Over 60. Disch. M.	Over 60. Disch. F.	Over 60. Died M.	Over 60. Died F.
MISCELLANEOUS DISEASES.																																									
Abdominal Tumour	2	2																								1															
" Wall, Sinus of	1		1																			1																1			
" Section, Sequelae of	1																																								
Abscess, Alveolar	1		1																							1															
Anasarca	1		1																							1															
Arthritis (Tuberculous)	1		1																																					1	
Breast, Malignant Growth of	1			1	1																											1									
Cellulitis	1		1																				1																		
Chilblain	1																						1											1							
Debility	3	3								1													2											1							
Elephantiasis	1	1																																1							
Epistaxis	1	1																					1																		
Glands—																																									
Tuberculous	2	1	1			1													1																1						
Malignant Growth in	2	1	1	1	1														1													1								1	
Enlarged	1	1													1																										
Intrathoracic Tumour	1	1																																							
Ilium, Malignant Growth of	1		1		1																					1		1				1									
Lumbago	1	1																					1																		
Malingering...	3	2	1																				1				1								2						

TABLE I. (continued).

DISEASE	Total	Discharged M.	Discharged F.	Died M.	Died F.
MISCELLANEOUS DISEASES—(continued).					
Mediastinum, Malignant Growth of...	5	1	...	3	1
Myalgia	4	4	...	...	...
Obesity	1	...	1	...	...
Otitis Media	1	1	1	...	...
" Externa	1	...	...	...	...
Parotid Tumour	1	1	1	...	...
Prematurity	8	...	...	5	3
Raynaud's Disease	2	...	1	...	...
Rhinitis	2	1	...	...	...
Ulcer of Foot	1	2	1	...	...
Unclassified...	7	4	3	...	...
Total	**59**	**28**	**15**	**10**	**6**

TABLE I. (continued).

DISEASE.	Total	Discharged M.	Discharged F.	Died M.	Died F.
LOCAL DISEASES.					
DISEASES OF THE NERVOUS SYSTEM.					
General.					
Amnesia	1	1	...	...	...
Amentia	1	1	...	...	...
Chorea	46	15	31	...	...
Convulsions	2	1	1	...	...
Delirium Tremens	2	1	...	...	1
Epilepsy	15	12	3	...	...
Hysteria	14	2	12	...	...
Hypochondriasis	1	...	1	...	...
Insanity	9	4	5	...	...
Megalencephaly	1	1	...	...	...
Muscular Hypertonicity	1	1	...	...	...
Myasthenia Gravis	1	...	1	...	...
Neurasthenia	10	1	9	...	...
Neuromimesis	3	1	2	...	...
Paralysis Agitans	4	4	...	...	...
Sclerosis, Disseminated	4	2	2	...	...
Tremor	3	3	...	...	...
Torticollis (Spasmodic)	2	2	...	...	...

TABLE I. (continued).

DISEASE	Total	Discharged M	Discharged F	Died M	Died F
DISEASES OF THE NERVOUS SYSTEM (continued).					
Cranial.					
Cerebellar Tumour...	1	1			
Cerebral Abscess ...	1				1
" Haemorrhage	20	7	1	12	1
" Syphilis ...	6	4	1	1	
" Tumour ...	6	4	2		
Cranial Nerves, Paralysis of	2		2		
Diplegia, Cerebral ...	1		1		
Headache ...	2	1	1		
Optic Atrophy	1	1			
" Neuritis ...	1	1			
Hemiplegia ...	24	20	3	1	
Hydrocephalus ...	1		1		
Meningitis ...	2	2			
" Post-Basal	9	2	2	5	
" Pseudo ...	1	1			
" Purulent ...	8			5	3
" Tuberculous ...	18			9	9
" Spinal, Purulent	1				1
Pons, Disease of ...	1	1			

TABLE I. (continued).

19

DISEASE	Total	Discharged M	Discharged F	Died M	Died F	Under 5 Disch. M	Under 5 Disch. F	Under 5 Died M	Under 5 Died F	—10 Disch. M	—10 Disch. F	—10 Died	—15 Disch.	—15 Died	—20 Disch.	—20 Died	—30 Disch. M	—30 Disch. F	—30 Died	—40 Disch. M	—40 Disch. F	—40 Died	—50 Disch. M	—50 Disch. F	—50 Died M	—50 Died F	—60 Disch. M	—60 Disch. F	—60 Died M	—60 Died F	Over 60 Disch.	Over 60 Died
DISEASES OF THE NERVOUS SYSTEM (continued).																																
Spinal.																																
Atrophy, Progressive Muscular	6	2	3	1													2	1		2	1											
Friedreich's Ataxy	2	1	1														1	1		1												
Myelitis, Acute	2	1		1																1					1							
Paralysis, Infantile	5	2	3			1	2			1										1			2	1				2		1		
Paraplegia, Ataxic	3	3																		1			2	1			2	1				
" Spastic	8	6	2				3			1			1																			
Sclerosis, Amyotrophic Lateral	1		1														1										2	1				
" Combined Lateral and Posterior	3	3		1																2	3		2				1					
" Lateral	2	2															2			3			1	1			2		2	1		
Tabes Dorsalis	13	8	4	1		3															1		1	1				1		1		
Tetany	3		3			1																						1				
Peripheral.																																
Neuralgia	3	3																		3	1											
Neuritis, Local	2	1	1																	1			1	1				1		1		
" Alcoholic	3	1	1	1																1			1	1								

TABLE I. (continued).

DISEASES.	Total	Discharged M.	Discharged F.	Died M.	Died F.
DISEASES OF THE NERVOUS SYSTEM. (continued).					
Peripheral (continued)—					
Neuritis, Diptheritic ...	4	2	2	...	...
" Influenzal ...	1	1	...	...	...
" Peripheral ...	2	1	...	...	**1**
Sciatica	6	5	1	...	...
Myopathies.					
Unclassified	2	2	...	...	...
Facio-scapulo Humeral ...	1	1	...	...	...
Pseudo-Hypertrophic Paralysis	1	1	...	...	...
Total	300	142	104	36	16

TABLE I. (continued).

DISEASE.	Total	Discharged M.	Discharged F.	Died M.	Died F.
DISEASES OF THE CIRCULATORY SYSTEM.					
Heart Disease—					
Asthenia ...	1	1	...	...	...
Congenital ...	3	1	1	...	1
Dilatation ...	8	4	2	1	1
Myocardial Degeneration ...	5	4	...	1	1
Palpitation ...	1	1	...	...	...
Tachycardia ...	2	2	...	...	...
Valvular—					
Aortic Regurgitation ...	12	8	1	3	1
" Double ...	4	3	1	...	...
Mitral Obstruction ...	16	4	10	2	3
" Regurgitation ...	34	15	16	4	1
" Double ...	34	12	17	5	2
" and Aortic ...	40	24	9	3	1
" and Tricuspid ...	5	1	...	...	1
" Tricuspid and Aortic ...	2	1	...	...	1
Pulmonary Regurgitation ...	1	1	...	...	...
Tricuspid " ...	1	1	...	...	...
Malignant Endocarditis ...	22	1	...	15	6
Pericarditis ...	6	1	3	...	2

TABLE 1. (continued).

DISEASE.	Total	Discharged M.	Discharged F.	Died M.	Died F.	Under 5. D M	Under 5. D F	Under 5. Dd M	Under 5. Dd F	—10.	—15. Died	—20.	—30. Disch	—40. Disch	—50. Disch	—60. Disch	—60. Died	Over 60. Disch
DISEASES OF THE CIRCULATORY SYSTEM (continued).																		
Aneurysm, Aortic—																		
Thoracic	17	14	1	2										4	2	6	1	2
Abdominal	2	2									1			1	1	1	1	
Arterio-sclerosis	4	3		1										2	1	1		2
Venous Thrombosis	6	3	3									1	2	1				
Total ...	226	107	63	37	19													

TABLE I. (continued).

DISEASE.	Total.	Discharged M.	Discharged F.	Died M.	Died F.
DISEASES OF THE RESPIRATORY SYSTEM.					
Bronchiectasis	3	3			
Bronchitis, Acute	22	4	15	2	3
„ Chronic	58	45	9	2	2
„ Plastic	1		1		
Bronchial Glands (Enlarged)	1		1		
Dyspnœa	1		1		
Emphysema	10	8	1	1	
Empyema	17	7	5	1	4
Hæmoptysis	4	3	1		
Laryngitis	5	4	1		
Laryngeal Obstruction	2	1		1	
„ Spasm	1				
Lung, Abscess of	1			1	
„ Fibrosis of	12	9	2	1	
„ Gangrene of	1			1	
„ Malignant Growth of	1			1	
Phthisis	64	41	6	12	5
Pleura, Malignant Growth of	1				1

TABLE I. (*continued*).

DISEASE.	Total.	Discharged.		Died.		Under 5.				— 10.				— 15.				— 20.				— 30.				— 40.				— 50.				— 60.				Over 60.			
						Discharged.		Died.		Discharged.		Died.		Discharged.		Died.		Discharged.		Died.		Discharged.		Died.		Discharged.		Died.		Discharged.		Died.		Discharged.		Died.		Discharged.		Died.	
		M.	F.	M.	F.	M.	F.	M.	F.	M.	F.	M.	F.	M.	F.	M.	F.	M.	F.	M.	F.	M.	F.	M.	F.	M.	F.	M.	F.	M.	F.	M.	F.	M.	F.	M.	F.	M.	F.	M.	F.
DISEASES OF THE RESPIRATORY SYSTEM (*continued*).																																								
Pleurisy	37	23	14	...	...	...	1	...	...	2	1	...	...	1	3	...	...	4	4	...	...	5	1	...	...	6	1	...	...	4	1	...	...	...	2	...	...	1	...	...	...
„ with Effusion ...	44	31	12	**1**	...	4	1	...	...	2	...	...	...	4	3	...	...	4	2	...	...	3	2	...	...	7	3	...	...	6	...	**1**	...	1	1	...	...	...	...	...	...
Pleurodynia	2	...	2	...	...	...	...	...	...	...	...	...	...	...	...	...	...	...	...	...	...	...	2	...	...	...	...	...	...	...	...	...	...	...	...	...	...	...	...	...	...
Pneumonia, Catarrhal ...	77	26	23	**16**	**12**	23	17	16	12	2	5	...	...	...	1	...	...	...	...	...	...	1	...	...	...	...	...	...	...	...	...	...	...	...	...	...	...	...	...	...	...
„ Croupous ...	190	133	47	**7**	**3**	28	11	**1**	**1**	21	15	...	...	14	3	...	...	27	5	**1**	...	23	6	**1**	...	2	2	...	**1**	8	2	**4**	**1**	...	3	...	...	...	...	...	...
Pyo-pneumo-thorax ...	1	...	...	**1**	...	...	...	...	...	...	...	...	...	...	...	...	...	...	...	...	...	...	...	**1**	...	...	...	...	...	...	...	...	...	...	...	...	...	...	...	...	...
Total	556	339	141	**44**	**32**	...	...	...	...	...	...	...	...	...	...	...	...	...	...	...	...	...	...	...	...	...	...	...	...	...	...	...	...	...	...	...	...	...	...	...	...

TABLE I. (*continued*). 25

DISEASE.	Total	Discharged.		Died.		Under 5.				— 10.				— 15.				— 20.				— 30.				— 40.				— 50.				— 60.				Over 60.			
						Discharged.		Died.		Discharged.		Died.		Discharged.		Died.		Discharged.		Died.		Discharged.		Died.		Discharged.		Died.		Discharged.		Died.		Discharged.		Died.		Discharged.		Died.	
		M.	F.	M.	F.	M.	F.	M.	F.	M.	F.	M.	F.	M.	F.	M.	F.	M.	F.	M.	F.	M.	F.	M.	F.	M.	F.	M.	F.	M.	F.	M.	F.	M.	F.	M.	F.	M.	F.	M.	F.
DISEASES OF THE DIGESTIVE SYSTEM.																																									
Abdominal Pain	6	4	2	...	...	1								1								1	...			1	1			1											
,, Tumour ...	5	1	4	...	...																	1				1	2			1			1		1						
Appendicitis	9	5	2	**1**	**1**			**1**	...	1				1		**1**	1									1	2			1											
Ascites	1	1	...	...	...																					1															
Colic	7	7	...	...	...							3				1				2					1																
Colitis	1	1	...	...	...																				1															
,, Mucous ...	2	1	1	...	...														1			1																			
Constipation	9	3	6	...	...					1				1				1				2	4			1															
Diarrhœa	6	4	1	**1**	**3**	3	1	**1**	**1**	1																															
,, and Vomiting ...	10	5	...	**2**	**3**	5	...	**2**	**3**	**3**																							1							
Duodenum, Ulcer of ...	1	...	...	**1**	...																																				
,, Malignant Growth of	1	...	...	...	**1**																	1																			
Dysentery	3	2	1	...	...							1								2					1																
Dyspepsia	18	7	11	...	...									1				2	2			2	6			1	2			1	1										
Dysphagia	1	1	...	...	...																													1							
Enteritis	5	4	1	...	...					2				1				1				1																			
Enteralgia	1	1	...	...	...																	1																			
Gall Stones	3	...	3	...	...																						1			2											
Gastric Ulcer	67	12	51	**3**	**1**											8	...			1	30			3	10	**1**		3	4	**3**	...			2				2			
Gastritis	29	10	19	...	...							2				2	1	...		1	10			2	4			1	1			2	2					1		
Gastro-enteritis	27	10	11	**3**	**3**	5	6	3	3			2	1			1	2			1				1				1						2			

TABLE I. (*continued*).

DISEASE	Total	Discharged		Died		Under 5 Disch.		Under 5 Died		-10 Disch.		-10 Died		-15 Disch.		-15 Died		-20 Disch.		-20 Died		-30 Disch.		-30 Died		-40 Disch.		-40 Died		-50 Disch.		-50 Died		-60 Disch.		-60 Died		Over 60 Disch.		Over 60 Died	
		M	F	M	F	M	F	M	F	M	F	M	F	M	F	M	F	M	F	M	F	M	F	M	F	M	F	M	F	M	F	M	F	M	F	M	F	M	F	M	F
DISEASES OF THE DIGESTIVE SYSTEM (*continued*).																																									
Gastrodynia	4		4																			2	1				1						1								
Hæmatemesis	5	2	2		1												1					1	1			1			1			1								
Intestinal Ulceration (Tuberculous)	2			1	1			1									1								1															
Icterus Gravis	1				1																			1																
Jaundice	10	7	3																					2	2			3		1			2							
Liver, Abscess of	1	1																								1														
„ Cirrhosis of	34	21	2	9	2				3												1	1	2	5	1	2	1	4	1	1	1	10	3	1	2	1			
„ Enlarged	3	2	1	1						1															1	2		2	1			1		1					
„ Malignant Disease of	6	3	2	1	2																				1	1	2	1				1			1				
Œsophagus— Malignant Disease of	2	1		1																					1			1			1								
Stricture of	3	3																								1		1				1								
Rupture of	1			1																												2								
Pancreas, Malignant Growth of	1			1																										1										
Peritonitis— Chronic	1			1			1					1																												
Tuberculous	18	7	6	3	2	1	2	3	1	1	1				1				1		1	1		2	2			1			1	1			1				1

TABLE I. (continued).

DISEASE	Total	Discharged M	Discharged F	Died M	Died F	Under 5 Disch. M	Under 5 Disch. F	Under 5 Died M	Under 5 Died F	−10 Disch.	−10 Died	−15 Disch. M	−15 Disch. F	−15 Died	−20 Disch. M	−20 Disch. F	−20 Died	−30 Disch. M	−30 Disch. F	−30 Died	−40 Disch. M	−40 Disch. F	−40 Died M	−40 Died F	−50 Disch. M	−50 Disch. F	−50 Died	−60 Disch. M	−60 Disch. F	−60 Died	Over 60 Disch.	Over 60 Died
DISEASES OF THE DIGESTIVE SYSTEM (continued).																																
Rectum, Prolapse of	3	2	1	...	...	1							1																			
Sphincter Ani, Spasm of	1		1	...	...																	1										
Spleen, Enlargement of	3	3		...	...										1			1			1											
Sprue	2		2	...	...										1						1											
Stomatitis	1	1		...	...	1																										
Stomach, Dilated	2	2		...	...							1									1				1			1				
" Malignant Growth of	14	8	1	3	2				**1**			3			1			1		**1**	2	2	**2**	**2**	1	1		5	1		1	
Tonsillitis	12	5	7	...	...							2			2			1			1				1	1		1				
Tonsillar Abscess	1	1		...	...																											
Typhlitis	1	1		...	...																											
Vomiting	2	1		...	1	1			**1**																							
Total ...	346	150	145	31	20																											

TABLE I. (continued).

DISEASE.	Total	Discharged M.	Discharged F.	Died M.	Died F.
DISEASES OF THE URINARY SYSTEM.					
Albuminuria	1	...	1	...	...
Bladder, Contracted	1	...	1	...	...
" New Growth of	1	...	1	...	...
Calculus, Renal	3	3	...	...	...
Colic, Renal	9	2	1	...	...
Cystitis	4	1	3	...	...
Hæmaturia	5	4	1	...	...
Hydro-nephrosis	2	1	1	...	...
Kidney, Movable	8	...	3	...	...
" Tuberculous	1	...	1	...	...
Nephritis, Acute	11	10	1	1	...
" Chronic Interstitial	16	1	5	7	3
" " Parenchymatous	28	18	10	3	2
" " Mixed	14	8	1	4	1
Pyo-nephrosis	1	...	1	...	...
Pyuria	1	...	1	...	...
Urethra, Stricture of	2	1	...	1	...
Urine, Incontinence of	1	...	1	...	...
Total ...	98	44	32	16	6

TABLE I. (*continued*).

29

DISEASE.	Total.	Discharged M.	Discharged F.	Died M.	Died F.	Under 5. Disch. M.	Under 5. Disch. F.	Under 5. Died M.	Under 5. Died F.	−10 Disch. M.	−10 Disch. F.	−10 Died M.	−10 Died F.	−15 Disch. M.	−15 Disch. F.	−15 Died M.	−15 Died F.	−20 Disch. M.	−20 Disch. F.	−20 Died M.	−20 Died F.	−30 Disch. M.	−30 Disch. F.	−30 Died M.	−30 Died F.	−40 Disch. M.	−40 Disch. F.	−40 Died M.	−40 Died F.	−50 Disch. M.	−50 Disch. F.	−50 Died M.	−50 Died F.	−60 Disch. M.	−60 Disch. F.	−60 Died M.	−60 Died F.	Over 60 Disch. M.	Over 60 Disch. F.	Over 60 Died M.	Over 60 Died F.
DISEASES OF THE FE-MALE GENERATIVE SYSTEM.																																									
Vulva, Cyst of ...	2		2																								2														
" Hypertrophy of	1		1																								1														
" Lipoma of ...	1		1																								1														
" Malignant Growth of	2		2																												1								2		
" Ulceration of	1		1																												1										
" Warts on ...	1		1																																1						
" Vulvo-vaginal Cyst	1		1																												1										
Urethra, Caruncle of	12		12																	1			2							1				5					3		
" Malignant Disease of	1		1																															1							
" Stricture of ...	2		2																				1											1							
Urethritis ...	2		2																												1								1		
Urethrocele ...	2		2																				1								1								1		
Vagina, Cystocele ...	8		8																				1				4				1			2							
" Lupus Minimus of	5		5																								5														
" Fistula, Recto-vaginal	1		1																												1										
" Vesico-vaginal	2		2																								1				1										
" Foreign Body in	1		1																																						
" Haemorrhage from	1		1																																						
" Injury to ...	3		3																				1																		
" Prolapse of ...	8		8																				3				3				1										
" Rectocele	2		2																				2								1										
Vaginismus ...	3		3																				2				1														

TABLE I. (*continued*).

DISEASE	Total	Discharged M	Discharged F	Died M	Died F	–20 Disch. F	–30 Disch. F	–40 Disch. F	–50 Disch. F	–60 Disch. F	Over 60 Disch. F
DISEASES OF THE FEMALE GENERATIVE SYSTEM (continued).											
Vaginitis	6	...	6	...	...	3	3				
Uterus, Cervix—											
Adenoma of	1	...	1	...	...				1		
Catarrh of	1	...	1	...	...				1		
Cyst of	1	...	1	...	...			1			
Erosion of	3	...	3	...	...		2	1			
Fibroid Tumour of	1	...	1	...	...		1		1		
Malignant Growth of	20	...	20	...	...			10	4	5	1
Polypus of	3	...	3	...	...			1		1	
Uterus, Body—											
Amenorrhœa	3	...	3	...	...	1	1	1			
Dilatation of	1	...	1	...	...			1			
Dysmenorrhœa	12	...	12	...	...	3	6	3			
Dysparennia	1	...	1	...	...		1				
Menorrhagia	4	...	4	...	...		3	1			
Endometritis	13	...	12	...	1		2	3	6	1	
Fibroid Tumour of	32	...	32	...	...		1	11	20	1	
Leucorrhœa	1	...	1	...	...			1			
Haemorrhage from	12	...	12	...	...	1	2	4	5		
Malignant Growth of	7	...	7	...	...		1		2	4	
Polypus of	2	...	2	...	...			1	1		
Prolapse of	9	...	9	...	...		3	3		3	
Retroversion of	6	...	6	...	...		2	3	1		2

TABLE I. (*continued*).

31

DISEASE.	Total	Discharged. M.	Discharged. F.	Died. M.	Died. F.	Under 5. Discharged. M.	Under 5. Discharged. F.	Under 5. Died. M.	Under 5. Died. F.	— 10. Discharged. M.	— 10. Discharged. F.	— 10. Died. M.	— 10. Died. F.	— 15. Discharged. M.	— 15. Discharged. F.	— 15. Died. M.	— 15. Died. F.	— 20. Discharged. M.	— 20. Discharged. F.	— 20. Died. M.	— 20. Died. F.	— 30. Discharged. M.	— 30. Discharged. F.	— 30. Died. M.	— 30. Died. F.	— 40. Discharged. M.	— 40. Discharged. F.	— 40. Died. M.	— 40. Died. F.	— 50. Discharged. M.	— 50. Discharged. F.	— 50. Died. M.	— 50. Died. F.	— 60. Discharged. M.	— 60. Discharged. F.	— 60. Died. M.	— 60. Died. F.	Over 60. Discharged. M.	Over 60. Discharged. F.	Over 60. Died. M.	Over 60. Died. F.
DISEASES OF THE FE- MALE GENERATIVE SYSTEM (*continued*). *Uterine Appendages*— Broad Ligament, Cyst of	4	...	4	...	...																		1				2								1						
„ „ Inflam- mation of	2	...	2	...	...																		1				1														
Hydro-salpinx	2	...	2	...	...																1		1																		
Pyo-salpinx	3	...	3	...	...																		2																1		
Salpingitis	19	...	19	...	...																1		9				5				4										
Ovaries, Cyst of	2	...	2	...	...																1		1				1														
„ Dermoid Tumour of	4	...	4	...	...																		1				3														
„ Malignant Growth of	6	...	6	...	...																2		2				1				1										
„ Suppuration of	1	...	1	...	...																		1																		
„ Tumour of	19	...	19	...	...																2		5				3				4				4				1		
„ Abscess in ...	5	...	5	...	...																		1				3				1										
Pelvis, Deformity of	1	...	1	...	...																																		1		
„ Inflammation in ...	2	...	2	...	...																		1				1														
„ „ Sequelæ of	3	...	3	...	...																						2				1										
„ Pain in	12	...	12	...	...																2		5								4				1						
„ Tumour in ...	3	...	3	...	...																		1				2														
Parametritis	6	...	6	...	...																		3				3														
„ Sequelæ of ...	1	...	1	...	...																		1																		
Perimetritis	11	...	10	...	**1**																		5				2	**1**			3										
„ Sequelæ of ...	8	...	8	...	...																1		4				2				1										
Sterility	1	...	1	...	...																		1																		
Total	311	...	309	...	**2**																																				

TABLE I. (*continued*).

DISEASE	Total	Discharged M.	Discharged F.	Died M.	Died F.	—30 Disch. F.	—30 Died M.	—40 Disch. F.	—50 Disch. F.
DISEASES CONNECTED WITH PREGNANCY AND PARTURITION.									
Pregnancy	3	...	3	...	...	2			1
Pregnancy complicated with—									
Abdominal Pain	4	...	4	...	...	1		2	1
Bronchitis	1	...	1	...	...			1	
Contracted Pelvis	5	...	5	...	...	2		2	1
Hæmorrhage	7	...	7	...	...	3		3	1
Hysterical Convulsions	1	...	1	...	...	1			
Heart Disease ...	3	...	3	...	...	1		2	
" and Phthisis	1	...	...	...	1		1		
Nephritis ...	3	...	2	...	...	2		1	
Retroversion of Uterus	1	...	1	...	...			1	
Tumour (Ovarian)	4	...	4	...	...	4			
Vomiting ...	1	...	1	...	...	1			
Molar Pregnancy—									
Carneous Mole ...	1	...	1	...	...	1			
Hydatidiform Mole	3	...	3	...	...	3			

TABLE I. (*continued*).

DISEASE	Total	Discharged M	Discharged F	Died M	Died F	Under 5	—10	—15	—20	—30	—40	—50	—60	Over 60
DISEASES CONNECTED WITH PREGNANCY AND PARTURITION (*continued*).														
Pregnancy, Extra-uterine—														
Tubal Gestation	7		7						3	3	3	1		
Tubal Rupture	4		4						2	2	2			
Tubal Abortion	2		2							1		1		
Tubal Mole	2		2						1	1	1	1		
Abortion—														
Incomplete	13		13						7	7	5	1		
Inevitable	20		20						9	9	9	2		
Repeated	1		1							1	1			
Sequelae of	2		2						1	1	1			
Threatened	16		16						4	4	7	4		
Parturition—	2		2								2			
Labour—														
Normal	1		1								1			
Abnormal—														
Caesarian Section	1				1					1				
Placenta Previa	5		5						2	2	3			
Prolonged	2		2						1	1				
Transverse Presentation	2		2						1		1			

D

TABLE I. (continued).

34

DISEASE	Total	Discharged		Died		Under 5.				− 10.				− 15.				− 20.				− 30.				− 40.				− 50.				− 60.				Over 60.			
		M.	F.	M.	F.	M.	F.	M.	F.	M.	F.	M.	F.	M.	F.	M.	F.	M.	F.	M.	F.	M.	F.	M.	F.	M.	F.	M.	F.	M.	F.	M.	F.	M.	F.	M.	F.	M.	F.	M.	F.
DISEASES CONNECTED WITH PREGNANCY AND PARTURITION (continued).																																									
Parturition (continued)—																																										
Labour (continued)—																																										
Sequelæ of ...																																										
,, Perineum, Rupture of ...	2		2																								2														
,, Placenta Retained	12		12																				5				5				1				1						
,, Pyæmia after ...	1				1																				1																
,, Sapræmia after ...	1				1																				1																
,, Septicæmia after ...	4		2		2																		2						2												
,, Uterus, Subinvolution of...	2		2																												2											
	3		3																												1				2						
Total	143		137		6																																				

TABLE I. (continued).

DISEASE.	Total	Discharged M.	Discharged F.	Died M.	Died F.
DISEASES OF THE CUTANEOUS SYSTEM.					
Darier's Disease	1	...	1	...	...
Dermatitis	1	...	1	...	...
Dermatitis Exfoliativa	1	...	1	...	...
Eczema	8	6	2	...	...
Erythema	3	1	2	...	...
Erythema Multiforme	1	...	1	...	...
Erythema Haemorrhagicum	2	...	2	...	...
Erythema Nodosum	9	2	7	...	...
Favus	1	...	1	...	...
Impetigo Contagiosa	1	...	1	...	...
Lichen Pilaris	1	1	...	...	...
Lupus Vulgaris	3	1	2	...	...
Pemphigus	2	...	2	...	...
Psoriasis	3	2	1	...	...
Purpura	5	1	2	1	1
Tuberculous disease of Skin	1	...	1	...	...
Xeroderma	1	...	1	...	...
Scleroderma	1	1	...	...	...
Urticaria	1	1	...	...	...
Keratosis Pilaris	1	1	...	...	...
Total	**47**	**17**	**28**	**1**	**1**

TABLE I. (*continued*).

POISONS.	Total.	Discharged M.	Discharged F.	Died M.	Died F.
Carbon-bisulphide ...	1	1			
Creolin ...	1	1			
Lead	4	3	1		
Nitric Acid ...	1				1
Opium	2	2			
Oxalic Acid ...	2	2			
Ptomaine ...	2	2			
Total ...	13	11	1	...	1

ABSTRACT OF TABLE I.

With Average Duration of Stay of Medical Patients in the Hospital.

DISEASES.	Total Number of Cases completed during the Year 1904.	Number of Cases discharged.		Deaths.		Remaining in the Hospital at the end of the Year 1904.
		M.	F.	M.	F.	
GENERAL DISEASES, A ...	185	90	63	18	14	
Do. B ...	310	132	153	15	10	
MISCELLANEOUS DISEASES	59	28	15	10	6	
LOCAL DISEASES—						
Diseases of the Nervous System	300	142	104	36	18	
,, Circulatory System	226	107	63	37	19	
,, Respiratory System	556	339	141	44	32	
,, Digestive System	346	150	145	31	20	
,, Urinary System	98	44	32	16	6	
,, Female Generative System	311	...	309	...	2	
,, connected with Pregnancy	143	...	187	...	6	
,, of the Cutaneous System	47	17	28	1	1	
DISEASES NOT NECESSARILY ASSOCIATED WITH GENERAL OR LOCAL DISEASES—						
POISONS	13	11	1	...	1	
	2,594	1,060	1,191	208	135	240
		2,251		343		
		2,594				

AVERAGE STAY OF—
Men ... ... 32·47 days.
Women ... ... 30·06 ,,

INDEX

OF THE DISEASES AND CHIEF SYMPTOMS OF PATIENTS IN THE MEDICAL WARDS DURING THE YEAR 1904.

N.B.—The mark (†) signifies that a case terminated fatally; a number in brackets, e.g. ‡ (82), indicates the page in the Post-mortem Register, Vol. XXXI., on which the notes of the autopsy will be found; (s) that a Surgical Post-mortem was made.

ABDOMINAL—
    Influenza—Males, II., 18.
    Malignant Growth—Females, V., 168; VI., 171, 473.
    Pain—Males, I., 89; II., 2, 14, 24; IV., 32, 63, 162; V., 74A, 223.
        Females, III., 100; IV., 92, 100; VI., 13.
    Tumour—Males, III., 73‡ (7); IV., 131; V., 66.
        Females, II., 88; III., 68; VI., 171.
ABORTION—Females, I., 74, 97, 157; VI., 29, 113, 220, 221A, 224, 287, 314, 316,
    319, 372, 379, 452.
    Incomplete—Females, VI., 1, 20, 83, 88, 207, 243, 269, 282, 304, 307, 326,
        330, 335, 360, 373, 374, 411, 416, 420, 459.
    Induced—Females, VI., 72, 198.
    Inevitable—Females, VI., 329.
    Recent—Females, VI., 145, 341, 431.
    Repeated—Females, VI., 47, 259,
    Sequelæ of—Females, VI., 2, 5, 84, 100, 129, 253, 297, 366, 378, 382, 413,
        427, 449.
    Threatened—Females, VI., 201, 317.
    Tubal—Females, VI., 165, 204.
ABSCESS—
    Alveolar—Females, I., 25.
    Cerebral—Females, II., 2A‡ (73).
    Cerebellar—Females, II., 2A‡ (73).
    Ischio-Rectal—Males, V., 70.
    Labial—Females, VI., 387.
    Liver—Males, I., 76, 211‡ (s); IV., 85; V., 210‡ (s).
    Lung—Males, II., 109†; IV., 117‡ (211).
    Parotid—Females, III., 132; V., 157.
    Pelvic—Females, V., 166‡ (212); VI., 211, 244, 350‡ (s), 429, 434, 478.
    Sterno-clavicular Joint—Females, VI., 328†.
    Subdiaphragmatic—Males, I., 78‡ (s); IV., 139.
    Submaxillary—Females, I., 151A.
    Thigh—Females, VI., 328†.
    Tonsil—Males, II., 44; Females, II., 50.
ADDISON'S DISEASE—Males, I., 4, 204‡ (59); V., 191. Females, II., 68†.
ADENOID VEGETATIONS—Males, II., 31, 44. Females, III., 4; V., 97†.
ALBUMINURIA—Males, II., 124B; III., 177; V., 175. Females, II., 26; IV., 167.
ALCOHOLISM—Males, III., 21, 132‡ (112), 183, 263; V., 215‡ (179). Females,
    III., 146.

AMENORRHŒA—Females, VI., 438.

AMENTIA—Males, V., 197.

AMNESIA, Males, V., 190.

AMYLOID DISEASE—Males, I., 192.

ANÆMIA—Males, I., 108 ; II., 22, 94, 180, 150, 212, 223‡ (126) ; III., 10 ; V., 101,
157. Females, I., 37, 62, 113, 164 ; II., 17, 61, 77, 99, 104, 110, 115 ;
III., 21, 42, 54, 104‡ (175), 133 ; IV., 12, 153 ; V., 3, 41, 49, 50, 124,
144, 148 ; VI., 393.
Pernicious—Males, II., 196‡ (325) ; III., 220‡ (256). Females, I.,
148‡ (198) ; V., 90.

ANÆSTHESIA—Females, III., 53.
Of Face—Females, I., 12.

ANASARCA—Males, II., 33‡ (36), 124, 124A, 124B ; III., 43 ; V., 40‡ (42).
Females, I., 17†, 28 ; II., 26 ; III., 24, 74, 156‡ (313) ; IV., 2 ; V., 1 ;
VI., 235.

ANEURYSM—
Aortic, Abdominal—Males, I., 169, 234‡ (s) ; II., 79, 186, 231‡ (s), 244‡
(74).
——— Thoracic—Males, I., 30, 157, 178, 190, 221 ; II., 175, 189 ; III., 74,
127, 151 ; IV., 9, 9A, 82†, 132 ; V., 33, 226‡ (294), 336. Females, I., 124.
Brachial Artery—Female, III., 158‡ (240).
Cerebral Artery—Males, II., 57‡ (19) ; IV., 10‡ (35).

ANGINA—Males, V., 79.

ANUS, Prolapse of—Males, II., 72.

APHASIA—Males, I., 25, 51, 153, 189 ; II., 19, 150 ; III., 293 ; IV., 21. Females,
I., 42 ; II., 5‡ (4).

APPENDICECTOMY—Males, II., 67 ; III., 273 ; IV., 62, 229. Females, I., 92, 196,
III., 151 ; V., 147, 169† ; VI., 309.

APPENDICITIS—Males, I., 219, 244 ; II., 1, 62, 67, 108, 111, 200‡ (162) ; III., 273,
291 ; IV., 62, 229. Females, I., 92, 196 ; III., 151 ; IV., 73, 155‡ (262) ;
VI., 309.

APPENDIX, Congestion of—Males, V., 37.

ARTERIES—
Arterio-sclerosis—Males, I., 22, 112, 145 ; III., 116‡ (130), 164, 201, 240‡
(267). Females, II., 145‡ (279) ; III., 156‡ (313) ; IV., 175‡ (328).
Embolism of—
Basilar—Females, I., 103‡ (108).
Brachial—Females, II., 23‡ (15).
Middle Cerebral—Females, II., 23‡ (15) ; V., 137.
Puncture of Intercostal—Males, III., 114‡ (94).
Thrombosis of Basilar—Males, III., 240‡ (267).

ARTERIO-SCLEROSIS—See Arteries.

ARTHRITIS—Males, I., 174 ; IV., 164 ; V., 97.
Gonorrhœal—Males, II., 63 ; III., 3, 33 ; V., 9 ; Females, III., 41 ; V., 80.
Hæmophilic—Males, I., 174.
Multiple—Males, V., 231 ; Females, I., 86, 198 ; IV., 120, 170 ; V., 86,
88, 88A.
Rheumatoid—Males, III., 31, 58 ; V., 177.
Suppurative—Males, V., 52‡ (79).
Syphilitic—Males, III., 98.
Tuberculous—Females, I., 67.
See also Osteo-arthritis.

ASCARIS LUMBRICOIDES—II., 78.

ASCITES—Males, I., 114‡ (257), 122, 147‡ (160), 148‡ (215), 193 ; II., 34, 61, 103
103A, 103B, 103E†, 124, 124A, 124B, 136†, 181, 235‡ (248) ; III., 53†,
114‡ (94), 144, 222, 262 ; IV., 1, 29, 137‡ (113) ; V., 105, 152.
Females, I., 48‡ (51) ; II., 3, 4, 4A‡ (92), 143, 148‡ (125) ; IV., 97 ;
V., 7‡ (5) ; VI., 171, 242.

ASTHMA—Females, I., 140, 161 ; II., 130‡ (258), 134.

ATROPHY, Muscular—Males, III., 229. Females, I., 40 ; III., 53.
    ,,   Progressive—See Myelitis, Chronic Anterior Polio-.

ATHEROMA—See Arterio-sclerosis.

ATHETOSIS—Males, III., 110.

BEDSORE—Females, V., 164‡ (275).

BLADDER—
    Contracted—Females, VI., 68.
    Foreign Body in—Females, I., 152.
    Malignant Growth of—Females, IV., 177 ; VI., 349.

BRAIN—See Cerebral.

BREAST, Malignant Growth of—Females, IV., 70‡ (119).

BRONCHIECTASIS—Males, I., 231‡ (136) ; II., 112, 139 ; III., 161 ; IV., 4 ; V., 125;
Females, I., 199‡ (324) ; II., 84‡ (140) ; III., 147A ; V., 75‡ (77).

BRONCHITIS—Males, I., 13, 31, 33, 45, 50, 56, 88, 96, 98, 113, 171, 176, 210, 218,
230 ; II., 8, 20, 28, 41, 43, 48, 51, 52, 70‡ (67), 88‡ (56), 96, 237†, 238 ;
III., 19, 20‡ (20), 38, 43, 46, 47, 76, 78, 82, 88, 92, 96, 105, 107, 109, 113,
134, 169, 203, 215‡ (186), 236, 266, 281 ; IV., 15, 59, 67, 91, 143, 147,
149, 151, 153, 168, 218 ; V., 43, 48, 78, 89, 107, 144, 145, 153, 173, 179,
192‡ (290), 200‡ (299), 218. Radcliffe—7. Females, I., 4, 9, 10, 81, 86,
94, 96, 110‡ (154), 116, 140, 161, 167, 172‡ (280), 183 ; II., 55‡ (95), 58,
65, 100†, 109, 130‡ (258), 133, 134, 144 ; III., 47, 52, 80, 115, 145, 156‡
(313) ; IV., 6, 6A, 27, 32, 33, 53, 63, 71, 140, 185 ; V., 6, 12, 14, 18, 19,
22‡ (58), 24, 38, 52, 60‡ (103), 67, 102†, 105, 122, 128, 150, 152, 153,
173‡ (320) ; VI., 59, 301, 437‡ (282). Radcliffe—40‡ (324).
    Fœtid—Females, V., 37.
    Plastic—Females, V., 61.

BRONCHO-PNEUMONIA—See Pneumonia, Catarrhal.

BRONCHUS, Rupture of Empyema into—Females, I., 132.

BUBO, Inguinal—Males, II., 8.

CÆSARIAN SECTION—Females, VI., 435‡ (312).

CALCULUS—
    Biliary—Males, I., 202‡ (s). Females, II., 117 ; V., 146, 172.
    Renal—Males, II., 242 ; III., 218, 220‡ (256), 272‡ (305) ; IV., 52, 125.
      Females, IV., 181 ; VI., 28A‡ (54).
    Vesical—Females, VI., 399.

CANCER—See Malignant Growth.

CARBUNCLE—Females, I., 91.

CARCINOMA—See Malignant Growth.

CARDIALGIA—Females, I., 37 ; III., 7.

CATARRH, Universal—Females, I., 60.

CELLULITIS—
    Foot—Males, II., 209.
    Hand—Females, I., 153.
    Leg—Females, IV., 186.
    Neck—Males, Radcliffe, 4‡ (3), 20. Females, III., 120. Radcliffe—20.

CEREBELLAR—
　　Abscess—Females, II., 2A‡ (73).
　　Cyst—Males, III.. 216.
　　Tumour—Males, III., 67.

CEREBRAL—
　　Abscess—Females, II., 2A‡ (73).
　　Diplegia—Females, V., 78.
　　Embolism—Males, I., 25, 246‡ (146) ; II., 57, 287‡ (234) ; IV., 116.
　　　　Females, I., 42 ; II., 5‡ (4), 23‡ (15), 149† ; V., 137.
　　Hæmorrhage—Males, I., 38‡ (30), 42, 110, 199, 209‡ (284), 227 ; II., 19, 87,
　　　　234 ; III., 8, 116‡ (130), 178‡ (304), 181‡ (295), 225‡ (307), 295‡ (235);
　　　　IV., 10‡ (35), 65†, 154‡ (268) ; V., 16†.　Females, II., 145‡ (279) ;
　　　　VI., 480.
　　Sinus, Thrombosis of—Females, I., 7‡ (25).
　　Syphilis—Males, I., 168 ; V., 65†, 132, 156.　Females. I., 187.
　　Thrombosis—Males, I., 153 ; IV., 21.
　　Tumour—Males, I., 44, 116 ; III., 81, 255‡ (283), 278 ; V., 62.　Females,
　　　　III., 92 ; IV., 75.

CHILBLAIN—Females, III., 18.

CHOLECYST-ENTEROSTOMY—Males, II., 195‡ (s).

CHOLECYSTOTOMY—Females, III., 157† ; V., 146, 172.

CHOREA—Males, I., 6, 75, 84, 103, 137, 160, 191 ; II., 13, 126, 177 ; III., 14, 83, 111,
　　　　185 ; V., 68, 147, 158.　Females, I., 2, 50, 53, 73, 89, 160, 173, 185 ;
　　　　II., 20, 59, 97, 126, 142 ; III., 3, 26, 102, 116 ; IV., 15, 22, 36, 69, 85, 95,
　　　　96 ; V., 2, 5, 9, 20, 33, 52, 71, 116, 126.　*Radcliffe*—28.

COLIC, Biliary—Males, III., 150.　Females, II., 62, 157.
　　Intestinal—Males, II., 153 ; III., 102 ; IV., 87, 112 ; V., 134.
　　Lead—Males, IV., 148, 183.
　　Renal—Males, II., 240 ; IV., 33 ; V., 46.　Females, IV., 181.

COLITIS—Males, II., 190.
　　Membranous—Females, III., 71.
　　Mucous—Males, II., 18.　Females, IV., 68, 179.
　　Ulcerative—Males, III., 190‡ (s).　Females, I., 197.

COLLAPSE—Females, I., 142.

COLOTOMY—Females, I., 197 ; III., 125‡ (s).

COLPORRAPHY—Females, VI., 8, 34, 247, 250, 268, 286, 377, 381.

COLPOTOMY—Females, VI., 12, 28, 36, 86, 112, 155, 165, 170, 204, 211, 283, 313
　　　　403, 421, 429, 434, 457.

COMA—Males, II., 160 ; III., 44‡ (14) ; IV., 154‡ (268) ; V., 215‡ (179).
　　Diabetic—Males, V., 140‡ (63), 174.

CONDYLOMATA—Females, IV., 1.

CONJUNCTIVITIS—Males, I., 12‡ (1).

CONSTIPATION—Males, III., 160 ; V., 180.　Females, I., 64, 68, 77, 84, 109, 135,
　　　　170 ; II., 7, 37 ; III., 100, 101 ; VI., 92, 96, 439, 470.

CONVULSIONS—Males, III., 56, 103, 132‡ (112), 200 ; IV., 153.　Females, IV., 63,
　　　　65, 109‡ (173), 125, 180‡ (319).

CYCLITIS—Males, V., 62.

CYST, Tubo-ovarian—Females, VI., 332.

CYSTITIS—Males, I., 95 ; II., 174‡ (255), 223‡ (126) ; III., 235.   Females, I., 152 ;
    III., 29, 95 ; IV., 93 ; V., 166‡ (212) ; VI., 338.

CYSTOCELE—Females, VI., 24, 50, 231, 247, 250, 268, 381, 401.

CYSTOTOMY, Supra-pubic—Females, I., 152.

DACTYLITIS, Tuberculous—Males, III., 69.

DEAFNESS—Males, I., 230.

DEBILITY—Males, III., 131 ; IV., 2, 6.   Females, I., 65 ; VI., 130, 400.

DELIRIUM—Males, I., 110 ; IV., 98, 98A.†   Females, IV., 175‡ (328).

DELIRIUM TREMENS—Males, II., 232.   Females, II., 109 ; V., 99‡ (241).

DEMENTIA—See Insanity.

DENTAL CARIES—Males, III., 283.

DERMATITIS—Males, I., 43, 43A.   Females, II., 25 ; V., 145.
    Exfoliativa—Females, V., 76.
    Hæmorrhagica—Females, I., 49.

DIABETES—
    Mellitus—Males, I., 73, 207 ; III., 27, 239, 267† ; IV., 121, 188 ; V., 71,
        140‡ (96), 168‡ (263).   Females, I., 91 ; II., 38, 88, 136, 151 ; III., 55,
        141, 143 ; IV., 59.
    Insipidus—Males, III., 170.   Females, I., 107 ; III., 22 ; V., 44.

DIARRHŒA—Males, I., 88 ; II., 225 ; III., 60, 234 ; IV., 64, 112, 133, 134‡ (129),
    156‡ (128), 159, 178 ; V., 206.   Females, I., 183 ; III., 30, 69, 83, 109 ;
    IV., 17, 72‡ (121), 125, 132‡ (222), 168, 185 ; V., 10†, 69‡ (76), 91.

DIPHTHERIA—Males, III., 198 ; IV., 180 ; V., 11‡ (34).   Radcliffe—6, 7, 10‡ (88),
    15, 30‡ (87), 31‡ (250), 32, 35, 39, 42, 40‡ (324).   Females, I., 199‡
    (324) ; II., 89.   Radcliffe—13, 16, 17, 18, 22‡ (89), 27‡ (213) 30, 40‡
    (324), 45.

DISSEMINATED SCLEROSIS—See Sclerosis.

DUODENUM—
    Dilatation of—Females, I., 114, 114A‡ (74) ; VI., 285.
    Malignant growth of—Females, I., 114, 114A‡ (74) ; VI., 285.
    Ulcer of—Males, I., 233, 243‡ (72).
        With Hæmatemesis—Males, I., 243‡ (72).

DYSENTERY—Males, III., 140 ; V., 135.   Females, I., 101.

DYSMENORRHŒA—Females, VI., 6, 49, 102, 150, 173, 174, 185, 189, 208, 210, 228,
    228A, 237, 274, 278, 394.

DYSPAREUNIA—Females, VI., 276, 394.

DYSPEPSIA—Males, II., 207 ; III., 106, 251, 260 ; IV., 119, 163 ; V., 95.   Females,
    I., 15, 31, 78, 84, 87 ; II., 83, 91, 119 ; III., 78 ; V., 3.

DYSPHAGIA—Males, III., 16.

DYSPNŒA—Females, IV., 83, 139.

ECTHYMA —Cachecticum—Females, II., 121.

ECZEMA—Males, I., 54 ; II., 115 ; V., 58, 64, 131, 186.   Females, I., 39, 86 ;
    III., 4 ; V., 99‡ (241).

ELEPHANTIASIS—Males, I., 150.

EMANSIO MENSIUM—Females, VI., 99, 438.

EMPHYSEMA—Males, I., 13, 96, 112 ; II., 43, 48, 96 ; III., 82, 109, 113, 134, 209, 281 ; IV., 15, 77‡ (99), 147, 149, 150, 227‡ (327) ; V., 99, 145. *Radcliffe*—31‡ (250). Females, I., 81 ; III., 115, 156‡ (313) ; IV., 33 ; V., 18, 24, 173‡ (320).

EMPYEMA—Males, I., 33, 78‡ (8), 149, 224‡ (266), 240 ; II., 38‡ (9) ; III., 162, 245‡ (285), 248‡ (116) ; IV., 14, 110, 117‡ (211) ; V., 3, 117, 143, 210‡ (8), 221. Females, I., 132 ; II., 60‡ (118) ; III., 17‡ (10), 138‡ (310); IV., 102‡ (122), 112‡ (177) ; V., 75‡ (77) ; VI., 437‡ (282).
    Sequelæ of—Females, II., 2A‡ (73), 13A.
    With Resection of Rib—Males. I., 59 ; II., 122, 224 ; IV., 181‡ (200) ; V., 47. Females, I., 36, 106 ; II., 2, 13 ; III., 107, 224.

ENDOCARDITIS –
    Acute Simple—Males, I., 103, 105, 137 ; III., 40, 87, 277 ; IV., 155, 174‡ (276), 221‡ (311) ; V., 52‡ (79), 161‡ (243), 220‡ (105). Females, I., 103‡ (108), 117‡ (102) ; II., 156‡ (270) ; III., 112‡ (230), 136‡ (293); V., 164‡ (275). *Radcliffe*—28.
    Ulcerative, Infective, or Malignant—Males, I., 32‡ (33), 242‡ (214), 246‡ (146) ; II., 11‡ (38), 30‡ (17), 57‡ (19), 65‡ (18), 160‡ (85) ; III., 72‡ (6), 73‡ (7), 287‡ (234), 300‡ (28) ; IV., 30, 226‡ (264) ; V., 76‡ (135), 240‡ (127). Females, I., 147‡ (195); II., 23‡ (15), III., 158‡ (240); IV., 66‡ (98) ; V., 95‡ (226) ; VI., 64‡ (13), 292‡ (195).

See also Heart.

ENDOMETRITIS—Female, VI., 80, 189, 200, 211, 241, 261, 274, 305, 308, 311, 333, 396, 410, 463.
    Hypertrophic—Females, VI., 387.
    Septic—Females, VI., 64‡ (13), 435‡ (312), 437‡ (282).

ENTERALGIA—Males, I., 214.

ENTERITIS—Males, I., 49, 151 ; II., 171 ; III., 130 ; V., 214. Females, II., 78 ; III., 107‡ (224).

EPILEPSY—Males, I., 52, 123, 168, 238 ; II., 6, 118, 148 ; III., 32 ; IV., 5, 126, 144 ; V., 174, 175. Females, I., 43, 63, 151A, 157 ; IV., 80.
    Jacksonian—Males, IV., 68 ; V., 104.

EPIPHYSITIS—Males, III., 247.

EPISTAXIS—Males, I., 11. Females, I., 72 ; III., 104‡ (175) ; IV., 107 ; V., 159‡ (153).

ERYSIPELAS—Males, III., 193 ; V., 239. Females, I., 192, 194 ; V., 167.

ERYTHEMA—Males, I., 173 ; IV., 20. Females, I., 30 ; IV., 119, 141.
    Hæmorrhagicum—Females, IV., 41.
    Marginatum—Females, I., 117‡ (102).
    Multiforme—Females, I., 112, 125 ; IV., 17.
    Nodosum—Males, I., 181 ; III., 211. Females, III., 39 ; IV., 20, 38, 54, 147, 158, 169 ; V., 27, 56.

EXOPHTHALMIC GOÎTRE—Males, II., 170 ; III., 5, 155 ; IV., 197 ; V., 73. Females, II., 4, 4A‡ (92), 30, 36, 90, 154 ; III., 30, 84, 87 ; IV., 58, 86, 163 ; V., 51, 97†, 109.

FAVUS—Females, I., 111.

FEBRICULA—Males, I., 16, 80, 126 ; IV., 39 ; V. 4. Females, I., 72, 130.

FÆCAL IMPACTION—Males, V., 116.

FEVER—Males, I., 188, 188A ; II., 71, 247 ; III., 143 ; IV., 18, 54 ; V., 178. Females, I., 137, 145, 166 ; IV., 128 ; V., 86, 107.

FISTULA—
  Anal—Females, I., 197.
  Fæcal—Females, I., 26‡ (s) ; VI., 30‡ (s).
  Recto-vaginal—Females, VI., 103.
  Vesico-vaginal—Females, VI., 399, 403, 406.
FLATULENCE—Females, VI., 397, 448.
FRIEDREICH'S ATAXY—Males, I., 37. Females, I., 23.

GALL-BLADDER, Empyema of—Males, IV., 137‡ (113).
GASTRIC EROSION—Females, II., 150.
GASTRIC ULCER—Males, I., 78‡ (s), 228‡ (s) ; II., 12†, 94, 106, 127 ; III., 4, 84‡ (106),
  122‡ (152), 207, 289 ; IV., 11, 175, 187 ; V., 38, 42, 51, 59, 228. Females,
  I., 21, 22, 60, 66, 70, 108, 122, 156, 159, 190‡ (s) ; II., 21, 24, 27†, 29, 35,
  37A, 44, 61, 77, 81, 89, 96, 137, 147 ; III., 6, 20, 48, 56, 72, 111, 130, 132,
  134 ; IV., 8, 16, 26, 42, 50, 62, 90, 114, 116, 130, 135, 160, 174, 178, 182,
  V., 16, 21, 26, 41, 42, 46, 53, 54, 63, 79, 157.
GASTRITIS—Males, I., 60, 87, 185, 194 ; II., 36, 219 ; III., 36, 184, 259 ; V., 137,
  163. Females, I , 74, 77, 155, 169, 171 ; III., 8, 36, 46, 97, 121, 139 ;
  IV., 14, 103, 142, 161, 184 ; V., 64, 87, 112, 153, 160.
GASTRODYNIA—Females, II., 69, 80, 114 ; V., 124.
GASTRO-ENTERITIS—Males, II., 39, 59, 191, 206‡ (209) ; III., 154, 158, 194‡ (207),
  196, 197, 256, 265 ; IV., 95, 157‡ (170). Females, I., 102, 134, 141, 142 ;
  II., 127 ; III., 76, 93, 96 ; IV., 89, 105‡ (142), 109‡ (173), 118, 140 ;
  V., 92‡ (219), 115†, 140.
GASTRO-ENTEROSTOMY—Males, V., 208. Females, I., 88‡ (s), 191‡ (s); III., 152‡ (s).
GASTROTOMY—Females, I., 190‡ (s) ; II., 27†.
GERMAN MEASLES—Females, V., 78.
GESTATION, Tubal—See Pregnancy, Extra-uterine.
GLANDS, LYMPHATIC—
  Enlarged—Males, V., 23. Females, III., 66 ; V., 4.
  Malignant Growth in—Males, I., 97‡ (83) ; V., 144. Females, III., 154‡
    (321) ; IV., 21‡ (27).
  Tuberculous—Males, I., 36‡ (23), 86‡ (101), III., 69. Females, III, 66 ;
    V., 82‡ (141), 161.
GLYCOSURIA—Males, III., 85 ; V., 213. Females, III., 50, 86.
GONORRHŒA—Males, III., 8. Females, VI., 175.
GOUT—Males, I., 52, 135, 145 ; II., 4, 239 ; III., 85, 157, 237 ; IV., 23, 47, 147,
  217 ; V., 5, 126, 145, 194. Females, IV., 144.
GUMS, Hæmorrhage from—Females, I., 24.

HÆMATEMESIS—Males, II., 116 ; III., 4, 44‡ (14), 84‡ (106), 122‡ (152), 269, 289 ;
  IV., 11, 29, 100, 100A, 104 ; V., 51, 59, 87‡ (205), 228. Females, I., 20,
  66, 70, 108, 122, 159, 190‡ (s) ; II., 21, 24, 29, 70‡ (139), 81, 137, 150 ;
  III., 20, 130, 132 ; IV., 42, 50, 62, 90, 116, 178 ; V., 21, 58‡ (109).
HÆMATOCELE, Pelvic—Females, VI., 9, 193, 204, 283, 313, 384.
HÆMONEPHROSIS—Males, I., 236.
HÆMATURIA—Males, I., 203 ; II., 21, 174‡ (255) ; IV., 42, 111, 231 ; V., 46.
  Females, I., 17†, 48‡ (51), 62, 152 ; III., 91 ; IV., 46 ; VI., 48.

HÆMOGLOBINURIA—Males, II., 76 ; III., 264.

HÆMOPHILIA—Males, I., 174, 206 ; IV., 164.

HÆMOPTYSIS—Males, I., 23, 81, 152‡ (197) ; II., 23, 89, 113 ; III., 49‡ (45), 101† ; III., 163, 189, 227, 268 ; IV., 28, 115 ; V., 100, 220‡ (105). Females, I., 95 ; III., 45‡ (75), 144 ; IV., 88.

HÆMORRHOIDS—Males, IV., 61. Females, VI., 294, 338.

HEADACHE—Males, III., 283. Females, I., 75 ; IV., 136.

HEART DISEASE—
    Arythmia—Males, II., 104. Females, III., 11.
    Asthenia—Males, IV., 40. Females, IV., 144.
    Bradycardia—Males, II., 82, 134.
    Congenital—Males, III., 20‡ (20) ; IV., 102. Females, II., 60‡ (118) ; IV., 101.
    Dilatation—Males, I., 6, 13, 22, 112, 122, 171 ; II., 9, 9†, 11‡ (38), 33‡ (36), 52, 88‡ (56), 124B, 173‡ (167) ; III., 6, 184, 219, 222 ; IV., 77‡ (99), 218 ; V., 43, 109‡ (201), 130, 158, 218. Females, I., 17†, 51, 54, 131, 150, 151♠ ; II., 92 ; IV., 19‡ (29), 30‡ (37), 93 ; V., 22‡ (58), 56, 164‡ (275), 173‡ (320).
    Fatty Degeneration—Males, IV., 66, 160†. Females, 124‡ (149) ; II., 156‡ (270) ; V., 164‡ (275), 173‡ (320) ; VI., 334‡ (144).
    Fatty Infiltration—Females, V., 173‡ (320) ; VI., 334‡ (144).
    Fibroid Degeneration—Females, III., 156‡ (313).
    Hypertrophy—Males, II., 178 ; III., 51.
    Myocardial Degeneration—Males, I., 70, 162 ; III., 147.
    Myocarditis—Males, II., 222 ; III., 277 ; IV., 221‡ (311).
    Palpitation—Males, III., 214.
    Tachycardia—Males, II., 82, 105.
        Paroxysmal—Males, IV., 120‡ (145).

VALVULAR DISEASE—
    Aortic, Regurgitation—Males, I., 23, 30, 39, 146, 152‡ (197), 178, 198, 235, 242‡ (214), 246‡ (146) ; II., 1, 7, 27, 27A, 65‡ (18), 73, 75, 79, 90, 100, 121, 140, 154, 156, 161 ; III., 2, 22, 39, 50, 51, 62, 68, 128, 179, 203, 300‡ (28) ; IV., 12, 19, 24, 30, 44, 90, 109, 120‡ (145), 146†, 200, 208 ; V., 18, 77, 79, 97, 109‡ (201), 118, 129, 152, 161‡ (243), 170, 172. Females, VI., 334‡ (144).
    ———— Obstruction—Males, I., 146, 178, 198, 235 ; II., 156 ; III., 128, 300‡ (28) ; V., 152, 172. Females, III., 91.
    ———— Double—Males, III., 72‡ (6), 73‡ (7). Females, III., 44, 158‡ (240) ; IV., 173.
    Mitral, Regurgitation—Males, I., 6, 9, 23, 25, 26, 30, 39, 71, 72, 122, 138, 178, 191, 242‡ (214) ; II., 7, 27, 46, 65‡ (18), 73, 75, 77, 90, 100, 110, 121, 136†, 150, 222, 228 ; III., 2, 6, 11, 14, 22, 23, 28, 35, 39, 50, 51, 54, 62, 68, 71, 72‡ (6), 95, 104, 107, 108, 176, 191, 292‡ (295) ; IV., 12, 19, 24, 30, 44, 46, 71, 75, 80, 90, 106, 109, 127, 130, 149, 155, 175, 185, 198, 208, 220 ; V., 18, 29, 30, 31‡ (48), 40‡ (42), 43, 44, 76‡ (135), 79, 84, 92, 97, 103, 161‡ (243). Females, I., 2, 5, 28, 47, 59, 64, 83, 89, 90, 117‡ (102), 128, 129, 131, 138, 143, 151A, 185, 196 ; II., 55‡ (95), 56, 59, 92, 124‡ (149), 126, 128, 131, 149†, 154, 156‡ (270) ; III., 1, 12, 21, 27, 49, 59, 63, 85, 94, 110, 116, 119, 137, 149, 156‡ (313) ; IV., 11, 52, 67, 69, 76, 77†, 85, 99, 104, 107, 124, 131†, 133, 139, 151, 157, 171 ; V., 28, 30, 68, 98, 105, 110, 111, 120, 125, 126, 128, 147 ; VI., 432.
    ———— Obstruction—Males, I., 17, 147‡ (160), ; II., 162‡ (159), 238 ; III., 140, 179 ; V., 56, 220‡ (105). Females, I., 85, 127, 182 ; II., 5‡ (4), 10, 20, 23‡ (15), 45, 47 ; IV., 6, 6A, 31, 46, 108, 126, 129 ; V., 217.
    ———— Double—Males, I., 129, 146, 163, 235 ; II., 5, 27A, 57‡ (19), 145‡ (229) ; III., 25, 37, 40, 83, 144, 145, 177, 213‡ (186), 221, 238, 252, 287‡ (234) ; IV., 98, 98A†, 116, 120‡ (145), 179 ; V., 17, 109‡ (201), 152, 161‡ (243), 169, 172, 183, 192‡ (290). Females, I., 54, 125, 167 ; II., 3, 9 ; III., 5, 7, 26, 33, 58, 112‡ (230), 118, 148 ; IV., 27, 64, 78, 150, 166 ; V., 11, 13, 23, 73, 137 ; VI., 175, 292‡ (195).

HEART DISEASE—*continued.*

   VALVULAR DISEASE—*continued.*
      Mitral and Aortic—Females, I., 57, 108‡ (108), 184 ; II., 8, 41, 73, 99 ;
         III., 37, 39, 51, 57, 113, 127, 136‡ (293) ; IV., 18, 35, 66‡ (98), 149 ;
         VI., 1, 7‡ (5), 95‡ (226), 131.
      Mitral and Tricuspid—Males, II., 9† ; IV., 172, 226‡ (264). Females, II.,
         118‡ (203).
      Mitral, Aortic and Tricuspid—Males, II., 27A, 162‡ (159), 216‡ (317), 238 ;
         III., 80, 215‡ (186), 221, 238, 252 ; V., 56, 161‡ (243). Females, I.,
         48‡ (51) ; III., 87 ; IV., 23‡ (24).
      Tricuspid Regurgitation—Males, II., 136† ; V., 15.
      Pulmonary Regurgitation—Males, IV., 26.

HEMIANÆSTHESIA—Males, I., 15. Females, V., 29.

HEMIPLEGIA—Males, I., 15, 25, 51, 69, 153, 189, 199, 246‡ (146) ; II., 78, 84‡ (56),
   87, 150, 236 ; III., 8, 32, 66, 98, 110, 152, 224, 240, 293 ; IV., 21, 116,
   122, 154‡ (242) ; V., 2, 93. Females, I., 12, 42 ; II., 2, 5‡ (4) ; III.,
   53 ; V., 95‡ (226), 100, 158.

HERNIA—
   Inguinal—Males, V., 199, 209. Females, VI., 301.
   Ventral—Females, VI., 144.

HERPES—Males, I., 62, 179. Females, II., 103 ; IV., 176.

HIP DISEASE—Females, II, 135.
   Ankylosis of Hip—Females, VI., 258.

HODGKIN'S DISEASE—*See* Lymphadenoma.

HYDROCEPHALUS—Males, V., 204. Females, V., 134.

HYDRONEPHROSIS—Males, V., 49. Females, VI., 28A‡ (54), 89.

HYDROSALPINX—Females, VI., 254, 302.

HYMEN, Imperforate—Females, VI., 27.

HYPERÆSTHESIA—Females, V., 103.

HYPERPYREXIA—Males, IV., 65†. Females, V., 164‡ (275).

HYPOCHONDRIASIS—Females, III., 101.

HYSTERECTOMY—
   Abdominal—Females, VI., 38, 53A, 56, 124, 184, 206, 327, 358, 446, 478.
   Vaginal—Females, VI., 25, 157, 158, 340, 380.

HYSTERIA—Females, I., 1 ; II., 52 ; III., 29 ; IV., 56, 123 ; V., 29, 43, 149.
   Convulsions—Females, I., 39 ; VI., 426.
   Dyspnœa—Females, I., 71.
   Paralysis—Females, IV., 117 ; V., 103, 158.

   See also Paraplegia, Functional.

HYSTEROPEXY, Abdominal—Females, VI., 6.

ICTERUS GRAVIS—Females, V., 159‡ (153).

ILIUM, Malignant disease of—Females, III., 104‡ (175).

IMPETIGO CONTAGIOSA—Males, III., 60, 173. Females, III., 120. *Radcliffe*—20.

INFARCTION—*See* Various Organs.

INFLUENZA—Males, I., 184, 246‡ (146) ; II., 45B, 123, 188 ; IV., 50, 192, 210 ; V.,
   22, 74A, 182, 184. Females, I., 93, 94 ; II., 11 ; IV., 61, 159, 164 ; V.,
   35, 59, 93, 133.
   Endocarditis, due to Influenza bacillus—Males, I., 246‡ (146).

INSANITY—
    Alcoholic—Males, I., 68.
    Dementia—Males, I., 110, 123 ; II., 76, 93. Females, I., 42 ; II., 109, 145‡
        (279) ; III., 19 ; IV., 74.
    Epileptic—Males, II., 118. Females, III., 89.
    Mania—Females, III., 64.
    Melancholia—Males, II., 29. Females, I., 8.

INSANE, General Paralysis of—Males, I., 75 ; V., 85.

INTESTINE—
    Hæmorrhage from—Males, II., 4, 12†, 72‡ (6), 292‡ (295). Females, III.,
        135, 136‡ (293) ; IV., 138‡ (223) ; V., 19.
    Malignant Growth of—Females, III., 125‡ (s), 126‡ (s).
    Obstruction of—Males, III., 190‡ (s), 274‡ (s). Females, III., 125‡ (s),
        126‡ (s).
    Perforation of, in Typhoid Fever—Males, II., 246‡ (s) ; IV., 60† ; V., 233‡
        (264). Females, I., 195‡ (s) ; V., 32.
    Resection of—Females, VI., 230.
    Ulceration of—Females, IV., 23‡ (24).
            Tuberculous—Males, I., 86‡ (101) ; III., 55‡ (46) ; V., 91‡ (178).
                Females, I., 7‡ (25) ; II., 46‡ (65).

    See also Duodenum, Jejunum, Colon, Rectum, &c.

INTUSSUSCEPTION—Males, III., 210‡ (s).

IRITIS—Males, III., 287.

IRIDO-CYCLITIS—Females, I., 125.

JAUNDICE—Males, I., 93, 152‡ (197) ; III., 42, 90, 150, 264, 270 ; IV., 55, 131 ;
        V., 31‡ (48), 54‡ (63), 178. Females, I., 109, 136 ; II., 117, 140, 157 ;
        III., 50, 83, 157† ; IV., 98; V., 60‡ (103), 89, 159‡ (153).

KERATITIS—Females, I., 125.

KERATOSIS PILARIS—Males, I., 28.

KIDNEY—
    Congenital Cystic Disease of—Females, II., 101‡ (169).
    Moveable—Males, II., 2, 21. Females, II., 114 ; IV., 3, 52 ; V., 85 ; VI., 98,
        278, 312.
    Tuberculous Disease of—Males, III., 178‡ (304) ; V., 107, 113‡ (206).
    Tumour of—Females, II., 13.

KYPHOSIS—Males, II., 146.

LABIUM—
    Abscess of—Females, VI., 387.
    Cyst of—Females, VI., 428.
    Hypertrophy of—Females, VI., 442.

LABOUR—Females, III., 144 ; VI., 11, 55, 76, 114, 148, 177‡ (82), 195, 217, 236B,
        284.
    Induced—Females, I., 114, 114A‡ (74) ; VI., 125, 132, 285, 317, 318, 364,
        460.
    Obstructed by Contracted Pelvis—Females, VI., 306.
    Premature—Females, I., 147‡ (195); VI., 205, 289 292‡ (195).
    Prolonged—Females, VI., 189, 459.
    Sequelæ of—Females, VI., 417, 424.
    With Transverse Presentation—Females, VI., 293, 318.

LAPABOTOMY—Males, II., 67, 68‡ (s), 245‡ (s) ; III., 77‡ (s), 190‡ (s), 210‡ (s).
  Females, I., 26‡ (s), 92, 195‡ (s) ; II., 27†, 93‡ (182) ; III., 32‡ (s), 123‡
  (s) ; V., 82, 147, 165‡ (s) ; VI., 9, 30‡ (s), 42‡ (s), 89, 90, 144, 154, 230,
  240, 252, 254, 295, 802, 346, 348, 350‡ (s), 362, 385, 891, 435‡ (312).
  Sequelæ of—Females, VI., 466.
  See also Appendicectomy, Cholecystotomy, Hysterectomy, Hysteropexy,
  Ovariotomy, &c.

LARYNGITIS—Males, V., 119‡ (150), 139. *Radoliffe*—7, 11, 26‡ (315), 29, 38, 43, 44.
  Females, I., 198 ; II., 155 ; IV., 82†. *Radoliffe*—37.
  Tuberculous—Males, I., 192† ; II., 183†, 215 ; III., 65‡ (52).

LARYNGEAL OBSTRUCTION—Males, *Radoliffe*—14 ; Females, *Radoliffe*—8†.

LARYNGEAL SPASM—Males, V., 21A.

LEAD POISONING—Males, I., 375 ; III., 159 ; IV., 183 ; V., 98. Females, I., 97.

LEUCORRHŒA—Females, VI., 464.

LEUKÆMIA—
  Lymphatic—Males, II., 149‡ (199) ; IV., 37‡ (57).
  Myelogenic—Males, I., 197 ; II., 147 ; III., 133, 253.

LICHEN, Pilaris—Males, I., 14.

LIVER—
  Abscess of—Males, I., 76, 211‡ (s) ; IV., 85 ; V., 210‡ (s).
  Cirrhosis—Males, I., 148‡ (215), 193, 205 ; II., 22, 34, 103, 103A, 103B, 103C,
    103D, 103E†, 181, 235‡ (248) ; III., 21, 44‡ (14), 90, 144, 222, 262, 269 ;
    IV., 1, 29, 52‡ (62), 100, 100A, 187‡ (113), 222‡ (247) ; V., 7, 11‡ (34),
    25‡ (31), 54‡ (63), 70, 87‡ (205). Females, II., 70‡ (139), 148‡ (125) ;
    III., 83, 106 ; V., 22‡ (58), 99‡ (241).
  Enlargement of—Males, II., 11‡ (38), 46, 61 ; III., 27, IV., 76, 165.
    Females, II., 4, 19 ; III., 80 ; V., 60‡ (103), 88, 89, 91.
  Floating lobe of—Females, I., 136.
  Hydatid of—Males, II., 195‡ (s) ; V., 210‡ (s).
  Malignant Growth of—Males, III., 114‡ (94), 184A ; IV., 76, 166. Females,
    II., 140 ; IV., 70‡ (119), 98 ; VI., 256.

LOCOMOTOR ATAXY—*See* Tabes Dorsalis.

LUMBAGO—Males, II., 172.

LUNGS—
  Abscess of—Males, II., 109† ; IV., 117‡ (211). *Radoliffe*—34‡ (233).
    Females, II., 84‡ (140).
  Collapse of—Males, III., 78. Females, V., 75‡ (77).
  Fibrosis of—Males, I., 1, 121, 125, 183, 201 ; III., 92, 139, 168, 284‡ (228) ;
    IV., 4, 79, 99. Females, III., 103 ; IV., 37.
  Gangrene of—Males, III., 26. Females, I., 7‡ (25).
  Infarction of—Males, V., 31‡ (48). Females, V., 7‡ (5).
  Malignant Growth of—Males, I., 97‡ (83) ; III., 59‡ (53). Females, III.,
    154‡ (321).
  Œdema of—Males, I., 136 ; IV., 146†. Females, V., 68.
  Passive Congestion of—Females, I., 182.

LUPUS—
  Minimus—Females, VI., 127, 138, 272, 277, 447.
  Vulgaris—Males, I., 67. Females, II., 40, 40A.

LYMPHADENOMA—Males, II., 26 ; III., 52 ; IV., 181‡ (200), 228‡ (271) ; V., 128.
  Females, III., 88.

LYMPHATIC GLANDS—*See* Glands, Lymphatic.

MALARIA—Males, I., 61, 167, 220 ; II., 86, 101, 107, 230 ; III., 125, 166 ; IV., 118 ;
    V., 57.
MALIGNANT GROWTH OF—
    Abdomen—Females, V., 168 ; VI., 171, 473.
    Bladder—Females, IV., 177 ; VI., 349.
    Breast—Females, IV., 70‡ (119).
    Duodenum—Females, I., 114, 114A‡ (74) ; VI., 285
    Glands, Lymphatic—Males, I., 12‡ (1), 97‡,(83) ; V., 144. Females, III., 154‡
        (321) ; IV., 21‡ (27).
    Ilium—Females, III., 104‡ (175).
    Intestine—Females, III., 125‡ (s), 126‡ (s).
    Liver—Males, I., 12‡ (1) ; III., 114‡ (94). Females, II., 140 ; IV., 70‡ (119),
        98 ; VI., 256.
    Lung—Males, I., 97‡ (83) ; III., 59‡ (53). Females, III., 154‡ (321).
    Mediastinum—Males, I., 97‡ (83), 204‡ (59) ; III., 34, 34A‡ (39). Females,
        III., 154‡ (321).
    Muscle (Leio-myoma)—Males, III., 77 (s).
    Œsophagus—Males, II., 68‡ (s) ; III., 279‡ (s) ; IV., 113‡ (131), 145.
    Ovary—Females, VI., 42‡ (s), 60, 60A, 152, 256, 273.
    Peritoneum—Males, IV., 230 ; Females, VI., 240.
    Pelvis—Females, II., 94.
    Pleura—Females, V., 66‡ (151)
    Rectum—Females, IV., 179.
    Stomach—Males, I., 91, 119‡ (237), 212, 213 ; II., 64‡ (49), 57, 245‡ (s) ; IV.,
        7, 150, 176‡ (185), 205 ; V., 146, 208. Females, I., 88‡ (s), 118, 191‡ (s) ;
        III., 152‡ (s) ; IV., 60‡ (60).
    Suprarenals—Males, II., 12.
    Testis—Males, I., 237‡ (s).
    Urethra—Females, VI., 161.
    Uterine Cervix—Females, VI., 25, 33, 39, 107, 141, 157, 158, 160, 166, 169, 242,
        245, 279, 340, 375, 390, 472, 475, 478.
    Uterus—Females, VI., 153, 155, 159, 265, 275, 380, 422.
    Vagina—Females, VI., 472.
    Vulva—Females, VI., 183, 215.
MALINGERING—Males, I., 106 ; IV., 184. Females, I., 163.
MALTA FEVER—Females, II., 135.
MARASMUS—Males, III., 294‡ (91) ; IV., 189, 196, 216 ; V., 231. Females, III.,
    128‡ (281) ; V., 69‡ (76), 92‡ (219), 140.
MEASLES—Males, I., 241 ; II., 202, 226 ; III., 198, 258. *Radcliffe*—1, 2, 15, 26‡
    (315), 38, 39, 46†. Females, I., 56, 198 ; III., 60 ; V., 153 ; VI., 398.
    Radcliffe—37.
MEDIASTINUM, Malignant Growth of—Males, I., 97‡ (83), 204‡ (59). Females,
    III., 154‡ (321).
MEGALENCEPHALY—Males, I., 29.
MELANCHOLIA—*See* Insanity.
MENINGES, Hæmorrhage into—Males, III., 296‡ (308).
MENINGITIS—
    Post Basal—Males, I., 57‡ (41) ; II., 237† ; IV., 203, 207, 211, 219‡ (21) ;
        V., 236†. Females, I., 99 ; IV., 140.
    Purulent—Males, II., 91‡ (69), 109† ; III., 232‡ (204) ; IV., 213 ; V., 45‡
        (61), 235‡ (107). Females, I., 119‡ (117) ; II., 123‡ (236) ; III., 98‡
        (168) ; IV., 102‡ (122), 106‡ (147).
    Pseudo—Males, III., 288.
    Tuberculous—Males, I., 36‡ (23), 158‡ (143), 239‡ (114) ; III., 199†, 206‡
        (231), 276‡ (176), 212‡ (137) ; IV., 152‡ (181), 173‡ (292), 223‡ (273) ;
        V., 60‡ (68), 91‡ (178), 202‡ (134). Females, 33‡ (44), 149† (278) ; III.,
        38‡ (70) ; IV., 51‡ (93) ; V., 65‡ (155), 70‡ (174), 77‡ (131), 118‡ (239);
        VI., 28A‡ (54). *Radcliffe*—33‡ (84).
    Spinal, Purulent—Females, V., 166‡ (212).

MENORRHAGIA—Females, VI., 133, 237, 388, 388A.

MENSES, Retention of—Females, VI., 27.

MENSTRUATION, Profuse—Females, VI., 436, 476.

METEORISM—Females, IV., 175‡ (328).

METRORRHAGIA—Females, VI., 459.

MICTURITION, Painful—Females, I., 52.

MIGRAINE—Females, III., 54.

MONOPLEGIA, Crural—Males, V., 89.

MORBUS COXÆ—Males, IV., 27. Females, II., 135.

MUSCLE, Malignant Growth of (Leio-myoma)—Males, III., 77‡ (s).

MUSCULAR ATROPHY—Males, II., 119 ; V., 90.

MUSCULAR HYPERTONICITY—Females, I., 32.

MYASTHENIA GRAVIS—Females, I., 46.

MYELITIS—
    Acute—Males, I., 94 ; II., 174‡ (255).
    „ Ant. Polio—Males, I., 161 ; V., 217. Females, I., 123 ; V., 96, 135.
    Chronic Ant. Polio—Males, II., 70‡ (67) ; III., 93. Females, I., 169 ; IV., 25, 113.

MYALGIA—Males, I., 64, 117 ; II., 50, III., 75.

MYOCARDITIS—See Heart.

MYXŒDEMA—Females, I., 104, 153 ; II., 53, 120.

NASAL POLYPI—Females, I., 161.

NEPHRITIS—
    Acute—Males, I., 136 ; II., 117 ; III., 45, 54, 142, 187, 205, 275 ; IV., 141 ;
    V., 237. Females, I., 34 ; VI., 177‡ (82).
    Chronic—
        Parenchymatous—Males, I., 20‡ (22), 74, 131, 172, 193 ; II., 93, 95‡ (55),
        133, 145‡ (229), 151† ; III., 63, 95 ; IV., 22, 63 ; V., 28, 67, 155, 179,
        240‡ (127). Females, I., 3, 27, 104 ; II., 12, 122† ; III., 24, 28, 74 ;
        IV., 2, 146‡ (274), 165 ; V., 38, 139, 147 ; VI., 195, 336.
        Interstitial—Males, I., 92‡ (86), 114‡ (257), 199 ; II., 33‡ (36), 84, 88‡
        (56), 157 ; III., 21, 85, 116‡ (130), 182‡ (291), 201, 228 ; IV., 42, 58‡
        (62), 82†, 154‡ (268) ; V., 108, 126. Females, I., 35, 48‡ (51), 115 ;
        II., 5‡ (4), 28‡ (2), 55‡ (95), 130‡ (258) ; III., 2, 91, 156‡ (313) ; IV.,
        81, 134‡ (202) ; V., 15, 99‡ (241), 173‡ (320) ; VI., 177‡ (82).
        Mixed—Males, I., 134, 180 ; II., 109†, 185‡ (191), 229, 235‡ (248) ; III.,
        88, 92, 138, 185† ; V., 229‡ (251). Females, I., 139‡ (218) ; II., 143.

NEPHRECTOMY—Males, V., 49.

NEPHRORRHAPHY—Males, V., 46.

NEPHROTOMY—Males, II., 242. Females, IV., 156‡ (s).

NEURALGIA—Males, II., 128 ; V., 159.
    Sacral—Males, I., 40.
    Brachial—Males, II., 155.

NEURASTHENIA—Males, I., 132. Females, I., 75 ; III., 145 ; IV., 121, 152 ; V.,
    45 ; VI, 35, 40, 203.

NEURITIS—
    Local—Females, III., 62.
    Multiple—Males, IV., 97 ; V., 98.
        Alcoholic—Males, I., 87 ; V., 215‡ (179). Females, IV., 84 ; V., 60‡ (103).
        Lead—Females, I., 97.

NEUROMIMESIS—Males, IV., 56. Females, II., 49, 67 ; III., 102.
NEUROSIS—Females, VI., 19, 228, 228A.
NODULES, Rheumatic—Males, III., 212 ; IV., 174‡ (276).
NYSTAGMUS—Males, II., 143.

OBESITY—Females, I., 81 ; VI., 197, 464.
ŒSOPHAGUS—
    Malignant Growth of—Males, II., 68‡ (s), 279‡ (s) ; IV., 113‡ (131), 145.
    Rupture of—Males, IV., 227‡ (327).
    Stricture of—Males, I., 115 ; III., 261 ; V., 162.
OPTIC ATROPHY—Males, III., 138 ; IV., 207.
OPTIC NEURITIS—Males, III., 81, 165 ; V., 52. Females, I., 187 ; III., 53, 92.
OSTEO-ARTHRITIS—Males, II., 142 ; III., 164. Females, I., 63, 79, 127 ; II., 51, 54,
    107, 108 ; III., 15, 70, 150 ; IV., 13 ; V., 90.
OTITIS EXTERNA—Females, IV., 4.
OTITIS MEDIA—Males, I., 57‡ (41), 74 ; II., 184 ; III., 223 ; V., 45‡ (61). Females,
    III., 4 ; V., 43.
OVARIOTOMY—
    Abdominal—Females, VI., 12, 16, 36, 60, 71, 85, 152, 154, 184, 234, 246, 254,
        273, 288, 295, 327, 347, 351, 352, 353, 371, 415, 423, 468, 477.
    Vaginal—Females, VI., 233, 263.
OVARY—
    Cystic—Females, VI., 16, 421.
    Dermoid Tumour of—Females, II., 153 ; VI., 71, 233, 263, 358, 468.
    Malignant Growth of—Females, IV., 97 ; VI., 42‡ (s), 60, 60A, 152, 256, 273.
    Prolapse of—Females, VI., 6, 185.
    Suppuration of—Females, II., 12, 391.
    Tumour of—Females, III., 126‡ (s) ; IV., 44 ; VI., 36, 85, 184, 192, 234, 236,
        236A, 236B, 246, 280, 288, 295, 347, 351, 352, 353, 371, 415, 423, 432, 477.
OXALURIA—Males, IV., 111.

PANCREAS—
    Malignant Growth of—Males, II., 81‡ (66).
    Inflammation of, Chronic—Males, I., 202‡ (s).
PARALYSIS—
    Agitans—Males, II., 3 ; III., 48, 297 ; IV., 194.
    Cranial Nerves, of—Females, I., 12 ; II., 72.
    Diphtheritic—Males, III., 204, 249. Females, IV., 122 ; V., 40.
    Facial—Males, IV., 225 ; V., 108.
    Hysterical—Females, IV., 117 ; V., 103.
    Infantile—See Myelitis, Acute Ant. Polio-
    Pseudo-Hypertrophic—Males, I., 143.
PARAMETRITIS—Females, VI., 143, 223, 238, 244, 310, 366, 403, 407, 431, 445.
    Sequelæ of—Female, VI., 162, 409.
PARAPLEGIA—
    Ataxic—Males, II., 129, 146 ; V., 20, 34.
    Functional—Males, I., 154, 159.
    Spastic—Males, I., 35, 164, 165 ; V., 123. Females, I., 6.

PAROTID GLAND—
    Parotitis—Females, IV., 42, 50.
      ,,   Suppurative—Females, III., 132 ; V., 157.
    Tumour—Males, I., 99.

PELVIC—
    Abscess—Females, VI., 211, 244, 346, 350‡ (s), 403, 429, 434, 478.
    Adhesions—Females, VI., 218.
    Deformity (See also Pelvis Contracted)—Females, VI., 258.
    Inflammation—Females, VI., 14, 75.
      ,,   Sequelæ of—Females, VI., 4, 188.
    Malignant Growth of—Females, II., 94.
    Pain—Females, VI., 32, 43, 57, 96, 105, 120, 123, 140, 146, 149, 219, 365, 412.
    Tumour—Females, VI., 81, 87.

PELVIS, Contracted—Females, VI., 11, 76, 125, 132, 306.

PEMPHIGUS—Females, III., 25 ; V., 151.

PERICARDITIS—Males, I., 32‡ (33), 147‡ (160) ; II., 93, 145‡ (229), 167, 193 ; III.,
    25, 128, 215‡ (186), 248‡ (116) ; IV., 174‡ (276), 221‡ (311) ; V., 52‡ (79),
    62, 118, 192‡ (290), 238‡ (53).   Females, I., 117‡ (102), 176† (261) ;
    II., 47, 92, 122†, 126, 143, 152‡ (303) ; III., 17‡ (10), 33, 37, 112‡ (230),
    116, 137 ; IV., 77†, 81 ; V., 28, 73.
    Purulent—Females, I., 119‡ (117), 193‡ (s) ; IV., 102‡ (122) ; V., 75‡ (77).

PERICARDIUM, Adherent—Males, V., 17, 109‡ (201).   Females, II., 4▲‡ (92), 156‡
    (270) ; III., 156‡ (313) ; V., 13.

PERIHEPATITIS—Females, I., 48‡ (51).

PERIMETRITIS—Females, VI., 51, 54, 70, 193, 202, 257, 350† (s), 359, 404, 429.
    Encysted—Females, VI., 252.
    Sequelæ of—Females, VI., 61, 63, 70▲, 93, 106, 162, 225, 369, 395.

PERIOSTITIS—Males, IV., 140.   Females, I., 193‡ (s) ; IV., 120.

PERINEUM—
    Ruptured—Females, IV., 47.
      ,,   and Repaired—Females, VI., 8, 31, 50, 58, 67, 104, 119, 291, 294,
    381, 401, 406, 410, 419, 431, 441, 450, 458, 471.

PERITONEUM—
    Malignant Growth of—Males, IV., 230.   Females, VI., 240.
    Hæmorrhage into—Males, I., 237‡ (s).

PERITONITIS—
    Acute—Females, III., 32‡ (s), 125‡ (s), 138‡ (310); IV., 60‡ (60) ; VI., 437‡
    (282).
    Chronic—Females, I., 48‡ (51) ; II., 4▲‡ (92) ; IV., 97.
      ,,   With Hæmorrhagic Effusion—Females, II., 148‡ (125).
    Purulent—Males, I., 78‡ (s) ; II., 185‡ (191).   Females, I., 195‡ (s) ; III.,
    17‡ (10), 123‡ (s) ; IV., 112‡ (177), 155‡ (262) ; V., 75‡ (77), 165‡ (s),
    166‡ (212), 169† ; VI., 64‡ (13), 435‡ (312).
    Tuberculous—Males, I., 208, 223, 245 ; II., 137, 165 ; III., 53†, 55‡ (46), 195†;
    IV., 107, 191, 222‡ (247); V., 91‡ (178), 133, 209, 238‡ (53).   Females, I.,
    26‡ (s); II., 42, 74 ; III., 13, 69 ; IV., 91 ; V., 114‡ (221), 162 ; VI., 28▲‡
    (54), 30‡ (s), 474.

PERTUSSIS—Males, I., 229 ; II., 138, 211, 218 ; III., 88 ; IV., 43, 67, 70.   Females,
    I., 110‡ (154), 174 ; II., 65 ; III., 67 ; IV., 29 ; V., 67, 136.

PHARYNGITIS—Males, V., 51.   Radcliffe—5.

PHLEGMASIA ALBA DOLENS—Females, I., 120 ; II., 1.

PHTHISIS PULMONALIS—Males, I., 55, 81, 90, 104, 107, 117, 124, 141, 179, 192†, 206, 215, 231‡ (136) ; II., 6, 53, 85, 89, 97, 141, 144, 176†, 215 ; III., 18, 30, 49‡ (45), 65‡ (52), 70, 89, 94, 101†, 163, 189, 189A‡ (80), 213, 227, 268 ; IV., 28, 81, 96, 115, 122, 123, 124, 195 ; V., 51, 91‡ (178), 100, 102, 119‡ (150), 127, 139, 185, 194, 196‡ (298), 211‡ (311). Females, I., 95, 116 ; II., 28‡ (2), 39, 71, 75†, 98‡ (190) ; III., 45‡ (75), 122‡ (326), 147, 147A ; IV., 87†, 88, 146‡ (274) ; V., 48, 82‡ (141) ; VI., 217, 232.

PLACENTA—
    Prævia—Females, VI., 11, 94, 114, 289, 364, 460.
    Retained—Females, VI., 386.

PLEURA, Malignant Disease of—Females, V., 66‡ (151).

PLEURISY—Males, I., 141, II., 6, 43, 53, 92, 104, 143, 152 ; III., 25, 76, 79, 97, 107, 139, 168, 170, 217, 254, 290 ; IV., 8, 13, 35‡ (47), 53, 123, 204 ; V., 1, 3, 41, 75, 120, 135, 189, 193. Females, I., 121, 176‡ (261), 177 ; II., 15, 83 ; III., 23, 32‡ (s), 67 ; IV., 9, 24, 39, 43, 45, 55, 57, 124, 146‡ (274), 180‡ (319) ; V., 90, 105, 117.
    With Effusion—Males, I., 18, 27, 32, 58, 63, 99, 107, 109, 114‡ (257), 118, 124, 127, 130, 144, 147‡ (160), 152‡ (197), 231‡ (136), 245 ; II., 17, 30‡ (17), 31, 124A, 137, 154, 183†, 205†, 224 ; III., 61, 86, 105, 117, 124, 127, 133, 146, 156, 174, 285 ; IV., 94, 96, 129, 193 ; V., 53, 74, 96, 136, 185, 201, 224. Females, I., 27, 44, 55, 69, 105, 117‡ (102), 119‡ (117) ; II., 42, 59, 113, 121, 125 ; III., 105, 140 ; IV., 40, 47, 150 ; V., 34, 37, 94, 104 ; VI., 435‡ (312).
    With Hæmorrhagic Effusion—Males, I., 130. Females, II., 148‡ (125) ; V., 66‡ (151).

PLEURODYNIA—Females, I., 58 ; IV., 94.

PNEUMONIA—
    Catarrhal—Males, I., 200‡ (302), 222, 224‡ (266), 225, 232 ; II., 38‡ (9), 42, 91‡ (69), 124, 124A, 139, 217‡ (166) ; III., 78A. 103, 148, 167, 172, 173, 186, 198, 208, 210‡ (s), 233‡(246), 243‡ (249), 247, 248‡ (116), 272‡ (305) ; IV., 34, 35‡ (47), 67, 70, 142, 158, 180, 182†, 202, 206† ; V., 19, 21, 26, 110, 164, 198, 199, 207, 235‡ (107). Radcliffe—15, 19‡ (259), 23‡ (253), 26‡ (315), 31‡ (250), 34‡ (233), 38, 41‡ (316). Females, I., 119‡ (117), 139‡ (218), 154, 158, 162, 165, 168‡ (269), 189, 198, 199‡ (324), 200 ; II., 18, 43‡ (64), 57, 60‡ (118), 79‡ (100), 84‡ (140), 101‡ (169), 130‡ (258), 132, 138 ; III., 60, 107‡ (224), 109, 112‡ (230), 114, 116, 117, 128‡ (281), 138‡ (310), 147, 147A ; IV., 10, 29, 30‡ (37), 34, 48, 82‡, 102‡ (122), 155‡ (262), 180‡ (319) ; V., 8, 8A, 31, 74‡ (111), 92‡ (219), 101†, 114‡ (221), 118‡ (239), 138, 141, 150, 170‡ (323). Radcliffe—22‡ (89), 27‡ (213), 40‡ (324), 47.
    Croupous—Males, I., 7, 48, 59, 66, 79, 82, 85, 100, 111, 120, 128, 140, 142, 155, 156, 170, 175, 182, 183, 186, 187, 216, 217, 226, 240, 242‡ (214) ; II., 35, 55, 56, 58, 80, 83, 98, 99, 102, 112, 114, 125, 131, 132, 158, 159, 163, 168, 173‡ (167), 178, 179, 180, 182, 187, 193‡ (97), 197, 203, 204, 210, 213, 218, 220 ; III., 1, 12, 20‡ (20), 23, 26, 28, 41, 64, 91, 99, 112, 115, 119, 123, 126, 129, 135, 137, 162, 171, 180†, 188, 233, 238, 241, 242, 243, 257, 271, 275, 282, 284‡ (228), 286 ; IV., 16, 31, 36, 41, 43, 69, 72, 73, 74, 86, 103, 108, 114, 136, 190, 199, 201, 214†, 215 ; V., 11‡ (34), 35, 39, 52‡ (79), 55, 72, 78, 80, 81, 82, 83, 94, 97, 106, 111‡ (165), 114, 115, 122, 138, 141, 143, 145, 154, 160, 161‡ (243), 168‡ (263), 171, 181, 195, 200‡ (299), 201, 203, 212, 214, 219, 220‡ (105), 222, 227, 230, 232, 240‡ (127). Females, I., 80, 82, 106, 133, 151, 180, 181, 186, 196 ; II., 11, 32, 48, 76, 82, 85, 95, 103, 105, 106, 112, 116, 152‡ (303) ; III., 9, 34, 61, 65, 79, 81, 94, 99, 108, 113, 131, 142, 153 ; IV., 19‡ (29), 49, 110, 111, 115, 137, 154, 176, 183 ; V., 47, 72, 81, 83, 102†, 121, 129, 130, 136, 156 ; VI., 469†.

PNEUMO-THORAX—Males, V., 117. Females, I., 7‡ (25).
    See also Pyo-pneumothorax.

POISONING BY—
  Arsenic—Males, I., 103.
  Carbon Bisulphide—Males, II., 49.
  Creolin—Males, I., 2.
  Heroin—Males, I., 75.
  Lead—Males, I., 3, 75 ; III., 159 ; IV., 183 ; V., 98.   Females, I., 97.
  Nitric Acid—Females, V., 39‡ (104).
  Opium—Males, III., 141 ; V., 194.
  Ptomaine—Males, III., 231 ; IV., 89.   Females, II., 127.
  Thyroid Extract—Females, I., 153.

PONS, Disease of—Males, V., 205.

PREGNANCY—Females, I., 74, 114, 114A‡ (74), 147‡ (195); II., 14 ; III., 154‡ (321);
      IV., 85, 100, 108, 126, 143 ; V., 73, 80 ; VI., 11, 18, 59, 94, 118, 175, 191,
      192, 195, 196, 198, 205, 217, 219, 221, 221A, 226, 236, 236A, 236B, 271,
      285, 299, 336, 357, 368, 385, 426.
  ———— With Abdominal Pain—Females, VI., 168.
  ———— With Nephritis—Females, VI., 177‡ (82).
  ———— With Painful Contraction of Uterus—Females, VI., 117.
  ———— With Vomiting—Females, VI., 148.
  ———— Molar—Females, VI., 29.
  ————.———— Carneous—Females, VI., 323.
  ————————— Hydatidiform—Females, VI., 45, 69, 91.
  ———— Extra-uterine—Tubal Gestation—Females, VI., 17, 41, 136, 321, 322, 408.
  ———— ————————— Rupture—Females, VI., 9, 230, 283, 311.
  ———— ————— ————— —— Mole—Females, VI., 249, 290.

PREMATURITY—Females, VI., 115†, 126‡ (32), 453†, 454†, 461†, 462†, 479†.

PRURITUS—Females, IV., 59 ; VI., 308.

PSILOSIS—Females, I., 144 ; II., 141.

PSORIASIS—Males, I., 46 ; III., 13.   Females, I., 13 ; IV., 181.

PURPURA—Males, II., 110, 120, 160 ; III., 72‡ (6), 107, 182‡ (291); IV., 27, 30, 93;
      V., 206.   Females, I., 35 ; II., 23‡ (15); III., 43 ; IV., 28 ; V., 10†, 99‡
      (241), 101†.

PYÆMIA—Males, III., 230‡ (230).
  Puerperal—Females, VI., 328†.

PYELITIS—Males, II., 242.   Females, III., 14, 124.

PYELO-NEPHRITIS—Males, III., 220‡ (256).

PYO-NEPHROSIS—Males, II., 223‡ (126).   Females, II., 146 ; IV., 156‡ (s).

PYO-PNEUMOTHORAX—Males, I., 195‡ (289) ; II., 38‡ (9).   See also Pneumo-
      thorax.

PYO-SALPINX—Females, VI., 71, 211, 332, 348, 391.

PYURIA—Males, I., 134, 161; IV., 26.   Females, II., 13 ; III., 14 ; IV., 177.

PYREXIA—See Fever.

RAYNAUD'S DISEASE—Males, V., 188.   Females, I., 11.

RECTOCELE—Females, VI., 34, 222, 401.

RECTUM—
  Malignant Growth of—Females, IV., 179.
  Polypi of—Females, VI., 354.
  Prolapse of—Males, IV., 170.
  Stricture of—Females, VI., 395, 470.

RETINITIS—Males, I., 145 ; V., 108.
    Albuminuric—Females, I., 35, 139‡ (218) ; II., 122† ; IV., 81.
RHEUMATISM—
    Acute and Sub-acute—Males, I., 10, 24, 72, 105, 163, 173, 177 ; II., 5, 25, 54
        92, 110, 121, 167, 192, 194, 208, 221, 228 ; III., 11, 23, 25, 35, 62, 68, 71,
        87, 100, 104, 108, 128, 136, 149, 175, 179, 212, 221, 277‡ (306), 280 ; IV.,
        12, 45, 83, 84, 105, 106, 127, 130, 155, 174‡ (276), 209, 220, 221‡ (311) ;
        V., 8, 12, 29, 30, 44, 56, 77, 88, 92, 103, 148, 149, 151, 166, 170, 176, 187 ;
        Females, I., 5, 18, 29, 41, 45, 53, 57, 59, 76, 83, 90, 105, 112, 117‡ (102),
        125, 126, 129, 138, 143, 146, 177 ; II., 10, 22, 63, 66, 92, 99, 128, 131, 156‡
        (270) ; III., 5, 27, 37, 39, 58, 59, 77, 82, 85, 110, 127, 129, 137, 149, 150,
        155 ; IV., 18, 64, 67, 76, 77†, 79, 124, 127, 145, 151, 153, 157, 162, 166,
        171, 172, 173 ; V., 30, 55, 98, 108, 110, 111, 120, 125, 154, 164‡ (275); VI.,
        255, 410.
        With Chorea—Males, III., 23 ; V., 44. Females, I., 53, 59.
        With Erythema—Males, I., 177 ; V., 187. Females, I., 112, 117‡
            (102), 125 ; III., 39.
        With Nodules—Males, III., 212 ; IV., 174‡ (276). Females, III., 37.
        With Pericarditis—Males, III., 25, 277‡ (306) ; V., 88 ; Females, I.,
            105, 117‡ (102) ; II., 92 ; III., 37, 137 ; IV., 77†.
        With Pleurisy—Males, III., 25. Females, I., 177 ; IV., 124.
        With Pleurisy with Effusion—Females, I., 105, 117‡ (102).
        With Relapse—Females, II., 22.
        With Tonsillitis—Males, V., 151. Females, IV., 76.
    Chronic—Males, I., 133, 196 ; IV., 38, 44, 101. Females, II., 102.
    Muscular—Males, I., 198.
RHINITIS—Males, II., 185. *Radcliffe*—5.
RHINORRHŒA—Females, III., 120.
RIB, Resection of—*See* Empyema.
RICKETS—Males, I., 31 ; II., 38‡ (9), 41, 42, 201, 210, 214 ; III., 192‡ (301) ; IV.,
    34, 168, 169‡ (133), 180, 206† ; V., 198. Females, I., 10, 119‡ (117); II.,
    26, 31‡ (43), 46‡ (65), 58, 60‡ (118), 105 ; III., 80 ; IV., 5, 30‡ (37), 63,
    65, 105‡ (142) ; V., 25, 91.
RINGWORM—Males, II., 158.

SALPINGITIS—Females, V., 114‡ (221) ; VI., 21, 38, 65, 73. 95, 95A, 111, 170, 194,
        212, 260, 295, 296, 298, 325, 339. 342, 376, 388, 388A, 392, 402, 437‡ (282).
    Tuberculous—VI., 28, 28A‡ (54), 154, 232.
SAPRÆMIA, Uterine—Females, VI., 22, 364, 414, 433, 469†.
SCABIES—Males, I., 93 ; II., 25, 48, 159 ; V., 30. Females, II., 98‡ (190) ; V., 99‡
    (241).
SCARLET FEVER—Males, III., 29, 236. Females, II., 111 ; IV., 133 ; V., 163.
    Radcliffe—21, 25, 36, 48.
SCIATICA—Males, II., 74 ; IV., 78, 224 ; V., 121, 124. Females, IV., 52.
SCLERODERMA—Males, II., 134.

SCLEROSIS—
    Amyotrophic Lateral—Females, I., 40.
    Combined—Males, II., 135 ; III., 244 ; IV., 8.
    Disseminated—Males, I., 62 ; III., 15. Females, II., 129 ; IV., 123 ; V., 17.
    Lateral—Males, III., 202, 250. Females, I., 98.
SCURVY, Infantile—Males, IV., 169‡ (133).

SEPTICÆMIA—Females, I., 27 ; V., 159‡ (153).
    Puerperal—Females, VI., 64‡ (13), 264†, 266†.

SKIN—
    Darier's Disease of—Females, V., 62.
    Papilloma of—Females, I., 43.
    Tuberculous Disease of—Females, V., 57.

SPINAL MENINGITIS—*See* Meningitis.

SPLEEN—
    Abscess of—Females, VI., 64‡ (13).
    Enlargement of—Males, II., 22, 32, 134 ; III., 10, 73‡ (7) ; IV., 165 ; V., 127,
        182, 230, 234. Females, I., 10, 42 ; III., 80 ; V., 14, 88, 91, 132.

SPRUE—*See* Psilosis.

STERILITY—Females, VI., 185, 189, 208, 394, 465.

STOMACH—
    Dilated—Males, I., 119‡ (237) ; II., 69‡ (s), 164, 199. Females, I., 88‡ (s),
        114, 114A‡ (74) ; VI., 285.
    Malignant Growth of—Males, I., 91, 119‡ (237), 212, 213 ; II., 64‡ (49),
        245‡ (s) ; III., 57 ; IV., 7, 150, 176‡ (185), 205. Females, I., 88‡ (s),
        118, 191‡ (s) ; III., 152‡ (s) ; IV., 21‡ (27), 60‡ (60).
    Perforation of—Females, IV., 60‡ (60).
    Ulcer of—*See* Gastric Ulcer.

STOMATITIS—Males, IV., 192 ; V., 165. Females, I., 56.

SUBDIAPHRAGMATIC INFLAMMATION—Females, L, 121. *See also* Abscess, sub-
    diaphragmatic.

SUPRA-RENAL CAPSULES, Hæmorrhage into—Females, VI., 480.

SYPHILIS—Males, I., 83 ; V., 55. Females, IV., 1.
    Cerebral—Males, I., 168.
    Congenital—Females, I., 125, 187 ; V., 88, 88A, 141.

TABES DORSALIS—Males, I., 8, 65, 102, 166 ; II., 166 ; III., 120 ; IV., 167† ; V., 69,
        86. Females, I., 184 ; II., 64 ; V., 84, 143.
    With Gastric Crises—Males, I., 65, 102. Females, V., 143.
    With Perforating Ulcer—Males, I., 166.

TESTIS—
    Tuberculosis of—Males, I., 95.
    Malignant Disease of—Males, I., 237‡ (s).

TETANUS—Males, I., 101.

TETANY—Males, II., 91‡ (69). Females, I., 114, 114A‡ (74) ; III., 80 ; IV., 5 ; V.,
    25 ; VI., 285.

THROMBOSIS—*See* Arteries and Veins.

TINEA VERSICOLOR—Males, I., 50.

TONSIL—
    Abscess of—Females, II., 50.
    Hypertrophy of—Females, V., 97†.
    Tonsillitis—Males, II., 10, 43, 47, 117, 139 ; III., 193, 278 ; IV., 51 ; V., 22,
        24, 151. Females, I., 23, 62, 175 ; II., 20, 34, 50, 91 ; IV., 76, 148 ;
        V., 8, 123, 127. *Radcliffe*—33‡ (84).

TORTICOLLIS—Males, III., 226 ; V., 150.

TRACHEA, Papilloma of—Females, II., 130‡ (258).

TRACHEOTOMY—Males, III., 105. *Radcliffe*—14, 30‡ (87), 26‡ (315), 35, 39, 42, 44. Females, V., 97†. *Radcliffe*—3, 8, 12, 24, 27‡ (213).

TREMORS—Males, III., 200. Females, V., 149.
    Alcoholic—Males, III., 24.
    Functional—Males, III., 118.

TUBERCULOSIS—
    Acute Miliary—Males, I., 148‡ (215), 158‡ (143) ; III., 192‡ (301), 206‡ (231), 255‡ (283), 276‡ (176) ; IV., 152‡ (181), 173‡ (292), 177‡ (148), 212‡ (137) ; V., 25‡ (31), 27†, 60‡ (68), 196‡ (298), 202‡ (134), 211‡ (314). *Radcliffe*—40‡ (34). Females, I., 33‡ (44), 100‡ (184), 179‡ (278), 199‡ (324) ; II., 31‡ (43) ; III., 38‡ (70), 122‡ (326) ; IV., 7‡ (12), 51‡ (93) ; V., 65‡ (155), 74‡ (111), 171‡ (300). *Radcliffe*—33‡ (84), 40‡ (324).
    Chronic Pulmonary—*See* Phthisis Pulmonalis.

TUMOURS—*See* Malignant Growths of Various Organs.

TYPHLITIS—*See* Appendicitis.

TYPHOID FEVER—
    FATAL CASES—Males, I., 139‡ (232) ; II., 246‡ (s) ; III., 292‡ (295) ; IV., 60† ; V., 233‡ (264). Females, I., 195‡ (s) ; III., 136‡ (293) ; IV., 138‡ (223), 175‡ (328).
    With Arterio-sclerosis—Females, IV., 175‡ (328).
    With Delirium—Females, IV., 175‡ (328).
    With Hæmorrhage—Males, V., 233‡ (264). Females, III., 136‡ (293) ; IV., 138‡ (223).
    With Hyperpyrexia—Males, I., 139‡ (232).
    With Laparotomy—Females, I., 195‡ (s).
    With Parotitis—Males, II., 246‡ (s).
    With Perforation—Males, II., 246‡ (s) ; IV., 60† ; V., 233‡ (264). Females, I., 195‡ (s).
    With Peritonitis, Suppurative—Females, I., 195‡ (s).
    With Pneumonia—Males, I., 139‡ (232).
    With Relapse—Males, I., 139‡ (232) ; IV., 60†.
    With Tympanites—Females, IV., 175‡ (328).

    RECOVERIES—Males, I., 5, 19, 21, 41, 53, 77 ; II., 15, 16, 37, 60, 66, 169, 198 ; III., 7, 9, 298, 299, 301' ; IV., 17, 25, 31, 48, 57, 161 ; V., 6, 13, 14, 32, 50, 167. Females, I., 14, 19, 38, 157, 178 ; II., 6, 14, 16, 86, 87 ; III., 11, 16, 31, 90, 140 ; IV., 120, 143 ; V., 19, 32, 106, 113, 119, 142.
    With Abortion—Females, I., 157.
    With Abscess—Females, II., 14.
    With Arthritis, multiple—Males, V., 6. Females, IV., 120.
    With Arythmia—Females, III., 11.
    With Bronchitis—Males, I., 19, 21 ; IV., 25. Females, V., 19.
    With Constipation—Males, I., 5. Females, I., 14.
    With Cystitis—Males, I., 77.
    With Delirium—Males, I., 19 ; IV., 17 ; V., 6.
    With Epilepsy—Females, I., 157.
    With Hæmorrhage—Males, I., 21, 77 ; II., 16 ; III., 9, 25. Females, II., 86 ; V., 19.
    With Lactation—Females, V., 119.
    With Perforation—Males, II., 66. Females, V., 32.
    With Perforation and Laparotomy—Females, V., 32.

TYPHOID FEVER—*continued.*

RECOVERIES—*continued,*

With Periostitis—Females, IV., 120.
With Pleurisy with Effusion—Females, III., 140.
With Pregnancy—Females, II., 14 ; IV., 143.
With Relapse—Males, I., 19, 21 ; II., 16 ; III., 9 ; IV., 48, 161 ; V., 6, 50.
   Females, I., 157, 178 ; II., 87 ; III., 11, 31 ; V., 82, 113.
With Rigors—Males, I., 21 ; II., 15.   Females, I., 178 ; III., 90.
With Thrombosis of Veins—Males, II., 15, 198 ; IV., 81.   Females, I., 178.
With Tympanites—Males, I., 5.

TYPHO-TOXIN INOCULATION—Males, II., 45, 45A.   Females, I., 149.

ULCER, of Leg—Males, V., 186.   Females, III., 35, 51.

URÆMIA—Males, I., 20‡ (22), 92‡ (86) ; II., 95‡ (55), 151†, 235‡ (248) ; III., 182‡
   (291) ; IV., 185† ; V., 229‡ (251).   Females, I., 139‡ (218) ; III., 28 ;
   IV., 134‡ (202).

URETHRA—
   Caruncle of—Females, VI., 44, 123, 131, 135, 182, 209, 213, 222, 227, 281, 345,
      355, 443.
   Inflammation of—Females, VI., 121, 156, 361, 463.
   Injury to—Females, VI., 52, 52A, 52B.
   Lupus of—Females, VI., 66.
   Malignant growth of—Females, VI., 161.
   Stricture of—Males, II., 223‡ (126) ; III., 235.   Females, VI., 121, 156.

URETHROCELE—Females, VI., 108, 262, 355.

URINE—
   Incontinence of—Females, VI., 147.
   Retention of—Females, VI., 53, 53A, 79, 179, 186, 191, 204.

URTICARIA—Males, III., 246.   Females, I., 140.
———— ————from Antitoxin injection—Females, I., 198.

UTERINE APPENDAGES—
   Inflammation of—Females, VI., 37, 425.
   Broad Ligament Cysts—Females, VI., 7, 86, 90, 144, 358.

UTERINE CERVIX—
   Adenoma of—Females, VI., 455.
   Catarrh of—Females, VI., 26, 182, 281.
   Cysts of—Females, VI., 182, 355, 467.
   Erosion of—Females, VI., 26, 172, 188, 261, 440.
   Fibroid Tumour of—Females, VI., 320.
   Hæmorrhage from—Females, VI., 93.
   Hypertrophy of—Females, VI., 430.
   Inflammation of—Females, VI., 270.
   Malignant Growth of—Females, VI., 25, 33, 39, 107, 141, 157, 158, 160, 166,
      169, 214, 242, 245, 279, 340, 375, 390, 472, 475, 478.
   Polypus of—Females, VI., 101, 122, 281, 334‡ (144), 456, 467.
   Splitting of—Females, VI., 430.
   Ulceration of (Simple)—Females, VI., 255, 441.

UTERINE HÆMORRHAGE—Females. VI., 2, 5, 10, 62, 77, 82, 84, 111, 116, 129, 134,
      137, 142, 164, 176, 180, 216, 253, 305, 308, 389, 405, 418, 449, 451.
   During Pregnancy—Females, VI., 94, 221, 221A, 236.
   Accidental—Females, VI., 72, 196, 198, 201. 205.
   — ————concealed—Females, VI., 284, 317.

UTERUS—
    Fibroid Tumour of—Females, VI., 10, 38, 46, 49, 56, 62, 66, 77, 82, 110,
        124, 142, 179, 184, 190, 206, 208, 248, 267, 296, 303, 324, 327, 358, 362, 370,
        383, 422, 444, 446, 478.
    ————— Impacted—Females, VI., 53, 53A, 79, 186.
    Hæmorrhage from—See Uterine Hæmorrhage.
    Hour-glass Contraction of—Females, VI., 435‡ (312).
    Malignant Growth of—Females, VI., 153, 155,‖159, 265, 275, 380, 422.
    Perforation of—Females, VI., 404.
    Polypus of—Females, VI., 3, 251.
    Prolapse of—Females, VI., 8, 15, 92, 109, 199, 301, 357, 377, 441, 450.
    Retroversion of—Females, VI., 6, 51, 63, 95A, 98, 106, 112, 172, 191, 299, 430,
        439, 457.
    Subinvolution of—Females, VI., 300, 315, 325, 343.

VAGINA—
    Foreign Body in—Females, VI., 181.
    Hæmorrhage from—Females, I., 24.
    Injury to—Females, VI., 52, 52A, 52B.
    Malignant Growth of—Females, VI., 472.
    Prolapse of—Females, VI., 118, 286, 344.

VAGINISMUS—Females, VI., 97, 102, 278.

VAGINITIS—Females, I., 127 ; VI., 167, 229, 363.
    Gonorrhœal—Females, VI., 18, 151.
    Senile—Females, VI., 178, 182, 281.

VALVULAR DISEASE—See Heart.

VARICELLA—Males, Radcliffe—38.

VARIOLOID—Females, Radcliffe—9.

VEINS—
    Iliac, Thrombosis of—Females, IV., 60‡ (60) ; V., 112.
    Innominate, Thrombosis of—Females, II., 60‡ (60).
    Limb, Thrombosis of—Males, I., 86‡ (101) ; II., 128, 205† ; V., 58, 112, 142.
        Females, I., 91, 120, 178 ; III., 20, 86 ; V., 34, 164‡ (275) ; VI., 385, 418.
    Renal, Thrombosis of—Females, IV., 60‡ (60).
    Varicose—Females, VI., 418.
    ————— Thrombosed—Females, V., 164‡ (275).

VERTIGO—Males, IV., 171.
    Auditory—Males, V., 10, 68, 86.

VITREOUS, Exudation into—Females, I., 187.

VISCERA, Transposition of—Males, II., 97.

VOMITING—Males, II., 64‡ (49) ; IV., 63 ; V., 61, 66.   Females, II., 93‡ (182) ;
    III., 118 ; IV., 17, 72‡ (121), 132‡ (222) ; V., 69‡ (76), 84, 91.
VULVA—
    Cyst of—Females, VI., 163, 294.
    Inflammation of, gonorrhœal—Females, VI., 151.
    Lipoma of—Females, VI., 337.
    Malignant Growth of—Females, VI., 183, 215.
    Ulceration of—Females, VI., 356.
    Warts of—Females, VI., 239.

VULVO-VAGINAL CYST—Females, VI., 78.

WHOOPING COUGH—See Pertussis.

XERODERMA—Males, II., 74.   Females, I., 16.

INDEX

TO REGISTER OF POST-MORTEM EXAMINATIONS

MEDICAL, Vol. XXXI., 1904.

ABNORMALITIES—
  Of Heart—20, 118.
  Of Liver—266.
  Of Intestine—8.
  Of Kidney—241, 245, 282.

ABSCESS—
  Muscles of Back—212.
  Retro-peritoneal—212.
  Subdiaphragmatic—262.
  Subpleural—212.
  Thigh—212.

ADDISON'S DISEASE—59.

ALCOHOLISM, Chronic—179, 299.

ANÆMIA, Pernicious—198, 256, 325.

ANASARCA—5, 22, 24, 42, 82, 95, 98, 99, 186, 271, 274, 290, 313.

ANEURYSM—
  Aortic Arch—90, 294.
  Basilar—267.
  Brachial—240.
  Cerebral Arteries—35, 267.
  Dissecting—294.
  Mitral Valve—240.
  Superior Mesenteric Artery—214.

AORTA—
  Aneurysm—*See* Aneurysm.
  Atheroma of—4, 11, 58, 62, 86, 90, 92, 103, 104, 110, 130, 139, 144, 149, 185, 197, 202, 235, 245, 251, 263, 280, 296, 304, 307, 313, 320, 328.
  Endarteritis, Syphilitic—48.
  Rupture of—294.

APPENDIX VERMIFORMIS—*See* Intestines.

ARTERIES—
  Aneurysm of—*See* Aneurysm.
  Arterio-sclerosis Diffuse—245, 279, 291, 313, 328.
  Basilar, Aneurysm of—267.
    „   Embolism of—108.
  Brachial, Embolism of—15.
  Cerebral—
    Atheroma of—4, 11, 30, 235, 267, 268, 284, 296, 304, 307, 313.
    Embolism of—4, 15, 28, 108, 146.
    Thrombosis of—267.
  Coronary, Atheroma of—313, 320, 328.
  Intercostal, Puncture of—94.
  Popliteal, Embolism of—28.
  Splenic, Atheroma of—313.

ARTHRITIS—*See* Joints.

ASCITES—5, 22, 24, 51, 58, 82, 90, 92, 95, 98, 99, 215, 230, 248, 274, 313.

ATHEROMA—*See* Aorta and Arteries.

BEDSORES—275.

BILE DUCTS—*See* Liver.

BLADDER—
    Cystitis—212.
    Malignant Growth of—175.
    Tubercle in—298, 314.

BRAIN—
    Cerebellum—
        Abscess of—73.
    Cerebrum—
        Abscess of—73.
        Atrophy of Cortex—40, 202, 297, 313.
        Congestion of—110.
        Cyst in, Calcified—11, 245.
        Embolism—4, 15.
        Hæmorrhage into, recent—11, 19, 30, 71, 130, 235, 245, 268, 279, 284,
            296, 304, 307, 308.
        Hæmorrhage into, old—30, 245.
        Hydrocephalus—41, 278, 283, 322.
        Pons Varolii, Softening of—267.
            Hæmorrhage into—245.
        Softening of—4, 245, 279.
        Tumour of—
            Tuberculous—283.

BREAST, Malignant Growth of—119.

BRONCHI—*See* Lung.

BROUGHT IN DEAD—16, 115, 172, 217, 227, 242, 277, 288, 309, 318.

CALCULUS—
    Biliary—125, 237, 280, 320.
    Renal—54, 266, 305.

CELLULITIS—3.

CEREBELLUM—*See* Brain.

CERVIX UTERI—*See* Uterine Cervix.

CHOROID, Tubercle of—70, 301, 326.

CYSTITIS—*See* Bladder.

DELIRIUM TREMENS—241.

DERMATITIS—126, 286.

DIABETES, Mellitus—96, 263.

DIPHTHERIA—34, 87, 88, 89, 115, 250, 252, 324.

DROWNING, Death from—110.

DUODENUM—*See* Intestines.

EAR, Suppuration of Middle—16, 21, 41, 50, 61, 64, 65, 100, 107, 115, 122, 170, 204,
    305.
    Tubercle of Middle—46, 134.

EMPHYSEMA, of Lung—*See* Lung.
  „   " Surgical "—327.
EMPYEMA—*See* Pleura.
ENDOCARDITIS—*See* Heart.
ENTERIC FEVER—*See* Typhoid Fever.
EPILEPSY—216.
EXOPHTHALMIC GOÎTRE—92.

FALLOPIAN TUBE—*See* Uterine Appendages.
FAUCES, Membrane on —115, 324.
FEMUR, Subperiosteal Hæmorrhage—133,

GALL BLADDER—*See* Liver.
GALLSTONES—*See* Calculus.
GLOTTIS—*See* Larynx.
GOUT—*See* Joints, Uratic Deposit in.

HEART—
    Abnormalities of (Congenital)—
        Deficient Cusps to Valves—18, 28, 146.
        Patent Ductus Arteriosus and Foramen Ovale—20.
              „   „   „   Rudimentary Septum between Auricles
          " and Ventricles—118.
    Aneurysm of—135.
    Atrophy of—237.
    Clots, Ante-mortem, in—240, 258.
    Coronary Arteries, Atheroma of—313, 320, 328.
    Endocarditis, Ulcerative or Infective—6, 7, 13, 15, 18, 28, 33, 38, 85, 95, 127,
        135, 146, 195, 214, 226, 229, 234, 240, 260, 317.
    Fatty Degeneration of—58, 60, 103, 120, 126, 132, 144, 149, 175, 198, 200,
        203, 270, 275, 311, 320, 325.
    Fatty Infiltration of—144, 245, 267, 320.
    Dilatation of—5, 18, 24, 29, 36, 37, 42, 55, 56, 58, 64, 80, 82, 86, 92, 95, 98,
        99, 100, 110, 124, 130, 149, 167, 171, 203, 226, 228, 230, 258, 270, 275,
        278, 280, 290, 306, 316, 319, 320.
    Hypertrophy of—5, 11, 18, 22, 24, 29, 30, 35, 36, 37, 42, 55, 56, 58, 62, 82, 92,
        95, 98, 99, 130, 149, 201, 202, 218, 226, 228, 230, 245, 251, 257, 260, 268,
        279, 280, 284, 290, 291, 296, 304, 317, 320.
    Fibroid Degeneration of—313.
    Hæmorrhage, Sub-endocardial—244.
    Malignant Growth of—321.
    Myocarditis—79, 97, 232, 261, 270, 306.
    Tubercle of—43, 300.
    Aortic Valve—
        Calcareous—5, 226, 240.
        Perforation of—240.
        Stenosis of—5, 6, 260.
        Thickened—5, 7, 24, 28, 42, 48, 51, 54, 90, 98, 108, 144, 145, 146, 149,
            160, 197, 201, 203, 240, 260, 290, 293, 317, 328.
        Vegetations on—56, 82, 98, 102, 108, 226, 270, 275, 276, 293, 306, 311.

HEART—*continued*.
    Mitral Valve—
        Aneurysm of—185, 240.
        Calcareous—51.
        Perforation of—240.
        Thickened—4, 5, 7, 13, 15, 24, 28, 42, 51, 92, 95, 98, 145, 149, 159, 160,
            186, 201, 203, 226, 229, 230, 234, 260, 290, 293, 295, 296, 311, 313,
            317.
        Vegetations on—4, 13, 15, 17, 19, 24, 29, 56, 98, 102, 105, 159, 160, 186,
            195, 230, 270, 276, 293, 306, 311.
    Mitral Orifice, Stenosis of—4, 5, 6, 13, 15, 24, 51, 98, 105, 108, 159, 160, 186,
        201, 203, 229, 243, 260, 313.
    Pulmonary Orifice, Vegetations on—79.
    Tricuspid Valve—
        Thickened—24, 42, 51, 203.
        Vegetations on—17, 159, 160, 270, 276, 311, 317.
    Tricuspid Orifice, Stenosis of—24, 51, 203.

HYDATID, of Liver—11.

HYDRO-THORAX—5, 24, 92, 95, 203, 313.

ILIUM, Malignant Growth of—175.

INFARCTS—*See* Various Organs.

INSANITY—202.

INTESTINES—
    Abnormalities of—
        Meckel's Diverticulum—8.
    Duodenum—
        Dilatation of—60, 74.
        Malignant Stricture of—74.
        Ulcer of—72.
    Small Intestine—
        Perforation of—264.
        Ulceration of—24, 131, 133, 137, 149.
            Tuberculous—12, 23, 25, 44, 46, 65, 75, 101, 134, 141, 174, 178, 184,
                190, 208, 231, 283, 300, 301, 326.
            Typhoid—223, 232, 264, 293, 295, 328.
    Cæcum—
        Ulceration of—24, 203.
            Tuberculous—25.
            Typhoid—223, 328.
    Appendix Vermiformis—
        Concretion in—162, 262.
        Gangrene of—262.
        Ulceration of—162.
            Tuberculous—300.
    Colon—
        Ulceration of—210, 286, 298.
            Tuberculous—23, 141, 208.
            In Typhoid Fever—328.

JAUNDICE—119, 153.
    Icterus Gravis—153.

JOINTS—
    Arthritis—79.
    Charcot's disease of—171.
    Uratic deposits in—11, 257, 284, 296, 307.

KIDNEY—
    Abnormality of—35, 241, 245, 282.
    Abscesses, Multiple, of—256.
    Calculus in—54, 266, 305.
    Cloudy Swelling—115, 223, 293, 306.
    Congestion, Chronic—201, 311, 317.
    Cystic Disease of—169.
    Fatty—18, 110, 275.
    Hæmorrhages under Capsule—132.
    Hydro-nephrosis—11, 54, 302.
    Infarction of—4, 7, 13, 15, 18, 38, 85, 95, 98, 127, 132, 226, 229, 230, 234, 240.
    Iron Reaction in—325.
    Malignant Growth in—27.
    Nephritis—
        Acute—51, 82, 195, 260, 297.
        Chronic Parenchymatous—22, 55, 127, 229, 274.
        Chronic Interstitial—2, 4, 7, 11, 30, 36, 51, 56, 62, 66, 82, 95, 104, 112,
            119, 130, 152, 165, 179, 185, 202, 241, 247, 248, 257, 258, 268, 284,
            296, 304, 313, 320.
        Mixed (Contracted White Kidney)—34, 86, 191, 218, 251, 291.
    Pyelitis—212.
    Pyelo-nephritis—126.
    Single—245.
    Thrombosis of Renal Vein—60, 273.
    Tuberculous Disease of—206.
    Tubercles, Miliary, in—8, 65, 68, 70, 134, 148, 184, 190, 208, 283, 298, 300,
        301, 314.
    Unequal size of—241.
    Uric Acid "infarcts"—158, 273, 302.

LARYNX—
    Corroded by Poison—104.
    Membrane in—115, 324.
    Œdema of—33, 252.
    Ulceration—
        Non-Tuberculous—33.
        Tuberculous—2, 52, 111, 141, 150, 190.

LEUKÆMIA, Lymphatic, Acute—57, 199.

LIVER—
    Abnormality of—266.
    Adenoma of—258.
    Cholangitis, Tuberculous—134, 184.
    Cirrhosis of—14, 30, 31, 58, 62, 63, 92, 103, 112, 113, 139, 152, 205, 215,
        241, 247, 248, 307.
    Fatty—2, 10, 27, 31, 62, 75, 95, 103, 110, 125, 141, 158, 240, 242, 267, 280,
        312, 320, 326.
    Gumma—34.
    Hæmorrhages in Capsule—153.
    Hydatid of—11.
    Icterus Gravis—153.
    Iron Reaction in—198, 325.
    Leukæmia—191.

LIVER—*continued*.

    Lymphadenoma—200.
    Malignant Growth of—1, 27, 66, 94, 119, 175, 194.
    Nutmeg—4, 5, 24, 80, 90, 95, 98, 102, 118, 149, 160, 201, 228, 270, 280, 290, 313.
    Perihepatitis—34, 51, 92, 179, 205, 248.
    Tubercles in—8, 12, 26, 43, 46, 50, 54, 65, 68, 70, 111, 123, 137, 143, 148,
        176, 181, 184, 208, 231, 283, 292, 298, 300, 301, 314, 324.

    Gall Bladder—
        Empyema of—63, 113.
        Gangrene of—66.
        Malformation of—266.

LUNG—
    Abscess of—140, 189, 211, 233, 258, 297.
    Atelectasis—32.
    Bronchiectasis—75, 77, 136, 140, 228, 271, 280.
    Bronchiolectasis—100, 228, 258, 316, 319, 324.
    Bronchitis—20, 56, 58, 88, 95, 100, 103, 133, 142, 181, 227, 238, 241, 258, 271,
        280, 282, 290, 292, 294, 302, 320.
    Bronchus—
        Compression of, by Caseous Gland—131.
        Frothy Fluid in (death from Drowning)—110.
        Malignant Growth of—321.
    Collapse of (partial or complete)—9, 10, 16, 20, 37, 69, 77, 83, 87, 88, 89,
        102, 107, 115, 124, 125, 128, 129, 131, 133, 137, 142, 154, 156, 157, 158,
        162, 163, 168, 170, 172, 181, 188, 192, 196, 207, 217, 221, 222, 238, 242,
        246, 249, 252, 253, 254, 259, 265, 266, 269, 270, 277, 285, 286, 288, 292,
        298, 302, 305, 309, 310, 313, 316, 319, 323.
    Congestion of—145, 160, 311.

    Emphysema—
        Vesicular—4, 95, 99, 115, 131, 154, 202, 203, 218, 228, 265, 269, 275, 284,
            299, 313, 314, 316, 319, 320.
        Interstitial—69, 76, 87, 89, 183, 196, 250, 280.
    Fibrosis of—75, 228.
    Frothy Fluid in (death from Drowning)—110.
    Gangrene of—25.
    Hæmorrhage into—25, 40, 117.
    Infarction of—5, 48, 95, 197, 203, 290.
    Malignant Growth in—53, 83, 321.
    Œdema of—5, 7, 15, 34, 55, 60, 82, 90, 98, 102, 103, 104, 109, 110, 120, 147,
        159, 165, 185, 195, 198, 201, 202, 203, 216, 226, 234, 235, 240, 241, 258,
        280, 282, 317, 318.

    Pneumonia—
        Catarrhal—9, 11, 21, 37, 47, 64, 69, 88, 89, 100, 107, 111, 115, 116, 117,
            118, 120, 122, 123, 124, 140, 166, 169, 181, 197, 218, 219, 224, 230,
            233, 239, 246, 249, 250, 252, 253, 258, 259, 262, 265, 266, 269, 270,
            281, 287, 298, 302, 305, 309, 310, 315, 316, 319, 323, 324.
        Lobar—29, 34, 79, 97, 105, 127, 163, 165, 167, 211, 214, 228, 229, 232,
            235, 243, 263, 299, 303.

    Tuberculosis of—
        Phthisis—2, 12, 25, 50, 52, 68, 75, 93, 111, 114, 123, 136, 141, 150, 178,
            190, 239, 274, 283, 289, 298, 314, 326.
        Acute Caseating—45, 80, 131, 134, 150, 154, 184.
        Miliary—8, 26, 31, 43, 46, 65, 68, 70, 101, 111, 137, 143, 148, 155,
            174, 176, 181, 184, 208, 278, 300, 301, 314, 324, 326.
        Obsolete—101, 126, 135, 139, 163, 165, 185, 202, 240, 241.

LYMPHADENOMA—200.

LYMPHATIC GLANDS—
    Abdominal—
        Leukæmic—57, 199.
        Lymphadenoma—200, 271.
        Malignant Growth of—1, 27, 119, 185.
        Tuberculous Disease of—8, 12, 23, 25, 26, 44, 46, 50, 65, 68, 93, 101
            123, 131, 134, 141, 150, 161, 176, 178, 184, 190, 208, 300.
    Bronchial and Tracheal—
        Malignant Growth of—175.
        Suppuration in—11.
        Tuberculous Disease of—8, 12, 25, 26, 43, 50, 65, 68, 70, 75, 93, 111, 114,
            116, 123, 131, 132, 134, 137, 141, 143, 148, 150, 154, 155, 174, 181,
            184, 190, 208, 239, 274, 278, 283, 298, 300, 301, 324.
            Calcareous—2, 132, 141, 163.
    Cervical—
        Malignant Growth of—27, 60.
        Suppuration in—11.
        Tuberculous Disease of—141, 150, 190, 283, 309, 321.
    Mediastinal—
        Malignant Growth of—321.
        Tuberculous Disease of—46, 111, 114, 208, 283, 298, 300, 301, 324.

MALIGNANT GROWTH—
    Of Bladder—175.
    Of Breast—119.
    Of Bronchus—321.
    Of Heart—321.
    Of Ilium—175.
    Of Intestine—74.
    Of Kidney—27.
    Of Liver—1, 27, 66, 94, 119, 175, 237.
    Of Lung—53, 83, 321.
    Of Lymphatic Glands—1, 27, 60, 119, 175, 321.
    Of Mediastinum—39, 59, 83, 321.
    Of Œsophagus—194.
    Of Ovary—175.
    Of Pancreas—66.
    Of Peritoneum—27, 237.
    Of Pleura—27, 66, 119, 151, 175, 321.
    Of Stomach—27, 49, 60, 185, 237.
    Of Suprarenal Capsule—1.
    Of Thoracic Duct—27.

MARASMUS—76, 91, 128, 156, 158, 183, 187, 192, 217, 281, 288, 298.

MEASLES—265, 315.

MEDIASTINUM—
    Inflammation of (Mediastinitis)—
        Acute—3, 306.
        Indurative—10.
    Malignant Growth of—39, 59, 83, 321.

MENINGES—
    Ependymitis—41, 61.
    Hæmorrhage into—11, 19, 32, 35, 112, 120, 225, 226, 244, 308.
    Tubercle in—*See* Meningitis, Tuberculous ; *also* Dura Mater, Tuberculous
        Tumour of.
    Dura Mater—
        Endothelioma of—313.
        Tuberculous Tumour of (obsolete)—102.
    Meningitis—
        Pachymeningitis Hæmorrhagic—40.
                „   Purulent—297.

MENINGES -*continued*.
  Leptomeningitis—
    Post-Basal—21, 41, 322.
    Purulent—61, 63, 69, 107, 117, 122, 147, 168, 188, 204, 236.
    Tuberculous—23, 26, 43, 44, 50, 54, 68, 70, 93, 114, 131, 134, 137, 143
      148, 155, 174, 176, 181, 208, 231, 239, 272, 278, 283, 292, 314.
    Spinal, Primary Purulent—212.

MYELITIS—*See* Spinal Cord.

NEPHRITIS—*See* Kidney.

NEURITIS, Peripheral—103.

NODULES, Rheumatic—102, 276, 311.

ŒSOPHAGUS—
    Corrosion by Mineral Acids—104.
    Enlarged Veins in—51, 139.
    Malignant Growth of—194.
    Rupture of—327.

OVARY—
    Cyst of—73, 139, 202.
    Malignant Growth of—175.

PANCREAS—
    Atrophy of—96.
    Malignant Growth of—66.
    Tubercle of—134, 184, 283.

PERICARDIUM—
    Adherent—22, 92, 150, 230, 270, 290, 303, 311, 313.
    Hæmo-pericardium—294.
    Hydro-pericardium—5, 82, 159.
    Pneumo-pericardium—14.
    Pericarditis—10, 17, 33, 79, 83, 97, 186, 214, 226, 229, 261, 276, 285, 299,
      306, 317.
      Hæmorrhagic—102.
      Purulent—9, 77, 116, 117, 122, 303.
      Tuberculous—150.
    Tubercles in—150, 208, 301.

PERIHEPATITIS—*See* Liver.

PERIMETRITIC ADHESIONS—5, 58, 103, 203.

PERISPLENITIS—*See* Spleen.

PERITONEUM—
    Adhesions of—5, 11, 25, 27, 40, 46, 51, 54, 60, 75, 119, 125, 134, 190, 195, 221,
      245, 274, 318.
    Malignant Growth of—27.
    Peritonitis—60, 162, 264, 282, 310.
      Chronic—51, 92, 296.
      Hæmorrhagic—125.
      Purulent—10, 13, 77, 177, 191, 212, 262, 312.
      Tuberculous—31, 46, 54, 247.
    Tubercles in—31, 46, 54, 134, 137, 141, 148, 150, 176, 178, 190, 221, 247.

Pertussis—16, 154.

Pharynx, Corrosion by Mineral Acids—104.

Phimosis—302.

Pleura—
    Adhesions—2, 10, 15, 22, 46, 51, 58, 64, 73, 75, 77, 98, 102, 103, 104, 122, 125,
        139, 140, 141, 145, 148, 150, 152, 154, 190, 194, 201, 206, 216, 224, 230,
        241, 244, 258, 266, 274, 283, 285, 298, 304, 314, 324, 326.
    Empyema—9, 10, 77, 116, 118, 122, 163, 165, 177, 189, 200, 211, 224, 233,
        266, 285, 303, 310.
    Hæmo-thorax—25, 94, 112, 199.
    Hydro-thorax—5, 24, 82, 90, 159.
    Malignant Growth of—27, 119, 151, 175, 321.
    Perforation of, from Gangrene—25.
    Pleurisy—5, 11, 12, 17, 25, 33, 37, 47, 54, 60, 102, 117, 123, 166, 186, 190, 219,
        221, 258, 261, 266, 274, 283, 299, 306, 309, 319,
        Definitely Tuberculous—190, 274, 283.
        With Effusion—127, 136, 141, 197, 214, 282, 287, 312, 327.
        With Hæmorrhagic Effusion—125, 151, 258.
    Pyo-pneumo-thorax—289.
    Sub-pleural Hæmorrhages—16, 40, 110, 117, 153, 244, 249, 252, 259, 277.
    Tubercles of—8, 12, 31, 50, 54, 65, 68, 70, 93, 137, 148, 150, 184, 208, 247,
        283, 300, 301, 324.

Poisoning—
    Nitric Acid—104.

Poly-Serositis—
    Simple—271, 296.
    Tuberculous—150.

Pons Varolii—See Brain.

Porencephalon—161.

Purpura—120.

Pyæmia—189.

Pyo-pneumo-thorax—See Pleura.

Rectum—See Intestines.

Retina—
    Albuminuric Retinitis—22.
    Hæmorrhages into—325.

Rib—
    Fracture of—17, 112.
    Necrosis of—73.
    Periostitis (Suppurative)—73.

Rickets—9, 37, 43, 65, 133, 142, 180, 277, 301.

Scurvy, Infantile—133.

Septicæmia—132, 153.

Sinuses, Cerebral, Thrombosis of—25, 46, 158.

Skin, Hæmorrhages into—18, 85, 153.

SKULL—
    Fracture—244.
    Thickening of—202.

SPINAL CORD—
    Malformation of—278.
    Myelitis—255.
    Poliomyelitis—67.
    Tabes Dorsalis—171.

SPINE—
    Lateral Curvature of—301.

SPLEEN—
    Abscess of—13.
    Cardiac—5, 24, 95, 98, 118, 160, 201, 270, 280, 290.
    Enlarged—198, 205, 293.
    Hæmorrhages into—286.
    Infarction of—13, 15, 18, 19, 38, 85, 127, 195, 226, 234, 260.
    Leukæmia—57, 191.
    Lymphadenoma—200.
    Perisplenitis—51, 62, 92, 139, 179, 205, 251, 304, 313, 317.
    Tubercles in—8, 12, 26, 43, 44, 50, 54, 65, 68, 70, 93, 114, 134, 137, 143,
        148, 174, 176, 181, 184, 190, 208, 231, 283, 292, 298, 300, 301, 314, 324.

STOMACH—
    Atrophy of—198.
    Corroded by Poisons—104.
    Dilatation of—74, 195, 237.
    Gastritis—179.
    Hæmorrhage into—104, 109.
    Hæmorrhage, Submucous, of—236.
    Hour-glass Contraction of—176.
    Lymphadenoma of—200.
    Malignant Growth of—27, 49, 60, 185, 237.
    Perforation of—60, 152.
    Ulcer of (simple)—106, 152.

SUPRARENAL CAPSULE—
    Atrophy of—59.
    Hæmorrhage into—225.
    Tubercle of—184.

SYPHILIS, Congenital—286.

TETANUS—78.

THORACIC DUCT, Malignant Growth of—27.

THYMUS GLAND—
    Enlarged—217.
    Inflammation of—118.
    Suppuration of—116.

TONGUE—
    Corroded by Poison—104.
    Ulcer of—5.

TOPHI, in Ear—284.

TRACHEA—
    Membrane in—115, 252, 324.
    Papilloma of—258.
    Tuberculous Ulceration of—2, 111, 141, 150, 190.

TRACHEOTOMY—87, 259.

TUBERCLE—
    Of Bladder—298, 314.
    Of Brain—134, 283.
    Of Choroid—70, 301, 326.
    Of Ear—46, 134.
    Of Heart—43, 300.
    Of Intestines—*See* Intestines.
    Of Kidney—8, 65, 68, 70, 134, 148, 184, 190, 208, 283, 298, 300, 301, 314.
    Of Larynx—2, 111, 141, 150, 190.
    Of Liver—8, 12, 26, 43, 46, 50, 54, 65, 68, 70, 111, 123, 137, 143, 148, 176, 181, 184, 208, 231, 283, 292, 298, 300, 301, 314, 324.
    Of Lung—*See* Lung.
    Of Lymphatic Glands—*See* Lymphatic Glands.
    Of Meninges—23, 26, 43, 44, 50, 54, 68, 70, 93, 102, 114, 131, 184, 137, 143, 148, 155, 174, 176, 181, 208, 231, 239, 272, 278, 283, 292, 314.
    Of Pancreas—134, 184, 283.
    Of Pericardium—150, 208 301.
    Of Peritoneum—31, 46, 54, 134, 137, 141, 143, 148, 150, 176, 178, 190, 221, 231, 247.
    Of Pleura—8, 12, 31, 50, 54, 65, 68, 70, 93, 137, 148, 150, 184, 208, 247, 283, 300, 301, 324.
    Of Suprarenals—184.
    Of Spleen—8, 12, 26, 43, 44, 50, 54, 65, 68, 70, 93, 114, 134, 137, 143, 148, 174, 176, 181, 184, 190, 208, 231, 283, 292, 298, 300, 301, 314, 324.
    Of Uterine Appendages—54, 221.

TUBERCULOSIS, Acute Miliary—8, 23, 26, 43, 44, 50, 54, 68, 70, 93, 114, 131, 134, 137, 143, 148, 155, 174, 176, 181, 184, 208, 215, 231, 239, 272, 283, 292, 298, 300, 301, 314, 324.

TYPHOID FEVER—223, 232, 264, 293, 295, 328.

URÆMIA—62, 82, 291.

URETER, Dilatation of—54, 302.

URETHRA, Stricture of—126.

UTERINE APPENDAGES—
    Fallopian Tube—
        Pyo-salpinx—147, 282.
        Tuberculosis of—54, 221.

UTERINE CERVIX, Erosion of—73.

UTERUS—
    Enlarged—13, 82, 132, 195, 282.
    Endometritis (Septic)—13, 275, 282, 312.
    Fibroid of—202.
    Mucous Polypus of—144.
    Subinvolution of—13, 74, 82, 132, 195, 282.

VEIN—
    Thrombosis of—
        Iliac—60, 101.
        Innominate—60.
        Jugular—60.
        Portal—14.
        Renal—60, 273.
        Veins of Leg—275.
    Varicose—275.

SURGICAL REPORT.

PREFACE TO THE SURGICAL REPORT.

The general arrangement of the Statistical Tables is the same as in previous years.

Table I. comprises all patients who left the Surgical Wards during the year ; each patient appears in this Table once only ; cases in which two or more injuries or diseases occurred in the same patient are entered only under the principal disease or injury. In the Library is kept a manuscript index in which all injuries and diseases are entered, irrespective of the number of patients. Thus, a patient with fracture of the base of the skull, fracture of the clavicle, and dislocation of the elbow would be entered in Table I. under the first heading only, but in the manuscript index under all three.

Table II. includes all operations upon the patients in Table I., and also operations performed upon patients in the Gynæcological and Medical Wards.

In the Appendix, the references to the volume and number of the notes of each case are given in brackets.

The bound volumes of notes are kept in the Library. They are numbered as follows :—

Mr. Langton ... ... Vol. I.
Mr. Harrison Cripps ... ... Vol. II.
Mr. Bruce Clarke ... ... Vol. III.
Mr. Bowlby ... ... Vol. IV.
Mr. Lockwood ... ... Vol. V.
Mr. Jessop and Mr. Holmes Spicer Vol. VI.

TABLE I.

Showing the Total Number of Cases under Treatment during the Year 1904, with the comparative Frequency and Mortality of each Disease at different Ages.

DISEASE.	Total.	Discharged. M.	Discharged. F.	Died. M.	Died. F.	Under 5. Disch. M.	Under 5. Disch. F.	Under 5. Died M.	Under 5. Died F.	−10. Disch. M.	−10. Disch. F.	−10. Died M.	−10. Died F.	−15. Disch. M.	−15. Disch. F.	−15. Died M.	−15. Died F.	−20. Disch. M.	−20. Disch. F.	−20. Died M.	−20. Died F.	−30. Disch. M.	−30. Disch. F.	−30. Died M.	−30. Died F.	−40. Disch. M.	−40. Disch. F.	−40. Died M.	−40. Died F.	−50. Disch. M.	−50. Disch. F.	−50. Died M.	−50. Died F.	−60. Disch. M.	−60. Disch. F.	−60. Died M.	−60. Died F.	Over 60. Disch. M.	Over 60. Disch. F.	Over 60. Died M.	Over 60. Died F.
DISEASES.																																									
GENERAL DISEASES.																																									
Actinomycosis ...	3	2	...	1	...																	1						1							1						
Anthrax ...	3	2	...	1	...																	1						1													
Enteric Fever ...	3	...	...	3	...											1				1				1				1		1											
Erysipelas ...	33	13	19	1	...	4				1	3			2					2			4	7			1				4	1			1							
Gangrene—																																									
Idiopathic	9	4	3	...	2			1																		1													1	3	3
Hæmophilia...	3	2	...	1	...	1			1											1																					
Snake bite ...	1	1	...	...	...	1																																			
VENEREAL DISEASES.																																									
Congenital Syphilis ...	1	1	...	...	...	1																																			
Gonorrhœal Vulvitis ...	1	...	1	...	...		1																																		

TABLE I. (*continued*). 74

DISEASE.	Total.	Discharged.		Died.		Under 5.				— 10.				— 15.				— 20.				— 30.				— 40.				— 50.				— 60.				Over 60.			
						Discharged.		Died.		Discharged.		Died.		Discharged.		Died.		Discharged.		Died.		Discharged.		Died.		Discharged.		Died.		Discharged.		Died.		Discharged.		Died.		Discharged.		Died.	
		M.	F.	M.	F.	M.	F.	M.	F.	M.	F.	M.	F.	M.	F.	M.	F.	M.	F.	M.	F.	M.	F.	M.	F.	M.	F.	M.	F.	M.	F.	M.	F.	M.	F.	M.	F.	M.	F.	M.	F.
MALFORMATIONS AND DEFORMITIES.																																									
Branchial Cyst	1	1	...	...	...	5	2			3	2			1				1	4							1															
Cleft Palate...	18	10	8	...	...	5	2			3	2			1				1	4							1															
„ „ with Hare Lip	10	5	4	**1**	...	5	4	**1**																																	
„ „ with Hare Lip previously closed	3	2	1	...	...	1	1			1																															
Contraction of Finger ...	5	3	2	...	...	1								1				2					1																		
Congenital Dislocation of Hip	7	1	6	...	...	1	1			4				1																											
Deformity of Arm	1	1	...	...	...													1																						
„ „ Leg	2	2	...	...	...	2																																		
„ „ Mouth ...	6	1	5	...	...	1	2											1					1					1												
„ „ Penis... ...	2	2	...	...	...	1				1																															
Fistula (Tracheal)	1	1	...	...	...																				1															
Genu Valgum	16	3	13	...	...	1	2			7				1	2			1	1			1																			
Genu Varum	1	...	1	...	...		1																																		
Hallux Valgus	6	3	3	...	...									2				1	1			1													1					
Hammer Toe	6	6	...	...	...					1				1	1			2				2																			
Hare Lip	4	...	4	...	...		4																																		
Rib (Accessory)	1	...	1	...	...									1																											
Spina Bifida...	5	1	...	**4**	...	1		**4**																																	
Spine, Lateral Curvature of	3	...	3	...	...					1								2																						
Supernumerary Fingers ...	2	...	2	...	...		2																																		

TABLE I. (continued).

DISEASE	Total	Discharged M	Discharged F	Died M	Died F	Under 5 Disch. M	Under 5 Disch. F	Under 5 Died M	Under 5 Died F	—10 Disch. M	—10 Disch. F	—10 Died M	—10 Died F	—15 Disch. M	—15 Disch. F	—15 Died M	—15 Died F	—20 Disch. M	—20 Disch. F	—20 Died M	—20 Died F	—30 Disch. M	—30 Disch. F	—30 Died M	—30 Died F	—40 Disch. M	—40 Disch. F	—40 Died M	—40 Died F	—50 Disch. M	—50 Disch. F	—50 Died M	—50 Died F	—60 Disch. M	—60 Disch. F	—60 Died M	—60 Died F	Over 60 Disch. M	Over 60 Disch. F	Over 60 Died M	Over 60 Died F
MALFORMATIONS AND DEFORMITIES (continued).																																									
Talipes—																																									
Cavus	2	2	…	…	…	…	…							1	1			1																							
Equinus	6	3	3	…	…	…	1			2	1			1				1				2	1			2															
Equino-Varus and Varus	14	7	7	…	…	5	2			2	1			2	1			2				1	1																		
Flat Foot	7	5	2	…	…	2					3			1				1				1																			
Webbed Fingers	2	2	…	…	…																																				
Wry Neck	6	1	5	…	…	1								1				1				1				1															
DISEASES OF THE NERVOUS SYSTEM.																																									
Epilepsy—																																									
Epilepsy, Jacksonian	4	3	…	1	…													1				1				1						1									
Neuralgia	3	2	1	…	…																					1	1			2	1										
Hysteria	4	1	3	…	…																																				
Paralysis—																																									
Infantile	7	4	3	…	…						1	1		1	1			2				2				3															
Old	2	2	…	…	…													2				2																			
Sciatica	3	2	1	…	…													1				1				1				1											
Brain and its Membranes—																																									
Cerebellar Cyst	1	1	…	…	…						1							1				1				1				1											
Tuberculous Meningitis	3	…	…	1	2	1		1					2																												

TABLE I. (continued).

DISEASE	Total	Discharged M	Discharged F	Died M	Died F	Under 5 Disch. M	Under 5 Disch. F	Under 5 Died M	Under 5 Died F	—10 Disch. M	—10 Disch. F	—10 Died M	—10 Died F	—15 Disch. M	—15 Disch. F	—15 Died M	—15 Died F	—20 Disch. M	—20 Disch. F	—20 Died M	—20 Died F	—30 Disch. M	—30 Disch. F	—30 Died M	—30 Died F	—40 Disch. M	—40 Disch. F	—40 Died M	—40 Died F	—50 Disch. M	—50 Disch. F	—50 Died M	—50 Died F	—60 Disch. M	—60 Disch. F	—60 Died M	—60 Died F	Over 60 Disch. M	Over 60 Disch. F	Over 60 Died M	Over 60 Died F
DISEASES OF THE EYE.																																									
Eyelids—																																									
Abscess	1	1																								1															
Blepharitis	1	1																				1																			
Chancre	1	1																1																							
Ectropion	5	3	2											2					1			1	1							1				1	1				1		
Entropion	6	1	5							1									1			2	2							1					1				1		
Ptosis	1	1								1																															
Tumours	4	3	1								1			1				1								1									1			1			
Wounds	2	2												1				1																							
Lachrymal Apparatus—																																									
Dacryo-cystitis & Abscess	9	3	6			1								1	2				1			1				1				1	1			1				2			
Obstruction	1	1																																							
Mucocele	1		1												1											1															
Conjunctiva—																																									
Conjunctivitis—																																									
Catarrhal	1		1								1												1												1				1		
Membranous	4	4				2																1													1						
Purulent	3	1	2			2				1					1																										
Trachoma	6	4	2			1								1					1				1				1				1										
Tumours	1		1											1																											
Injuries	3	3				1								1								1																1			

TABLE I. (continued).

DISEASE	Total	Discharged M	Discharged F	Died M	Died F	Under 5 Disch M	Under 5 Disch F	Under 5 Died M	Under 5 Died F	−10 Disch M	−10 Disch F	−10 Died M	−10 Died F	−15 Disch M	−15 Disch F	−15 Died M	−15 Died F	−20 Disch M	−20 Disch F	−20 Died M	−20 Died F	−30 Disch M	−30 Disch F	−30 Died M	−30 Died F	−40 Disch M	−40 Disch F	−40 Died M	−40 Died F	−50 Disch M	−50 Disch F	−50 Died M	−50 Died F	−60 Disch M	−60 Disch F	−60 Died M	−60 Died F	Over 60 Disch M	Over 60 Disch F	Over 60 Died M	Over 60 Died F
DISEASES OF THE EYE (c continued).																																									
Cornea—																																									
Keratitis—																																									
Superficial	2		2				2							1	1																										
Interstitial	9	4	5			2	3				3			1	1			2	2			1	1																		
Corneal Ulcers	17	9	8			1				1				1	1							5	1			2				1				1				3			
„ „ s Hypopyon	9	8	1							1				1								1												1							
Keratoconus	1		1							1												1				1				1				1							
Leucoma and Nebula	5	3	2			1				1								1																							
Staphyloma	1	1	1																																						
Wounds and Foreign Bodies	11	10	1			2				1				2				1				3				1															
Sclerotic—																																									
Wounds	6	5	1											1				1				2													1						
Iris—																																									
Iritis	18	15	3															1	1			5	1			3				3	1			2	1			2	1		
Irido-cyclitis	5	1	4																1			1								1				1	1			1	1		
Irido-dialysis	1	1																																1							
Lens—																																									
Dislocation	2		2																							1												1			
Cataract—																																									
Congenital	8	2	1			1												1	1																						
Diabetic	1	1																																1				1			
Lamellar	5	1	4				1				1							1				3																	1		

TABLE I. (continued).

78

DISEASE	Total	Discharged M	Discharged F	Died M	Died F	Under 5 Disch. M	Under 5 Disch. F	Under 5 Died M	Under 5 Died F	−10 Disch. M	−10 Disch. F	−10 Died M	−10 Died F	−15 Disch. M	−15 Disch. F	−15 Died M	−15 Died F	−20 Disch. M	−20 Disch. F	−20 Died M	−20 Died F	−30 Disch. M	−30 Disch. F	−30 Died M	−30 Died F	−40 Disch. M	−40 Disch. F	−40 Died M	−40 Died F	−50 Disch. M	−50 Disch. F	−50 Died M	−50 Died F	−60 Disch. M	−60 Disch. F	−60 Died M	−60 Died F	Over 60 Disch. M	Over 60 Disch. F	Over 60 Died M	Over 60 Died F
DISEASES OF THE EYE (continued).																																									
Cataract (continued)—																																									
Senile ...	40	24	16	...	...																										3			2	4			22	9		
Traumatic ...	10	5	5	...	...					2				1	5															1											
After Cataract...	31	17	14	...	...										1			2	1			1	4				3							7				7	5		
Glaucoma—																																									
Primary ...	11	4	7	...	...																					1				4	1				2			4	1		
Secondary ...	4	2	2	...	...																									1					1						
Retina and Choroid—																																									
Retinitis ...	10	5	5	...	...	2																1	3			1				2	2			1							
Glioma of Retina ...	2	2	...	...	...	2																																			
Detachment of Retina...	9	8	6	...	...																	2				3				1				1							
Choroiditis ...	1	1	...	...	...																	1				1												1			
Tumour of Choroid ...	1	1	1	...	...																																		1		
Optic Nerve—																																									
Papillitis ...	2	1	1	...	...									1				1																							
Orbit—																																									
Cellulitis ...	3	1	2	...	...					1				1								1				1								1							
Tumour ...	2	2	...	...	...									1																											
Fracture ...	1	1	...	...	...																																				
Vitreous Humour—																																									
Hemorrhage into Vitreous ...	1	1	...	...	...									1																											

TABLE I. (*continued*).

Disease	Total	Discharged M	Discharged F	Died M	Died F
DISEASES OF THE EYE (*continued*).					
Strabismus—					
Concomitant ...	46	22	24	...	...
Paralytic ...	4	3	1	...	...
General Diseases—					
Contracted Socket ...	1	1	...	...	...
Painful Blind Eye ...	8	4	4	...	...
Ruptured Eyeball ...	1	1	...	...	...
Pseudo-Glioma ...	1	1	...	...	...
Toxic-amblyopia ...	3	2	...	...	...
Dermoid of Scalp ...	1	1	...	...	...
Cysticercus of Eye ...	1	1	...	...	...
Amaurosis ...	1	...	1	...	...
Errors of Refraction—					
Myopia ...	10	1	9	...	...
Astigmatism ...	1	1	...	...	...
DISEASES OF THE EAR.					
Otitis Media... ...	87	44	39	2	2
" " with Cerebellar Abscess	1	1	...	1	...
" " with Cerebral Abscess	1	1	...	1	...

TABLE I. (continued).

DISEASE.	Total	Discharged M	Discharged F	Died M	Died F
DISEASES OF THE EAR (continued).					
Otitis Media (continued)—					
" " with Mastoid Abcess	31	11	20		
" " " Meningitis	3			2	1
" " " Sinus	2	1	1		
" " " Thrombosis	2		2		1
Cholesteatoma	1				
Aural Polypi	2				
Deformity of Ear following Complete Mastoid Operation	1		1		
DISEASES OF THE NOSE AND ANTRUM.					
Deformity of Nose	10	8	2		
Deviated Septum	7	6	1		
Empyema of Antrum (Superior Maxillary)	2	1	1		
Epistaxis	3	3			
Hypertrophied Turbinate Bone	5	4	1		
Nasal Spur	3	2	1		

TABLE I. (continued).

Disease	Total	Discharged M	Discharged F	Died M	Died F
DISEASES OF THE NOSE AND ANTRUM (continued).					
Tumours—					
Polypi (Nasal) ...	3	...	3	...	...
Polypi (Naso-Pharyngeal) ...	3	2	1	...	...
Sarcoma ...	1	...	1	...	...
Oscena ...	1	1	...	...	...
DISEASES OF THE LARYNX AND TRACHEA.					
Laryngitis ...	3	2	1	...	...
Old Tracheotomy ...	1	1	...	...	...
Tumours—					
Carcinoma ...	4	3	...	1	...
Papillous ...	1	...	1	...	...
DISEASES OF THE DUCTLESS GLANDS.					
Thyroid—					
Goitre—					
Adenomatous ...	6	1	5	...	...
Chronic Parenchymatous ...	4	2	2	...	...
Malignant ...	2	...	1	...	1

G

TABLE I. (continued).

DISEASE	Total	Disch. M	Disch. F	Died M	Died F	Under 5 Disch M	Under 5 Disch F	Under 5 Died M	Under 5 Died F	—10 Disch M	—10 Disch F	—10 Died M	—10 Died F	—15 Disch M	—15 Disch F	—15 Died M	—15 Died F	—20 Disch M	—20 Disch F	—20 Died M	—20 Died F	—30 Disch M	—30 Disch F	—30 Died M	—30 Died F	—40 Disch M	—40 Disch F	—40 Died M	—40 Died F	—50 Disch M	—50 Disch F	—50 Died M	—50 Died F	—60 Disch M	—60 Disch F	—60 Died M	—60 Died F	Over 60 Disch M	Over 60 Disch F	Over 60 Died M	Over 60 Died F
DISEASES OF THE DUCTLESS GLANDS (continued).																																									
Thyroid Cyst	3	1	2																				2			1															
Cretinism	1	1								1																															
Supra-renal Gland—																																									
Malignant Tumour	1			1																																				1	
DISEASES OF THE CHEST.																																									
Heart—																																									
Morbus Cordis	2			1	1																											1					1				
Pericarditis	1			1																												1									
Lungs—																																									
Broncho-Pneumonia	2			2				2																																	
Pleura—																																									
Empyema	5	4	1											1				1				1				1					1										
„ (Old)	2	2																												1								1			
Pleurisy	1	1																																				1			

TABLE I. (continued).

DISEASE.	Total	Discharged M	Discharged F	Died M	Died F	Under 5 Disch M	Under 5 Disch F	Under 5 Died M	Under 5 Died F	—10 Disch M	—10 Disch F	—10 Died M	—10 Died F	—15 Disch M	—15 Disch F	—15 Died M	—15 Died F	—20 Disch M	—20 Disch F	—20 Died M	—20 Died F	—30 Disch M	—30 Disch F	—30 Died M	—30 Died F	—40 Disch M	—40 Disch F	—40 Died M	—40 Died F	—50 Disch M	—50 Disch F	—50 Died M	—50 Died F	—60 Disch M	—60 Disch F	—60 Died M	—60 Died F	Over 60 Disch M	Over 60 Disch F	Over 60 Died M	Over 60 Died F
DISEASES OF THE VASCULAR SYSTEM.																																									
Arteries—																																									
Aneurysm—																																									
Aorta	2			2																								2													
Abdominal	1	1																								1															
Carotid	1	1																1																							
Popliteal	1		1																																						
Aneurysmal Varix...	1		1																																						
Veins—																																									
Phlebitis and Thrombosis	7	4	3																			2	2			2	1														
Varicose Veins...	87	54	33															8	2			28	18			12	9			5	4										
DISEASES OF THE LYMPHATIC SYSTEM.																																									
Glands—																																									
Inflamed & Suppurating—																																									
Axilla	3	1	2																																						
Neck	13	8	5																																						
Inguinal	4	1	3																																						
Pelvic	1	1																																							

TABLE I. (continued).

DISEASE	Total	Under 5 Disch. M.	Under 5 Disch. F.	Under 5 Died M.	Under 5 Died F.	—10 Disch. M.	—10 Disch. F.	—10 Died M.	—10 Died F.	—15 Disch.	—15 Died	—20 Disch. M.	—20 Disch. F.	—20 Died M.	—20 Died F.	—30 Disch. M.	—30 Disch. F.	—30 Died	—40 Disch.	—40 Died	—50 Disch.	—50 Died	—60 Disch.	—60 Died	Over 60 Disch.	Over 60 Died
DISEASES OF THE LYMPHATIC SYSTEM (continued).																										
Glands (continued)—																										
Tuberculous—																										
Axilla	1					1														1						
Inguinal	1											1				1										
Mesentery	2					3				2						1			1		2	3	2			
Neck	59	4	1			3	5			2		5	8			3	15		1	5						6
Tumours—																										
Lymphadenoma	3											1							1				1			
Carcinoma—																										
Axilla (Recurrent)	1																				1					
Mesentaric	1						1												1		2		1			
Neck (Secondary)	11			1			1												1		1	1	1		6	
Sarcoma	3		1																			1				
„ (Melanotic)	2		2																1		1					
Lymphatics—																										
Elephantiasis—																										
Pseudo-, of Leg	2									1									1							
Œdema—																										
Leg	2	1	1																			1	1			

TABLE I. (continued).

DISEASE.	Total	Discharged M.	Discharged F.	Died M.	Died F.	Under 5 Disch. M.	Under 5 Disch. F.	Under 5 Died M.	Under 5 Died F.	—10 Disch. M.	—10 Disch. F.	—10 Died M.	—10 Died F.	—15 Disch. M.	—15 Disch. F.	—15 Died M.	—15 Died F.	—20 Disch. M.	—20 Disch. F.	—20 Died M.	—20 Died F.	—30 Disch. M.	—30 Disch. F.	—30 Died M.	—30 Died F.	—40 Disch. M.	—40 Disch. F.	—40 Died M.	—40 Died F.	—50 Disch. M.	—50 Disch. F.	—50 Died M.	—50 Died F.	—60 Disch. M.	—60 Disch. F.	—60 Died M.	—60 Died F.	Over 60 Disch. M.	Over 60 Disch. F.	Over 60 Died M.	Over 60 Died F.
DISEASES OF THE DIGESTIVE SYSTEM.																																									
Mouth, Palate, and Fauces—																																									
Cancrum Oris	2		2							1																															
Stomatitis	2	1	1			1	1																																		
Hypertrophy of Gums	1	1				1	1																																		
" " Uvula	1	1												1																											
Tumours—																																									
Carcinoma—																																									
Fauces	2	2																																2							
Floor	6	5	1																							1						3		2							
Palate	2	2																																2							
Salivary Glands																																									
Parotid—																																									
Tumours	4	2	2															1								1					1			2							
" Recurrent	1		1																							1				1											
Abscess	1	1																																							
Pharynx—																																									
Tumour	1	1																								1								1							
Naso-pharynx—																																									
Adenoids	6	3	3			1	1			2	1			2				1																							
" & Enlarged Tonsils	8	3	5			1	1			2	1			2								1				1								1							
Tonsils—																																									
Inflamed	2	2																				2																			
Carcinoma	2	1	1																															1					1		

TABLE I. (*continued*)

DISEASE	Total	Disch. M	Disch. F	Died M	Died F	Under 5 Dis. M	Under 5 Dis. F	Under 5 Died M	Under 5 Died F	−10 Dis. M	−10 Dis. F	−10 Died M	−10 Died F	−15 Dis. M	−15 Dis. F	−15 Died M	−15 Died F	−20 Dis. M	−20 Dis. F	−20 Died M	−20 Died F	−30 Dis. M	−30 Dis. F	−30 Died M	−30 Died F	−40 Dis. M	−40 Dis. F	−40 Died M	−40 Died F	−50 Dis. M	−50 Dis. F	−50 Died M	−50 Died F	−60 Dis. M	−60 Dis. F	−60 Died M	−60 Died F	Over 60 Dis. M	Over 60 Dis. F	Over 60 Died M	Over 60 Died F
DISEASES OF THE DIGESTIVE SYSTEM (*continued*).																																									
Tongue—																																									
Inflammation	1		1																			1																			
Tumour	1	1																																							
Tumours—Carcinoma	32	28	2	2							1															1		1		7	1	1	1	9	1	3		12			
Oesophagus—																																									
Dysphagia	3	3									1																1			1				1				2			
Stricture (Fibrous)	1	1	1	1																																					
Carcinoma	22	10	1	10	1																		1			1				2		1		1	1	3		6	1	1	1
Stomach—																																									
Adhesions	2	2	2	3	2														1				1			1	1	1		1	1	1									
Dilatation	4	2	1																1			1	1			1															
Dyspepsia	5	4	1																																						
Fibrous Stricture of Pylorus	1	1										1				1										1	1	1		1		1		1							
Gastric Ulcer	10	1	4	3	2																	1	1	1		3		1		1	1	1			1	1					
" " & Perforation	19	8	4	3	4											1						5	3	2	3	3		1				1	1		1	1		6		1	1
" " (*Old*)	2		2		1																	1				1					2			1		1					
Gastritis	6	4										1														1		1						1		1		1		1	
Tumours	2																																								
Carcinoma	21	6	5	5	5																	1		2		1	1	1	1	1	1	1	1	2	1	1	1	2	1	1	2

TABLE I. (continued).

DISEASE.	Total	Discharged M.	Discharged F.	Died M.	Died F.
DISEASES OF THE DIGESTIVE SYSTEM (continued).					
Duodenum—					
Ulcer ...	1	1	...	...	...
" d perforation	4	...	...	4	...
Stricture ...	1	1	...	...	...
Liver—					
Abscess ...	2	1	...	1	...
Accessory Lobe ...	1	1	1	...	...
Hydatid Cyst ...	3	1	...	2	...
Jaundice ...	3	1	3	...	...
Malignant Disease	1	...	...	...	...
Gall Bladder and Ducts—					
Adhesions ...	1	...	2	...	1
Biliary Fistula ...	2	3	2	3	...
Gall Stones ...	25	8	16	3	3
Carcinoma ...	3	...	2	1	1
Sarcoma ...	1	...	...	1	...
Pancreas—					
Carcinoma ...	2	...	1	...	1
Cyst ...	1	1	...	...	...
Inflammation ...	1	1	...	...	...

TABLE I. (continued).

DISEASE.	Total	Discharged M.	Discharged F.	Died M.	Died F.	Under 5 Disch. M	Under 5 Disch. F	—10 Disch. M	—10 Disch. F	—15 Disch. M	—15 Disch. F	—20 Disch. M	—20 Disch. F	—30 Disch. M	—30 Disch. F	—30 Died M	—30 Died F	—40 Disch. M	—40 Disch. F	—50 Disch. M	—50 Disch. F	—50 Died M	—50 Died F	—60 Disch. M	—60 Disch. F	—70 Disch. M	—70 Disch. F	—70 Died M	Over 60 Disch. M	Over 60 Disch. F
DISEASES OF THE DIGESTIVE SYSTEM (continued).																														
Intestines—																														
Hernia—																														
Reducible—																														
Femoral ...	9	2	7																			1		2	1					
Inguinal ...	189	168	21			13		12	1	10	2	27	7	63		4	7	28	4	7				4		6				2
,, ♂ Partially descended Testis	14	14						1		5				4				1												
Interstitial ...	3	3				1				1																				
Umbilical ...	10	3	7			1														3						3				1
Irreducible—																														
Femoral ...	24	3	21									1		6		3		6	1	7				1	4	1			1	1
Inguinal ...	21	16	4	1				1		1		1		6		1		1		5		7			1	4		1	1	1
,, ♂ Partially descended Testis	1	1												1																
Umbilical ...	9		9					1						1		1		1		4				1		1			2	
Strangulated—																														
Femoral ...	13	2	11	2										2		2		1		1	1		1	1		2			1	5
Inguinal ...	14	11	1							1		1		1				1		4	1	1	1	1		1	1		1	1
Umbilical ...	4		4							2										1				1	1	1			1	1
Ventral ...	2		1	1	1									1										1		1				
Obstructed—																														
Inguinal ...	1		1	1																								1		
Umbilical ...	1		1																					1						
Pnæumatio Ventral ...	14	7	7			2	1	2	1	2		1		3	1			3		1	1									1
Hydrocele of Hernial Sac ...	1		1		1																								1	

TABLE I. (continued).

DISEASE.	Total	Discharged M.	Discharged F.	Died M.	Died F.	Under 5 Disch. M	Under 5 Disch. F	Under 5 Died M	Under 5 Died F	−10 Disch. M	−10 Disch. F	−10 Died M	−10 Died F	−15 Disch. M	−15 Disch. F	−15 Died M	−15 Died F	−20 Disch. M	−20 Disch. F	−20 Died M	−20 Died F	−30 Disch. M	−30 Disch. F	−30 Died M	−30 Died F	−40 Disch. M	−40 Disch. F	−40 Died M	−40 Died F	−50 Disch. M	−50 Disch. F	−50 Died M	−50 Died F	−60 Disch. M	−60 Disch. F	−60 Died M	−60 Died F	Over 60 Disch. M	Over 60 Disch. F	Over 60 Died M	Over 60 Died F
DISEASES OF THE DIGESTIVE SYSTEM (continued).																																									
Intestines (continued)—																																									
Abdominal Pain ...	28	14	14	…	…		1			1				1	2			2	3			3	5			5	2			1	1			1	4				1		
Constipation ...	11	3	8	…	…													1				1				3			2				1	2				1		
„ Tumour ...	10	4	6	…	…													1				2				2			1					2						
Enteritis ...	1	1	1	…	…	1																										1									
Faecal Fistula ...	3	1	…	**1**	**1**	1																		**1**			1														
Sarcoma, Small Intestine...	1	…	1	…	**3**																																				
Intestinal Obstruction ..	7	…	3	**3**	**3**			**1**	**1**										3	**3**	**1**					1	1	**1**													
Strangulation by Band	3	…	1	**4**	**1**	1	1	**1**											1	**3**	**1**						1								2					
Intussusception ...	7	1	1	**1**	**1**	1	1	**3**	**1**																																
Volvulus ...	1	1	…	**1**	…																						1														
Caecum—																																									
Carcinoma ...	4	1	1	**1**	**1**																					1			**1**						1				1	**1**	
Tubercle ...	1	…	…	**1**	…																																				
Omentum—																																									
Carcinoma ...	1	…	1	…	…																						1							1							
Inflammation ...	1	1	…	**1**	…	1																																			
Vermiform Appendix—																																									
Appendicitis—																																									
Acute cases without external suppuration ...	67	46	21	…	…		1			3	2			6	1			5	3			22	11			7	2			1	2				1						
Chronic relapsing cases without external suppuration ...	80	37	42	**1**	…		1			1	1			3	1			6	8			18	16			8 13	**1**			1	3				1						

TABLE I. (continued).

DISEASE.	Total.	Discharged M.	Discharged F.	Died M.	Died F.	Under 5 Disch. M.	Under 5 Disch. F.	Under 5 Died M.	Under 5 Died F.	—10 Disch. M.	—10 Disch. F.	—10 Died M.	—10 Died F.	—15 Disch. M.	—15 Disch. F.	—15 Died M.	—15 Died F.	—20 Disch. M.	—20 Disch. F.	—20 Died M.	—20 Died F.	—30 Disch. M.	—30 Disch. F.	—30 Died M.	—30 Died F.	—40 Disch. M.	—40 Disch. F.	—40 Died M.	—40 Died F.	—50 Disch. M.	—50 Disch. F.	—50 Died M.	—50 Died F.	—60 Disch. M.	—60 Disch. F.	—60 Died M.	—60 Died F.	Over 60 Disch. M.	Over 60 Disch. F.	Over 60 Died M.	Over 60 Died F.
DISEASES OF THE DIGESTIVE SYSTEM (continued).																																									
Intestines (continued)—																																									
Vermiform Appendix (cont.)																																									
Appendicitis (cont.)—																																									
Acute Gangrenous	10	2	4	2	2	1		1			1	1		1	1		1	1	3	1	1	2			2	1			1											1	
Acute, with Suppuration	56	23	18	6	9	5	5		1	5	4	1		3	3	1	1	3	3	2	2	5	5	2	3	4	4	1		2	1	1	1	1			1		1	1	
Acute, with Abscess	10	6	2	2		1				1				1				2	2			2		1		1												1	1	1	
Old Appendicitis, Abscess previously opened	1	1																				1																			
Old Appendicectomy	3	3																	1			1				1															
Colon—																																									
Carcinoma	9	1		4	4																					1		1	1		1	2	1			1	1				1
Colio	3	2	1												1			1	1				1																		
Colitis, Ulcerative	3			3																1				1								1									
Old Colotomy	2		2																												1									1	
Sigmoid Flexure—																																									
Carcinoma	3	1																									1						1			1					
Peritoneum—																																									
Adhesions	3	2	1		1				1																						1			2							
Ascites	1				1																																				
Hydatid Cyst	1	1									1																														
Peritonitis—																																									
Acute Suppurative	4		1	2	3		2	1	1																							2								1	
Tuberculous	7		4								1				1												1				1				1				1		
Subphrenic Abscess	3	2	1	2							1												1																	1	

TABLE I. (continued).

Disease	Total	Discharged M	Discharged F	Died M	Died F
DISEASES OF THE DIGESTIVE SYSTEM (continued)—					
Intestines (continued)—					
Rectum—					
Hemorrhoids ...	72	36	36	...	...
Prolapse ...	3	1	2	...	...
Stricture (Fibrous) ...	3	1	2	...	...
Ulceration—					
Tuberculous ...	1	...	...	...	1
Tumours—					
Polypus ...	5	2	3	...	...
Carcinoma ...	30	17	11	2	...
Hemorrhage ...	1	1	...	...	...
Anus—					
Fissure ...	5	3	2	...	...
Fistula ...	26	20	6	...	...
Imperforate ...	3	1	2	...	...
DISEASES OF THE GENITO-URINARY ORGANS.					
Bladder—					
Calculus ...	4	2	2	...	...
Cystitis ...	8	6	2	...	...

DISEASE.	Total	Discharged M.	Discharged F.	Died M.	Died F.	Under 5 Disch. M	Under 5 Disch. F	Under 5 Died M	Under 5 Died F	−10 Disch. M	−10 Disch. F	−10 Died M	−10 Died F	−15 Disch. M	−15 Disch. F	−15 Died M	−15 Died F	−20 Disch. M	−20 Disch. F	−20 Died M	−20 Died F	−30 Disch. M	−30 Disch. F	−30 Died M	−30 Died F	−40 Disch. M	−40 Disch. F	−40 Died M	−40 Died F	−50 Disch. M	−50 Disch. F	−50 Died M	−50 Died F	−60 Disch. M	−60 Disch. F	−60 Died M	−60 Died F	Over 60 Disch. M	Over 60 Disch. F	Over 60 Died M	Over 60 Died F
DISEASES OF THE GENITO-URINARY ORGANS (contd.).																																										
Bladder (continued)—																																										
Ectopion Vesice	2		1																			1																			
Foreign Body	1	1	1																1				1																			
Tubercle	8	4	4	2																			1			2	1														
Tumours—																																										
Carcinoma	8	5	1	1	1																						1	1		1	2			2				4	1	2	
Papilloma	6	6			2																	1								1				2							
Kidney—																																										
Calculus	11	6	3	1	1											1				1		1				2		1		5		1	1	1							
Hydro-nephrosis	7	2	5		1															2	1	2				2		1			1			1							
Nephritis	1		1																				1																			
Movable Kidney	16	3	13																	1		4				6				1	3			1							
Perinephric Abscess	2		2																			1				1															
Pyo-nephrosis	7		4	1									1									1				2		1													
Renal Colic	12	8	4	1			1			1												4	1			1	1			2				1				1			
Tubercle	2	1	1																			1				1								1							
Tumours	5	1	3	1	2		1				1															1			1												
Prepuce—																																										
Phimosis	5	5					2															2																			
Penis—																																										
Ulcer	1	1																																1							
Tumours—																																										
Carcinoma	7	7																								3				1				2				1			
Papilloma	1	1																				1																			

TABLE I. (continued).

DISEASE.	Total	Discharged M.	Discharged F.	Died M.	Died F.
DISEASES OF THE GENITO-URINARY ORGANS (contd.).					
Prostate—					
Calculus ...	1	1	...	...	...
Enlarged ...	11	10	...	1	...
Malignant Growth	2	1	...	1	...
Scrotum—					
Carcinoma ...	3	8	...	...	...
Syphilitic Ulceration	1	1	...	...	...
Spermatic Cord—					
Encysted Hydrocele	8	8	...	...	...
Varicocele ...	70	70	...	...	...
Testis—					
Orchitis and Epididymitis	5	5	...	...	...
Partially descended Testis ...					
Misplaced Testis	6	6	...	...	...
Hydrocele of Testis	1	1	...	...	...
Tertiary Syphilis	4	4	...	...	...
Tubercle ...	3	3	...	...	...
Tumours—	13	18	...	...	...
Carcinoma ...	1	...	...	1	...
Sarcoma ...	1	1	...	1	...
Teratoma ...	1	1	...	...	...

TABLE I. (continued).

DISEASE.	Total	Discharged M.	Discharged F.	Died M.	Died F.	Under 5. Disch. M/F	Under 5 Died	—10 Disch.	—10 Died	—15 Disch.	—15 Died	—20 Disch.	—20 Died	—30 Disch.	—30 Died	—40 Disch.	—40 Died	—50 Disch.	—50 Died	—60 Disch.	—60 Died	Over 60 Disch.	Over 60 Died
DISEASES OF THE GENITO-URINARY ORGANS (contd.).																							
Tunica Vaginalis—																							
Hæmatocele	1	1	…	…	…							3		8		12		6		3		1	
Hydrocele	38	38	…	…	…							3		8		12		4		4		1	
Urethra—																							
Calculus	5	5	…	…	…									1		1		1		1			
Caruncle	1	…	1	…	…																		
Fistula	1	1	1	…	…																		
Stricture	63	60	…	2	…					1		2		2		3 1		20 1	1	15		10	1
Urethritis	1	1	…	1	…													1					
Carcinoma	1	…	…	…	…																		1
Urine and Urination—																							
Extravasation	7	5	…	2	…			1						1				1	1	1	1	1	
Enuresis	2	2	…	…	…			1		2						1							
Glycosuria	1	1	…	…	…			1								1							
Hæmaturia	14	10	4	…	…			1		2		3		3		2 1		1		2			
Oxaluria	1	1	1	…	…							1											
Pyuria	4	3	1	…	…							3		1									
Retention	4	2	1	1	…							1				1				1			1
Ovary—																							
Cyst	15	…	13	…	3	1										4	2	3	1			1	
Carcinoma	1	…	…	…	1											1	1						
Vulva and Vagina—																							
Fistula (Recto-Vaginal)	2	…	2	…	…			1						1								1	
Vulvitis	2	…	2	…	…									1				4		1			

TABLE I. (continued).

DISEASE.	Total	Discharged M	Discharged F	Died M	Died F	Under 5				−10				−15				−20				−30 Disch. F	−30 Disch. M	−30 Died F	−30 Died M	−40 Disch. F	−40 Disch. M	−40 Died F	−40 Died M	−50 Disch. F	−50 Disch. M	−50 Died F	−50 Died M	−60 Disch. F	−60 Disch. M	−60 Died F	−60 Died M	Over 60 Disch. F	Over 60 Disch. M	Over 60 Died F	Over 60 Died M
DISEASES OF THE GENITO-URINARY ORGANS (contd.).																																										
Vulva and Vagina (cont.)—																																										
Tumours—																																										
Carcinoma of Vulva ...	4		4																										1								2			
Papilloma of Labium ...	1		1																						1								1							
Lipoma ...	1		1																						1															
Uterus and Appendages—																																										
Dysmenorrhœa ...	1		1																		1				1															
Erosion ...	2		2																		1				1															
Endometritis ...	1		1																		1																			
Menorrhagia ...	1		1																										1											
Pelvic Inflammation ...	5		5																		1				4															
Hæmatocele ...	2		2																		2																			
„ Pregnancy ...	2		2																		2																			
Prolapse ...	1		1																		1				1															
Pyo-Salpinx ...	6		6		4																1		1				1				1				1				1		
Ruptured Extra-Uterine Gestation ...	3		2		1																1		1		1		1													
Tumours—																																										
Fibro-Myoma ...	6		5																						5												2			
Carcinoma ...	3		3		1																				1		1													
Breast—																																										
Hypertrophy ...	1		1																		1																			

TABLE I. (*continued*).

DISEASE.	Total	Discharged M.	Discharged F.	Died M.	Died F.
DISEASES OF THE GENITO-URINARY ORGANS (contd.)					
Breast (*continued*)—					
Mastitis—					
Acute Suppurative	21	...	20	...	...
Chronic	12	...	12	...	...
Tubercle	6	...	6	...	...
Tumours—					
Adeno-Fibroma	20	...	20	...	...
Cysts	3	1	3	...	...
Carcinoma	66	...	62	...	3
Nipple "—					
Carcinoma (*Recurrent*)	1	...	1	...	...
DISEASES OF THE ORGANS OF LOCOMOTION.					
Bones—					
Caries—					
Tarsus	7	4	3	...	...
Teeth	2	...	2	...	...
Tibia	1	...	1	...	...
Spine	33	14	13	3	3

TABLE I. (continued).

DISEASE	Total	Discharged M	Discharged F	Died M	Died F
DISEASES OF THE ORGANS OF LOCOMOTION (continued).					
Bones (continued)—					
Necrosis—					
Femur	9	6	3	...	...
Humerus	2	1	1	...	...
Jaw	7	4	2	...	1
Malar	1	1	...	...	...
Metacarpus	2	2	...	...	...
Patella	1	1	...	...	...
Pelvis	2	1	1	...	...
Rib	1	1	...	...	...
Skull	4	... 3	...	1	...
Tibia	8	6	2	...	1
Ulna	2	1	1	...	...
Periostitis and Osteitis—					
Acute—					
Femur	4	8?	...	...	1
Tibia	7	3	3	...	1
Ulna	1	1	...	...	...
Chronic—					
Femur	1	1	...	...	...
Hand Bones	4	2	2	...	...
Humerus	2	2	...	...	...

H

TABLE I. (continued).

DISEASE	Total	Discharged M	Discharged F	Died M	Died F
DISEASES OF THE ORGANS OF LOCOMOTION (continued).					
Bones (continued) —					
Periostitis and Osteitis (continued) —					
Chronic (continued) —					
Jaw	1	1	...	...	...
Rib	3	3	...	...	...
Scapula	1	1	...	...	...
Temporal Bone	1	...	1	...	...
Tibia	7	7	...	...	...
Ulna	1	...	1	...	...
Osteo-myelitis —					
Acute —					
Femur	1	1	...	...	...
Pelvis	1	1	...	...	...
Tibia	1	1	...	...	...
Epiphysitis —					
Acute —					
Humerus	1	1	...	...	...
Radius	1	1	...	...	...
Tibia	1	1	...	...	...
Tertiary Syphilis —					
Rib	1	1	...	...	...
Stumps	9	8	1	...	...

TABLE I. (continued).

DISEASE.	Total.	Discharged M.	Discharged F.	Died M.	Died F.	Under 1. Disch. M	F	Died M	F	—10. Disch. M	F	Died M	F	—15. Disch. M	F	Died M	F	—20. Disch. M	F	Died M	F	—25. Disch. M	F	Died M	F	—30. Disch. M	F	Died M	F	—40. Disch. M	F	Died M	F	—50. Disch. M	F	Died M	F	—60. Disch. M	F	Died M	F	Over 60. Disch. M	F	Died M	F
DISEASES OF THE ORGANS OF LOCOMOTION (continued).																																																
Bones (continued)—																																																
Tumours—																																																
Epulis ...	3	1	2																					1				1											1								
Jaw (Upper) ...	5	1	4																									4											1								
" (Lower) ...	2	1	1																	1																			1								
Exostosis—																																																
Femur ...	2	1													1													1																				
Fibula ...	1	1													1													1																				
Jaw ...	3	1	2																																													
Metatarsus ...	2		2																																													
Scapula ...	2	1	1													1												1																				
Multiple Exostosis	1	1																																														
Chondroma—	1	1																						1																								
Carcinoma—																																																
Jaw ...	3	2	1																																			1					1				
" (Recurrent) ...	1	1	1																									1											1								
Endothelioma ...	1	1																																				1									
Odontome ...	1	1																																														
Sarcoma—																																																
Clavicle ...	1		1																					1																								
Femur ...	5	3	2																					1				1									1	1							2	1
Jaw ...	7	5	2																					1				1								1	1	1									

TABLE I. (*continued*).

DISEASE.	Total	Discharged M.	Discharged F.	Died M.	Died F.
DISEASES OF THE DIGESTIVE SYSTEM (continued).					
Intestines (continued)—					
Vermiform Appendix(cont.)					
Appendicitis (cont.)—					
Acute Gangrenous ...	10	2	4	2	2
Acute, with Suppuration	56	23	18	6	9
Acute, with Abcess ...	10	6	2	2	
Old Appendicitis, Abcess					
previously opened ...	1	1	...	...	...
Old Appendicectomy ...	3	3	...	...	...
Colon—					
Carcinoma ...	9	1	1	4	4
Colia ...	3	2	1	...	...
Colitis, Ulcerative ...	3	...	...	3	...
Old Colotomy ...	2	...	2	...	...
Sigmoid Flexure—					
Carcinoma ...	8	1	...	...	2
Peritoneum—					
Adhesions ...	3	2	1	...	...
Ascites ...	1	...	...	1	1
Hydatid Cyst ...	1	1	...	...	...
Peritonitis—					
Acute Suppurative	4	...	1	2	3
Tuberculous ...	7	4	4	...	...
Subphrenic Abscess ...	3	2	1	...	...

TABLE I. (continued).

DISEASE.	Total	Discharged M	Discharged F	Died M	Died F	Under 5 Disch M	Under 5 Disch F	—10 Disch M	—10 Disch F	—10 Died M	—15 Disch F	—20 Disch M	—20 Disch F	—20 Died F	—30 Disch M	—30 Disch F	—40 Disch M	—40 Disch F	—50 Disch M	—50 Disch F	—60 Disch M	—60 Disch F	—60 Died M	Over 60 Disch M	Over 60 Disch F	Over 60 Died M
DISEASES OF THE DIGESTIVE SYSTEM (continued)—																										
Intestines (continued)—																										
Rectum—																										
Hæmorrhoids	72	36	36						1						8	11	7	12	13	7	8	4			1	
Prolapse	3	1	2															1	1	1						
Stricture (Fibrous)	3	1	2														1	1		1						
Ulceration—																										
Tuberculous	1				1									1												
Tumours—																										
Polypus	5	2	3												1	1	1	1		1						
Carcinoma	30	17	11	2													1		3	3	7	3		6	5	2
Hæmorrhage...	1	1	1												1	1										
Anus—																										
Fissure	5	3	2									1	1		1		1	1			1					
Fistula	26	20	6									7	3				7	5	1							
Imperforate	3	1	2			1	2																			
DISEASES OF THE GENITO-URINARY ORGANS.																										
Bladder—																										
Calculus	4	2	2								1							1	1	1	1					
Cystitis	8	6	2								1	3					1			1	1			2		

TABLE I. (continued).

DISEASE.	Total	Discharged M	Discharged F	Died M	Died F
DISEASES OF THE GENITO-URINARY ORGANS (contd.).					
Bladder (continued)—					
Ectopion Vesicæ	2	1	1	...	...
Foreign Body	1	...	1	...	...
Tubercle	8	4	4	...	...
Tumours—					
Carcinoma	8	5	1	2	...
Papilloma	6	6	...	...	...
Kidney—					
Calculus	11	6	3	1	1
Hydro-nephrosis	7	2	5	...	...
Nephritis	1	...	1	1	...
Movable Kidney	16	3	13	...	...
Perinephric Abscess	2	...	2	...	...
Pyo-nephrosis	7	...	4	1	2
Renal Colic	12	8	4	1	...
Tubercle	2	1	1	1	...
Tumours	5	...	3	...	...
Prepuce—					
Phimosis	5	5	...	...	...
Penis—					
Ulcer	1	1	...	...	...
Tumours—					
Carcinoma	7	7	...	...	...
Papilloma	1	1	...	...	...

TABLE I. (continued).

DISEASE.	Total	Discharged M	Discharged F	Died M	Died F	Under 5. Disch. M	Under 5. Disch. F	Under 5. Died M	Under 5. Died F	—10. Disch. M	—10. Disch. F	—10. Died M	—10. Died F	—15. Disch. M	—15. Disch. F	—15. Died M	—15. Died F	—20. Disch. M	—20. Disch. F	—20. Died M	—20. Died F	—30. Disch. M	—30. Disch. F	—30. Died M	—30. Died F	—40. Disch. M	—40. Disch. F	—40. Died M	—40. Died F	—50. Disch. M	—50. Disch. F	—50. Died M	—50. Died F	—60. Disch. M	—60. Disch. F	—60. Died M	—60. Died F	Over 64. Disch. M	Over 64. Disch. F	Over 64. Died M	Over 64. Died F
DISEASES OF THE GENITO-URINARY ORGANS (contd.).																																									
Prostate—																																									
Calculus ...	1	1																																				1			
Enlarged ...	11	10		1																						1				3				3				5		1	1
Malignant Growth	2	1		1																						1				1				1						1	
Scrotum—																																									
Carcinoma ...	3	3																2												1											
Syphilitic Ulceration ...	1	1																1																							
Spermatic Cord—																																									
Encysted Hydrocele	8	8								4				4												4				1				1							
Varicocele ...	70	70								4				34				30				1																			
Testis—																																									
Orchitis and Epididymitis ...	5	5												1				1				4								1											
Partially descended	6	6				2				1				1				1												1											
Testis ...	1	1																																							
Misplaced Testis	4	4												1												2				1				1							
Hydrocele of Testis	3	3																								3															
Tertiary Syphilis	13	13								1								6								3															
Tubercle ...	1																																								
Tumours—																																									
Carcinoma ...	1			1				1																				1													
Sarcoma ...	1			1																																					
Teratoma ...	1	1																								1												1			

TABLE I. (continued).

DISEASE	Total	Discharged M	Discharged F	Died M	Died F	Under 5 Disch. M	Under 5 Disch. F	Under 5 Died M	Under 5 Died F	—10 Disch. M	—10 Disch. F	—10 Died M	—10 Died F	—15 Disch. M	—15 Disch. F	—15 Died M	—15 Died F	—20 Disch. M	—20 Disch. F	—20 Died M	—20 Died F	—30 Disch. M	—30 Disch. F	—30 Died M	—30 Died F	—40 Disch. M	—40 Disch. F	—40 Died M	—40 Died F	—50 Disch. M	—50 Disch. F	—50 Died M	—50 Died F	—60 Disch. M	—60 Disch. F	—60 Died M	—60 Died F	Over 60 Disch. M	Over 60 Disch. F	Over 60 Died M	Over 60 Died F
DISEASES OF THE GENITO-URINARY ORGANS (contd.).																																									
Tunica Vaginalis—																																									
Hæmatocele	1	1																																				1			
Hydrocele	38	38				3				3				1				8				12				6				3				4				1			
Urethra—																																									
Calculus	5	5																				1								2				1							
Caruncle	1		1												1																										
Fistula	1	1	1								1																			1				1							
Stricture	63	60		2																						13	1			20		1		15		1		10			
Urethritis	1	1																												1											
Carcinoma	1			1																												1				1				1	
Urine and Urination—																																									
Extravasation	7	5		2						1								1								1		1		3		1		1		1					
Enuresis	2	2																1																							
Glycosuria	1	1																1																							
Hæmaturia	14	10	4			1	1							2				1				3								1				1				2			
Oxaluria	1	1	1							1								1																							
Pyuria	4	3	1							1																1												1			
Retention	4	2	1	1			1															1								1		1		1							
Ovary—																																									
Cyst	15		12		3														1								4	2			3	2			4						
Carcinoma	1				1																							1				1									
Vulva and Vagina—																																									
Fistula (Recto-Vaginal)	2		2																																3				1		
Vulvitis	2		2				1																																1		

TABLE I. (continued).

DISEASE	Total	Discharged M	Discharged F	Died M	Died F
DISEASES OF THE GENITO-URINARY ORGANS (contd.).					
Vulva and Vagina (cont.)—					
Tumours—					
Carcinoma of Vulva	4	...	4	...	...
Papilloma of Labium	1	...	1	...	...
Lipoma	1	...	1	...	...
Uterus and Appendages—					
Dysmenorrhœa	1	...	1	...	...
Erosion	2	...	2	...	...
Endometritis	1	...	1	...	...
Menorrhagia	1	...	1	...	...
Pelvic Inflammation	5	...	5	...	...
" Hæmatocele	2	...	2	...	...
Pregnancy	2	...	2	...	...
Prolapse	1	...	1	...	...
Pyo-Salpinx	6	...	2	...	4
Ruptured Extra-Uterine Gestation	3	...	2	...	1
Tumours—					
Fibro-Myoma	6	...	5	...	1
Carcinoma	8	...	3	...	...
Breast—					
Hypertrophy	1	...	1	...	...

The remaining columns of the table record the distribution of Discharged and Died cases (Male and Female) across the age groups: Under 5, –10, –15, –20, –30, –40, –50, –60, and Over 60.

TABLE I. (continued).

DISEASE.	Total	Discharged M.	Discharged F.	Died M.	Died F.
DISEASES OF THE GENITO-URINARY ORGANS (contd.)—					
Breast (continued)—					
Mastitis—					
Acute Suppurative ...	21	...	20	...	1
Chronic ...	12	...	12	...	...
Tubercle ...	6	...	6	...	...
Tumours—					
Adeno-Fibroma ...	20	...	20	...	...
Cyst ...	3	...	3	...	3
Carcinoma ...	66	1	62	3	3
Carcinoma (Recurrent)	20	...	20	...	...
Nipple—					
Carcinoma ...	1	...	1	...	...
DISEASES OF THE ORGANS OF LOCOMOTION.					
Bones—					
Caries—					
Tarsus ...	7	4	8	...	...
Teeth ...	2	...	2	...	...
Tibia ...	1	1	1	...	...
Spine ...	38	14	18	3	3

TABLE I. (continued).

DISEASE	Total	Discharged M.	Discharged F.	Died M.	Died F.	Under 5 Disch. M.	Under 5 Disch. F.	Under 5 Died M.	Under 5 Died F.	−10 Disch. M.	−10 Disch. F.	−10 Died M.	−10 Died F.	−1L Disch. M.	−1L Disch. F.	−1L Died M.	−1L Died F.	−20 Disch. M.	−20 Disch. F.	−20 Died M.	−20 Died F.	−30 Disch. M.	−30 Disch. F.	−30 Died M.	−30 Died F.	−40 Disch. M.	−40 Disch. F.	−40 Died M.	−40 Died F.	−50 Disch. M.	−50 Disch. F.	−50 Died M.	−50 Died F.	−60 Disch. M.	−60 Disch. F.	−60 Died M.	−60 Died F.	Over 60 Disch. M.	Over 60 Disch. F.	Over 60 Died M.	Over 60 Died F.
DISEASES OF THE ORGANS OF LOCOMOTION (continued).																																									
Bones (continued)—																																									
Necrosis—																																									
Femur	9	6	3			1	1			1								1	1			1				3	1			1											
Humerus	2	1	1							1					1			1																							
Jaw	7	4	2		1		1				1								1	1		3				1															
Molar	1	1				1																					1														
Metacarpus	2	2									1																			1											
Patella	1	1								1																															
Pelvis	2	1	1							1			1	1								1																			
Rib	1	1																	2								1														
Skull	4	3	2	1	1			1							1				2				3			1				1											
Tibia	8	6	1												1			1	1							1				1											
Ulna	2	1				1												1	1																						
Periostitis and Osteitis—																																									
Acute—																																									
Femur	4	3		1	1			1	1			1		1				1																							
Tibia	7	3	3			1	1							2				2								1															
Ulna	1	1												1																											
Chronic—																																									
Femur	1	1				1													1																						
Hand Bones	4	2	2															1	1											1											
Humerus	2	2																	1							2															

H

TABLE I. (*continued*).

DISEASE	Total	Discharged M.	Discharged F.	Died M.	Died F.
DISEASES OF THE ORGANS OF LOCOMOTION (*continued*).					
Bones (*continued*)—					
Periostitis and Osteitis (*continued*)—					
Chronic (*continued*)—					
Jaw	1	1			
Rib	8	8			
Scapula	1	1			
Temporal Bone	1		1		
Tibia	7	7			
Ulna	1		1		
Osteo-myelitis—					
Acute—					
Femur	1	1			
Pelvis	1	1			
Tibia	1	1			
Epiphysitis—					
Acute—					
Humerus	1	1			
Radius	1	1			
Tibia	1	1			
Tertiary Syphilis—					
Rib	1		1		
Stumps	9	8	1		

TABLE I. (continued).

DISEASE.	Total	Discharged M.	Discharged F.	Died M.	Died F.	Under 5 Disch. M	Under 5 Disch. F	Under 5 Died M	Under 5 Died F	—10 Disch. M	—10 Disch. F	—10 Died M	—10 Died F	—16 Disch. M	—16 Disch. F	—16 Died M	—16 Died F	—20 Disch. M	—20 Disch. F	—20 Died M	—20 Died F	—30 Disch. M	—30 Disch. F	—30 Died M	—30 Died F	—40 Disch. M	—40 Disch. F	—40 Died M	—40 Died F	—50 Disch. M	—50 Disch. F	—50 Died M	—50 Died F	—60 Disch. M	—60 Disch. F	—60 Died M	—60 Died F	Over 60 Disch. M	Over 60 Disch. F	Over 60 Died M	Over 60 Died F
DISEASES OF THE ORGANS OF LOCOMOTION (continued).																																									
Bones (continued)—																																									
Tumours—																																									
Epulis ...	3	1	2																1				1								1										
Jaw (Upper) ...	5	1	4																			1	4																		
,, (Lower) ...	2	1	1																1																				1		
Exostosis—																																									
Femur ...	2	1	1								1												1																		
Fibula ...	3	1	...												1								1				1												1		
Jaw ...	1	1	2																				1																1		
Metatarsus ...	2	...	...				1																																		
Scapula ...	1	2	...				1												1				1																		
Multiple Exostosis	1	1	...											1													1								1						
Chondroma ...	3	1	1																							1					1								1		
Carcinoma—																																									
Jaw ...	1	2	1																1																				1		
,, (Recurrent) ...	1	1	...																																				1		
Endothelioma ...	1	...	1																				1				1				1										
Odontoma ...	1	1	...																																						
Sarcoma—																																									
Clavicle ...	1	...	1																			1	1																1		
Femur ...	5	3	2																1				1												1				1		
Jaw ...	7	5	2																				1							1									2	1	

TABLE I. *(continued)*.

DISEASE	Total	Discharged M	Discharged F	Died M	Died F	Under 5 Disch. M	Under 5 Disch. F	Under 5 Died M	Under 5 Died F	−10 Disch. M	−10 Disch. F	−10 Died M	−10 Died F	−15 Disch. M	−15 Disch. F	−15 Died M	−15 Died F	−20 Disch. M	−20 Disch. F	−20 Died M	−20 Died F	−30 Disch. M	−30 Disch. F	−30 Died M	−30 Died F	−40 Disch. M	−40 Disch. F	−40 Died M	−40 Died F	−50 Disch. M	−50 Disch. F	−50 Died M	−50 Died F	−60 Disch. M	−60 Disch. F	−60 Died M	−60 Died F	Over 60 Disch. M	Over 60 Disch. F	Over 60 Died M	Over 60 Died F
DISEASES OF THE ORGANS OF LOCOMOTION (continued).																																									
Bones (continued)—																																									
Tumours (continued)—																																									
Sarcoma *(continued)*—																																									
Pelvis	2		1		1									1		1																									
Rib	1	1																												1											
Scapula	3	3																1				2								1											
Tibia	1	1																												1											
Cyst—																																									
Jaw	1	1																1																							
Joints—																																									
Adhesions—																																									
Ankle	1	1																												1											
Elbow	1	1																								1				1											
Hip	1	1																												1											
Knee	3	1	2																			1																			
Ankylosis—																																									
Elbow	2	2	2																1				1				1				1								1		
Hip	10	8	2					2	1		2	1							5	1			1	1			1			1											
Knee	3	2	1												1								1												1						
Shoulder	1	1																																							
Synovitis—																																									
Ankle	1		1			1																																			
Knee	12	7	5											1								2	2			2	1			1								1			
Wrist	1	1																								1															

TABLE I. (continued).

DISEASE	Total	Discharged M.	Discharged F.	Died M.	Died F.
DISEASES OF THE ORGANS OF LOCOMOTION (continued).					
Joints (continued)—					
Arthritis—					
Gonorrhœal—					
Knee	1	1	...	...	...
Osteo-Arthritis—					
Ankle	1	1	...	...	...
Knee	7	4	3	...	...
Polyarticular	3	...	3	...	...
Suppurative—					
Hand	1	1	1	...	...
Hip	1	1	...	1	...
Multiple	1	...	...	1	...
Syphilitic—					
Acquired	1	1	1	...	...
Congenital	3	2	...	...	...
Intermittent Hydrops Articuli	1	...	1	...	...
Tuberculous Disease—					
Ankle	5	1	4	...	...
Elbow	8	8	5	...	...
Hip	53	26	24	2	1
Knee	29	20	9	...	...
Sacro-Iliac	4	1	3	...	...
Shoulder	1	1	...	...	...
Wrist	2	1	1	...	...

TABLE I. (continued).

DISEASE	Total	Disch. M	Disch. F	Died M	Died F	U5 D.M	U5 D.F	U5 Di.M	U5 Di.F	-10 D.M	-10 D.F	-10 Di.M	-10 Di.F	-15 D.M	-15 D.F	-15 Di.M	-15 Di.F	-20 D.M	-20 D.F	-20 Di.M	-20 Di.F	-30 D.M	-30 D.F	-30 Di.M	-30 Di.F	-40 D.M	-40 D.F	-40 Di.M	-40 Di.F	-50 D.M	-50 D.F	-50 Di.M	-50 Di.F	-60 D.M	-60 D.F	-60 Di.M	-60 Di.F	60 D.M	60 D.F	60 Di.M	60 Di.F	Over 60 D.M	Over 60 D.F	Over 60 Di.M	Over 60 Di.F
DISEASES OF THE ORGANS OF LOCOMOTION (continued).																																													
Joints (continued)—																																													
Charcot's Disease—																																													
Hip	1	1	…	…	…																					1																			
Loose and Displaced Semilunar Cartilage	17	13	4	…	…													3	1			8	3			1				1															
Dislocation—																																													
Pathological—																																													
Hip	2	1	1	…	…					1	1																																		
Old Excision—																																													
Astragalus	1	1	…	…	…																					1																			
Knee	1	…	1	…	…																						1																		
DISEASES OF BURSÆ, FASCIÆ, TENDONS AND MUSCLES.																																													
Bursæ—																																													
Inflamed and Suppurating—																																													
Prepatellar	8	2	6	…	…													1	2				1							1	2													1	
Sub-deltoid	1	…	1	…	…										1																														
Simple Enlargement—																																													
Prepatellar	13	2	11	…	…													1	1				5			1	1				4														
Ischial	1	1	…	…	…																					1																			
Semi-membranosus	3	1	2	…	…														1			1	1																						

DISEASES OF BURSÆ, FASCIE, TENDONS AND MUSCLES (continued).									Total
Bursæ (continued)—									
Tuberculous Disease ...									3
Syphilitic									1
Fascia—									
Dupuytren's Contraction of Palmar Fascia ...	1								6
Contractions—									
Hand	1			2					2
Fingers				1	1				3
Calcification ...				1					1
Tendons—									
Ganglia—									
Simple		1				1			4
Compound ...	1								1
Teno-synovitis—									
Tuberculous ...						2			2
Contracted... ...						1			2
Muscles—									
Hypertrophy									1
Tumours—									
Carcinoma (secondary) ...							1		1
Sarcoma							1		1

DISEASE	Total	Discharged M	Discharged F	Died M	Died F	Under 5 Disch. M	Under 5 Disch. F	Under 5 Died M	Under 5 Died F	—10 Disch. M	—10 Disch. F	—10 Died M	—10 Died F	—15 Disch. M	—15 Disch. F	—15 Died M	—15 Died F	—20 Disch. M	—20 Disch. F	—20 Died M	—20 Died F	—30 Disch. M	—30 Disch. F	—30 Died M	—30 Died F	—40 Disch. M	—40 Disch. F	—40 Died M	—40 Died F	—50 Disch. M	—50 Disch. F	—50 Died M	—50 Died F	—60 Disch. M	—60 Disch. F	—60 Died M	—60 Died F	—80 Disch. M	—80 Disch. F	—80 Died M	—80 Died F	Over 80 Disch. M	Over 80 Disch. F	Over 80 Died M	Over 80 Died F
DISEASES OF THE CELLULAR TISSUE.																																													
Absces, Inflammation and Suppuration—																																													
Abscess—																																													
Abdominal Wall	7	3	4				1				1								1				1				1				1														
Arm	7	1	6				2					1							1	1			1	2			1	1				1				3				3					
Axilla	13	10	3				2				1	1			1	1			2	2			2	2			2				1				1				1				1		
Back	2	1	1								1								1				1	1																					
Chest Wall	4	3	1								1				1				1				3	1			1				1														
Dental	9	5	4				1				1								1	1			3				1	1																	
Face	3	1	2							1									1				2				1																		
Foot	1	1																																											
Gluteal	1	1	..							1																																			
Groin	8	5	3				1				2								1				2	2			2	1																	
Hand	1	1	1																																										
Iliac	3	1	1																1								2	1																	
Ischio-Rectal	13	8	5				1				3	2				1							2	2			1	1																	
Leg	15	8	6		1		1		1		2	1	1			2			1				2	6			3	2			2				3				3					
Lumbar	12	15	4				5				2	1				1			1				3	2			2	1			1				1				1					
Neck	29	3	14				3				2	1			2	1			1				2	6			2	1			1				1				1				1		
Perineal	3	1	..	1			1				1																1																		
Peri-urethral	1	3	1												1								1																						
Popliteal	4	1	1								2												1									1				1				1				1
Psoas	1	..	1								1								1												1														

DISEASE	Total	Discharged M	Discharged F	Died M	Died F	Under 5 Disch M	Under 5 Disch F	Under 5 Died M	Under 5 Died F	−10 Disch M	−10 Disch F	−10 Died M	−10 Died F	−15 Disch M	−15 Disch F	−15 Died M	−15 Died F	−20 Disch M	−20 Disch F	−20 Died M	−20 Died F	−30 Disch M	−30 Disch F	−30 Died M	−30 Died F	−40 Disch M	−40 Disch F	−40 Died M	−40 Died F	−50 Disch M	−50 Disch F	−50 Died M	−50 Died F	−60 Disch M	−60 Disch F	−60 Died M	−60 Died F	Over 60 Disch M	Over 60 Disch F	Over 60 Died M	Over 60 Died F
DISEASES OF THE CELLULAR TISSUE (continued).																																									
Abscess, Inflammation and Suppuration (continued)—																																									
Abscess (continued)—																																									
Retro-pharyngeal	1	1	...	...	...	1																																			
Scalp	1	1	...	...	...	1																																			
Scrotum	1	1	1	...	...															1																					
Submental	1	...	1	...	...																		1																		
Whitlow	1	...	...	...	...																	1																		
Multiple	1	1	...			1																		1			1														
Cellulitis	91	54	28	6	1	1	2	3	1	3	...	1	...	3	...	1	...	7	3	...	...	16	7	7	1	...	2	2	2	8	...	4	1	5	1	...	1	2	6	...	1
DISEASES OF THE CUTANEOUS SYSTEM.																																									
Boils	2	2	...	...	...																	2																			
Carbuncle—																																									
Back	5	4	1	...	...																									1	...							2	...		
Neck	6	5	1	...	...							1											1				1			1					1			4	1		
Cicatrix	4	...	4	...	...					1																1												1			
Keloid	1	...	1	...	...																																				
Eczema	3	...	3	...	...													1				1				1				1				1							
Lupus	7	1	6	...	...	...				1				1				1				1				1												1			

TABLE I. (continued).

DISEASE	Total	Discharged M	Discharged F	Died M	Died F	Under 5 — Discharged M	Under 5 — Discharged F	Under 5 — Died M	Under 5 — Died F	-10 Disch. M	-10 Disch. F	-10 Died M	-10 Died F	-15 Disch. M	-15 Disch. F	-15 Died M	-15 Died F	-20 Disch. M	-20 Disch. F	-20 Died M	-20 Died F	-30 Disch. M	-30 Disch. F	-30 Died M	-30 Died F	-40 Disch. M	-40 Disch. F	-40 Died M	-40 Died F	-50 Disch. M	-50 Disch. F	-50 Died M	-50 Died F	-60 Disch. M	-60 Disch. F	-60 Died M	-60 Died F	Over 60 Disch. M	Over 60 Disch. F	Over 60 Died M	Over 60 Died F
DISEASES OF THE CUTANEOUS SYSTEM (continued).																																									
Lupus Erythematosus	1	..	1	..	..																						1														
Sinuses	18	11	7	..	..														1			6		1		1	5			2	2	2			1				1		
Tuberculous Disease	3	..	3	..	..										1				1			1		1						2										
Ingrowing Toe-nail	1	..	1	..	..														1			1		1																
Ulcers—																																									
Chronic and Varicose	11	4	7	..	..										1				1			3		3			1			2	4			1				1		
Perforating	4	3	1	..	..														1			1		1		1	1			1	1			2				1		
Simple	16	9	7	..	..										1				1			1				1	1			3				2	2			2		
Syphilitic	1	..	1	..	..																					1														
Tuberculous	2	1	1	..	..										1				1																					
AFFECTIONS OF THE HEAD.																																									
Hypertrophy—																																									
Cheek	1	..	1	..	..					1														1																
Lip	1	1	..	..	..																																				
Cysts—																																									
Lip	1	..	1	..	..														1																						
Sebaceous Cysts—																																									
Scalp	2	2	..	..	..																	1									1										
Dermoid Cysts—																																									
Nose	1	..	1	..	..	1																																			
Scalp	2	2	..	..	..	1													1																						

TABLE I. (continued.)

DISEASE.	Total	Discharged M.	Discharged F.	Died M.	Died F.
AFFECTIONS OF THE HEAD *(continued)*—					
Fibroma—					
Face ...	1	1	...	...	...
Lipoma—					
Face ...	2	2	...	...	...
Mole—					
Cheek ...	1	...	1	...	...
Nævus—					
Face ...	2	2	2	1	...
Rodent Ulcer ...	9	8	...	1	...
Carcinoma—					
Ear ...	3	1	1	...	...
Face ...	3	2	1	...	...
Lip ...	6	6	...	...	...
„ *(recurrent)*	4	4	...	...	...
Nose ...	3	1	1	1	...
AFFECTIONS OF THE NECK.					
Cysts—					
Dermoid ...	1	1	...	...	...
Hydatid ...	1	1	...	...	...
Sebaceous ...	2	2	...	...	...
Lipoma ...	5	2	3	...	...
Nævus ...	1	...	1	...	...
Sarcoma ...	3	2	...	1	...
Tumour (? Cause) ...	1	1	...	...	...

TABLE I. (*continued*).

DISEASE.	Total.	Discharged. M.	Discharged. F.	Died. M.	Died. F.	Under 5.	— 10.	— 15.	— 20.	— 30.	— 40.	— 50.	— 60.	Over 60.
AFFECTIONS OF THE TRUNK.														
Cysts—														
Sacral ...	1	1	...	...	...									
Sebaceous	2	...	2	...	...					1 ... 2				
Fibroma—														
Buttock ...	1	...	1	...	...									
Leio-myoma—	2	...	1	1	...							1 ... 1 1		
Nævus—														
Retro-peritoneal														
Nævus—														
Back	1	...	1	...	...	1								
Papilloma—														
Back	1	1	...	...	...					1				
Anus ...	1	1	...	...	...				1					
Rodent Ulcer—														
Back ...	1	1	...	...	...								1	
Sacro-coccygeal Tumour	1	...	1	...	...	1								
AFFECTIONS OF THE UPPER EXTREMITY.														
Angeio-Neuroma—														
Arm ...	1	...	1	...	...				1					
Lipoma—														
Arm ...	3	2	1	...	...				1			2 1	1 1	
Shoulder ...	5	2	3	...	...									

DISEASE.	Total	Discharged M.
AFFECTIONS OF THE UPPER EXTREMITY (*continued*).		
Hairy Mole— *Hand* ...	1	...
Carcinoma (recurrent)	1	1
Sarcoma (recurrent)— *Arm* ...	1	...
Melanotic— *Axilla* ...	1	1
AFFECTIONS OF THE LOWER EXTREMITY.		
Fibroma— *Leg* ...	1	...
Lipoma— *Thigh* ...	2	...
Lymphangeioma— *Leg* ...	2	...
Gumma— *Leg* ...	1	...
Nevus— *Leg* ...	2	2
Nevo-Lipoma ...	1	1

TABLE I. (continued).

DISEASE.	Total	Discharged M	Discharged F	Died M	Died F
AFFECTIONS OF THE LOWER EXTREMITY (continued).					
Neuroma— Leg	1	...	1	...	...
Carcinoma— Foot	1	1	...	...	...
Sarcoma— Leg	1	1	...	...	...
INJURIES.					
Burns	29	14	11	1	3
Scalds	16	5	8	2	1
INJURIES OF THE HEAD AND FACE.					
Contusions	8	6	2	...	...
Wounds— Incised	3	2	1	...	...
Lacerated	9	5	4	...	...
Concussion	26	23	3	...	...

TABLE I. (*continued*).

INJURY	Total	Discharged M.	Discharged F.	Died M.	Died F.	Under 5. Dis. M.	Under 5. Dis. F.	Under 5. Died M.	Under 5. Died F.	—10. Dis. M.	—10. Dis. F.	—10. Died M.	—10. Died F.	—15. Dis. M.	—15. Dis. F.	—15. Died M.	—15. Died F.	—20. Dis. M.	—20. Dis. F.	—20. Died M.	—20. Died F.	—30. Dis. M.	—30. Dis. F.	—30. Died M.	—30. Died F.	—40. Dis. M.	—40. Dis. F.	—40. Died M.	—40. Died F.	—50. Dis. M.	—50. Dis. F.	—50. Died M.	—50. Died F.	—60. Dis. M.	—60. Dis. F.	—60. Died M.	—60. Died F.	Over 60. Dis. M.	Over 60. Dis. F.	Over 60. Died M.	Over 60. Died F.
INJURIES OF THE HEAD AND FACE (*continued*).																																									
Fractures— Skull— Base	11	5		6		1		1														3	1	1		3		2				1				1				2	
Vault	5	3	1	1	1									1								1	1	1				1		1											
Jaw— Lower	2	1		1																		1		1																	
Skull— Old	1	1																1																							
INJURIES OF THE NECK.																																									
Contusions	2	1	1															1				1																			
Wounds— Gunshot	2	1	1															1	1			1												1		1					
Incised	10	5	1	4						1								1				2	1	1		1				1		1		1		1			1	1	
INJURIES OF THE THORAX.																																									
Contusions	3	3																				1				1				1											
Wounds— Punctured	5	4	1											1				3				1				1													1		

TABLE I. (continued).

Injury	Total	Discharged M	Discharged F	Died M	Died F
INJURIES OF THE THORAX *(continued)*—					
Foreign Bodies—					
Œsophagus	2	2	…	…	…
Trachea	1	1	…	…	…
Fracture—					
Rib	20	16	2	2	…
INJURIES OF THE ABDOMEN.					
Contusions	6	6	…	…	…
Intestine—					
Laceration	2	…	…	2	…
Foreign body	1	1	…	…	…
Kidney, Ruptured	1	1	…	…	…
Muscle, Ruptured	1	1	…	…	…
Liver, Laceration	3	…	1	3	…
Spleen, Laceration	2	…	…	1	1
INJURIES OF THE BACK.					
Contusions	2	1	1	…	…
Fracture—					
Dislocation of Spine	1	1	…	…	…

Age distribution (Discharged / Died, M and F) for the above rows:

Injury	Under 5	— 10.	— 15.	— 20.	— 30.	— 40.	— 50.	— 60.	Over 60.
Œsophagus						Disch. 1		Disch. 1	
Trachea								Disch. 1	
Rib	Disch. 1	Disch. 1		Disch. 2	Disch. 3	Disch. 1	Disch. 3, Died 1	Disch. 5 1	Disch. 3 1
Contusions (abd.)				Disch. 3	Disch. 1	Disch. 1	Disch. 1		
Intestine *Laceration*					Died 1		Died 1		
Foreign body					Disch. 1				
Kidney, Ruptured				Disch. 1					
Muscle, Ruptured							Disch. 1		
Liver, Laceration			Died 1	Died 2					
Spleen, Laceration									Died 1 1
Contusions (back)				Disch. 1					
Dislocation of Spine							Disch. 1		

TABLE I. (continued).

INJURY.	Total	Discharged M	Discharged F	Died M	Died F	Under 5 D.M	Under 5 D.F	Under 5 Di.M	Under 5 Di.F	−10 D.M	−10 D.F	−10 Di.M	−10 Di.F	−15 D.M	−15 D.F	−15 Di.M	−15 Di.F	−20 D.M	−20 D.F	−20 Di.M	−20 Di.F	−30 D.M	−30 D.F	−30 Di.M	−30 Di.F	−40 D.M	−40 D.F	−40 Di.M	−40 Di.F	−50 D.M	−50 D.F	−50 Di.M	−50 Di.F	−60 D.M	−60 D.F	−60 Di.M	−60 Di.F	Over 60 D.M	Over 60 D.F	Over 60 Di.M	Over 60 Di.F
INJURIES OF THE PELVIS AND GENITALS.																																									
Contusions ...	4	4												2								1				1															
Wounds—																																									
Incised, of Penis	1	1										1																													
Fractures—																																									
Pelvis ...	6	2		4								1										1			2													1			
Ruptured Perineum	2		2																					1				1													
INJURIES OF THE UPPER EXTREMITY.																																									
Foreign Body in ...	5	1	4				1							1						1		2								1											
Wounds—																																									
Incised ...	2	2																				1								1											
Lacerated ...	11	11			1									1						1		2				4				2				1							
Punctured Wound of Artery	1	1	1																							1															
Injuries of Nerve ...	6	5	1																			3				1								1							
Tendons Divided ...	5	3	2																	1		2		3	2	1								1							
Fractures—																																									
(Simple)—																																									
Clavicle	2	2	1											1												3				1								1			
Humerus	10	9	1																							1				1				3				1			
Metacarpus	1	1																				1		1		1															
Olecranon	4	3	1																			1				1				1											
Radius ...	4	2	2																			1		1		1				1								1			
Scapula ...	1	1																				1																			

TABLE I. (continued).

INJURY	Total	Discharged M.	Discharged F.	Died M.	Died F.	Under 5 Disch. M.	Under 5 Disch. F.	Under 5 Died M.	Under 5 Died F.	—10 Disch. M.	—10 Disch. F.	—10 Died M.	—10 Died F.	—15 Disch. M.	—15 Disch. F.	—15 Died M.	—15 Died F.	—20 Disch. M.	—20 Disch. F.	—20 Died M.	—20 Died F.	—30 Disch. M.	—30 Disch. F.	—30 Died M.	—30 Died F.	—40 Disch. M.	—40 Disch. F.	—40 Died M.	—40 Died F.	—50 Disch. M.	—50 Disch. F.	—50 Died M.	—50 Died F.	—60 Disch. M.	—60 Disch. F.	—60 Died M.	—60 Died F.	Over 60 Disch. M.	Over 60 Disch. F.	Over 60 Died M.	Over 60 Died F.
INJURIES OF THE UPPER EXTREMITY (continued).																																									
Fractures (continued)—																																									
(Compound)—																																									
Humerus ...	3	3																								1															
Metacarpus	3	2	1				1											1												1				1	1			1			
Radius and Ulna	3	2	1															1												1					1			1			
Ulna ...	1	1																												1											
(Old)—																																									
Humerus ...	2	1	1							1																								1							
Mal- or Ununited—																																									
Humerus ...	2	2								1								1								1															
Ulna ...	7	5	2							2				1				1				3	1	1						1	1			1				1			
Radius and Ulna	3		3												1			1				1				1															
Dislocations—																																									
(Simple)—																																									
Humerus ...	4	:2	4												1							1								1				2				2			
" (Old)...	2	2																																							
Separation of Epiphysis—																																									
Humerus ...	1	1												1																											
Radius ...	1	1																1												1											
INJURIES OF THE LOWER EXTREMITY.																																									
Contusions ...	7	4	8																			1				1				1				1				1	1		

TABLE I. (continued).

INJURY.	Total	Disch. M	Disch. F	Died M	Died F	Under 5 Disch. M	Under 5 Disch. F	−10 Disch. M	−10 Disch. F	−15 Disch. M	−15 Disch. F	−20 Disch. M	−20 Disch. F	−30 Disch. M	−30 Disch. F	−40 Disch. M	−40 Disch. F	−50 Disch. M	−50 Disch. F	−60 Disch. M	−60 Disch. F	Over 60 Disch. M	Over 60 Disch. F	Died (various)
INJURIES OF THE LOWER EXTREMITY (continued).																								
Foreign body in ...	7	1	6	...	...							1	1		1		1		1				1	
Wounds—																								
Gunshot (Old) ...	1	1	...	...	...														1					
Incised ...	2	2	...	...	...																			
Lacerated ...	7	4	3	...	...			3	2								1							
Injury to Nerve ...	1	1	...	...	...					1														
Fracture—																								
(Simple)—																								
Astragalus ...	1	...	...	...	**1**																			
Femur—																								
Neck (Extracapsular)	3	1	2	...	...									2		2								
" *(Intracapsular)*	4	1	3	...	...									1		3	1						1	
Shaft ...	36	28	7	**1**	...	5	4	9		2		3		4		4	1	9	1	3	1	1	1	
Fibula ...	5	4	1	...	...									3		1		6	2	3				
Patella ...	23	20	3	...	...									4		6	3	3		3	1	1	1	
Pott's ...	22	18	4	...	...									5	1	3	1	3		3	1	3	1	
Tibia ...	21	17	4	...	...									5		3	1	12	3	7		11	2	
Tibia and Fibula ...	65	50	15	...	...			2		5		2				6	3			4				
(Compound)—																								
Tibia ...	2	1	1	...	...							1				1				1				
Tibia and Fibula ...	15	12	2	**1**	...							2				2		3		1		3		
Femur ...	3	2	...	**1**	...											2						1		

TABLE I. (continued).

INJURY.	Total.	Discharged.		Died.		Under 5.				-10.				-15.				-20.				-30.				-40.				-50.				-60.				Over 60.			
		M.	F.	M.	F.	Dis. M	Dis. F	Died M	Died F	Dis. M	Dis. F	Died M	Died F	Dis. M	Dis. F	Died M	Died F	Dis. M	Dis. F	Died M	Died F	Dis. M	Dis. F	Died M	Died F	Dis. M	Dis. F	Died M	Died F	Dis. M	Dis. F	Died M	Died F	Dis. M	Dis. F	Died M	Died F	Dis. M	Dis. F	Died M	Died F
INJURIES OF THE LOWER EXTREMITY (continued).																																									
Fractures (continued)—																																									
(Old)—																																									
Femur	1	1	...	...	...																	1				1															
Patella	1	...	1	...	...																	1																1			
(Malunited)—																																									
Femur	2	2	...	...	...																						1												1		
Tibia	1	1	...	...	...																1				1							1							1		
Tibia and Fibula	2	2	...	...	...																1																		1		
(Ununited)—																																									
Patella	1	1	...	...	...																	1																			
Tibia	4	3	1	...	...													1				2	1																		
Tibia and Fibula	1	...	1	...	...																																				
Dislocations—																																									
Femur	4	4	...	...	...					1				1				1				1								1				1							
Synovitis, Traumatic—																																									
Ankle	3	3	...	...	...																1	3 1			1				1												
Knee	4	3	1	...	...																																				
Separation of Epiphysis—																																									
Tibia	1	...	1	...	...													1				1																			
Admitted for Examination	4	2	2	...	...									1												1												1			
Cases UNCLASSIFIED	10	6	4	...	...																																				

ABSTRACT OF TABLE I.

With average duration of stay of Surgical Patients in the Hospital.

Discharged, Cured or Relieved ... ... $\left\{\begin{array}{l}\text{M. 2,237}\\ \text{F. 1,493}\end{array}\right\}$ 3,730

Died ... ... $\left\{\begin{array}{l}\text{M. 168}\\ \text{F. 93}\end{array}\right\}$ 261

*Remaining in, December 31st, 1904 :—

Male ... ... 188 $\left.\right\}$ 318

Female 130

Average stay of—

Men ... ... 28·45 days.

Women ... ... 29·08 ,,

* These cases are not included in Table I. or II.

TABLE II.

SURGICAL OPERATIONS PERFORMED.

OPERATIONS	TOTAL		Discharged		Died		Under 5 Years		—10		—20		—30		—40		—50		—60		—70		Over 70	
	M.	F.	M.	F.	M.	F.	M.	F.	M.	F.	M.	F.	M.	F.	M.	F.	M.	F.	M.	F.	M.	F.	M.	F.
REMOVAL OF TUMOURS.																								
(NON-MALIGNANT.)																								
Cysts—																								
Dermoid	3	…	3	…	…	…	1	…	1	…	1	…	…	…	…	…	…	…	…	…	…	…	…	…
Hydatid	1	…	1	…	…	…	…	…	1	…	…	…	…	…	…	…	…	…	…	…	…	…	…	…
Lip …	…	1	…	1	…	…	…	…	…	1	…	…	…	…	…	…	…	…	…	…	…	…	…	…
Sebaceous	5	2	5	2	…	…	…	…	…	…	2	2	1	…	…	…	1	1	1	…	…	…	…	…
Fibroma—																								
Face	1	1	1	1	…	…	…	…	…	…	1	…	…	1	…	…	…	…	…	…	…	…	…	…
Leg	…	1	…	1	…	…	…	…	…	…	…	…	…	1	…	…	…	…	…	…	…	…	…	…
Trunk	1	1	1	1	…	…	…	…	…	…	…	…	1	1	…	…	…	…	…	…	…	…	…	…
Lipoma—																								
Arm …	2	1	2	1	…	…	…	…	…	…	…	…	…	…	1	…	2	1	…	…	…	…	…	…
Face …	2	…	2	…	…	…	…	…	…	…	…	…	…	…	…	…	1	…	1	…	…	…	…	…
Neck …	1	2	1	2	…	…	…	…	…	…	…	1	…	…	…	…	…	1	…	1	…	1	…	…
Shoulder	3	3	3	3	…	…	…	…	…	…	…	…	…	…	…	…	1	1	2	1	…	…	…	…
Thigh	…	2	…	2	…	…	…	…	…	…	…	…	…	…	…	…	…	2	…	…	…	…	…	…
Leio-myoma …	1	1	…	1	1	…	…	…	…	…	…	…	…	…	…	…	…	…	…	…	…	…	…	…
Lymphangeioma—																								
Leg … …	…	1	…	1	…	…	…	1	…	…	…	…	…	…	…	…	…	…	…	…	…	…	…	…

* See also Various Organs.

TABLE II. *(continued)*.

OPERATIONS	Total M	Total F	Discharged M	Discharged F	Died M	Died F	Under 5 Years M	Under 5 Years F	—10 M	—10 F	—20 M	—20 F	—30 M	—30 F	—40 M	—40 F	—50 M	—50 F	—60 M	—60 F	—70 M	—70 F	Over 70 M	Over 70 F
REMOVAL OF TUMOURS *(continued)*.																								
(NON-MALIGNANT) *(contd.)*—																								
Mole—																								
Cheek		1		1																1				
Nævus—																								
Back...		1		1				1																
Cheek		2		2				1																
Leg ...	2		2				1						1											
Neck ...		1		1						1														
Nævo-Lipoma—																								
Leg ...	1		1				1																	
Neuroma—																								
Leg ...		1		1												1								
Papilloma—																								
Anus...	1	1	1	1				1																
Sacro-coccygeal Tumour		1		1				1																
(MALIGNANT.)																								
Bodent Ulcer—																								
Face ...	6		5		1												1		1		2		2	
Back ...	1		1																1					
Squamous-celled Carcinoma—																								
Ear ...	1		1														1							
Face ...	2	1	2	1														1	1					
Lip ...	6		6																2		2		1	
„ (recurrent)	4		4																		2		1	
Nose ...	1	1	1	1																			1	1

TABLE II. (*continued*).

OPERATIONS.	TOTAL M	TOTAL F	Discharged M	Discharged F	Died M	Died F	Under 5 Years M	Under 5 Years F	−10 M	−10 F	−20 M	−20 F	−30 M	−30 F	−40 M	−40 F	−50 M	−50 F	−60 M	−60 F	−70 M	−70 F	Over 70 M	Over 70 F
REMOVAL OF TUMOURS (*contd.*) (**MALIGNANT**) (*contd.*)—																								
Sarcoma—																								
Neck	3	..	2	..	..	..	..	..	..	..	..	..	..	..	..	..	..	..	2	..	1	..	..	..
Thigh	1	..	1	..	1	..	..	..	..	..	..	..	..	..	..	..	1	..	..	..	..	..	..	..
PLASTIC OPERATIONS.																								
For Cleft Palate ...	10	6	10	6	..	..	5	3	4	1	1	2	..	..	..	..	..	..	..	..	..	..	..	..
" Deformity of Cheek	..	1	..	1	..	..	..	..	..	..	..	..	..	1	..	..	..	..	..	..	..	..	..	..
" " Ear	1	1	1	1	..	..	..	..	..	..	..	..	1	1	..	..	..	..	..	..	..	..	..	..
" " Mouth	1	2	1	2	..	..	1	..	..	..	..	..	..	1	..	1	..	..	..	..	..	..	..	..
" " Nose	3	1	3	1	..	..	..	..	..	..	2	..	1	1	..	..	..	..	..	..	..	..	..	..
" Ectopion Vesicæ	5	4	4	4	1	..	5	4	..	..	..	..	..	..	..	..	..	..	..	..	..	..	..	..
" Hare-Lip ...	1	1	1	1	..	..	1	1	..	..	..	..	..	..	..	..	..	..	..	..	..	..	..	..
" Hypospadias ...	1	..	1	..	..	..	..	..	1	..	..	..	..	..	..	..	..	..	..	..	..	..	..	..
" Old Burns ...	..	2	..	2	..	..	..	1	..	..	..	1	..	..	..	..	..	..	..	..	..	..	..	..
" Recto-Vaginal Fistula	..	3	..	3	..	..	..	..	..	..	..	..	..	1	..	1	..	1	..	..	..	..	..	..
" Ruptured Perineum*	..	21	..	21	..	..	..	..	..	..	..	1	..	7	..	6	..	5	..	2	..	..	..	..
" Webbed Fingers ...	2	..	2	..	..	..	2	..	..	..	..	..	..	..	..	..	..	..	..	..	..	..	..	..
" Umbilical Fistula	..	1	..	1	..	..	..	1	..	..	..	..	..	..	..	..	..	..	..	..	..	..	..	..
OPERATIONS ON THE NERVOUS SYSTEM.																								
Division of Nerve—																								
Inferior dental ...	1	..	1	..	..	..	..	..	..	..	..	..	..	..	..	..	1	..	..	..	..	..	..	..
Supra-orbital ...	1	..	1	..	..	..	..	..	..	..	..	..	..	..	..	..	1	..	..	..	..	..	..	..

* In 19 of these cases the operation was performed in a Gynæcological Ward.

OPERATIONS.	TOTAL M	TOTAL F	Discharged M	Discharged F	Died M	Died F	Under 5 Years M	Under 5 Years F	-10 M	-10 F	-20 M	-20 F	-30 M	-30 F	-40 M	-40 F	-50 M	-50 F	-60 M	-60 F	-70 M
OPERATIONS ON THE NERVOUS SYSTEM (continued).																					
Exploration of Nerve— *Ulnar*	1	...	1	...	...	...	...	...	...	...	...	...	1	...	...	...	...	...	...	...	...
Stretching of Nerve— *Great Sciatic*	1	...	1	...	...	...	...	...	...	...	...	...	1	...	...	...	...	...	...	...	...
Suture of Nerve— *Median*	1	...	1	...	...	...	...	...	...	...	...	...	1	...	...	...	...	...	...	...	...
Medium and Ulnar	...	1	...	1	...	...	...	...	...	...	...	...	...	1	...	1	...	...	...	...	...
Musculo-spiral	1	...	1	...	...	...	...	...	...	...	1	...	1	...	...	...	...	...	...	...	...
Excision of Spinal Meningo-cele	1	...	1	...	...	...	1	...	...	...	...	...	...	...	...	...	...	...	...	...	...
OPERATIONS ON THE NOSE AND ANTRUM.																					
For Deviated Septum	5	1	5	1	...	...	...	...	1	...	2	...	2	...	...	1	...	...	...	...	...
Drainage of Superior Maxillary Antrum	1	...	1	...	...	...	...	...	...	...	...	...	...	...	...	...	...	...	1	...	...
Excision of Cyst of Antrum	...	1	...	1	...	...	...	...	...	...	...	1	...	...	...	...	...	...	...	...	...
Injection of Paraffin Wax for Deformity of Nose	4	1	4	1	...	...	...	...	1	...	2	...	1	1	...	...	...	...	...	...	...
Removal of Nasal Spur	2	1	2	1	...	...	...	...	...	...	1	1	...	...	...	...	1	...	...	...	...
Removal of Turbinated Bones	5	...	5	...	...	...	...	...	...	...	2	...	3	...	...	...	1	...	...	...	...
Removal of Tumours— *Polypi**	...	3	...	3	...	...	...	...	...	...	...	...	...	1	...	1	...	1	...	...	...
Naso-pharyngeal Polypi	2	1	2	1	...	...	...	...	...	...	1	...	...	1	1	...	...	...	...	...	...

* In one of these cases the operation was performed in a Medical Ward.

TABLE II. (continued).

AGE AND SEX

OPERATIONS	TOTAL		Discharged		Died		Under 5 Years		-10		-20		-30		-40		-50		-60		-70		Over 70	
	M.	F.	M.	F.	M.	F.	M.	F.	M.	F.	M.	F.	M.	F.	M.	F.	M.	F.	M.	F.	M.	F.	M.	F.
OPERATIONS ON THE EYE.																								
Lids—																								
Abscess	1		1												1									
Cyst		1		1								2												
For Ectropion	3	2	3	2							2			1		1				1	1			
" Entropion	1	4	1	4				1	1		1	1								1			1	
" Expression	4	1	4	1					1												1			
Ptosis	1		1						1															
Tumours	2		2				1												1					
Lachrymal Apparatus—																								
Abscess, &c.	3	6	3	6			1				1	3	1			1								
Sclerotic—																								
Scleral Puncture	1	2	1	2										2				1						
" Suture	1		1																1					
Cornea—																								
Cauterisation	5	2	5	2							1		1								2			
Paracentesis	1		1								1													
Tattooing	1		1																					
Iris—																								
Iridectomy	9	10	9	10			3			1	1	1	2	1		4			1	3	2			
Lens—																								
Simple Extraction	13	8	9	8					1					8		3		1	1	8	3		3	1
Extraction with Irideo-tomy	12	10	12	10							8	6	1	8		1		3	8	8	3		3	2
Discission	5	13	5	13							2	2	1	8	6				8	5	4	1	1	
" for After Cataract	15	13	15	13					1	1		2	1	8		3				5	4	1	1	1
" " Myopia	1	7	1	7				2																

TABLE II. (*continued*).

OPERATIONS.	TOTAL M	TOTAL F	Discharged M	Discharged F	Died M	Died F	Under 5 Years M	Under 5 Years F	—10 M	—10 F	—20 M	—20 F	—30 M	—30 F	—40 M	—40 F	—50 M	—50 F	—60 M	—60 F	—70 M	—70 F	Over 70 M	Over 70 F
OPERATIONS ON THE EYE (*continued*).																								
Orbit—																								
Removal of Growths	2	1	2	1	…	…	…	…	…	…	1	…	…	…	…	…	1	…	1	…	…	1	…	…
Cellulitis	1	1	1	1	…	…	…	…	…	…	1	…	…	…	…	1	…	…	…	…	…	…	…	…
Strabismus—																								
Advancement	22	20	22	20	…	…	…	…	8	3	8	11	6	6	…	…	…	…	…	…	…	…	…	…
Tenotomy	1	3	1	3	…	…	…	…	…	2	…	1	1	1	…	…	…	4	…	…	…	…	…	…
Excision	15	13	15	13	…	…	1	…	3	…	3	1	4	1	2	…	…	…	…	…	3	4	…	1
Dermoid Cyst	1	…	1	…	…	…	…	…	…	…	…	…	…	…	…	…	…	…	…	…	…	…	…	…
EXCISIONS OF BONES AND JOINTS.																								
Astragalus	2	…	2	…	…	…	…	…	…	…	…	…	1	…	…	…	…	…	1	…	…	…	…	…
Ankle	1	1	…	1	…	…	…	…	…	…	…	…	…	1	…	…	…	1	…	…	…	1	…	…
Elbow	1	1	1	1	…	…	…	…	…	…	1	…	1	1	…	…	…	…	…	…	1	…	…	…
Hip	3	1	3	1	…	…	…	…	3	…	1	…	1	…	1	…	…	…	1	…	…	…	…	…
Jaw	2	1	2	1	…	…	…	…	1	…	1	1	1	…	…	…	…	…	…	…	…	…	…	…
Knee	4	4	4	4	…	…	…	…	…	…	1	1	2	2	…	…	…	1	…	…	…	…	…	…
Metatarsal (Head of)	2	2	2	2	…	…	…	…	…	1	1	1	…	…	…	…	…	…	1	…	1	…	…	…
Phalanx (Head of)	5	2	5	2	…	…	…	…	…	…	2	2	2	…	1	…	…	…	1	…	…	…	…	…
Rib*	18	7	12	7	1	…	3	3	…	…	1	1	3	2	3	…	2	…	…	…	…	…	…	…
Scapula	1	…	1	…	…	…	3	…	…	…	…	…	…	…	…	…	1	…	1	…	…	…	…	…
Shoulder	2	…	2	…	…	…	4	1	…	…	…	…	…	…	…	…	…	…	…	…	…	…	…	…
Tarsus	6	2	6	2	…	…	4	…	2	…	…	…	…	…	…	1	…	1	1	…	…	…	…	…
Wrist	1	1	1	1	…	…	…	…	…	…	…	…	…	…	…	…	…	1	…	1	…	…	…	…

In 11 of these cases the operation was performed in a Medical Ward.

TABLE II. (*continued*).

OPERATIONS.	Total		Discharged		Died		Under 5 Years		—10		—20		—30		—40		—50		—60		—70		Over 70	
	M	F	M	F	M	F	M	F	M	F	M	F	M	F	M	F	M	F	M	F	M	F	M	F
OPERATIONS ON THE LARYNX AND TRACHEA.																								
Laryngectomy	1				1												1							
Thyrotomy	1		1														1							
Tracheotomy	11	6	5	3	6	3	7	6		2	1						3							
Scarification	1	1	1								1					1								
Removal of Papilloma		1		1																				
OPERATIONS ON THE THYROID GLAND.																								
Partial removal for Goitre	2	2	2	2							2			1		1				1		1		
Removal of Tumours—																								
Adenoma	2	5	2	5										2	2	1		1				1		
Cyst		2		2										2		1								
Sarcoma		1		1												1								
OPERATIONS ON THE CHEST.																								
Incision and Drainage of Empyema		1		1												1		1						
OPERATIONS ON THE VASCULAR SYSTEM.																								
Arteries—																								
Exploratory Laparotomy for Aneurysm	2				2										2									
Ligature of Arteries	4	1	4	1										1	3		2							

TABLE II. (continued).

OPERATIONS	TOTAL		Discharged		Died		Under 5 Years		—10		—20		—30		—40		—50		—60		—70		Over 70	
	M	F	M	F	M	F	M	F	M	F	M	F	M	F	M	F	M	F	M	F	M	F	M	F
OPERATIONS ON THE VASCULAR SYSTEM (continued).																								
Veins—																								
Ligature, or Ligature and Excision, of Varicose Veins	55	32	55	32	...	...	...	...	...	...	8	2	28	17	13	3	6	4	...	...	...	...	...	...
OPERATIONS ON THE LYMPHATIC SYSTEM.																								
Excision of Lymphatic Glands—																								
Axilla—																								
For Carcinoma ...	1	..	1	..	..	..	..	..	..	..	..	..	..	..	..	..	1	..	..	..	..	..	..	..
,, Inflammation	1	2	1	2	..	..	..	..	..	..	..	..	..	1	..	..	..	..	..	..	..	..	..	..
,, Tubercle ...	1	..	1	..	..	..	..	..	..	1	..	..	..	..	..	..	..	..	..	..	..	..	..	..
,, Sarcoma ...	1	..	1	..	..	..	..	..	..	..	..	..	..	..	..	..	..	..	..	..	..	..	..	..
,, Melanotic ...	1	1	1	1	..	..	..	..	..	..	..	..	..	..	..	1	..	..	1	1	..	..	..	..
Groin—																								
For Inflammation ...	..	2	..	2	..	..	..	..	..	..	..	..	..	..	..	1	..	..	..	1	..	..	..	..
,, Lymphadenoma	1	..	1	..	..	..	..	..	..	..	1	..	..	..	..	..	..	..	1	..	..	..	..	..
,, Sarcoma, Melanotic...	1	..	1	..	..	..	..	..	..	..	..	..	..	..	..	1	..	..	1	..	..	..	..	..
,, Tubercle ...	1	1	1	1	..	..	..	..	..	..	..	..	..	..	..	1	..	..	..	..	..	..	..	..
Mesentery—																								
For Laparotomy ...	3	1	3	1	..	..	..	..	..	..	..	..	..	..	2	1	1	..	..	..	..	..	..	..
Neck—																								
For Carcinoma (secondary)	9	..	9	..	..	..	..	..	..	..	1	..	..	..	1	..	2	..	..	..	4	..	1	..
,, Inflammation ...	4	..	4	..	..	..	..	..	1	..	1	..	..	..	2	..	..	..	..	..	..	..	..	..
,, Lymphadenoma ...	2	..	2	..	..	..	..	..	..	..	1	..	..	..	1	..	..	..	..	..	..	..	..	..

TABLE II. (*continued*).

OPERATIONS	TOTAL M	F	Discharged M	F	Died M	F	Under 5 Years M	F	−10 M	F	−20 M	F	−30 M	F	−40 M	F	−50 M	F	−60 M	F	−70 M	F	Over 70 M	F
OPERATIONS ON THE LYMPHATIC SYSTEM (*contd.*).																								
Excision of Lymphatic Glands (*continued*)—																								
Neck (*continued*)—																								
For Sarcoma	1	1	1	1					1	1					1									
" *Tubercle*	19	35	19	35			4	2	3	4	6	8	3	14	1	3	2	2		2				
Erasion of Lymphatic Glands	2	3	2	3						1	1	1	1	1										
OPERATIONS ON THE EAR.																								
Incision of Abscess	5	4	5	4			2	2	1	1	1			1	1									
Complete Mastoid Operation	34	44	31	41	3	3	2	4	5	7	11	13	7	14	4	5	4	1	1					
Erasion of Middle Ear	7	11	7	11					1	2	3	1	3	5		1		1		1				
OPERATIONS ON BONES.																								
Erasion or Gouging of Carious Bones—																								
Femur	2		2								1		1											
Rib	2		2								1		1											
Tarsus	2	2	2	2							1	1	1			1								
Temporal		1		1								1												
Tibia	5	1	5	1					2	1	1		1		1									
For Old Fracture	3		3				1						1		1									
Incision of Bone—																								
For Periostitis—																								
Femur	5	2	5	1	1				1	1	8				1	1								
Malar	1		1								1													
Tarsus	1	1	1	1						1	1													

TABLE (II. *continued*).

OPERATIONS	TOTAL		Discharged		Died		Under 5 Years		AGE AND SEX −10.		−20.		−30.		−40.		−50.		−60.		−70.		Over 70.	
	M.	F.	M.	F.	M.	F.	M.	F.	M.	F.	M.	F.	M.	F.	M.	F.	M.	F.	M.	F.	M.	F.	M.	F.
OPERATIONS ON BONES (*continued*).																								
Incision of Bone (*continued*)—																								
For Periostitis (*continued*)—																								
Tibia	5	4	5	3	..	..	..	2	..	..	3	2	1	..	1	..	..	..	..	..	..	..	..	..
Ulna	1	..	1	..	..	..	..	..	..	..	1	..	..	..	..	..	..	..	..	..	..	..	..	..
For Epiphysitis—																								
Radius	1	..	1	..	..	..	1	..	..	..	..	..	..	..	..	..	..	..	..	..	..	..	..	..
Tibia	1	..	1	..	..	..	..	..	..	..	1	..	..	..	..	..	..	..	..	..	..	..	..	..
For Tuberculous Dactylitis	1	1	1	1	..	..	..	..	..	..	1	..	..	1	..	..	..	..	..	..	..	..	..	..
Laminectomy	2	..	1	..	1	..	..	..	1	..	1	..	..	..	..	..	..	..	..	..	..	..	..	..
Osteoclasia—																								
Radius and Ulna	..	1	..	1	..	..	..	..	..	1	..	..	..	..	..	..	..	..	..	..	..	..	..	..
Osteotomy—																								
Femur—																								
Infra-trochanteric—																								
For Ankylosis	4	2	4	2	..	..	..	..	1	1	2	1	1	..	..	..	..	..	..	..	..	..	..	..
Supra-condyloid—																								
For Genu Valgum	3	11	3	11	..	..	1	2	..	5	2	3	..	1	..	..	..	..	..	..	..	..	..	..
" *Malunion*	1	..	1	..	..	..	..	..	..	..	1	..	..	..	..	..	..	..	..	..	..	..	..	..
" *Tibia*	1	1	..	..	..	..	1	1	..	..	..	..	..	..	..	..	..	..	..	..	..	..	..	..
" *Tibia and Fibula*	..	1	..	1	..	..	..	1	..	..	..	..	..	..	..	..	..	..	..	..	..	..	..	..
Sequestrotomy—																								
Femur	6	3	6	3	..	..	..	..	..	..	1	1	1	..	3	1	..	1	1	..	..	..	..	..
Humerus	1	1	1	1	..	..	..	..	..	..	1	1	..	..	..	..	..	..	..	..	..	..	..	..
Jaw	4	2	4	2	..	..	..	..	1	..	..	..	3	..	..	1	..	..	..	..	..	..	..	..
Metatarsus	1	1	..	1	..	..	..	..	..	..	..	..	1	..	..	1	..	..	..	..	..	1	..	..
Patella	1	..	1	..	..	..	..	..	..	..	..	..	..	..	..	..	..	..	..	..	..	..	..	..
Pelvis	1	1	1	1	..	..	..	..	..	..	1	1	1	..	..	..	..	..	..	..	..	..	..	..

TABLE II. (continued).

OPERATIONS.	TOTAL		Discharged.		Died.		AGE AND SEX. Under 5 Years		—10.		—20.		—30.		—40.		—50.		—60.		—70.		Over 70.	
	M.	F.	M.	F.	M.	F.	M.	F.	M.	F.	M.	F.	M.	F.	M.	F.	M.	F.	M.	F.	M.	F.	M.	F.
OPERATIONS ON BONES (*continued*).																								
Sequestrotomy (*continued*)—																								
Sacrum	1	…	1	…	…	…	…	…	…	…	1	…	…	…	…	…	…	…	…	…	…	…	…	…
Scapula	1	…	1	…	…	…	…	…	…	…	…	…	…	…	1	…	…	…	…	…	…	…	…	…
Skull	3	…	2	…	1	…	1	…	…	…	…	…	…	…	1	…	1	…	…	…	…	…	…	…
Tibia	7	2	7	2	…	…	…	…	…	…	…	2	4	…	…	…	…	1	…	…	…	…	…	…
Ulna	1	1	1	1	…	…	…	…	…	…	1	…	…	…	…	…	…	1	…	…	…	…	…	…
Trephining—																								
Skull—																								
For Cerebral Abscess	1	…	…	…	1	…	…	…	…	…	1	…	…	…	…	…	…	…	…	…	…	…	…	…
„ *Cerebral Hemorrhage*	2	…	1	…	1	…	1	…	…	…	…	…	…	…	2	…	…	…	…	…	…	…	…	…
„ *Cerebellar Abscess*	1	…	…	…	1	…	…	…	1	…	…	…	…	1	…	…	…	…	…	…	…	…	…	…
„ *Cerebellar Cyst*	1	…	1	…	…	…	…	…	…	…	…	…	…	…	…	1	…	…	…	…	…	…	…	…
„ *Epilepsy*	2	…	1	…	1	…	…	…	…	…	1	…	…	…	…	…	2	…	…	…	…	…	…	…
„ *Meningitis*	…	1	…	…	…	1	…	…	…	1	1	…	…	…	…	…	…	…	…	…	…	…	…	…
Wiring or Suture of Fractured Bones—																								
Femur	1	…	1	…	…	…	…	…	…	…	…	…	…	…	1	…	…	…	…	…	…	…	…	…
Humerus	3	1	3	1	…	…	…	…	…	…	1	…	…	…	2	…	…	…	…	1	…	…	…	…
Olecranon	3	2	3	2	…	…	…	…	…	…	1	…	2	1	1	…	…	…	…	1	…	…	…	…
Patella	14	…	14	…	…	…	…	…	…	…	…	…	3	…	4	1	4	…	3	…	1	…	…	…
Tibia	2	…	2	…	…	…	…	…	…	…	1	…	…	…	1	…	…	…	…	…	…	…	…	…
Tibia and Fibula	5	…	5	…	…	…	…	…	…	…	1	…	…	…	1	…	2	…	1	…	…	…	…	…
Removal of Wire from Old Fracture—																								
Patella	1	…	1	…	…	…	…	…	…	…	…	…	…	…	…	…	1	…	…	…	…	…	…	…

TABLE II. (continued).

OPERATIONS.	Total M.	Total F.	Discharged M.	Discharged F.	Died M.	Died F.	Under 5 Years M.	Under 5 Years F.	—10 M.	—10 F.	—20 M.	—20 F.	—30 M.	—30 F.	—40 M.	—40 F.	—50 M.	—50 F.	—60 M.	—60 F.	—70 M.	—70 F.	Over 70 M.	Over 70 F.
OPERATIONS ON BONES (continued).																								
Local Removal of Tumours—																								
Chondroma—																								
Pelvis	1	...	1	...	...	...	...	...	...	...	...	...	...	...	...	...	1	...	...	...	...	...	...	...
Cyst—																								
Jaw	1	...	1	...	...	...	...	...	...	...	...	...	...	...	...	...	1	...	...	...	...	...	...	...
Epulis—																								
Upper Jaw	1	2	1	2	...	...	...	...	...	...	...	1	1	...	...	...	...	1	...	...	...	...	...	...
Lower Jaw	1	4	1	4	...	...	...	...	...	...	...	...	...	4	...	...	...	...	1	...	...	...	...	...
Exostosis—																								
Femur	1	1	1	1	...	...	...	...	...	1	1	...	...	...	...	...	...	...	...	...	...	...	...	...
Fibula	1	...	1	...	...	...	...	...	...	...	...	...	1	...	...	...	...	...	...	...	...	...	...	...
Jaw	2	2	1	2	...	...	1	...	...	...	...	...	1	1	...	...	...	1	...	...	...	...	...	...
Metatarsus	1	1	1	1	...	...	...	...	...	...	...	...	...	1	...	...	...	...	...	...	...	...	...	...
Scapula	2	...	2	...	...	...	...	...	...	...	...	...	...	...	...	...	...	...	...	...	...	...	...	...
Carcinoma—																								
Upper Jaw	3	...	3	...	...	...	...	...	...	...	...	...	...	1	...	...	...	...	1	...	...	...	2	...
Endothelioma—																								
Jaw	...	...	...	...	...	...	...	...	...	...	...	...	...	...	...	...	...	...	...	...	...	...	...	...
Odontoma—																								
Jaw	1	...	1	...	...	...	...	...	...	...	...	...	...	...	...	...	1	...	...	...	...	...	...	...
Sarcoma—																								
Clavicle	...	...	...	...	...	...	...	...	...	...	...	...	...	1	...	...	...	...	...	...	...	...	...	...
Upper Jaw	1	...	1	...	...	...	...	...	...	...	...	...	...	...	...	...	1	...	...	...	...	...	...	...

K

TABLE II. (*continued*).

OPERATIONS.

AMPUTATIONS.

Primary—
- Arm
- Finger
- Leg
- Thigh (Middle Third)
- Toes

Secondary—
- Arm
- Leg

For Disease—

Arm—
- *For Angeio Neuroma*
- " *Deformity*
- " *Tubercle*
- " *Sarcoma*

Fingers

Forearm—
- *For Deformity*

Leg—
- *For Carcinoma*
- " *Gangrene*
- " *Infantile Paralysis*
- " *Tubercle*
- " *Ulcer*
- " *Ununited Fracture*

	—40.		—50.		—60.		—70.		Over 70.	
	M.	F.	M.	F.	M.	F.	M.	F.	M.	F.

TABLE II. (*continued*).

OPERATIONS.	TOTAL M	TOTAL F	Discharged M	Discharged F	Died M	Died F	Under 5 Years M	Under 5 Years F	—10 M	—10 F	—20 M	—20 F	—30 M	—30 F	—40 M	—40 F	—50 M	—50 F	—60 M	—60 F	—70 M	—70 F	Over 70 M	Over 70 F
AMPUTATIONS (*continued*).																								
For Disease (*continued*)—																								
Thigh—																								
(At Hip Joint)—																								
For Infantile Paralysis	1	..	1	..	..	..	..	..	..	..	..	..	..	..	1	..	..	..	..	..	..	..	..	..
„ Tubercle ...	..	1	..	1	..	..	..	..	..	..	..	..	..	..	..	..	..	..	..	..	..	1	..	..
Shaft—																								
For Chronic Ulcer ...	1	1	1	1	..	..	..	..	..	..	..	..	..	..	..	..	..	1	..	..	1	..	..	..
„ Deformity ...	1	1	1	1	..	..	..	..	..	..	..	..	..	..	..	..	..	1	1	..	..	..	..	..
„ Gangrene ...	2	..	2	..	..	..	..	..	..	..	..	..	..	..	..	..	..	..	1	..	1	..	..	..
„ Infantile Paralysis	2	..	2	..	..	..	..	..	..	..	1	..	1	..	2	..	..	..	..	..	..	..	..	..
„ Osteo-myelitis ...	1	1	1	1	..	..	1	..	..	..	1	..	1	..	..	..	1	1	2	..	..	..	..	..
„ Sarcoma ...	4	..	4	..	..	..	..	..	..	..	..	..	..	..	..	..	1	..	..	..	..	..	..	..
„ Suppuration ...	1	1	1	1	..	..	..	..	..	..	..	..	1	..	..	..	1	1	1	..	..	..	..	..
„ Tubercle ...	3	2	3	2	..	..	1	..	1	..	1	..	1	..	1	..	1	..	..	..	..	1	..	..
Toes	6	..	6	..	..	..	..	..	..	..	..	..	1	..	..	..	..	..	..	..	..	..	..	..
Upper Extremity—																								
For Sarcoma ...	1	..	1	..	..	..	..	..	..	..	..	..	1	..	..	..	..	..	..	..	..	..	..	..
OPERATIONS ON JOINTS.																								
Arthrotomy—																								
Hip—																								
For Acute Suppurative Arthritis ...	1	..	1	..	..	..	1	..	..	..	..	..	1	..	..	..	..	..	..	..	..	..	..	..
Knee—																								
For Chronic Synovitis ...	2	..	2	..	..	..	..	1	..	..	..	..	..	..	..	..	..	..	1	..	..	..	..	..
Multiple Septic Arthritis ...	1	..	..	..	1	..	1	..	..	..	..	..	..	..	..	..	..	..	..	..	..	..	..	..

TABLE II. (*continued*).

OPERATIONS.	TOTAL		Discharged.		Died.		Under 5 Years.		—10.		—20.		—30.		—40.		—50.		—60.		—70.		Over 70.	
	M.	F.	M.	F.	M.	F.	M.	F.	M.	F.	M.	F.	M.	F.	M.	F.	M.	F.	M.	F.	M.	F.	M.	F.
OPERATIONS ON JOINTS (*continued*).																								
Incision or Erasion of Tuberculous Joints—																								
Elbow		8		3	1							3							1	1				
Hip	10	6	9	6	1				4	4	5	1				1	1							
Knee	2		2											1										
Sacro-iliac		2		2								2												
Removal of Loose Bodies or Displaced Semi-lunar Cartilage	12	2	12	2							3	1	7	2	1									
Removal of Tumours— Cysts— Knee	1		1						1															
Lorens Operation for Congenital Dislocation of Hip	1	3	1	3			1			2		1	1											
OPERATIONS ON BURSÆ, FASCIÆ, MUSCLES AND TENDONS.																								
Bursæ— Bursæ Incised or Removed—																								
Ischial	1	1	1									4	1			1			1					
Prepatellar	4	16	4	16			1				1	4		5		1		6	1	6	1			
Semi-membranous	1	2	1	2			1					1		1										
Sub-deltoid		1		1								1												
Trochanteric		1		1										1										

TABLE II. (continued).

OPERATIONS.	TOTAL		Discharged.		Died.		AGE AND SEX																
							Under 5 Years.		−10.		−20.		−30.		−40.		−50.		−60.		−70.		Over 70.	
	M.	F.	M.	F.	M.	F.	M.	F.	M.	F.	M.	F.	M.	F.	M.	F.	M.	F.	M.	F.	M.	F.	M.	F.
OPERATIONS ON BURSÆ, FASCIÆ, MUSCLES AND TENDONS (continued).																								
Fasciæ—																								
Excision for Contractions ...	4	2	4	2								1			1		2	1			1			
Excision of Calcified Fasciæ	1	1	1	1													1	1						
Division of Fasciæ ...	1	1	1	1											1					1				
Muscles—																								
For Carcinoma ...		1		1								2												
„ Hypertrophy ...	1		1								1													
Tendons—																								
Ganglia Incised or Removed	1	3	1	3								2							1					
Suture of Tendons—																								
Primary ...	3	2	3	2							1		1						1	1				
Secondary ...	2		2								1								1	1				
Incision for Teno-synovitis	1		1																1					
Tenotomy—																								
For Contractions ...	1		1				1																	
„ Talipes ...	5	11	5	11			1	1		3	4	4												
Plastic Operation for Flat-foot	1		1								1													
OPERATIONS ON THE CUTANEOUS SYSTEM.																								
Erasion or Excision of Carbuncle—																								
Back	4	1	4	1															2		1			1
Neck	5	1	5	1															4	1				

TABLE II. (*continued*).

184

AGE AND SEX

OPERATIONS.	TOTAL.		Discharged.		Died.		Under 5 Years.		—10.		—20.		—30.		—40.		—50.		—60.		—70.		Over 70.	
	M.	F.	M.	F.	M.	F.	M.	F.	M.	F.	M.	F.	M.	F.	M.	F.	M.	F.	M.	F.	M.	F.	M.	F.
OPERATIONS ON THE CUTANEOUS SYSTEM (*cont.*)—																								
Erasion of Lupus ...	1	1	1	1									1							1				
Erasion or Excision of Ulcers	6	4	6	4							2		1	2	1		2		1					
Excision of Scar ...	9	6	9	6							1	1		1	1		1	2						
Erasion of Sinuses ...	9	6	9	6					1		1	1	5	3	1	1	1	1	1					
Skin Grafting ...	4	5	4	5					1		1	1		1	1		1		1					
Ligature of Veins for Varicose Ulcer ...		3		3														3						
OPERATIONS ON THE CELLULAR TISSUE.																								
Incision of Abscesses—																								
Abdominal Wall ...	2	3	2	3							1		1				1							
Alveolar ...	5	4	5	4							1	1	3	3	1									
Arm ...	2	6	2	6			1			1	1	3	2	2	1									
Axilla ...	9	3	9	3			2		1	1	1	1	1		2		1		1					
Back ...	2	1	2	1									1											
Chest ...	2	1	2	1								1												
Face ...	1	3	1	3									1					1						
Foot ...		1		1																				
Gluteal ...	2	1	1	1					2		1	2	1	2	2		1							
Groin ...	5	3	5	3							1			2				1	1					
Hand ...	1		1				1																	
Iliac ...	1	4	1	4	1	2					1	2	2											
Ischio-rectal ...	9	6	9	6			1				1	2	2	2	1		3							

TABLE II. (continued).

OPERATIONS.	TOTAL. M	TOTAL. F	Discharged. M	Discharged. F	Died. M	Died. F	Under 5 Years. M	Under 5 Years. F	—10. M	—10. F	—20. M	—20. F	—30. M	—30. F	—40. M	—40. F	—50. M	—50. F	—60. M	—60. F	—70. M	—70. F	Over 70. M	Over 70. F
OPERATIONS ON THE CELLULAR TISSUE (cont.)—																								
Incision of Abscesses (cont.)—																								
Leg	5	1	5	1					3		1		2	1		1	1							
Lumbar	7	8	7	3			5			1	1		3	1	2	1	1							
Neck	15	11	15	11			1	4		2	2	1	2	5	8					1	1	3		
Perineal	4	..	4	..							1				1									
Peri-urethral	1	..	1	..							1													
Popliteal	3	1	3	1							2		1					1						
Post-pharyngeal	1	..	1	..																				
Psoas	6	8	6	8		1	1		2		4	2		1				1	5					
Retro-pharyngeal	2	1	2	1		1	1	1	1			1								1				
Scalp	2	..	2	..							1													
Scrotum	1	..	1	..							1													
Submaxillary	..	4	..	4		1		2																
Thigh	2	8	2	7		1		1	1	1	3	1	1	1	1	1	1			1	2	3		
Incisions for Cellulitis	54	21	47	20	7	1	4	2	2	2	8	5	16	2	12	1	10	2	5	2	2	3		3
OPERATIONS ON GENITO-URINARY ORGANS.																								
Bladder—																								
Cystotomy—																								
(Supra-pubic)—																								
For Calculus	3	2	3	2					1				1							1				
" Carcinoma	3	..	2	..	1																2			
" Foreign Body	..	1	..	1								1							1		1			
" Papilloma	3	..	3	..													1		1		1			
" Retention	1	..	..	..	1																1			

TABLE II. (continued).

OPERATIONS.	TOTAL M	TOTAL F	Discharged M	Discharged F	Died M	Died F	Under 5 Years M	Under 5 Years F	-10 M	-10 F	-20 M	-20 F	-30 M	-30 F	-40 M	-40 F	-50 M	-50 F	-60 M	-60 F	-70 M	-70 F	Over 70 M	Over 70 F
OPERATIONS ON GENITO-URINARY ORGANS (continued)																								
Bladder (continued)—																								
Lithotrity ...	1	:	1	:	:	:	:	:	:	:	1	:	:	:	:	:	:	:	:	:	:	:	:	:
Kidney—																								
Nephrectomy—																								
(Abdominal)—																								
For Carcinoma ...	1	:	1	:	1	:	:	:	:	:	:	:	:	:	1	:	:	:	:	:	:	:	:	:
" Hydro-nephrosis*	1	1	1	1	:	:	:	:	:	:	:	:	:	:	1	1	:	:	:	:	:	:	:	:
" Tubercle ...	1	:	1	:	:	:	:	:	:	:	:	:	:	:	1	:	:	:	:	:	:	:	:	:
(Lumbar) ...	2	3	2	3	:	:	:	:	:	:	:	:	2	:	:	2	2	:	:	1	:	:	:	:
Nephrotomy—																								
For Haematuria ...	2	:	2	:	:	:	:	:	:	:	1	:	:	:	:	:	:	:	:	:	:	:	:	:
" Hydro-nephrosis	1	2	1	2	1	:	:	:	:	:	:	:	:	2	1	1	:	1	1	:	:	:	:	:
" Pyo-nephrosis	1	3	:	2	1	1	:	:	:	:	:	:	3	:	1	:	:	1	:	:	:	2	:	:
" Renal Colic ...	4	1	4	1	:	:	:	:	:	:	:	:	1	1	1	1	:	:	:	:	:	:	:	:
" Tubercle ...	1	1	:	:	1	1	:	:	:	:	:	:	:	1	1	:	:	:	:	:	:	:	:	:
Nephro-Lithotomy ...	3	3	3	2	:	1	:	:	:	:	:	:	1	1	1	1	2	1	:	:	:	:	:	:
Nephrorraphy ...	3	8	3	8	:	:	:	:	:	:	1	:	1	2	:	4	1	:	:	:	:	:	:	:
Incision of Perinephric Abscess ...	:	2	:	2	:	:	:	:	:	:	:	:	:	1	1	:	:	:	:	:	:	:	:	:
Abdominal Section—																								
Exploratory—																								
For Malignant Growth	:	1	:	1	:	:	:	:	:	:	:	:	:	:	:	:	:	1	:	:	:	:	:	:
" Moveable Kidney	:	1	:	1	:	:	:	:	:	:	:	:	:	:	:	:	1	1	:	:	:	:	:	:
Prepuce—																								
Circumcision ...	10	:	10	:	:	:	1	:	2	:	1	:	5	:	:	:	:	:	:	:	1	:	:	:

* In one of these cases the operation was performed in a Gynæcological Ward.

TABLE II. (*continued*).

OPERATIONS.	TOTAL.		Discharged.		Died.		Under 5 Years.		—10.		—20.		—30.		—40.		—50.		—60.		—70.		Over 70.	
	M.	F.	M.	F.	M.	F.	M.	F.	M.	F.	M.	F.	M.	F.	M.	F.	M.	F.	M.	F.	M.	F.	M.	F.
OPERATIONS ON GENITO-URINARY ORGANS (*continued*).																								
Penis—																								
Amputation (Complete)— *For Carcinoma of Urethra*	1				1														1					
Amputation (Partial)— *For Carcinoma*	6		6												1		1		3		1			
„ *Wound*	1		1																		1			
Local Removal of Papilloma	1		1												1									
Prostate—																								
Prostatectomy— (Supra-pubic)	5		4		1														2		3			
Scrotum— *For Carcinoma*	3		3								3													
Spermatic Cord— Removal of Encysted Hydrocele	7		7						4		3													
Excision of Varicocele	69		69								34		30											
Testis—																								
Excision— *For Inflammation*	1		1						1															
„ *Partially Descended Testis*	3		3								2				1									
„ *Syphilis*	1		1												1									
„ *Teratoma*	1		1				1																	
„ *Tubercle*	8		8				1				1		3		2						1			
Transplantation of Partially Descended Testis	3		3								2		1											

TABLE II. (continued).

OPERATIONS.	TOTAL M	TOTAL F	Discharged M	Discharged F	Died M	Died F	Under 5 Years M	Under 5 Years F	-10 M	-10 F	-20 M	-20 F	-30 M	-30 F	-40 M	-40 F	-50 M	-50 F	-60 M	-60 F	-70 M	-70 F	Over 70 M	Over 70 F
OPERATIONS ON GENITO-URINARY ORGANS (continued).																								
Testis (continued)—																								
Hydrocele of Testis ...	4		4												1		1		1				1	
Erasion of Testis—																								
For Syphilis ...	1		1										1											
,, *Tubercle* ...	2		2				1				1													
Exploratory Laparotomy—																								
For Carcinoma ...	1				1								1											
,, *Retained Testis*	1		1										1											
Tunica Vaginalis—																								
Excision of Haematocele ...	1		1												1									
Excision of Sac of Hydrocele	40		40						3		9		18		6		4							
Urethra—																								
Urethrotomy—																								
External ...	21		20		1						1		3		3		7		3		3		1	
Internal* ...	27	1	26	1	1								1		5	1	9		6		6			
Incision for Extravasation of Urine ...	9		7		2										1		6		2					
Removal of Caruncle ...		1		1														1						
Ovary—																								
Ovariotomy—																								
For Cystoma ...		17		13		4								7		7		2		1				1
Oöphorectomy—																								
For Dysmenorrhœa ...		1		1								1												
,, *Hernia* ...		1		1												1								
,, *Carcinoma* ...		2		2												2								

* In one of these cases the operation was performed in a Medical Ward.

TABLE II. (continued).

OPERATIONS	TOTAL		Discharged		Died		Under 5 Years		—10.		—20.		—30.		—40.		—50.		—60.		—70.		Over 70.	
	M.	F.	M.	F.	M.	F.	M.	F.	M.	F.	M.	F.	M.	F.	M.	F.	M.	F.	M.	F.	M.	F.	M.	F.
OPERATIONS ON GENITO-URINARY ORGANS (*continued*).																								
Vulva and Vagina—																								
Removal of Carcinoma of Vulva	…	4	…	4	…	…	…	…	…	…	…	…	…	…	…	…	…	1	…	1	…	2	…	…
Removal of Lipoma of Vulva	…	1	…	1	…	…	…	…	…	…	…	…	…	…	…	1	…	…	…	…	…	…	…	…
Removal of Papilloma of Labium	…	1	…	1	…	…	…	…	…	…	…	…	…	…	…	1	…	…	…	…	…	…	…	…
Colpotomy	…	1	…	1	…	…	…	…	…	…	…	…	…	1	…	…	…	…	…	…	…	…	…	…
Uterus and Appendages—																								
Hysterectomy—(Abdominal)—																								
For Carcinoma	…	1	…	1	…	…	…	…	…	…	…	…	…	…	…	1	…	…	…	…	…	…	…	…
,, *Fibroid*	…	7	…	6	…	1	…	…	…	…	…	…	…	…	…	5	…	…	…	1	…	1	…	…
Hysteropexy	…	1	…	1	…	…	…	…	…	…	…	…	…	…	…	…	…	…	…	1	…	…	…	…
Abdominal Section—																								
For Extra-uterine Gestation	…	3	…	2	…	1	…	…	…	…	…	…	…	2	…	1	…	…	…	…	…	…	…	…
,, *Pyo-salpinx*	…	7	…	2	…	5	…	…	…	…	…	…	…	3	…	1	…	…	…	…	…	…	…	…
Incision for abscess	…	2	…	2	…	…	…	…	…	…	…	…	…	…	…	2	…	…	…	1	…	…	…	…
Breast—																								
Incision of Mammary Abscess	…	21	…	20	…	1	…	…	…	…	…	4	…	9	…	6	…	2	…	…	…	1	…	…
Incision of Suppurating Carcinoma	…	2	…	2	…	…	…	…	…	…	…	…	…	1	…	…	…	…	…	1	…	…	…	…

TABLE II. (continued).

OPERATIONS	TOTAL		Discharged		Died		Under 5 Years		AGE AND SEX −10.		−20.		−30.		−40.		−50.		−60.		−70.		Over 70.	
	M.	F.	M.	F.	M.	F.	M.	F.	M.	F.	M.	F.	M.	F.	M.	F.	M.	F.	M.	F.	M.	F.	M.	F.
OPERATIONS ON GENITO-URINARY ORGANS (continued).																								
Breast (continued)—																								
Amputation of Whole Breast (with Removal of Axillary Glands)—																								
For Carcinoma ...	1	53	1	53												5		23		13		11		1
„ Mastitis ...		3		3												1		1		1				
(Without Removal of Axillary Glands)—																								
For Carcinoma ...		3		2		1														1		2		
„ Fibro-Adenoma		2		2														1		1				
„ Tubercle ...		3		3												2		1						
Partial Amputation—																								
For Chronic Mastitis		7		7								7												
„ Tubercle...		1		1														1						
Local Removal of Tumour—																								
Carcinoma (Recurrent)		15		15												4		6		3		2		
Cyst		2		2														2						
Fibro-Adenoma ...		17		17								8		7		2								
Nipple—																								
Carcinoma, Excision		1		1																1				
Operations performed in the Gynæcological Wards—																								
Ovary and Appendages—																								
Ovariotomy		36		36								8		5		8		8		6		1		
Exploratory Laparotomy—																								
For Malignant Disease		2		1		1												2						
„ Pyo-salpinx ...		1		1																		1		

OPERATIONS ON GENITO-URINARY ORGANS (continued).

Operations performed in the Gynaecological Wards (continued)—

Uterus—		
Hysterectomy (Abdominal) ...	13	13
" (Vaginal) ...	5	5
Local Removal of Carcinoma of Cervix ...	8	8
Hysteropexy ...	1	1
Abdominal Section—		
For Extra-uterine Gestation ...	2	2
Caesarian Section ...	1	
Vulva and Vagina—		
Colporrhaphy ...	8	8
Colpotomy ...	17	17
Removal of Urethral Caruncle ...	13	13
Removal of Imperforate Hymen ...	1	1
Removal of Carcinoma of Vulva ...	2	2
Abdominal Section—		
For Abdominal Tumour ...	1	1

TABLE II. (continued).

OPERATIONS.	TOTAL		Discharged.		Died.		Under 5 Years.		—10.		—20.		—30.		—40.		—50.		—60.		—70.		Over 70.	
	M.	F.	M.	F.	M.	F.	M.	F.	M.	F.	M.	F.	M.	F.	M.	F.	M.	F.	M.	F.	M.	F.	M.	F.
OPERATION ON GENITO-URINARY ORGANS (continued).																								
Operations performed in the Gynaecological Wards (continued)—																								
Abdominal Section (cont.)—																								
For Appendicitis ...	..	1	..	1	..	..	..	..	..	..	..	..	..	..	..	..	..	2	..	..	..	..	..	..
„ *Pelvic Abscess* ...	..	3	..	1	..	2	..	..	..	..	..	..	..	..	..	..	..	..	..	..	..	..	..	..
„ *Tuberculous Perito-nitis* ...	..	1	..	..	..	1	..	..	..	..	..	1	..	..	..	..	..	..	..	..	..	..	..	..
Injection of Paraffin for Prolapse ...	..	1	..	1	..	..	..	..	..	..	..	..	..	..	..	..	..	..	..	..	..	1	..	..
Lithotomy—Vaginal ...	..	1	..	1	..	..	..	..	..	..	..	..	..	..	..	1	..	..	..	..	..	..	..	..
OPERATIONS UPON THE ALIMENTARY CANAL.																								
Mouth, Palate and Fauces—																								
Erasion for Cancrum Oris ...	1	..	..	2	..	..	1	..	1	..	..	..	..	..	..	..	1	..	..	..	..	..	..	..
Removal of Enlarged Uvula	..	1	1	..	..	..	..	..	..	..	..	..	..	..	..	..	..	..	..	..	..	..	..	..
Removal of Tumours— Carcinoma—																								
Fauces ...	2	1	2	..	..	..	..	..	..	..	..	..	..	..	1	1	1	..	..	..	..	..	1	..
Floor ...	3	1	3	1	..	..	..	..	..	..	..	..	..	..	..	1	..	..	2	1	..	..	..	..

OPERATIONS	TOTAL		Discharged		Died		Under 5 Years		—10.		—20.		—30.		—40.		—50.		—60.		—70.		Over 70.	
	M.	F.	M.	F.	M.	F.	M.	F.	M.	F.	M.	F.	M.	F.	M.	F.	M.	F.	M.	F.	M.	F.	M.	F.
OPERATIONS UPON THE ALIMENTARY CANAL (*continued*).																								
Mouth, Palate and Fauces (*continued*)—																								
Salivary Glands—																								
Parotid—																								
Incision of Abscess* ...	1	2	1	2	...	...			...	...	...	...												
Removal of Tumour— *Mixed Tumour* ...	1	3	1	3	...	...			...	...	...	...												
Naso-pharynx—																								
Removal of Adenoids† ...	5	3	5	3	...	...			4	1	...	...												
Removal of Tonsils and Adenoids ...	5	6	5	6	...	...			2	2	1	2												
Enucleation of Tonsils ...	1	1	1	1	...	...			...	...	...	...												
Incision for Abscess ...	1	...	1	...	...	...			...	...	...	...												
Removal of Tumour— *Carcinoma* ...	1	...	1	...	...	...			...	...	...	...												
Tongue—																								
Partial Excision— With Removal of Glands— *For Carcinoma* ...	12	1	12	1	...	...			...	...	...	...												
Partial Excision— Without Removal of Glands *For Carcinoma* ...	11	...	10	...	1	...			...	...	...	...												
Local Excision— *For recurrent Carcinoma*	1	1	1	1	...	...			...	...	...	...												

* In two of these cases the operation was performed in a Medical Ward.

† In one of these cases the operation was performed in a Medical Ward.

TABLE II. (continued).

144

OPERATIONS	TOTAL M	TOTAL F	Discharged M	Discharged F	Died M	Died F	Under 5 Years M	Under 5 Years F	-10 M	-10 F	-20 M	-20 F	-30 M	-30 F	-40 M	-40 F	-50 M	-50 F	-60 M	-60 F	-70 M	-70 F	Over 70 M	Over 70 F
OPERATIONS UPON THE ALIMENTARY CANAL (continued).																								
Stomach—																								
Gastrostomy—																								
For Carcinoma of Œsophagus ...	10	1	2	..	8	1	..	..	..	..	..	..	..	..	2	..	..	..	3	..	5	1	..	..
Gastrotomy—																								
For Gastric Ulcer ...	..	1	..	..	..	1	..	..	..	..	..	..	..	..	..	..	..	1	..	..	..	..	..	..
" Hæmatemesis	..	1	..	..	..	1	..	..	..	..	..	..	..	..	..	..	..	1	..	..	..	..	..	..
Gastro-Enterostomy—																								
For Dilatation ...	2	..	2	..	..	..	..	..	..	..	..	..	..	..	1	1	1	..	..	..	..	..	..	..
" Gastric Ulcer ...	1	3	1	3	..	..	..	..	..	..	..	1	..	1	1	1	..	..	..	..	..	..	..	..
" Pyloric Stenosis (non-malignant)	2	..	1	..	1	..	..	..	..	..	1	..	1	..	..	..	..	..	2	1	1	1	..	..
" Duodenal Ulcer	1	..	1	..	..	..	..	..	..	..	1	..	..	..	1	..	..	..	..	..	..	..	..	..
" Stricture ...	1	..	1	..	..	..	..	..	..	..	..	..	..	..	1	1	..	..	..	..	..	..	..	..
" Carcinoma of Stomach	1	1	2	..	2	1	..	..	..	..	..	1	..	..	1	2	1	..	2	..	1	1	..	..
" " Pylorus	4	4	2	2	..	2	..	..	..	..	..	..	..	..	..	1	..	..	1	..	..	..	..	..
Pylorectomy	1	1	1	..	..	1	..	..	..	..	..	..	..	..	..	..	..	..	1	1	..	..	..	..
Abdominal Section—																								
For Perforated Gastric Ulcer ...	12	8	8	4	4	4	..	..	..	..	6	1	6	1	4	1	..	5	..	..	..	..	..	..
" Perigastric Adhesions	1	3	..	2	1	1	..	..	..	..	..	..	..	..	..	1	..	..	..	..	..	..	..	..
(Exploratory)—																								
For Carcinoma of Stomach	6	1	4	1	2	..	..	..	..	..	..	..	..	..	2	..	2	..	1	1	..	..	..	..
" " Œsophagus	1	..	..	..	1	1	..	..	..	..	..	..	..	..	..	..	..	..	1	..	8	1	..	..
" Gastric Ulcer ...	..	1	1	..	..	..	..	..	..	..	..	..	..	..	..	..	..	1	..	1	..	..	..	..
" Gastritis ...	1	..	1	..	..	..	..	..	..	..	..	..	..	..	1	..	..	..	..	..	..	..	..	..

TABLE II. (continued).

OPERATIONS.	TOTAL		Discharged.		Died.		Under 5 Years.		—10.		—20.		—30.		—40.		—50.		—60.		—70.		Over 70.	
	M.	F.	M.	F.	M.	F.	M.	F.	M.	F.	M.	F.	M.	F.	M.	F.	M.	F.	M.	F.	M.	F.	M.	F.
OPERATIONS UPON THE ALIMENTARY CANAL (*continued*).																								
Liver—																								
Abdominal Section—																								
With Removal of Accessory Lobe		1		1														1						
For Abscess	2		1		1						1		1											
" Hydatid Cyst	2		1		1						1		1											
" Rupture	2				2						2													
Gall Bladder and Ducts—																								
Cholecystotomy		12		10		2								3	4				3		1			
Cholecystectomy—																								
For Carcinoma	2	1	1		1								1		1	1	1							
" Gall Stones	1	2		2							1		1			1		1						
Choledochotomy	1	1		1	1								1											
Cholecyst-enterostomy	1					1		1					1											
Exploratory Laparotomy—																								
For Carcinoma	2		1	1	1	1									1		1	1						
" Gallstones	1		1		1												1		1	1	1	1		
" Sarcoma	1																							
Pancreas—																								
Abdominal Section—																								
For Cyst (Exploratory)—	1		1												1									
For Carcinoma		1		1																		1		

L

TABLE II. *(continued).*

OPERATIONS.	TOTAL.		Discharged.		Died.		AGE AND SEX.																	
							Under 5 Years.		—10.		—20.		—30.		—40.		—50.		—60.		—70.		Over 70.	
	M.	F.	M.	F.	M.	F.	M.	F.	M.	F.	M.	F.	M.	F.	M.	F.	M.	F.	M.	F.	M.	F.	M.	F.
OPERATIONS UPON THE ALIMENTARY CANAL *(continued)*.																								
Intestines—																								
Operations for Hernia—																								
Radical Cure—																								
(Reducible)—																								
Femoral ...	...	7	...	7	...	...	...	...	...	...	1	1	...	1	1	1	...	1	...	...	...	...	...	...
Inguinal ...	152	20	152	20	...	...	8	...	11	1	38	8	59	7	26	4	5	...	5	...	...	...	...	...
" with Excision of partially descended Testis ...	7	...	7	...	...	...	...	...	...	...	5	...	2	...	...	...	...	...	...	...	...	...	...	...
" Fixation of partially descended Testis ...	3	...	8	...	...	...	...	...	1	...	1	...	1	...	...	...	...	...	...	...	...	...	...	...
Interstitial ...	2	3	2	3	...	...	1	...	...	...	2	...	1	...	...	1	...	2	...	...	...	...	...	...
Umbilical ...	2	2	2	...	...	...	...	...	2	1	1	1	1	...	...	2	...	1	...	1	...	...	...	...
(Traumatic)—																								
Ventral ...	4	6	4	6	...	...	...	...	...	...	...	...	...	...	...	...	...	...	...	...	...	...	...	...
(Irreducible)—																								
Femoral ...	3	21	3	21	...	...	...	...	...	...	1	2	...	6	...	7	3	1	8	4	...	1	...	...
Inguinal ...	11	4	11	4	...	...	...	...	...	...	...	...	5	...	1	...	...	...	...	...	1	...	1	...
" with Excision of partially descended Testis ...	1	...	1	...	...	...	...	...	...	...	...	...	1	...	...	1	...	...	...	...	...	...	...	...
Umbilical...	...	8	...	8	...	...	...	...	...	1	...	...	...	...	...	8	...	...	...	1	...	2	...	...

TABLE II. (*continued*).

OPERATIONS.	TOTAL M	TOTAL F	Discharged M	Discharged F	Died M	Died F	Under 5 Years M	Under 5 Years F	-10 M	-10 F	-20 M	-20 F	-30 M	-30 F	-40 M	-40 F	-50 M	-50 F	-60 M	-60 F	-70 M	-70 F	Over 70 M	Over 70 F
OPERATIONS UPON THE ALIMENTARY CANAL (*continued*).																								
Intestines (*continued*)—																								
Herniotomy, or Radical cure for Strangulated Hernia—																								
Femoral ...	2	11	2	11										2		1	1	1		2		1	1	4
Inguinal ...	13	1	12	1	1		1				2		1		1		5	1	2				1	
Umbilical ...		4		4												1		1		1		1		
Ventral ...		2		1		1								1				1						
Herniotomy for Incarcerated Hernia ...	1				1																1			
Hydrocele of Femoral Sac Removed ...		1		1										1										
Duodenum—																								
Abdominal Section—																								
With Suture of Perforated Ulcer ...	4				4								1		2				1					
Caecum—																								
Caecotomy—																								
For Carcinoma ...		1				1														1				
Excision of Caecum—																								
For Tubercle ...	1				1								1											
Exploratory Laparotomy—																								
For Carcinoma ...	1																				1			
Intestinal Anastomosis—																								
For Carcinoma ...	1		1														1							

TABLE II. (*continued*).

OPERATIONS	TOTAL		Discharged		Died		Under 5 Years		−10		−20		−30		−40		−50		−60		−70		Over 70	
	M	F	M	F	M	F	M	F	M	F	M	F	M	F	M	F	M	F	M	F	M	F	M	F
OPERATIONS UPON THE ALIMENTARY CANAL (*continued*).																								
Intestines (*continued*)— Vermiform Appendix— For Appendicitis— I. (Acute cases, without external suppuration)— *Free Incision, with removal of Appendix**	27	17	27	17	…	…		…	4	2	6	3	12	8	5	3	…	1					…	…
II. (Chronic, relapsing cases without external suppuration)— *Free Incision, removal of Appendix*	38	38	34	38	1	…	…	…	1	1	8	9	18	15	8	10	…	3					…	…
III. (Acute, gangrenous)— *Free Incision and drainage. No search for Appendix*	…	1	…	…	…	1	…	…	…	…	…	1	…	1	…	…	…	…					…	…
Free Incision, removal of Appendix and drainage	4	5	2	4	2	1	…	…	…	…	1	2	2	1	1	…	…	1					…	1
IV. (Acute c̄ Suppuration)— *Free incision into general Peritoneal cavity, removal of Appendix and drainage*	9	12	7	7	2	5	…	1	3	…	1	1	3	8	1	3	1	…					…	…
Free Incision and drainage, Appendix not removed	20	14	16	11	4	3	1	…	3	4	7	4	4	1	3	2	2	1			…	1	…	…

AGE AND SEX.

* In one of these cases the operation was performed in a Medical Ward.

TABLE II. (*continued*).

OPERATIONS.	TOTAL		Discharged		Died		AGE AND SEX																
							Under 5 Years.		—10.		—20.		—30.		—40.		—50.		—60.		—70.		Over 70.	
	M.	F.	M.	F.	M.	F.	M.	F.	M.	F.	M.	F.	M.	F.	M.	F.	M.	F.	M.	F.	M.	F.	M.	F.
OPERATIONS UPON THE ALIMENTARY CANAL (*continued*).																								
Intestines (*continued*)—																								
Vermiform Appendix (*continued*)—																								
For Appendicitis (*contd.*)—																								
V. (Chronic with Abscess)—																								
Free Incision, removal of Appendix	2	...	2	...	...	...	...	...	1	...	1	...	...	...	...	...	...	...	...	...	...	...	...	...
Free Incision and Drainage, Appendix not removed	6	2	5	2	1	...	...	...	1	...	1	...	1	...	2	...	1	1	...	1	...	...	...	...
Appendicectomy—																								
With Intestinal Ulceration	1	...	...	...	1	...	...	...	...	...	...	...	1	...	...	...	1	...	...	...	...	...	...	...
Colon and Sigmoid Flexure—																								
Abdominal Section—																								
(Exploratory)—																								
For Carcinoma	...	1	...	...	...	1	...	...	...	...	...	...	1	...	...	1	...	...	...	...	...	...	...	...
Laparotomy and formation of Fecal Fistula—																								
For Carcinoma	1	...	1	...	...	...	...	...	...	...	...	...	...	...	...	...	...	...	1	...	...	...	...	...
Excision of Colon—																								
For Carcinoma	3	...	...	...	3	...	...	...	...	...	1	...	...	...	...	...	...	...	1	...	...	...	...	...
Excision of Sigmoid Flexure—																								
For Carcinoma	...	2	...	...	...	2	...	...	...	...	...	...	...	...	...	...	...	1	1	...	1	1	...	...

TABLE II. (continued).

OPERATIONS.	TOTAL		Discharged		Died.		Under 5 Years.		—10.		—20.		—30.		—40.		—50.		—60.		—70.		Over 70.	
	M.	F.	M.	F.	M.	F.	M.	F.	M.	F.	M.	F.	M.	F.	M.	F.	M.	F.	M.	F.	M.	F.	M.	F.
OPERATIONS UPON THE ALIMENTARY CANAL (continued).																								
Intestines (continued)—																								
Colon and Sigmoid Flexure (continued)—																								
Colotomy—																								
(Inguinal)—																								
For Carcinoma of Peritoneum ...	1	…	…	…	1	…	…	…	…	…	…	…	…	…	1	…	…	…	…	…	…	…	…	…
" Carcinoma of Sigmoid Flexure ...	1	1	1	1	…	…	…	…	…	…	…	…	…	…	…	…	…	…	…	…	1	1	…	…
" Colitis (Ulcerative)...	2	1	…	1	2	…	…	…	…	…	…	…	2	…	…	…	…	1	…	…	…	…	…	…
" Intestinal Obstruction...	2	…	2	…	…	…	…	…	…	…	…	…	…	…	…	…	…	…	…	…	2	…	…	…
(Transverse)—																								
For Carcinoma ...	1	2	…	…	1	2	…	…	…	…	…	…	…	1	…	…	…	…	1	…	…	1	…	…
" Intestinal Obstruction	…	2	…	…	…	2	…	…	…	…	…	…	…	…	…	1	…	1	…	…	…	…	…	…
Colotomy—																								
For Carcinoma of Rectum	14	6	13	6	1	…	…	…	…	…	…	…	…	…	1	…	3	1	4	3	6	2	…	…
" Stricture of Rectum	1	1	1	1	…	…	…	…	…	…	…	…	…	…	1	…	…	1	…	…	…	…	…	…
Excision of Prolapse from Old Colotomy Wound ...	…	2	…	2	…	…	…	…	…	…	…	…	…	…	…	1	…	1	…	…	…	…	…	…
Peritoneum—																								
Abdominal Section—																								
For Acute Suppurative Peritonitis ...	…	4	…	1	…	3	…	1	…	…	…	…	…	2	…	…	…	1	…	…	…	…	…	…
" Hydatid Cyst ...	1	1	1	1	…	…	…	…	…	…	1	…	…	…	…	1	…	…	…	…	…	…	…	…
" Tuberculous Peritonitis*	8	2	2	2	1	…	1	1	…	…	1	1	1	…	1	…	1	…	…	1	…	…	…	…

* In one of these cases the operation was performed in a Medical Ward.

TABLE II. (*continued*).

OPERATIONS	TOTAL		Discharged		Died		Under 5 Years		—10		—20		—30		—40		—50		—60		—70		Over 70	
	M.	F.	M.	F.	M.	F.	M.	F.	M.	F.	M.	F.	M.	F.	M.	F.	M.	F.	M.	F.	M.	F.	M.	F.
OPERATIONS UPON THE ALIMENTARY CANAL (*continued*)—																								
Intestines (continued)—																								
Peritoneum (*continued*) —																								
(Exploratory)—																								
For Adhesions ...	1	..	1	..	..	..	..	..	..	..	..	..	..	..	..	..	1	..	..	..	..	..	..	..
„ *Ascites* ...	..	1	..	..	..	1	..	1	..	..	..	..	..	..	..	..	..	..	..	..	..	..	..	..
„ *Carcinoma* ...	..	2	..	1	..	1	..	..	..	..	..	..	..	..	..	..	..	..	..	..	..	1	..	1
Subphrenic Abscess—																								
Drainage of ...	2	1	2	1	..	..	..	..	1	..	..	..	..	..	..	..	1	..	..	..	..	1	..	..
Rectum—																								
Hæmorrhoids—																								
Ligature or Excision	35	31	35	31	..	..	..	..	..	..	..	..	8	9	7	11	14	7	6	3	..	1	..	..
Excision of Rectum	4	2	3	2	1	..	..	..	..	..	..	..	..	..	..	..	..	1	4	..	..	1	..	..
Enteropexy—																								
For Prolapse ...	1	..	1	..	..	..	..	..	..	..	..	..	..	..	1	..	..	..	..	..	..	..	..	..
Proctotomy—																								
(Linear)—																								
For Stricture ...	..	1	..	1	..	..	..	..	..	..	..	..	..	..	..	..	..	1	..	..	..	..	..	..
Removal of Polypi ...	..	2	..	2	..	..	..	..	..	..	..	..	..	1	..	1	..	..	..	..	..	..	..	..
Anus—																								
Anal Fissure Incised	2	1	2	1	..	..	..	..	..	..	..	..	..	..	..	1	1	..	1	..	..	..	..	..
Anal Fistula Incised	19	5	19	5	..	..	..	..	..	..	..	..	5	2	4	1	5	1	5	..	..	1	..	..
Imperforate—																								
Anus Incised ...	1	..	1	..	..	..	1	..	..	..	..	..	..	..	..	..	..	..	..	..	..	..	..	..

TABLE II. (continued).

OPERATIONS	TOTAL M	TOTAL F	Discharged M	Discharged F	Died M	Died F	Under 5 Years M	Under 5 Years F	—10 M	—10 F	—20 M	—20 F	—30 M	—30 F	—40 M	—40 F	—50 M	—50 F	—60 M	—60 F	—70 M	—70 F	Over 70 M	Over 70 F
OPERATIONS UPON THE ALIMENTARY CANAL (*continued*).																								
Intestines (continued)—																								
Abdominal Section—																								
With Reduction of Intussusception	2	2	1	1	...	**1**	2	2	...	...	...	...	...	...	...	...	...	...	...	...	...	...	...	...
With Excision of Intussusception	3	...	...	...	**3**	...	2	...	...	...	1	...	...	1	...	...	...	...	...	...	...	...	...	...
For Faecal Fistula	...	1	...	...	...	**1**	...	...	...	...	...	...	...	...	...	...	...	...	...	...	...	...	...	...
" Intestinal Obstruction (*Strangulation by band*)	3	...	...	...	**3**	...	2	...	...	...	1	...	1	...	...	...	...	...	...	...	...	...	...	...
With Suture of Perforating Typhoid Ulcer	3	2	1	1	**3**	**1**	...	...	1	1	1	...	1	...	1	...	...	...	...	...	...	...	...	...
For Laceration of Intestine	3	...	...	...	**3**	...	1	...	1	...	...	...	1	...	...	...	...	...	...	...	...	...	...	...
" Perforating Ulcer	2	1	...	...	**2**	**1**	...	...	...	...	...	...	...	...	...	...	1	...	...	...	...	...	...	...
(*Exploratory*)—																								
For Abdominal Pain	4	...	4	...	...	...	...	...	...	...	...	...	...	...	...	...	...	...	...	3	...	...	...	...
" Intestinal Obstruction	1	...	...	1	...	**1**	...	...	...	...	1	...	1	...	1	...	...	...	...	...	...	...	...	...
" Sarcoma of Intestine	1	...	1	...	...	...	...	...	...	...	...	...	...	...	...	...	...	...	...	...	...	...	...	...
Complicated by Diseases of Chest	3	1	...	...	**3**	**1**	1	...	...	...	2	...	...	...	...	...	...	...	...	1	...	...	...	...
For Fractured Pelvis	1	...	...	...	**1**	...	...	...	...	...	...	...	...	...	1	...	...	...	...	...	...	...	...	...
MISCELLANEOUS OPERATIONS.																								
Erasion of Actinomycosis	2	...	1	...	**1**	...	...	...	...	...	...	...	...	...	1	...	...	...	...	...	...	...	...	...

TABLE II. (continued).

OPERATIONS	TOTAL		Discharged		Died		Under 5 Years		—10		—20		—30		—40		—50		—60		—70		Over 70	
	M.	F.	M.	F.	M.	F.	M.	F.	M.	F.	M.	F.	M.	F.	M.	F.	M.	F.	M.	F.	M.	F.	M.	F.
MISCELLANEOUS OPERATIONS (*continued*)—																								
Excision of Anthrax ...	2	...	1	...	1	...	...	...	...	...	...	...	1	...	...	...	1	...	...	...	...	...	...	...
Excision of Branchial Cyst ...	1	1	1	1	...	...	...	...	...	...	...	1	1	...	...	...	...	...	...	...	...	...	...	...
For Macroglossia ...	...	1	...	1	...	...	...	1	...	...	...	...	...	...	...	...	...	...	...	...	...	...	...	...
Insertion of Gold Shield under Scalp ...	1	...	1	...	...	...	...	...	...	...	1	...	...	...	...	...	...	...	...	...	...	...	...	...
Removal of Foreign Bodies ...	3	10	3	10	...	...	...	...	...	...	2	1	...	5	1	2	...	2	...	...	...	...	...	...

Number of Surgical Operations performed upon In-Patients during the Year.

Males	...	...	...	...	...	...	...	1,628
Females	...	...	...	...	...	...	...	1,272
								2,900

STATISTICS OF ANÆSTHETICS.

During 1904, Anæsthetics were administered on 7,966 occasions, as follows :—

Chloroform	...	...	...	...	...	...	2,694	times.
Gas and Ether	...	...	...	...	...	...	1,806	„
Gas	...	...	...	...	...	...	1,688	„
Gas, Ether and Chloroform	...	...	...	...	731	„
Somnoform	...	...	...	...	...	...	287	„
Chloroform and Ether ...	...	...	...	...	217	„
Ethyl Chloride, Ether and Chloroform	...	...	175	„
Ethyl Chloride and Ether	...	...	...	...	138	„
Ethyl Chloride ...	...	...	...	...	...	68	„
Gas and Oxygen	...	...	...	...	...	59	„
A. C. E. Mixture	...	...	...	...	...	37	„
Somnoform and Ether ...	...	...	...	...	34	„
Somnoform, Ether and Chloroform	...	...	...	18	„
Ether	...	...	...	...	...	...	...	14	„
			Total	...	...	7,966	times.

There was one casualty :—

A female, aged 23, suffering from exophthalmic goitre, was anæsthetised by gas and ether, preparatory to operation on naso-pharynx (tonsils and adenoids). The tonsils were removed and considerable bleeding followed. During this period, a small amount of chloroform was administered by means of Junker's apparatus. In the course of the removal of the adenoids the complexion became white, and the pulse was found to have disappeared. Death was due to cardiac syncope.

APPENDIX.

GENERAL DISEASES.

Actinomycosis.

Three patients suffering from this disease came under observation during the course of the year. In two of these cases the disease appeared to have originated in the abdominal wall, and in the third case in the jaw. Two of these cases recovered.

The patient who died was a farm labourer, aged 38, who five weeks before admission had noticed a small lump in the right side of the abdomen, close to the umbilicus. This swelling quickly increased, and appeared to change its place, travelling lower down towards the pubes. On admission the general condition of the patient appeared good, except for slight jaundice. In the right side of the abdomen was a large fluctuating swelling, the skin over which was red and œdematous. This swelling was incised and a large quantity of pus evacuated, and in the pus were granules visible to the naked eye, which, on microscopical examination, proved to be nodules of mycelium. No communication was found between the abscess cavity and the interior of the abdomen. Large and increasing doses of potassium iodide were administered, and for a time the patient appeared to be considerably relieved. Later, signs of deep-seated suppuration supervened, accompanied by rise of temperature and rigors, and the patient finally died seven weeks after admission. During this time the jaundice had become considerably deeper. Post-mortem : The wound in the abdominal wall did not communicate with the peritoneal cavity, but at this situation were many adhesions and a few beads of pus. In the liver were two large abscesses containing granules of mycelium. One of these abscesses had burst, and was tracking towards the spleen. (Male, iv. 1256.)

The other cases were : Male, i. 16, iv. 794.

Anthrax.

Three patients, all males, were admitted on account of malignant pustule about the face or neck. Of these three patients, two recovered and one died.

The fatal case occurred in a horse-hair dresser. Seven days previous to admission he had had a small pimple behind the ear ; only eighteen hours before admission had he complained of feeling ill and of his neck swelling. On examination he appeared very ill, with a temperature of 103°, the right side of the neck was very much swollen, and there was a small abrasion of the right pinna, but there was no sign of the usual malignant pustule. Incisions were made into the cellular tissues, and cultures revealed the presence of anthrax bacilli. The patient became rapidly worse, and died within two days with symptoms of asphyxia. Post-mortem : The signs of a general septicæmia were present, and also œdema of the glottis. The heart's blood and also the pleural fluid contained both anthrax bacilli and streptococci, the latter in superior numbers. (Male, i. 2044.)

Of the two cases that recovered, one was in a general labourer, who had a malignant pustule on the face. The pustule was excised in the usual way, and the patient made a rapid and uneventful recovery. (Male, iv. 2459.)

The third case occurred in a horse-hair sorter, aged 31, and is of extreme interest, because it was the first case at this hospital treated by means of Sclavo's anti-anthrax serum. The pustule, which was on the face, was of three days' standing. Anthrax bacilli were abundant in the vesicular fluid. 40 c.c. of the serum were injected subcutaneously, and a dry dressing of antiseptic gauze applied to the pustule ; no other treatment being given. After two days the vesicles had disappeared, and the pustule was not increasing and the surrounding œdema was diminishing. After three days no anthrax bacilli were demonstrable in the fluid. The temperature rapidly fell and the general condition improved. On the eighteenth day after the injection a small slough separated, and on the twenty-first day after admission the patient was discharged with only a small scar remaining. (Male, v. 3155.)

Enteric Fever.

Five patients suffering from enteric fever with perforation were submitted to operation, the abdomen being opened and the perforation sutured in each case. One of these cases recovered and the other four died.

These four cases all developed signs of general peritonitis, and in one of them a second perforation was found. (Male, ii. 1253, 3421, iv. 3458 ; Female, iv. 2660.)

A woman, aged 38, was admitted on December 2nd in the fourteenth day of the disease suffering from enteric fever. The disease ran the usual course till December 24th, when signs of perforation appeared. On the same day the abdomen was opened and an ulcer in the ileum found and sutured. The general condition rapidly improved, though the wound suppurated. Four weeks later the patient had a relapse and was transferred to a Medical Ward, where she eventually recovered. (Female, iv. 2791.)

Snake Bite.

On August 24th, while in the Isle of Wight, a man of 35 was bitten in the thumb by a large adder. The finger smarted and began to swell immediately. On August 27th he was admitted in a very collapsed condition ; the whole of the arm and the left side of the chest were enormously swollen, so much so that the skin looked as if ready to burst. A large number of free incisions were made into the arm and strychnine and brandy were freely administered. The patient rapidly recovered from his collapse, and thenceforward made an uneventful recovery. (Male, iv. 2445.)

Malta Fever.

In December, 1903, a girl, aged 6, was admitted, suffering from supposed Malta fever. In March, 1904, the hip joint was opened and four ounces of straw-coloured fluid drawn off. A skiagram showed that the head of the femur was dislocated on to the dorsum ilii. Under an extension the dislocation was permanently reduced, and in June, 1904, the patient was discharged wearing a Thomas' hip splint. (Female, ii. 2855*.)

Hæmophilia.

Three males were admitted with this condition, all of whom had a family history of " bleeding " on the maternal side.

Two of these cases came to the hospital on account of continued bleeding from a small cut on the lip. In both instances the bleeding was after a time arrested and the patients discharged cured. (Male, ii. 2107, iii. 2321.)

The third case occurred in a boy, aged 4 months, who came to the hospital on account of phimosis. Circumcision was performed in the Surgery. There was considerable oozing after the operation, so the wound was again dressed and all bleeding points carefully tied and the skin surfaces sutured ; adrenalin was also applied. In spite of these measures the bleeding still continued, so the boy was admitted to the hospital. Slow bleeding continued for three days, and on the fourth day he died. It was found afterwards that the maternal uncle nearly died from hæmorrhage after extraction of a tooth. Post-mortem : Nothing abnormal was found, but cultures from the heart's blood showed the presence of streptococci. (Male, iii. 3564.)

Gangrene.

Nine patients suffering from gangrene were admitted.

Four were cases of diabetic gangrene. In two cases only the toes were affected, and these both recovered without operation (Female, i. 508, v. 1128). One with gangrene of the foot recovered after amputation through the leg (Female, i. 336). One suffering from gangrene of both feet died two days after admission, without any operation being performed. This case was complicated with advanced arterio-sclerosis (Female, v. 1730).

MALFORMATIONS AND DEFORMITIES.

Branchial Cyst.

One case showing this deformity was noticed during the year.

This was in a man, aged 34, who fifteen years previously had noticed a small swelling in the left side of the neck. This had steadily increased, so that on admission the swelling was about five inches in diameter, and occupied both the anterior triangles of the neck. The skin over the swelling was reddened, but it was not tender. A long incision was made over the swelling, and the sterno-mastoid muscle cut through and a large cyst containing thick yellow material dissected out. The patient made an uneventful recovery. (Male, v. 165.)

Accessory Cervical Ribs.

A female, aged 20, gave a history of having had for the last four months pain and tingling sensations in the right arm and hand ; the hand also at times became very cold and the fingers blue. On examination a hard, bony swelling was found in the left side of the neck, above the clavicle ; this, it was stated, had been present from birth. A skiagram revealed the presence of a cervical rib on both sides of the neck, the one on the right side being the larger. The right arm and hand appeared normal, except for the fact that the radial pulse was very small.

A two-inch incision was made along the anterior border of the trapezius muscle above the clavicle, and the brachial plexus exposed ; the nerve cords were found spread out over the accessory rib ; these were pulled aside and the rib sawn through at its base. The wound healed by first intention, and the patient was discharged relieved of most of her discomfort, though she still complained of an aching sensation in the arm on much exertion. (Female, v. 924.)

Congenital Dislocation of the Hip.

Four of these cases are of interest, for the reason that they were treated by means of Lorenz's bloodless operation. In none was the treatment highly satisfactory, and in three the operation was a failure.

One female, aged 8, had a double dislocation. On October 28th, 1903, the operation was performed and the legs put up in plaster with the thighs widely abducted, flexed and externally rotated. In April, 1904, the plaster was removed, and the thighs gradually came down from their position of abduction. On her discharge in July she could walk a few steps with assistance, though her thighs were still somewhat abducted. (Female, iv. 2315*.)

Another female, aged 11, had a congenital dislocation on the right side only. An attempt was made to forcibly abduct the thigh in the usual manner, but failed owing to the strength of the abductor longus tendon; this, therefore, was divided subcutaneously, and the leg put up in plaster in a position of extreme abduction and external rotation. An unsatisfactory result was obtained, because it was found impossible to fix the head of the femur in the too shallow acetabulum for any length of time. (Female, ii. 1037.)

Another female, aged 5, with a double dislocation of the hips, was treated in a similar manner and was finally discharged with the legs in plaster. A skiagram showed that even after prolonged treatment the heads of the femora were lying on the dorsum ilii, though at the time of operation they were felt to enter the acetabulum. (Female, i. 1536 and 2182.)

The other case was Male, v. 1686*.

Spina Bifida.

Five infants were admitted suffering from spina bifida in the lumbo-sacral region. Four out of the five died, all with suppurative meningitis.

A male infant, 7 days old, had a fluctuating translucent swelling, about the size of a tangerine orange, in the upper sacral region, connected to the trunk by a fine pedicle. Beyond a condition of double calcaneus talipes, the baby appeared healthy and well-nourished. The sac became less tense and the skin over it firmer, so four weeks after admission it was removed. The sac was lined by epithelium, but no communication was found between it and the sub-dural space. The child made a good recovery. (Male, i. 204.)

Congenital Absence of the Femur.

This was a case of a boy, aged 4, who appeared in all other respects to be perfectly normal. The right leg was normal and very well developed; the left leg was very much shorter, and by means of a skiagram it could be seen that the femur was represented only by a small knob of bone; the fibula of the same side was absent. The boy could get about well and even run, carrying the normal limb with the knee flexed to a right angle. The treatment adopted was to put a high patten on to the deformed limb, so that the patient could walk making use of his full height. (Male, iv. 1663.)

Macrostoma with Accessory Auricles.

One case of a boy, aged 10 months, presented some points of considerable rarity. The mouth was very large, and extended a quarter of an inch further to the right than the left. There was also a small pedunculated body on the right cheek, one inch from the angle of the mouth, and two other similar bodies near the tragus of the right ear, and a fourth on the right concha close to the external auditory meatus. These bodies were supposed to be accessory auricles. A plastic operation was performed on the mouth to reduce it to proper dimensions, and the accessory auricles were cut away. (Male, i. 887.)

DISEASES OF THE NERVOUS SYSTEM.

Epilepsy.

A man, aged 47, was found unconscious in the street. It was stated that he had had a fall on the head three years previously, and that since that time been subject to fits of an epileptiform nature. After admission the patient had a number of rapidly recurring fits, which commenced with conjugate deviation of the head and eyes to the right, immediately followed by twitching of the left side of the face, then of the left arm and leg, and then of the whole body. During the fits patient was unconscious. As the fits were increasing in frequency and severity, the skull was trephined over the left occipital region. The brain was found to be œdematous, but nothing more. Shortly after operation the fits recurred almost without interval, and six hours after the patient died comatose. Post-mortem : No sign of fracture of the skull was visible. At the anterior end of the right frontal lobe and in the lower part of the right occipital lobe were small collections of fluid between the pia mater and brain ; the fluid was possibly old blood. (Male, i. 388.)

Jacksonian Epilepsy.

Two patients suffering from epileptiform fits were subjected to operation.

A man, aged 22, was shot in the head during the Boer war. After waiting a period of five months, some operation, he knows not what, was performed on him. After the operation he was able to resume his duties with the regiment. He looked on admission ill and starved ; his gait was unsteady and his general mental capacity appeared below average. His hearing has been impaired since the operation. In the occipital region of the skull was a circular hole, the size of a two-shilling piece, through which the brain could be felt to pulsate. The patient complained of dull, aching pain over the whole of the head. The optic discs were normal, and the special senses of taste, touch, and smell were unimpaired. While in the Ward patient had two fits, accompanied with rigidity of the muscles, twitching, and loss of consciousness. The patient avers that the fits begin with tingling in the right arm, which spread to the rest of the body and are followed by complete unconsciousness. In such fits he has fallen down and received such injuries as a broken nose and scalp wounds. The hole in the skull was exposed and a small arachnoid cyst removed and the gap covered in by means of a gold plate, which was slipped in under the scalp. The patient remained in the hospital for three weeks after the operation, and no more fits occurred. He returned, however, some months later in no way improved, and having had a second operation in some other hospital, in which the gold plate had been removed. (Male, ii. 3251*.)

Cerebellar Cyst.

A boy, aged 5, with the following history, was admitted to a Medical Ward.

In September, 1903, he was found to stagger in walking, and occasionally to fall, always falling towards the left side. In October, 1903, his arms were sensibly weak, and he was unable to sit up in bed owing to weakness of the trunk muscles. About this time also some prominence of the occipital region of the skull was noticed. Patient was admitted in February, 1904, when a globular protrusion of the occipital region of the skull was noticed. He complained of feeling giddy, and was constantly sick : the pupils were widely dilated, and there was no evidence that he had any power of vision. The skull was trephined over the swelling ; the bone was exceedingly thin and seemed to have undergone atrophy from pressure of an underlying cerebellar cyst. The cyst was not opened till ten days later, when it was easy to puncture it and draw off the clear fluid contained in it. There was only a slight temporary improvement in the general condition. (Male, iv. 164.)

DISEASES OF THE EYE.

Conjunotivitis.

Three cases of membranous conjunctivitis ; all three cases showed a grey membrane adherent to the palpebral conjunctiva. The first case differed from the two others in giving a pure culture of the diphtheria bacillus, and in the presence of definite ulceration beneath the patches of membrane ; 6,000 units of anti-diphtheritic serum were injected on admission ; the case was discharged cured after twelve days. From the other two cases cocci were obtained, which were not identified. These cases were cured by local treatment in ten and fourteen days respectively. (Male, vi. 373, 2635, 2834.)

Syphilis.

A case of primary syphilitic sore on the eyelid showed a secondary rash within a fortnight of the appearance of the sore. The eye was well at the end of two months, with a small scar at the outer canthus ; secondary manifestations, namely, papular rash, and mucous condylomata in the mouth and throat, continued for six months. (Male, vi. 2021.)

Hysterical Blindness.

Two cases of hysterical blindness, both females, were treated by assumption of indifference to their condition, and a small amount of normal suasion. The first case started with a scald, eight years ago, which injured both eyes. The left eye had to be excised three years ago, the right eye became blind three months before admission. The only objective sign was a certain amount of conjunctival inflammation. The cure occupied one month, and was complete.

In the second case, a woman, aged 40, the predisposing cause was alcohol. When first seen she had been blind for five weeks, her pupils were dilated and did not react to light. On admission, a week later, she could distinguish light from dark, and the pupils reacted to light. The cure was complete in four days. (Female, vi. 1893, 2525.)

Sympathetic Ophthalmia.

Recovery. This was the case of a boy, aged 11, with no history of tubercle or rheumatic fever, and no family history of syphilis. On April 6th patient received a blow in the right eye from a hammer ; there was a linear wound in the lower part of the cornea, extending into the sclera on the nasal side, and prolapse of the iris. Four hours after this injury, the prolapsed iris was removed ; the rest of the iris appeared to be free after the operation. The right eye did not quiet down satisfactorily, and the left eye became irritable, and on May 2nd the right eye was excised. On May 14th keratitis punctata was observed for the first time in the left eye. On June 1st there was diffuse retinitis, and more than a millimetre swelling of the disc. He left hospital on July 1st, the left eye being much better and the vision nearly normal ($\frac{6}{9}$ partly). On December 13th the left eye was quite quiet, vision good ($\frac{6}{6}$), a few spots of the old keratitis punctata remained on the cornea, and the eye was slightly flushed after examination. (Male, vi. 1005.)

Oysticerous.

Bilateral cysticercus cellulosæ in the choroid. A man, aged 30, a civil servant in South Africa, noticed some pain in the right eye, with gradual loss of vision and the appearance of muscæ volitantes in July, 1903. The left eye was affected in September, and he lost all vision suddenly, and subsequently suffered from recurring attacks of pain. After operation for detachment of the retina in the right eye, in South Africa, a cysticercus was diagnosed and removed from the eye at Moorfields, but all vision was lost (May, 1904). In August the pain in the left eye became so bad that the eye was excised in this hospital, and a cysticercus was found lying between the retina and choroid, and causing an extensive retinal detachment. (Male, vi. 2386.)

Papillitis with complete loss of Vision.

Recovery. A girl, aged 19, a bank note registrar, had been suffering from headaches for three months. On September 27th, 1904, the headache was worse than ever, on the 28th the vision of the right eye was dim, on the 29th she was blind in the right eye. On October 6th she was found to have no perception of light in the right eye, the vision of the left eye was nearly normal ($\frac{6}{9}$). The pupils were equal, but the direct light reflex was absent from the right, and the consensual reflex from the left pupil. There was papillitis in the right eye, with much exudation and more than a millimetre swelling of the disc (more than 4. D.) She is the youngest of a family of twelve, all quite healthy, she had had no illness, and was not anæmic. After admission she improved quickly. On October 8th she could see large objects with the right eye, on the 18th the swelling of the disc was less than a quarter of what it had been, on November 4th the fields of vision of the two eyes for 10 m.m. white square were equal, on November 16th the vision of the right eye was equal to that of the left ($\frac{6}{9}$ in each); there was no swelling of the disc, but it was pale, and opaque with edges soft and ill-defined. The treatment consisted in purging and leeching on the day of admission (October 5th), and subsequently in general inunctions of mercury, and the local application of mercury ointment to the right brow. (Female, vi. 2194.)

DISEASES OF THE EAR.

Otitis Media.

Many cases of otitis media were admitted during the year. Two of these developed a cerebellar abscess, and both died (Male, i. 476, ii. 1702). In one case a cerebral abscess of the tempero-sphenoidal lobe was discovered post-mortem. (Male, iii. 2412.)

A female, aged 13, was admitted suffering from a discharge from the right ear and vomiting. There was tenderness over the mastoid region and double optic neuritis. The mastoid process was incised and found to contain carious bone, which was scooped out. Patient did not improve at all after the operation, but became gradually comatose, and died nine days after admission with symptoms pointing rather to meningitis. Post-mortem : Nothing abnormal was found in the brain. The lateral sinus, however, contained a breaking-down clot. The left sterno-clavicular articulation contained pus, and there was also purulent pericarditis and recent vegetations on the mitral valves. (Female, ii. 2397.)

DISEASES OF THE NOSE AND ANTRUM.

Naso-pharyngeal Polypi.

Three tumours growing from the naso-pharynx are of interest.

A boy, aged 15, gave a history of nasal obstruction and epistaxis for a period of six months. The left nostril was completely obstructed by a large rounded swelling, which appeared to be attached by a broad pedicle to the base of the

M

skull and to extend forward into the nasal cavities. Microscopical examination revealed the tumour to be a fibro-angeioma, and indeed this was suspected at the operation, for the hæmorrhage was profuse. A preliminary laryngotomy was performed, and an incision was made, as for removal of the upper jaw, and the nose detached from the face. Through the nasal apertures the tumour was attacked with a raspatory and removed from its base and delivered through the mouth. The result was eminently satisfactory. (Male, ii. 1562.)

A similar tumour was found in a man, aged 31, who had a fifteen months' history of difficulty of breathing through the nose and occasional attacks of epistaxis. The soft palate was bulged downwards by a large rounded tumour, which could easily be felt by the finger to be attached to the base of the skull. After a preliminary laryngotomy, a gutter was made in the hard palate, through which opening the tumour was removed in pieces without much difficulty and without much bleeding. After the operation there was a considerable amount of subcutaneous emphysema, but the patient eventually made a good recovery. (Male, v. 1762.)

The third case was that of a female, aged 21. In this patient the tumour was not so large as in the preceding cases, and it was removed without much difficulty through the anterior nares. The swelling was attached to the base of the skull and was torn away by means of a pair of forceps. Very little bleeding followed. (Female, ii. 264.)

Sarcoma.

One case of a rapidly-growing sarcoma of the naso-maxillary region was met with in a girl of 15. The growth was so extensive that the unanimous opinion expressed at consultations was that the condition was quite beyond operation. (Female, iv. 1455.)

DISEASES OF THE LARYNX AND TRACHEA.

Malignant Growths.

Four cases of this disease were met with. In two of these the growth was extensive, and the patients were discharged without any operation being performed and without experiencing much relief. (Male, i. 1025, iii. 3235*.)

There were two cases of intrinsic epithelioma of the larynx.

A baker, aged 45, had had symptoms for three months. It was seen that the right half of the epiglottis and the right arytenoid cartilage were infiltrated with growth. One hard, enlarged lymphatic gland was found on the right side of the neck. A preliminary tracheotomy was performed and a Hahn's tube inserted. The thyroid cartilage was then split in the middle line and the right half removed. No growth was found in the opposite side of the larynx. Patient died eight days after operation with septic broncho-pneumonia. Post-mortem a small amount of growth was found remaining in the larynx. (Male, i. 1025.)

The second case occurred in a man, aged 48. He was admitted suffering from severe dyspnœa, for which a tracheotomy was performed. Later on a thyrotomy was undertaken, and an intrinsic epithelioma removed. On patient's discharge some three months later a recurrence of the growth could already be seen. (Male, ii. 1684.)

Papilloma of Larynx.

Two small papillomata were removed under cocaine from the vocal cords of a female, aged 30. Patient's voice had been hoarse for fourteen years and absent for one week. Much relief was experienced after the operation. (Female, v. 2327.)

DISEASES OF THE DUCTLESS GLANDS.

Thyroid Gland.

CYSTS AND CYSTIC ADENOMA.—Nine cases in all were admitted for this disease, seven females and two males. In all a successful operation was performed, the operation being either an enucleation or a partial excision of the thyroid gland. (Male, i. 2819, iv. 1795 ; Female, i. 1066, 2140, 2680, ii. 1274, iv. 385, 1522, v. 493.)

PARENCHYMATOUS GOÎTRE.—Four cases were admitted, in all of whom partial thyroidectomy was successfully performed. (Male, ii. 173, 899 ; Female, iv. 2228, v. 2281.)

Sarcoma.

Two cases.

Four months previous to admission, a woman, aged 60, noticed a swelling in the region of the thyroid gland. On admission the patient appeared somewhat distressed with dyspnœa, and in the region of the thyroid was a swelling, which was firmly fixed, did not move on swallowing, and appeared to pass down below the sternum. A few days later the patient died suddenly. Post-mortem a large malignant growth of the thyroid was found, with very large secondary deposits in the lungs and pleural cavities. (Female, i. 2165.)

In 1903 the left half of the thyroid gland was removed for a "malignant growth." The patient remained well for twelve months, when the growth recurred. An operation was undertaken to remove this recurrence with only partial success. (Female, v. 2449.)

Supra-renal Gland.

A very interesting pathological condition was noted in connection with a rope-worker, aged 63. In 1902 one half of the tongue was removed for epithelioma. In 1903 the abdomen began to swell, and shortly after the glands in neck became much enlarged. In the abdomen was a large swelling which was thought to be a malarial spleen. The patient died without any operation being performed. Post-mortem it was found that there were in the patient two entirely different malignant tumours. In the first place there was an epithelioma of the tongue with its secondary deposits in the cervical lymphatic glands. The abdominal swelling proved to be a tumour of the kidney, a carcinoma of the type arising from the supra-renal gland. This tumour infiltrated the kidney, and had invaded and distended the renal vein, and even extended up into the inferior vena cava. (Male, iii. 120.)

DISEASES OF THE CHEST.

Empyema.

Five cases of empyema were treated, four by resection of a rib and one by incision. In all a successful result was obtained. (Male, iii. 1008 and 1084, v. 2673 and 2983 ; Female, i. 1903.)

DISEASES OF THE VASCULAR SYSTEM.

Aneurysm.

Four patients suffering from aneurysm were admitted. In two of these the abdominal aorta was the artery affected, in one the popliteal artery and in the third the external carotid. Both the patients with the abdominal aneurysm died.

A man, aged 39, an ex-stoker in the Royal Navy, had complained of vague abdominal pains for the last two years. In the epigastric region there was a pulsating swelling presenting all the ordinary characters of an aneurysm. An exploratory operation was undertaken to see whether it could be ligatured or wired. On opening the abdomen, a flattened liver was found spread out over a large fusiform aneurysm of the aorta, and any idea of further operative interference was abandoned. Six days later the aneurysm suddenly burst, the patient dying in a few minutes. The autopsy revealed a large aneurysm of the descending thoracic aorta and the upper part of the abdominal aorta, which had caused extensive erosion of the vertebræ. The aneurysm had burst into the right pleural cavity. ' (Male, ii. 911.)

The second case occurred in a male, aged 33, who had been employed in the Chinese custom house. He had had syphilis and had been in the habit of consuming large quantities of alcohol. Two months previous to admission he had noticed a swelling in the upper part of the abdomen. The abdomen was opened in the middle line and a large aneurysm found, which was not amenable to surgical treatment. At one point the aneurysm was bulging and looked as if it was on the point of bursting. Four days later the aneurysm did burst, and the patient died in a few moments from hæmorrhage. Post-mortem a large fusiform aneurysm of the lower part of the abdominal aorta was found, which had ruptured into the sub-peritoneal tissue. (Male, ii. 873.)

An aneurysm of the popliteal artery was found in a man, aged 42, a boot finisher by occupation. He owned to be of very intemperate habits, and had had syphilis and several attacks of gout. The superficial femoral artery was tied in the apex of Scarpa's triangle, with the result that the pulsation in the swelling stopped immediately. Six days later the pulse reappeared in the posterior artery and not in the sac. (Male, ii. 976.)

Six months previous to admission, a carman, aged 39, noticed a small swelling behind the jaw on the right side. On admission this swelling was about two and a half inches in diameter, and had a distinct expansile pulsation. A soft systolic bruit could be heard over it ; the pulse in the right superficial temporal and facial arteries was distinctly weaker on the affected side. On February 6th the right common carotid artery was tied, the operation being followed by no complication. On February 23rd the patient was discharged, the aneurysm then being much smaller, measuring only one inch in diameter and not pulsating. He was seen again on March 16th in the Out-Patient room, when the aneurysm was found to be no larger, but pulsating again. (Male, iii. 364.)

Arterio-venous Aneurysm.

A girl, aged 19, gave a history of having had a soft swelling in the palm of the left hand for the last five years. At different times the radial and ulnar arteries had been tied in both the lower and the upper thirds of the arm, but with only temporary relief. The swelling was pulsatile, and there seemed to be communication of pulsation between the arteries and the dilated veins on the surface. On this occasion the brachial artery was tied and a dissection made to remove the palmar swelling, which was found to be intimately connected with the median nerve and even to follow the distribu-tion of that nerve. No improvement followed this operation, and the patient came in again, when an amputation through the forearm was performed. (Female, iv. 1351.)

Thrombosis.

Several cases of thrombosis of veins were admitted. Two of these were submitted to operation.

In one instance the affected veins were excised (Male, iii. 3023) ; and in the other the internal saphenous vein was ligatured below the saphenous opening (Male, iv. 1255). Both cases made a good recovery.

DISEASES OF THE LYMPHATIC SYSTEM.

Tuberculous Mesenteric Glands.

Two cases of tuberculous disease of the mesenteric glands are of interest for the reason that in each case the condition was diagnosed as appendicitis.

A man, aged 32, was admitted to a Medical Ward complaining of severe pain in the right iliac fossa ; associated signs were vomiting, constipation and fever. The patient stated that he had had four similar attacks in the last six months. The condition was diagnosed as appendicitis, and after the acute symptoms had disappeared the patient was transferred to the Surgical side, the only signs remaining being a distinct resistance in the right iliac fossa. At the operation the appendix was found to be healthy, but the mesenteric glands close to the cæcum were found caseous and in part calcareous. The patient made an uneventful recovery, and while in the hospital had no return of pain. (Male, i. 1145.)

Another man, aged 30, was admitted for what was taken to be an attack of appendicitis. A fortnight before admission he had a sudden acute attack of pain in the abdomen. On admission there was slight tenderness and a small hard lump in the right iliac fossa. The abdomen was opened, and a caseating mesenteric gland removed. The appendix was not seen. Patient had had no previous attacks. (Male, iv. 3264*.)

Malignant Disease.

Two cases of advanced inoperable malignant disease of the glands of the neck were treated by means of Otto Schmidt's anti-cancer serum. No improvement whatever was obtained. (Male, i. 3178.)

One man with an inoperable epithelioma of the tongue had, in addition to Otto Schmidt's serum. injections of sodium cinnamate. In this case the patient died without any improvement being noted. (Male, i. 3174*.)

DISEASES OF THE DIGESTIVE SYSTEM.

Parotid Gland.

Five patients were admitted suffering from tumour of the parotid gland. In four of these the tumours were successfully removed, the remaining patient refusing operation. In one instance the tumour had recurred after removal by Mr. Butlin in 1898 ; microscopically the tumour showed the ordinary structure of a mixed parotid tumour (Female, ii. 2315).

The other cases were : Male, i. 2230, iii. 2230 ; Female, i. 615, v. 2442.

Tongue.

Twenty-eight patients, of whom two were females, suffering from epithelioma of the tongue were submitted to operation. In most of these cases the cervical lymphatic glands were removed as well as the tongue, and in some cases a preliminary laryngotomy was performed. Only one case died after operation (Male, iii. 2198), the cause being septic broncho-pneumonia.

A man, aged 41, was admitted with a very extensive and inoperable epithelioma of the tongue and floor of mouth. The lymphatic glands were extensively infiltrated, and later suppurated. The patient finally died from repeated hæmorrhages from the tongue. (Male, ii. 1189.)

Epithelioma of the Floor of the Mouth.

An iron-moulder, aged 71, was admitted with a very rapidly-growing epithelioma of the floor of the mouth. An extensive operation was performed, in which the anterior part of the lower jaw, the anterior part of the tongue and the floor of the mouth were removed. The patient was making a good recovery from the operation, but three weeks later had an attack of apoplexy, followed by right hemiplegia, and became semi-conscious, in which condition he remained until his removal. (Male, iii. 2657.)

Epithelioma of the Tonsil.

A man, aged 67, was admitted with an extensive malignant ulceration affecting the left tonsil, part of the soft palate, and the wall of the pharynx. He had been quite well until four months previously, when he complained of sore throat. Three months ago the left tonsil was cauterised several times. After a preliminary laryngotomy, the cheek was split and an extensive operation performed, in which the tonsil, part of the soft palate, the pillar of the fauces, and part of the base of the tongue were removed. Three weeks later a second operation was performed to remove the glands in the neck. The patient made a good recovery, but he had some recurrence in the glands in the neck a few months later. (Male, iv. 639.)

Epithelioma of the Fauces.

Four months previous to admission, an indigo planter, aged 53, noticed some soreness of the throat. On examination he was found to have a small shallow ulcer, the size of a shilling, on the anterior pillar of the fauces. No enlarged glands could be felt, and the only trouble experienced by the patient was some difficulty in swallowing. After splitting the cheek the growth was removed locally ; no glands were removed. Two months later the patient was re-admitted with a small recurrent growth on the anterior pillar of the fauces and with very definite enlargement of the lymphatic glands. The recurrence was removed locally, and an extensive dissection made to remove the glands, which were much involved. The patient made a satisfactory recovery. (Male, iii. 2046.)

Œsophagus.

Fibrous Stricture.— On June 21st an engine cleaner, aged 20, accidentally drank some caustic potash solution instead of some tea. He suffered much pain, and was very collapsed for some hours. On admission in August the patient, who was very emaciated, could only swallow fluids, and that with difficulty. Several attempts were made to pass a bougie, but nothing would pass further than six inches from the teeth. Without any definite treatment the dysphagia became less, and the man was discharged in October very much improved and able to swallow soft solids. (Male, iv. 2292.)

Carcinoma.—Twenty males and two females were admitted suffering from carcinoma of the œsophagus. Of the two females, one was discharged without operation (Female, v. 879). The other died after a gastrostomy (Female, v. 2073).

Ten males were submitted to gastrostomy, and only two of these recovered (Male, i. 2134) and (Male, iii. 2435), a bricklayer, aged 40, who, after the operation, had a severe attack of hæmatemesis, and likewise developed an abscess in the parotid gland.

A labourer, aged 64, had been suffering for six months from loss of flesh and with increasing difficulty in swallowing. He was very anæmic : red blood cells, 1,952,000 ; white blood cells, 14,000 ; hæmoglobin, 26 %. There was obstruction to the passage of a bougie fourteen inches from the teeth.

There was a loud systolic murmur heard all over the cardiac area. A gastrostomy was performed, and everything appeared satisfactory until two days later, when the patient suddenly died. The post-mortem revealed a large carcinoma of the lower end of the œsophagus and cardiac end of the stomach, and also a sacculated aneurysm of the descending thoracic aorta. (Male, i. 985.)

Stomach.

ADHESIONS.—In several instances, in the course of operations on the stomach, perigastric adhesions were met with. The following case is conducive to the belief that adhesions may be the cause of great trouble.

A woman, aged 39, gave a distinct history of having had a gastric ulcer two years previously ; since that time she had had continual pain in the region of the stomach. On examination, nothing was found but some tenderness in the epigastric region ; the stomach was not dilated, there was no vomiting, but the patient constantly complained of attacks of pain which bore no relation to her meals. The abdomen was opened, and two long slender adhesions found between the abdominal wall and the anterior surface of the stomach. These were divided, and while the patient remained in the hospital she had no further attacks of pain. (Female, iii. 646.)

DILATATION.—Four cases, three males and one female, were admitted for dilatation of the stomach, the exact cause for which was not obvious.

The female was discharged without operation. (Female, i. 2868.)

Two males recovered after a gastro-enterostomy. (Male, i. 3226, iii. 2368.)

On the third case, a male, aged 29, an exploratory laparotomy was performed ; a few adhesions about the stomach were divided, but nothing further done. After the operation the patient had persistent vomiting, and died three days later. Post-mortem : Many adhesions were found about the stomach, and in the lungs advanced phthisis and also tuberculous ulceration of the intestine. (Male, ii. 115.)

FIBROUS STRICTURE OF THE PYLORUS.—Only one case of obvious fibrous stricture of the p lorus was admitted, though several of the cases entered under the heading of dilatation of the stomach may have had a similar condition.

A railway porter, aged 39, had a history of a gastric ulcer thirteen years previously. Since that time patient suffered much from attacks of pain and vomiting, and to gain relief had been in the habit of washing out his stomach. The condition had been such as to prevent him following any regular employment. A gastro-enterostomy was performed with an eminently successful result ; all pain disappeared, and on his discharge he could take solid food with comfort. (Male, iii. 1336.)

GASTRIC ULCER.—Out of a total of ten cases that were admitted for simple gastric ulcer without perforation, five died.

Out of the ten cases six were females. Of these, two were relieved without operation (Female, i. 2547, v. 629).

Four were submitted to operation and two died.

Recoveries.—In June, 1904, a female, aged 20, was operated on for what was thought to be a perforated gastric ulcer. The abdomen was opened and an ulcer found, not perforated, but apparently on the point of perforating ; the area of the stomach involved was inverted by means of Lembert's sutures. Shortly after this another severe attack of abdominal pain occurred. On June 30th a posterior gastro-enterostomy was performed. The morning after the operation the patient was very sick, and vomited two large round worms (ascaris lumbricoides), and was occasionally sick during the next few days. On July 14th there was another severe attack of abdominal pain attended with collapse. Patient was discharged on July 23rd without any further complications occurring. (Female, i. 1485.)

A woman, aged 49, was admitted with symptoms of gastric ulcer, which had extended over a period of four years. The abdomen was opened, and a large chronic ulcer found on the posterior wall of the stomach near the pylorus. Gastro-enterostomy was performed, and the patient made an excellent recovery, being relieved of most of her symptoms. (Female, iii. 1469.)

Fatal Cases.—A cook, aged 34, was transferred to the Surgical side from a Medical Ward, where she had had prolonged treatment for a gastric ulcer without success. The abdomen was opened in the middle line and the stomach drawn out of the wound and examined. Nothing abnormal was seen, so an incision was made into the stomach so as to examine the mucous membrane. A small superficial ulcer about the size of a sixpenny piece was found, which bled freely when touched. The mucous membrane was stitched over this denuded area with fine silk. The stomach was finally closed with Lembert's sutures. Vomiting continued after the operation, and resisted all treatment; the patient became steadily weaker, and died eight days after the operation. There was no post-mortem examination. (Female, ii. 2254*.)

The other fatal case was Female, iii. 186.

Of the four male cases with gastric ulcer, two had a gastro-enterostomy performed. One recovered (Male, v. 2318) and one died (Male, v. 554).

Both the other two cases died; one as the result of severe hæmatemesis (Male, v. 762); and the other with peritonitis and subphrenic abscess (Male, i. 335).

PERFORATED GASTRIC ULCER.—Nineteen cases altogether came under observation during the year, eleven males and eight females. In each case laparotomy was performed and the ulcer sutured. Eight of the males and four of the females recovered.

A window-cleaner, who had had dyspepsia for two years, was taken on the morning of admission with acute abdominal pain, which was not localised in any particular region. On admission the abdomen was hard, but not motionless. The pulse was 64 and the temperature 98·2°, but a few hours later the pulse had risen to 94 and the temperature to 101·6°. The abdomen was opened in the middle line, and a perforated ulcer found on the anterior wall of the stomach and sutured. Patient made an uneventful recovery. (Male iii. 1550.)

A man, aged 26, was admitted in a collapsed conditon, and complaining of pain in the abdomen; the abdomen was not distended, but it was rigid, resonant and tender all over; the liver dulness was absent. The abdomen was opened in the middle line, and two small perforations found on the anterior surface of the stomach near the pylorus; these were sutured and the abdomen sponged out. The patient made an excellent recovery, and was discharged twenty days after the operation. (Male, i. 3182.)

The other males that recovered were : Males, i. 587, iii. 2878, v. 912, 1268, 1635. 1786.

Fatal Cases.—A skin-dresser was seized while at work with acute pain in the abdomen. He did not come up for treatment till twenty-four hours later. By this time he was acutely ill, with a frequent pulse and a distended and tender abdomen. Immediate laparatomy was performed, and a perforation on the anterior wall of the stomach close to the pylorus sutured. Patient died five hours after the operation. The post-mortem revealed much peritonitis. (Male, i. 3506.)

The other fatal cases were : Male, v. 2014, 2777.

Of the eight female cases, four recovered.

Fatal Cases. – Female, iv. 2982*, v. 1213, 1726, 2190.

All these cases developed general septic peritonitis, and one case also a sub-diaphragmatic abscess (Female, iv. 2982*).

Recoveries.—The following cases recovered after operation : Female, ii. 1230, iv. 709, 1435, 2302.

CARCINOMA.—Twenty-one cases in all were recognised as suffering from this disease. In comparison with previous years this is a very considerable increase in numbers.

With one exception, all these cases were unsuitable, owing to the advanced nature of the disease, for a radical operation (Male, iii. 865).

Of the other male cases, gastro-enterostomy was performed in six cases, and in four cases an exploratory laparotomy showed the growth to be beyond the reach of surgical treatment.

Five out of the total of eleven males died.

Recoveries (Male) :—

COLLOID CARCINOMA.—A violinist, aged 46, was admitted on account of a swelling in the region of the stomach. He had suffered pain in the back and epigastrium for three months, but otherwise he seemed a healthy individual, and had very few symptoms referable to his stomach. On opening the abdomen a mass of growth was found along the lesser curvature and the cardiac end of the stomach : the glands in the meso-colon were enlarged. A portion of the growth removed for examination proved to be a colloid carcinoma. A second operation was undertaken a week later in order to attempt the removal of the whole stomach ; this, however, was found to be impossible, owing to the fixity of the stomach to the surrounding structures, especially the pancreas. A gastric fistula formed after this operation, but closed later before patient's discharge to Friedenheim. (Male, i. 2281.)

The other cases were : Male, iv. 1560, iii. 169, 865, v. 1054, 3356*.

Fatal Cases :—

A labourer, aged 30, was admitted complaining of pain in the abdomen and distension. He first complained of pain some eight weeks before admission, but he had no severe symptoms till a few days before admission, when he complained of pain and vomiting after food. He was a somewhat pale thin-looking man. The abdomen was slightly distended, and he complained of pain in the lower part. There were signs of free fluid in the abdomen, and nothing else abnormal was discovered. Per rectum a hard mass could be felt in Douglas' pouch, and even under an anæsthetic nothing was made out. The patient did not improve during his stay in the hospital, he vomited daily, and medicine was necessary to open the bowels. An exploratory operation was undertaken, and the abdomen opened in the middle line below the umbilicus. The intestines were found matted together, and covered with small nodules of what looked like new growth. A nodule was also found in the liver. The sigmoid flexure was found distended, and under the idea that the case was probably one of malignant disease of the rectum with multiple growths, a left inguinal colotomy was performed. The patient died shortly after the operation, and at the post-mortem examination the whole of the intestines were found covered with hundreds of small secondary growths, and also several nodules in the liver. The primary growth was found to be a large carcinomatous ulcer of the pyloric end of the stomach. The hard mass which was felt per rectum in life was found to be a portion of the peritoneum, which was thickened and infiltrated. (Male, v. 188.)

CARCINOMA OF THE PYLORUS.—A labourer, aged 50, was admitted to the hospital in May, 1904, under the idea that he might be suffering from a malignant tumour of the stomach. He then gave a four months' history of pain in the abdomen and loss of flesh, and occasional vomiting. He then had no tumour palpable, he was able to take his food fairly well, and had no vomiting. As his general condition considerably improved, he was discharged without any operation being performed. He was re-admitted in August, when it was found that there was an easily palpable tumour in the region of the pylorus ; he was very much thinner and was in continual pain ; he had, however, no vomiting and no melæna ; the stomach was somewhat distended. The abdomen was opened and an extensive growth found close to the pylorus, and too extensive for removal, so a gastro-enterostomy was performed. After the operation vomiting became almost constant, and the patient died a few days later. Post-mortem a large carcinomatous ulcer was found in the pyloric region of the stomach, and the pylorus itself was adherent to the under-surface of the liver. A few small glands were found enlarged along the lesser curvature of the stomach, but beyond this no other secondary growths were found. (Male, iv. 2328.)

The other fatal cases were : Male, i. 544, ii. 302, iii. 1744.

Of the ten females, four were considered to be beyond surgical treatment, and two of these died shortly after admission (Female, iv. 1386, v. 9).

In the other six cases, five were submitted to gastro-enterostomy, and three died, and in one case, after an exploratory laparotomy, the stomach was found to be hopelessly diseased (Female, ii. 2509).

Fatal Cases.—A woman, aged 48, was transferred to the Surgical side, suffering from collapse and vomiting. On opening the abdomen a large growth was found in the region of the pylorus. Patient died almost directly after the operation, and the post-mortem examination revealed a large malignant growth involving the whole circumference of the pylorus. The stomach was not greatly distended The lymphatic glands along the greater curvature were enlarged, but no other secondary deposits were found. (Female, v. 1978.)

The other fatal cases were : Female, i. 1395, iii. 2128.

The two cases relieved after gastro-enterostomy were : Female, iv. 326, v. 2030.

Liver.

ABSCESS.—Two cases were admitted during the year.

A farm labourer, aged 40, who had never been out of England, complained for some months of pain and swelling in the upper part of the abdomen. The abdomen was distended by a large liver which extended to half an inch below the umbilicus. Leucocytosis 24,000. The abdomen was opened and a very large loculated abscess found and drained. In the pus streptococci was found, but no other organisms. The patient was discharged after a prolonged convalescence. (Male, i. 2652.)

The other case occurred in a labourer, aged 28, who, while in China in August, 1904, had suffered from dysentery. In September, 1904, he was seized with colic accompanied with vomiting, rigors, and increasing pain in the abdomen. Leucocytosis 20,000. The abdomen was opened and a blood-stained peritoneal exudate found. The condition of the patient being so feeble nothing further was attempted, and the patient died a few hours later. The post-mortem revealed a large hepatic abscess eroding a branch of the hepatic artery, and the immediate cause of death was hæmorrhage. In the pus amœbæ were found. (Male, iii. 2531.)

ACCESSORY LOBE.—A woman, aged 47, gave a history of pain and swelling in the right epigastric region. To the right of the umbilicus could be felt a movable, rounded, rather tender swelling, which appeared to be continuous with the liver. On opening the abdomen, this swelling was found to be linguiform lobe of an otherwise healthy liver. The abdomen was closed without anything further being done. (Female, v. 1948.)

HYDATID CYST.—Three cases were admitted during the year.

A man, aged 26, was submitted to operation for a condition similating biliary colic. On opening the abdomen, the gall bladder was found to be distended with bile and mucus. It contained no stones and no obstruction could be felt in the common bile duct. A cholecyst-enterostomy was performed; the patient died five days later. At the post-mortem examination the following was discovered : The common bile duct was seen to be very much distended, and on opening the duodenum the opening of the duct was found much dilated, and through it was protruding a portion of the wall of a hydatid cyst, which completely blocked the lumen. The common hepatic duct was much dilated, and opened into a cyst cavity, situated in the inferior part of the left lobe of the liver, and containing disintegrated hydatid remains. In the right lobe was a second cyst containing fresh daughter cysts and brood capsules. (Male, ii. 1907.)

A chemist's assistant, aged 17, was found on operation to be suffering from a suppurating hydatid cyst of the liver. The abscess was drained through the pleural cavity. The patient died three weeks later from pneumonia. (Male, iii. 859.)

The other case was Male i. 764.

ADHESIONS ABOUT THE GALL BLADDER.—Eight weeks before admission a woman, aged 68, began to complain of pain and vomiting after food. On admission the patient was much collapsed and too ill for any operation to be attempted. Post-mortem examination : There were many dense adhesions uniting the pylorus and duodenum. The gall bladder was small and shrunken and contained a few stones. It was bound by firm adhesions to the duodenum, and these adhesions, in contracting, had given rise to a constriction of the duodenum about two inches beyond the pyloric orifice. As a result of the constriction the stomach was enormously dilated. (Female, iv. 340.)

Gall Bladder and Ducts.

GALL STONES.—Nineteen men and six women were admitted suffering from gall stones or their effects. In four cases the operation of cholecystectomy was performed, and in three cases it was eminently successful. The following cases present some points of interest :—

In 1908, a woman, aged 59, was in President Ward, suffering from an abscess in the right side of the abdomen. In this abscess was found a gall stone. The gall bladder was perforated and contained stones. The stones were removed and the gall bladder sewn up. At the beginning of this year the patient became jaundiced and ill. The abdomen was opened and the gall bladder found natural except for some adhesions. The common bile duct was found to contain two stones, which were removed through an incision in the wall of the duct, At the same time a radical cure of a ventral hernia, the result of the previous operation, was performed, and the patient made an uneventful recovery. (Female, ii. 2308.)

A woman, aged 54, with marked jaundice, was admitted in a moribund condition, and died the following day. Post-mortem examination : The gall bladder and bile ducts were much distended with thin bile. The ampulla of Vater was occupied by a large stone which projected into the duodenum ; another stone lay higher up in the duct, and another in the gall bladder. The pancreas was very hard, and on cutting across it, the pancreatic duct was much dilated and bile could be squeezed from the gall bladder, up the pancreatic duct. (Female, iii. 2745.)

CARCINOMA OF GALL BLADDER.—In July, 1904, a woman aged 53, was admitted suffering from jaundice and biliary colic. There was tenderness in the region of the gall bladder, but nothing obvious was felt. The abdomen was opened in the middle line, and the gall bladder exposed and opened ; six stones were found and removed. The wall of the gall bladder was found very brittle, exciting suspicion, so a portion was removed for a microscopic examination, which revealed a columnar-celled carcinoma. The gall bladder was stitched to the abdominal wall and a drain inserted. In October of this year the patient returned saying she had had attacks of pain and vomiting since the first operation. The abdomen was again opened and the whole gall bladder removed; no secondary deposits were found, and the patient made an uneventful recovery. (Female, v. 1659.)

SARCOMA OF GALL BLADDER.—A boy, aged 5, was admitted suffering from jaundice, which had lasted three months. In the upper part of the abdomen was a distinct swelling continuous with the liver. The superficial abdominal veins were dilated, his temperature was raised and there was a leucocytosis of 25,000 ; the case was thought to be one of cholecystitis. An incision was made into the swelling and about half a pint of pus removed. For a time the patient's condition improved, but the sinus did not close, the swelling increased, and the patient died seven weeks later. Post-mortem : Attached to the under-surface of the liver was a large swelling occupying a space between the liver and the pancreas. The gall bladder was not found, and this tumour was assumed to be arising from it. On incising the swelling a number of soft semi-gelatinous pedunculated masses attached to the capsule presented. There were several enlarged glands in the neighbourhood. A microscopic examination showed the tumour to be a spindle-celled sarcoma. (Male, i. 596.)

Pancreas.

CARCINOMA.—Two cases, both females, were admitted during the year.

A woman, aged 52, gave a history of eight weeks' duration of jaundice, associated with vomiting, constipation and loss of flesh. On admission she was markedly jaundiced, and a hard swelling could be felt in the region of the gall bladder. Laparotomy was performed and the gall bladder found distended ; it was opened, but no stone found ; a hard swelling, however, was discovered in the situation of the head of the pancreas, which was believed to be a malignant growth. An anastomosis was then made between the gall bladder and the transverse colon by means of a Murphy's button. Vomiting continued after the operation, and the patient died a few days later. A post-mortem examination was refused. (Female, v. 105.)

A woman, aged 63, was admitted suffering from deep jaundice, which had lasted for eleven weeks, commencing after a typical attack of biliary colic. On opening the abdomen the gall bladder was found distended; it was opened and found full of mucus, no stone being present. A hard mass, which was thought to be a carcinoma, could be felt in the region of the head of the pancreas. The gall bladder was stitched to the abdominal wall and a drainage tube inserted. The patient left the hospital somewhat improved, though with some jaundice still persisting and a biliary fistula patent. (Female, i. 1796.)

PANCREATIC CYST.—A waiter, aged 36, gave the following history. Up to three weeks before the date of admission he had been perfectly well, when he was taken with pain in the abdomen and vomiting. The pain at times being sufficiently severe as to prevent him working. He had suffered at various times from malaria, dysentery, tape worms and biliary colic. The general condition of the patient was good, no wasting, no jaundice. Between the umbilicus and ensiform cartilage was situated a distinct, rounded, tense swelling, in which no fluctuation could be obtained. On respiration no movement occurred ; there was no resonance percussion, and its dulness appeared continuous with the liver dulness. Blood count was normal. Operation : The abdomen was opened in the right linea semilunaris and a large elastic mass was found in the posterior part of the abdomen. This mass was found to be a large cyst containing turbid brown fluid. No attempt was made to remove it,

173

and the patient was discharged with a small sinus. Reaction of the fluid was alkaline. Specific gravity 1020, and there was present an amylolytic ferment. (Male v. 3473*.)

Hernia.

A total of three hundred and thirty cases of hernia, of all sorts, were admitted during the year. Of these, five died.

(REDUCIBLE FEMORAL).—Nine cases were admitted, seven females and two males, and on all these cases, except one of the males, a radical cure was performed.

(REDUCIBLE INGUINAL).—Of this variety, one hundred and eighty-nine cases were recognised, of which one hundred and sixty-eight were males. Of the twenty-one female cases, twenty were submitted to the radical operation. The operation of radical cure was performed in one hundred and fifty-seven of the one hundred and sixty-eight male cases, and four of these cases were for herniæ which had recurred after a previous operation for the cure. No deaths occurred amongst all these cases.

(REDUCIBLE INGUINAL WITH PARTIALLY DESCENDED TESTIS).—Fourteen cases were admitted during the year. In seven of these a radical cure was performed and the testis excised. In three cases radical cure was performed and the testis stitched to the bottom of the scrotum. In three cases the testis was left *in situ*, and in one case, a man, aged 39, no operation was performed.

(INTERSTITIAL).—Three cases of interstitial hernia with partially descended testis were admitted, and on two of these radical cure was performed. (Male, i. 2829 ; ii. 908.)

The other case was Male, v. 1853.

(REDUCIBLE UMBILICAL).—Ten cases were admitted, seven females and three males. The operation for cure was done in five cases.

(IRREDUCIBLE FEMORAL).—Twenty-four cases were admitted, three of which were males. All these cases were submitted to operation with successful results.

(IRREDUCIBLE INGUINAL).—Twenty-one cases were admitted during the year, four of whom were females. Amongst these was one fatal case. This was in a baker, aged 58, who had been ruptured for forty years. The scrotum was enormously distended by a large scrotal hernia, containing bowel and omentum. The bowel was reducible, the omentum irreducible. Owing to the confinement in bed the patient developed bronchitis and died. No post-mortem examination was made. (Male, i. 1721.)

(IRREDUCIBLE INGUINAL, WITH PARTIALLY DESCENDED TESTIS).—A butcher, aged 28, had had a rupture since the age of 13, and up to ten days before admission the rupture had always been easily reducible. On admission a large, tense, tender swelling was found distending the left side of the scrotum and extending into the inguinal canal. It was irreducible, and there was no impulse on coughing. The swelling was tapped and blood-stained fluid drawn off, when the testicle was found lying in the inguinal canal. Later the sac was laid freely open, and in it was found some inflamed adherent omentum and the testicle being in the inguinal canal. The case was taken to be one of hernia into the unclosed tunica vaginalis ; the testicle remaining in the inguinal canal, and the hernia descending into the scrotum. The operation of radical cure was performed and the testis was removed.

(REDUCIBLE UMBILICAL).—Nine cases were admitted, all females ; eight of these cases were submitted to operation.

(STRANGULATED FEMORAL).—Thirteen cases were admitted during the year, of which two were males. They were all submitted to operation, and all recovered.

A woman, aged 75, had a right femoral hernia for twenty years; for two days she had complained of constipation and pain. There was a small irreducible femoral hernia on the right side. The sac was opened and found to contain some adherent omentum which had become strangulated; there was no gut present. The omentum was removed and a radical cure performed. During her convalescence the patient had an epileptic fit, during which she dislocated her right shoulder; this was reduced under an anæsthetic. (Female, i. 1050.)

(STRANGULATED INGUINAL).—Fourteen cases were admitted during the year, one female and thirteen males. All were submitted to operation. Two males died.

Fatal Cases.

A metal-plate worker, aged 49, was admitted with an inguinal hernia of the right side, which had been strangulated for three days. The sac was opened in the usual situation and the contents found to be gangrenous. A second incision was then made in the right linea semi-lunaris, and the gangrenous gut, which proved to be a portion of the small intestine, was drawn out through this incision and resected. The intestines were united by an end-to-end anastomosis effected by suture. The patient developed general peritonitis and died. (Male, iii. 3439.)

A commercial traveller, aged 53, had suffered for the last four years from a reducible right inguinal hernia, which had always been retained by a truss. On January 12th, while bathing, the hernia came down and could not be reduced. At five a.m. on January 13th he sent for a doctor, who "reduced it." Vomiting and hiccoughing came on after this and persisted; constipation was not absolute. On admission he appeared very ill, constantly sick and hiccoughing, and with a greatly distended abdomen. There was no obvious hernia, but on coughing a protrusion immediately appeared through the right inguinal ring. The abdomen was opened in the middle line and a hernia found, which had been reduced *en masse* with its sac, and the intestine had become constricted by a band of omentum. This band was divided, and the intestine, which did not appear gangrenous, reduced. The patient died next day. (Male, v. 171.)

(STRANGULATED UMBILICAL).—Four cases were admitted during the year, females, and they all recovered.

Two cases of strangulated ventral hernia occurred, both women. One case occurred in a woman, aged 39, who had a ventral hernia subsequent to a laparotomy performed ten years previously. Herniotomy was performed, and the patient made an uninterrupted recovery. (Female, iv. 1811.)

Ten years ago a female, aged 49, developed a ventral hernia after childbirth. Eight years ago an operation for cure was performed, but the hernia recurred. She was admitted with symptoms of strangulation of seven days' duration. The abdomen was opened, the intestines returned and a radical cure performed. At the post-mortem a constriction was found in that part of the intestine which had been in the hernia. The liver was markedly cirrhotic. (Female, iii. 2144.)

(INCARCERATED INGUINAL.)—One fatal case occurred in a man, aged 67, after herniotomy. (Male, ii. 1502.)

(TRAUMATIC VENTRAL).—Nine out of the fourteen cases admitted were submitted for the operation of radical cure.

Duodenum.

DUODENAL ULCER.—There was one case in which an ulcer of the duodenum was diagnosed. This occurred in a painter, aged 31, who had had two severe attacks of hæmatemesis. A posterior gastro-enterostomy was performed, and gave great relief. (Male, i. 1205.)

DUODENAL ULCER WITH PERFORATION.—Four males suffering from this disease were admitted during the year. In all cases the abdomen was opened and the ulcers sutured, but all cases ended fatally : three at least dying of peritonitis. In three out of four cases the ulcer was on the superior aspect of the duodenum. In the fourth case the ulcer was on the anterior aspect.

A metal caster, aged 32, had been subject for four weeks to pain in the epigastric region, coming on about two hours after food ; there had been no vomiting or hæmatemesis. On the day of admission, while eating his dinner, the patient was seized with acute pain in the abdomen. The abdomen was rigid and retracted, with a tender spot just above the umbilicus. A few hours after the perforation the abdomen was opened and a perforation on the superior aspect of the duodenum was sutured. Four days later the patient died of general purulent peritonitis. Post-mortem : Immediately beyond the pylorus, which appeared natural, were two small deep ulcers on opposite sides of the duodenum. The ulcer on the wall continuous with the lesser curvature of the stomach had perforated. (Male, iv. 2472.)

The other cases were : Male, iii. 836, 1925, v. 3566*.

DUODENAL STRICTURE.—A male, aged 48, suffering from a much dilated stomach and continual vomiting, was submitted to operation, when a constriction of the duodenum was found close to the pylorus and many firm adhesions between the pylorus and neighbouring structures. Posterior gastro-enterostomy was performed, and the patient made a rapid and uneventful recovery, all the symptoms disappearing. (Male, i. 2184.)

UMBILICAL FISTULA.—A female child, aged 11 weeks, was admitted with a patent Meckel's diverticulum opening at the umbilicus. Four days after birth the cord separated and a small dark swelling was noticed at the umbilicus ; from this swelling urine and fæces were discharged. The fistula was closed by plastic operation. (Female, iv. 756.)

SARCOMA OF SMALL INTESTINE.—A gardener, aged 54, had noticed swelling of his abdomen for six weeks, and on examination a very large tumor could be felt in the right side of the abdomen. On opening the peritoneal cavity a tumour was presented and was found to contain a large quantity of what appeared to be altered blood clot. After this was washed out it was found that the tumour was connected through a small hole with the interior of the small intestine. The patient died twelve hours after the operation from collapse, and at the post-mortem examination a remarkable tumour was found in connection with the small intestine. Microscopically, this growth proved to be a sarcoma in which was black pigment, suggesting a melanotic growth. (Male, iii. 1049.)

Intestinal Obstruction.

HERNIA INTO PERITONEAL POUCH.—A woman, aged 36, had suffered for ten days with signs of intestinal obstruction. She was admitted in a very collapsed state, with a much distended abdomen and fæculent vomiting. The patient was too ill for any operation, and died shortly after admission. At the post-mortem examination it was found that about six inches of the ileum immediately above the cæcum had entered the pouch of peritoneum lying just above the angle formed by the junction of the ileum with the cæcum : this portion had become strangulated, and nowhere was it perforated, but general purulent peritonitis had supervened. (Female, iii. 72.)

A woman, aged 59, was admitted with the symptoms of intestinal obstruction. The abdomen was opened, but no obstruction found. The transverse colon was distended, and a transverse colotomy was performed. The temperature rose to 103°, and the patient died the following day. Post-mortem : There was no obstruction in any part of the alimentary canal. There was, however, suppuration in and about the pancreas—no cause for this suppuration was found ; there were no gallstones and no obstruction to the pancreatic duct. (Female, v. 1326.)

Another case, suffering from intestinal obstruction, on whom a transverse colotomy was performed, was found, post-mortem, to be suffering from a columnar-celled carcinoma of the descending colon. (Female, iii. 912.)

INTESTINAL OBSTRUCTION BY BAND.—Three males were admitted during the year suffering from intestinal obstruction by band. Two of these cases (iii. 3595, iv. 151) were the result of old appendicitis.

In the third case (iii. 9614), a coachman, aged 36, the origin of the band was not discovered. In this case a portion of the gut was gangrenous and needed resection.

All these cases ended fatally.

INTUSSUSCEPTION.—Six infants and one adolescent were admitted with this complaint. Laparotomy was performed, and the intussuscepted portion reduced or resected. Only two of these cases recovered.

A child, aged 6 months, was admitted with intussusception, the symptoms of which had been present for five days. The abdomen was opened and an ileo-colic intussusception found. Reduction was impossible on account of adhesions, so a resection was performed and a lateral anastomosis established. (Male, iv. 2432.)

A boy, aged 16, had a history of attacks of abdominal pain with sickness and constipation recurring constantly since childhood. In 1902 the appendix was removed, and for about a year the patient was free of the symptoms. Three weeks before admission he had a worse attack of pain associated with vomiting and constipation. On opening the abdomen an ileo-colic intussusception was found, necessitating, on account of adhesions, resection of two feet of ileum and cæcum. The patient died as a result of general peritonitis. (Male, iii. 634.)

The other cases were : Male, ii. 3045, v. 1278, 2493 ; Female, i. 337, 2529.

VOLVULUS.—One case was admitted. The chief interest in this case lies in the post-mortem examination.

A man, aged 32, was admitted with all the symptoms of acute intestinal obstruction, and he was so ill that any operation was considered inadvisable. He died shortly after admission. The cause of the obstruction was found in the small intestine about four feet above the cæcum. At this point the periphery of a loop of the gut was bound down to the inner side of the cæcum by firm adhesions. The lumen of the bowel was not much narrowed by these adhesions, but the upper part of the intestine had become twisted on itself, forming a sort of volvulus, and thus causing obstruction. The cause of the adhesions was old appendicitis, the appendix being found to be small and shrunken and surrounded by a mass of adhesions. The upper part of the small intestine was enormously distended and contained fluid fæcal material ; nothing else abnormal was noted. (Male, i. 2851.)

Cæcum.

CARCINOMA.—Four cases of this disease were admitted during the year.

CARCINOMA OF THE CÆCUM AND ILEO-COLIC ANASTOMOSIS.—This patient, a fairly healthy-looking man, aged 48, was suffering from a large rounded swelling in the right iliac region, which he had noticed for about three months. The mass was slightly tender, nodular on the surface and fixed to the abdominal wall. He suffered from obstinate constipation, which was only relieved by enemata, and the stools constantly contained much dark blood. At the operation this mass was found to be a large malignant growth of the cæcum, which was attached to and invading the abdominal wall. On account of its great extent no attempt was made to remove it, but a lateral anastomosis was made between the lower part of the ileum and the transverse colon. No secondary growths were found. The patient was much relieved by the operation and left the hospital four weeks later, his bowels acting naturally. After the operation a small fæcal fistula appeared for a few days, but this rapidly closed. (Male, iv. 28.)

The other cases were: Male, i. 2671 ; Female, iii. 1671, v. 86.

TUBERCLE.—An Italian ice cream vendor, aged 29, was admitted with symptoms of intestinal obstruction which had lasted three days. Per rectum a tender swelling could be felt high up on the right side. The abdomen was opened in the middle line, and the cæcum, which was enlarged and hard, was brought out of the wound for examination. A malignant growth was diagnosed, and a resection of the cæcum with a portion of the ascending colon carried out. The patient died with symptoms of peritonitis. No post-mortem examination was allowed. Microscopically, tuberculous disease of the cæcum was discovered.

INFLAMED OMENTUM.—In February, 1904, a male, aged 20, was submitted to operation for the cure of a right inguinal hernia. At the operation a large piece of omentum was ligatured and returned to the abdomen. There was some suppuration in the wound, slightly delaying convalescence. Patient went to Swanley, but returned on account of much abdominal pain and a large doughy swelling on the left side of the abdomen at the level of the umbilicus. The swelling at first sight simulated an abdominal aneurysm, but on further examination it was found to be the stump of inflamed omentum. (Male, ii. 1030.)

Vermiform Appendix.
Appendicitis.

(*Acute cases without external suppuration*).—Sixty-seven cases, forty-six males and twenty-one females, were admitted. Forty-one were successfully treated by removal of the appendix.

In a schoolboy, aged 10, whose abdomen was opened for the removal of the appendix, some enlarged, caseous mesenteric glands were discovered in the posterior aspect of the cæcum. The appendix, which was long and thickened, also the glands, were removed. Microscopically the glands proved to be tuberculous. The appendix was thickened, but showed no evidence of tubercle. Convalescence was only delayed by an attack of tonsillitis. (Male, v. 176.)

(*Chronic relapsing cases without external suppuration*).—Eighty cases, thirty-eight males and forty-two females, were admitted. Seventy-one were successfully treated by removal of the appendix. There was one fatal case.

A man, aged 39, had had recurring attacks of appendicitis. He was admitted in a very exhausted condition and apparently suffering from the effects of opium, and it was difficult to say far his symptoms were attributable to this cause. The abdomen was opened, and an appendix, showing old inflammation, removed. The patient died twelve hours after the operation, the symptoms being those of opium poisoning. (Male, i. 3324.)

'(*Acute Gangrenous*).—Four males and six females were admitted suffering from this complaint. All were submitted to operation and the appendix removed in all but one case. The fatal cases were: Male, i. 2824, v. 3326 ; Female, i. 1205, v. 1471. The cases which recovered were: Male, i. 3443*, ii. 3464* ; Female, i. 2589*, 2852*, iii. 1674, v. 1847.

(*Acute, with suppuration*).—Fifty-six cases, twenty-nine males and twenty-seven females, were admitted. Sixteen cases were successfully treated by incision without the removal of the appendix. Four cases treated in a similar manner died, three with general peritonitis (Male, iii. 3073 and 3255, v. 2314), one with subphrenic abscess. (Male, iii. 841).

A baker, aged 39, was admitted suffering from acute suppurative appendicitis. The abdomen was opened in the middle line and general purulent peritonitis found. A second incision was made in the right iliac fossa, but the appendix was not removed owing to the bad condition of the patient. A month later the patient was discharged to Swanley. (Male, iv. 1433.)

A blacksmith, aged 22, was admitted with general peritonitis as a result of suppurative appendicitis. The abdomen was freely drained, and the patient slowly recovered, though convalescence was delayed by the formation of an empyema, which necessitated resection of a rib. Patient was re-admitted later in the year with a ventral hernia. (Male, iv. 155.)

Seven males recovered from a similar condition after appendicectomy ; two died, each as the result of purulent peritonitis. (Male, ii. 994, 1501.)

Eleven females were successfully treated by incision and drainage, and four died. (Female, i. 144, 2758, iv. 712, v. 2373.)

Seven cases were successfully treated by removal of the appendix and five died. (Female, ii. 353, 1518, 1899, iii. 2814, v. 430.)

One case, after an operation at which an old abscess was found round the proximal end of the appendix, developed suppurative parotitis and pneumonia. (Female, i. 1705.)

(*Chronic, with abscess*).—Ten cases, eight males and two females, were admitted with this complaint. Six cases were successfully treated by incision and two by appendicectomy. There were two fatal cases.

In March, 1904, a book packer, aged 44, was admitted with an appendix abscess and was successfully treated by incision and drainage. A few days previous to re-admission in June, 1904, abdominal pain returned, with some symptoms of intestinal obstruction. The abdomen was opened and a piece of gut found strangulated between two bands of omentum. The patient did not rally from the operation, and died the following day. Post-mortem examination : There were many old peritoneal adhesions and much matting about the cæcum. The appendix was found lying in a small pocket of pus open at the end, and exuding fæcal matter. (Male, i. 1570.)

The other fatal case occurred in a joiner, aged 61, who died without operation. The post-mortem examination revealed a diseased appendix, with a narrow fistulous track running from it and communicating with a large subphrenic abscess. (Male, ii. 3233.)

(*Old Appendicectomy*).—Three cases were admitted for minor troubles following previous operations.

Colon.

CARCINOMA.—Out of nine cases admitted for this complaint only one patient survived (Male, iv. 1236). In this case an artificial anus was made.

Fatal cases :—

A man, aged 44, had suffered from abdominal pain and constipation for four months, and during that time had lost much weight. In the abdomen could be felt a small moveable swelling in the region of the sigmoid flexure. This swelling, which proved on microscopical examination to be a columnar-celled carcinoma of the sigmoid flexure, was resected and the intestines joined end-to-end by suture. The patient died from general peritonitis, the result of leakage from the join. (Male, v. 2533.)

A woman, aged 52, was transferred from the Medical side, suffering with the symptoms of chronic intestinal obstruction. There was marked abdominal distension, but no tumour could be felt. On opening the abdomen a small tense broad ligament cyst was discovered in the right side of the pelvis. The descending colon was found to be distended with fæces and fingers could be passed from the anus into the distended bowel ; the obstruction, therefore, was thought to be due to the cyst. The patient died ten hours later. Post-mortem : A large carcinomatous (columnar-celled) growth was found at the splenic flexure of the colon, constricting the lumen. (Female, iii. 876.)

The other cases were : Male, ii. 1524, iii. 2109, 3577 ; Female, i. 260, 1492, iv. 855.

ULCERATIVE COLITIS.—Three cases were admitted.

A man, aged 52, was admitted complaining of vomiting and some constipation, and passing " black fluid " at stool. The abdomen was much distended and tympanitic. In the left inguinal region was a large irreducible hernia. It was thought that the hernia was obstructed, so the sac was opened and an artificial opening made in a coil of the bowel. The patient, who was very weak, died the next morning. At the post-mortem no obstruction was found but extensive ulceration of the colon. (Male, i. 2814.)

The other cases were : Male iii. 2239, iv. 2919.

OLD COLOTOMY.—Two cases were admitted on account of great prolapse from an old colotomy wound. In each case the prolapsed portion was excised. (Female, i. 586, iv. 499.)

Peritoneum.

HYDATID CYST.—A schoolboy, aged 12, was transferred from the Medical side suffering from what was thought to be tuberculous peritonitis. In the abdomen could be felt an indefinite (slightly moveable) swelling, measuring about six inches in diameter. When the abdomen was opened a large cystic swelling bulged into the wound.. The swelling was incised and about one pint of thin whitish fluid containing small cysts evacuated. The cyst was drained and patient made a satisfactory recovery. (Male, v. 3132.)

SUBPHRENIC ABSCESS.—Three cases of subphrenic abscess, in which the cause was not definitely ascertained, are classified under this heading. None of these were fatal. (Male i. 946, v. 708 ; Female ii. 2010.)

Rectum.

FIBROUS STRICTURE.—A police-constable, aged 39, was admitted on account of pain and difficulty of defæcation. The ischio-rectal fossæ were hard, and apparently . infiltrated with inflammatory exudation ; around the anus was much redness and excoriation. Under an anæsthetic the rectum was found to be constricted and tubular like ; no new growth was found. A left inguinal colotomy was performed with successful result. (Male, iv. 1879.)

A domestic servant, aged 41, was admitted with a recurrent fibrous stricture of the rectum. Two previous operations had been performed in 1886 and 1887. On examination, a tight fibrous stricture was found, just admitting the tip of the finger, about one and a half inches above the anus. Below the stricture the rectum was ballooned, and there was a small cul-de-sac passing upwards in front of the true canal. In addition, patient had advanced osteo-arthritis in both knee-joints. A posterior linear proctotomy was performed, and the patient discharged much relieved. (Female, ii. 879.)

A female, aged 49, was admitted with a recurrence of a fibrous stricture. Two previous operations for the same complaint had been performed in 1888 and 1900. She had been in the habit of passing bougies, but the stricture had gradually recurred, and attacks of hæmorrhage occurred from time to time. There was an annular fibrous stricture of the rectum, with a lumen of about a quarter of an inch in diameter, about one inch from the anus. (Female, ii. 919.)

CARCINOMA.—Of the thirty cases admitted for this complaint, twenty-six were submitted to operation, eight females and eighteen males.

In twenty cases a left inguinal colotomy was performed. Amongst these cases only one was fatal.

A man, aged 57, suffering with an advanced carcinoma of the rectum, on whom a left inguinal colotomy had been performed, died as the result of peritonitis, resulting from a leakage from the colotomy wound. There were secondary deposits in the liver, and there was also old and recent tuberculosis in each lung (Male, i. 369.)

In two cases the high operation with excision of the coccyx was performed.

A labourer, aged 57, had been known to be suffering from carcinoma of the rectum in November, 1902. At that time a fixed nodular outgrowth could be felt, three inches from the anus, on the posterior wall of the rectum. On admission a large hard ulcerated mass could be felt on the posterior wall of the rectum. An extensive operation was undertaken, in which the coccyx and the lowest portion of the sacrum had to be removed before the growth could be reached. The patient died seven days later, the wound being in a sloughing condition. No secondary growths were found at the post-mortem examination. (Male, i. 319.)

The other case recovered (Male, iii. 826).

IMPERFORATE ANUS.—Three cases were admitted, one male and two females.

A male infant, 24 hours old, was admitted on account of imperforate anus. In the region of the anus was a dimple; there was no other deformity. An incision was made in the middle line below the coccyx, and the rectum found at a distance of a quarter of an inch from the skin. Patient made a good recovery. (Male, ii. 3560.)

A female infant, 6 weeks old, was admitted with a recto-vaginal fistula. The anus was represented by a small dimple. Other deformities were a cleft palate and a small tubercle in front of the tragus on each ear. A plastic operation was performed, the anus opened posteriorly and the fistula closed. (Female, v. 1521.)

In the third case, the opening of the rectum was in the perineum. No operation was performed. (Female, i. 1240.)

DISEASES OF THE GENITO-URINARY SYSTEM.

Bladder.

URINARY CALCULUS.—Two males and two females were admitted for this complaint.

In one case lithotrity was successfully performed (Male, iii. 568), in the other three supra-pubic cystotomy was performed. (Male, v. 2600, Female, iv. 47, 2025.)

VESICAL CALCULI FOLLOWING HYSTERECTOMY.—A woman, aged 50, on whom, in 1902, abdominal hysterectomy was performed for fibroids. During the operation the bladder, which was very adherent to the uterus, was torn across in the process of separation, and it was subsequently sutured with silk. A few weeks later she began to complain of pain and frequency of micturition, and on the bladder being opened, a vesical calculus was found, having embedded in it a piece of silk. For several months after this the patient remained well, then the bladder symptoms returned, and have remained up to the present time. Supra-pubic cystotomy was again performed, and two large calculi were removed from the bladder, and in the centre of one of them a piece of silk suture was found. No other pieces of silk could be found in the bladder, which was then sutured with catgut. The patient made a good recovery, and was discharged cured. (Female, iv. 47.)

ECTOPION VESICÆ.—Two cases were admitted.

One, a boy, aged 10, was admitted to be measured for an instrument. (Male, i. 3236.)

The other case was in a female, aged 25. The bladder was completely extroverted, and level with the abdominal wall. There was no symphysis pubis, the two halves of the pelvis being separated by about half an inch. No uterus could be felt. An attempt was made to make a bladder by freeing the mucous membrane from the abdominal wall, and turning it over. All the stitches gave way, and patient was in no way improved by the operation. (Female, v. 1775.)

FOREIGN BODY IN BLADDER.—A girl, aged 17, was admitted complaining of symptoms simulating vesical calculus. Cystoscopic examination revealed a hairpin, thickly encrusted with phosphates. The pin was successfully removed by the supra-pubic operation. (Female, i. 870.)

TUBERCULOUS CYSTITIS.—Eight cases, four males and four females, were admitted. No operation was performed in any of them. (Male, i. 983, ii. 2098, v. 2676, 2694 ; Female, i. 178, iii. 251, v. 1026, 1954.)

CARCINOMA OF BLADDER.—Eight cases were admitted ; in three cases an exploration was made by means of a supra-pubic incision. (Male, i. 3134, iii. 1710, iv. 2468.)

One case, in which no operation was performed, died. (Male, ii. 2711.)

PAPILLOMA.—Four cases were successfully treated by excision of the growth, through a supra-pubic incision. (Male, i. 1547, v. 518, 934, 2228.)

Two other cases were admitted, on whom the operation was not performed. (Male, v. 1390, 2081.)

Kidney.

CALCULUS.—Eleven cases, seven males and four females, were admitted.

There were two fatal cases.

A man, aged 41, underwent at this hospital in 1902 an operation for nephritic abscess, a lumbar incision being made and the abscess drained. He was re-admitted in February, 1902, with a sinus in the right side, discharging blood and urine and complaining of pain and tenderness in the right kidney region. The total amount of urine passed per diem was about two pints, and diminishing to one pint a few days before death, which occurred sixteen days after admission. The urine contained albumen, blood and pus. 7 °/₀ of urea was present. The patient rapidly became worse, symptoms of uræmia, vomiting, restlessness and twitching of the limbs coming on a week before death. No operation was performed. Postmortem : The right kidney was found firmly fixed in the loin by old and very dense adhesions. The sinus in the loin communicated with the interior of the kidney, which on section showed extensive fibrosis, especially of the capsule, and embedded in the substance of the kidney was a large irregularly shaped stone. There were many suppurating foci in the medulla and a large abscess cavity in that part of the pelvis which communicated with the sinus in the loin. The left kidney was small, shrunken and fibrotic, and contained a few small calculi and numerous small abscesses and cysts. (Male, v. 344.)

The other fatal case was Female, i. 657.

Nephrectomy was successfully performed in two cases.

A man who had suffered from many attacks of renal colic was submitted to operation. The urine contained a few pus cells and many amorphous phosphates and oxalates ; neither kidney was palpable. Through a lumbar incision the right kidney was exposed and removed with some difficulty, owing to many adhesions. The organ was small and shrunken ; in the upper front of the ureter were lying several small stones. The patient made a satisfactory recovery. (Male, ii. 1377.)

The other case of nephrectomy was Male, iv. 1605.

HYDRO-NEPHROSIS.—Seven cases. Four were successfully treated by nephrectomy. (Male, iii. 3191* ; Female, i. 386, iii. 920, iv. 1271.)

Three were discharged after nephrotomy. (Male, i. 2916 ; Female, i. 1868, iii. 1797.)

MOVABLE KIDNEY. — Thirteen cases were treated successfully by nephrorrhaphy, and in one case the appendix was removed as well. Four were discharged without operation.

PYO-NEPHROSIS.—Of the seven cases admitted for this complaint, three died. (Male, i. 774 ; Female, ii. 507.)

A female, aged 39, was transferred from the Medical side on account of lumbar pain and hæmaturia, which had occurred at intervals since 1899. In the right lumbar region was a large swelling, which extended forwards nearly to the middle line. A lumbar incision was made and a large abscess opened and drained. The following day the patient suddenly collapsed and died. Post-mortem : A large tuberculous pyo-nephrosis was found, the kidney substance being completely disorganised. The ureter was thickened, and there was a small ulceration in the bladder close to the ureteral opening. (Female, iv. 959.)

TUBERCULOUS DISEASE.—A clerk, aged 33, had suffered for twelve months from intermittent hæmaturia and frequency of micturition. The left kidney could be felt enlarged ; the urine contained blood and pus ; no tubercle bacilli were discovered. Abdominal nephrectomy was performed. The kidney was double its normal size and was a mere bag containing caseous material. Patient eventually made a satisfactory recovery. (Male, ii. 3072.)

Another case, diagnosed as tuberculosis of the kidney, was discharged without operation. (Female, i. 1861.)

CARCINOMA.—A man, aged 31, was admitted for pain and swelling in the right loin. In March, 1903, the right kidney had been explored and nothing abnormal found ; microscopically sections of the pelvis revealed no disease. The kidney was again exposed through a lumbar incision, and this time a large growth was found involving the lower part of the kidney and fixed to the intestine and the posterior abdominal wall. The kidney and growth were removed as freely as possible. The patient died five days later, and no post-mortem examination could be obtained. (Male, iii. 2275.)

Penis.

EPITHELIOMA.—Seven cases were admitted during the year. In five cases partial amputation was performed successfully. (Male, ii. 3523, iii. 72, 2036, v. 1127, 2218.)

Two cases were discharged without operation. (Male, i. 2840, iv. 280.)

Prostate.

CALCULI.—A vinegar maker, aged 70, was admitted with cystitis. The prostate was not enlarged, but a sound could be felt to grate on something in the prostatic urethra. An external urethrotomy was performed and several prostatic calculi removed. The wound healed slowly, but eventually the patient made a satisfactory recovery. (Male, v. 593.)

ENLARGED.—Eleven cases were admitted for this disease. Five cases were submitted to the operation of supra-pubic prostatectomy. Of these, four were successful (Male, i. 321, 1215, iii. 2284, 3175), and one died (Male, iv. 2074).

MALIGNANT DISEASE.—Two cases were admitted. A man, aged 66, was admitted with an enormously enlarged and painful prostate. For two years he had had catheters passed, and only three weeks before admission had begun to pass blood. On admission it was found that he could pass urine naturally, but slowly; the urine was alkaline and contained much blood, pus and albumen. Patient gradually passed less and less urine and died comatose. Post-mortem: The whole of the pelvis was occupied by a large hard mass (microscopically, a round-celled sarcoma) apparently originating in the prostate. The bladder was firmly adherent to this mass, and the walls were infiltrated with growth. The ureters were dilated and partially obstructed by the growth. The kidneys showed acute pyelo-nephritis. (Male, iv. 527.)

The other case was Male, iii. 27.

Scrotum.

EPITHELIOMA.—Three cases were admitted. One in a tobacco blender (Male, i. 508), another in a lead worker (Male, iv. 3208), and a third in a barge builder (Male, v. 1615).

Testis.

CARCINOMA.—A packer, aged 36, was transferred from a Medical Ward suffering from abdominal distension and jaundice. An exploratory laparotomy was performed and the liver found studded with nodules of new growth. Post-mortem: The right testis was found to be the seat of a breaking-down malignant growth. There were multiple secondary deposits in the liver, ribs, vertebræ and muscles. In one of the ribs a spontaneous fracture had occurred. (Male, i. 1878.)

SARCOMA.—A boy, aged 2, was admitted with an abdominal tumour rising up out of the pelvis to within two inches of the umbilicus, and it was thought to be a growth of the bladder. The tumour grew rapidly, and patient died much wasted two months after admission. Post-mortem: The abdominal tumour was found to be very much enlarged, secondarily involved malignant glands, the primary growth being a very small one, situated in the right testis. Microscopically it was found to be a round-celled sarcoma. (Male, ii. 3317.)

TERATOMA.—A man, aged 35, had suffered for twelve months from progressive painless enlargement of the testis. The testis was excised, and microscopically proved to be a teratoma. (Male, iv. 255.)

Urethra.

CARCINOMA.—Of the large number of cases admitted for stricture of the urethra, one proved of great interest.

For two years a carpenter, aged 67, had suffered with a stricture and difficulty of micturition, for which catheters had been used. In May of this year he was admitted with acute retention of urine, and subsequently internal urethrotomy was performed and patient apparently recovered. In November he was re-admitted with an impassable stricture 12½ cm. from the meatus. An external urethrotomy was performed and a lobulated hard swelling found at the site of the stricture. A portion was removed for examination, and proved to be a squamous-celled carcinoma. Later a complete amputation of the penis and crura was performed and some enlarged inguinal glands removed. The patient developed cystitis and suppurative pyelo-nephritis and died. Post-mortem : No secondary growths were discovered. (Male, v. 3063.)

Ovary.

CYSTS.—Fifteen cases of ovarian cysts were admitted into the General Wards, and all were submitted to operation. The following are worthy of note :—

For two months a woman, aged 38, had had recurring attacks of abdominal pain, associated with vomiting. On admission she was complaining of much pain in the abdomen, especially in the right iliac region. In the right side of the abdomen, rising out of the pelvis, could be felt a hard, tender swelling. Both temperature and pulse rate were raised. The abdomen was opened and an ovarian cyst found, the walls of which were black and friable ; the fluid in the cyst was the colour of claret ; the pedicle had a complete twist. The cyst was removed, and patient completely recovered. (Female, ii. 1304.)

Since 1903 a woman, aged 52, had noticed gradual enlargement of the abdomen. On one occasion the abdomen had been tapped and fluid drawn off. Menstruation had been regular up to the menopause, which occurred in 1901, and since then there had been no bleeding and no discharge. At the operation a large multilocular cyst was found, closely adherent to an enlarged fibroid uterus. The opposite ovary also contained a small cyst. Supra-vaginal hysterectomy was performed, and removal of both ovaries. Recovery was uninterrupted. (Female, ii. 1502.)

There were three fatal cases :—

A woman, aged 31, was admitted with a large multilocular ovarian cyst, reaching nearly to the ensiform cartilage. In addition there was an irreducible umbilical hernia. The operation for the removal of the cyst was very difficult on account of many dense adhesions, and on attempting to separate the upper part of the cyst from the transverse colon, this organ was cut. The two ends were stitched into the abdominal wall and left for a future operation. Later an unsuccessful attempt was made to close the intestine. Some six weeks after the first operation, patient developed bronchitis and died. No post-mortem was made. (Female, iii. 2446*.)

The two other fatal cases both proved to be malignant carcinoma, and died with secondary deposits in the omentum and peritoneum. (Female, iii. 1670, v. 2998*.)

CARCINOMA.—A woman, aged 39, was admitted with an abdominal swelling, which had been noticed twenty-one months. The abdomen was distended with fluid and a hard mass could be felt in the pelvis. The case was diagnosed as one of malignant disease and no operation was advised. A few days after admission she developed left hemiplegia, and died four weeks later. Post-mortem : Both ovaries were found to be malignant, and there were secondary deposits in the liver. In the left side and lower part of the pons was a small discoloured and softened area. The left femoral vein was thrombosed. (Female, ii. 2555.)

PYO-SALPINX.—Six cases were admitted to the General Wards with this complaint. One recovered after laparotomy (Female, iv. 2072), and four died after laparotomy (Female, ii. 1721, 2131, iii. 381, 1794), and one was discharged without operation (Female, ii. 1373).

RUPTURED EXTRA-UTERINE GESTATION.—Three cases were admitted, and were submitted to operation. Two recovered (Female, i. 1971, v. 1319), and one died (Female, iii. 382).

Uterus.

UTERINE FIBROID.—Six cases were admitted. In four abdominal hysterectomy was successfully performed. In one case (Female, ii. 1784) a subperitoneal fibroid was successfully enucleated. One woman died as the result of peritonitis after abdominal hysterectomy (Female, i. 547).

CARCINOMA OF UTERUS.—In one case abdominal hysterectomy was successfully performed for carcinoma of the cervix uteri. (Female, v. 792.)

Breast.

HYPERTROPHY.—A domestic servant, aged 21, stated that her left breast had been getting steadily larger since the age of fourteen. The left breast was flaccid, uniformly enlarged, and about three times the size of the right breast. The breast was a little tender, but the patient chiefly complained of the weight. She was given a bag to support the breast, and advised to return if this did not relieve the pain. (Female, ii. 2724.)

CHRONIC MASTITIS.—Out of the twelve cases admitted, three were discharged without operation ; seven were successfully treated by local removal of the affected breast, and in two cases the whole breast with the axillary glands were removed (Female, i. 1603, iii. 1583).

TUBERCULOUS DISEASE.—This disease was met with in six cases. Two were cases of chronic abscess of the breast (Female, i. 1470, v. 757).

A housewife, aged 41, had noticed a swelling in the right breast for nine months. On admission the breast was red, hot and swollen. The nipple was retracted. Two small abscesses could be felt in the breast and some induration around them, but no definite tumour. The axillary glands were slightly enlarged ; beyond this nothing abnormal was found. The diagnosis lay between carcinoma and tuberculous disease. After a few days abscesses burst, discharging pus. A local amputation of the breast was undertaken, and the patient made a good recovery. Microscopic examination of the breast proved it to be a case of tuberculous disease. (Female, v. 126.)

Three other cases were treated by local amputation of the breast, and all recovered. (Female, ii. 1038, iv. 586, 1960.)

CALCIFYING FIBRO-ADENOMA.—Of the twenty cases admitted for fibro-adenoma of the breast, one is of special interest.

A woman, aged 60, had noticed for many years a swelling in the breast under the nipple. The tumour was densely hard and freely movable, and shelled out easily. It was stone-like in consistency, and after decalcification showed on section the structure of a fibro-adenoma. (Female, ii. 2611.)

CARCINOMA.—Eighty-six cases of carcinoma were admitted during the year.

One case occurred in a male, a spinner, aged 72. He had noticed a swelling in the left breast for two months. In the breast could be felt a hard swelling, which was adherent to the pectoralis major muscle ; no enlarged glands could be felt. The complete breast operation was performed. (Male, iii. 1312.)

Three cases of columnar-celled carcinoma were met with. (Female, ii. 1296, 1498, 2316.)

In one case of recurrent carcinoma, injections of sodium cinnamate were tried, but without affording any relief. (Female, v. 19.)

There were three fatal cases.

One died with multiple secondary deposits, without any operation having been performed. (Female, i. 2595.)

One woman, aged 62, died after a local excision of the growth. Post-mortem: Many secondary deposits were found. (Female, i. 1703.)

A woman, aged 74, was admitted with an atrophic scirrhus of the breast and enormous distension of the abdomen, causing dyspnœa. The swelling simulated ovarian cyst, but on opening the abdomen multiple miliary secondary deposits were found on the peritoneum, and much ascites. The patient died directly after. (Female, iii. 1178.)

Nipple.

EPITHELIOMA.—One case of epithelioma of the nipple was met with. and was successfully treated by excision. (Female, iv. 935.)

DISEASES OF THE ORGANS OF LOCOMOTION.

Bones.

EXOSTOSIS.—Two cases of exostosis of the scapula were admitted. Both proved to be cancellous in nature, and both were successfully removed by local excision. (Male, iii. 2700, iv. 2520.)

MULTIPLE EXOSTOSES.— A boy, aged 16, was admitted complaining of pain and swelling of the right leg. On examination he was found to have a large number of exostoses, which had been present since early childhood. The exostoses were growing chiefly from the bones of the limbs, but these were not limited to the extremities of the bones. Patient stated that his father, three brothers and two sisters had similar exostoses. No operation was performed. (Male, iv. 3371.)

SARCOMA OF THE FEMUR AND SPONTANEOUS FRACTURE.—The patient a man, aged 55, while crossing the road, slipped and, without any actual injury to the leg itself, sustained a simple fracture of the right femur, On admission a fracture was found in the lower third of the femur, and as there was considerable swelling around and in the joint, it was suspected that the fracture had involved the knee-joint. On the assumption that the fracture was of the ordinary character it was put up in the usual way. It was found, however, that the bones did not unite, and the swelling about the lower end of the femur, instead of diminishing, rather increased, and the temperature was at times irregular. Some fourteen weeks after admission, fluid was withdrawn from the swelling with an exploring needle, which proved to be pure blood. Bacteriological examination proved it to be sterile. A skiagram showed the two ends of the bone ununited, lying in a slightly opaque substance. A suspicion was now entertained that the case might be one of sarcoma, either following as a result of the accident, or possibly preceding it. The case was shown at consultations, and the general opinion expressed was that an amputation should be performed. Sixteen weeks after admission the femur was amputated at the junction of the upper and middle thirds. On examination of the leg, a large malignant growth, probably periosteal in origin, was found involving the lower third of the femur, and the two united ends of the bone were completely surrounded by the growth. No attempt at repair had occurred, and it was evident that the growth must have existed prior to the accident, and that fracture had occurred at the point where the bone was weakened by the infiltration of the new growth, as a result of a very slight injury. Microscopical examination showed the growth to be a spindle-celled sarcoma. The patient made an excellent recovery. (Male, ii. 1681.)

Joints.

INTERMITTENT HYDROPS ARTICULI.—A married woman, aged 23, gave a history of intermittent swelling of the left knee every fourteen days. The condition had lasted thirteen months, and no cause for the onset was known. The patient was a delicate looking woman with much oral sepsis and a purulent discharge from the right ear. The patient was carefully watched in bed for a long period, and it was found that on every fifteenth day the left knee-joint commenced to swell ; the attack lasted five days, attaining its maximum on the second day. One attack would correspond with the menstrual period, and the alternate one midway between the two periods. During the attack the affected joint would become distended with fluid and slightly hotter than the other side, and caused the patient some dull pain. Nothing else abnormal could be discovered about the joint. During one attack some fluid was aspirated from the joint and cultivations for organisms made ; none were discovered. The blood count did not alter during the occurrence of an attack. Patient was discharged *in statu quo*. (Female, ii. 1214.)

DISEASES OF BURSÆ, FASCIÆ, TENDONS AND MUSCLES.

Fasciæ.

CALCIFICATION OF FIBROUS TISSUE OF THE LEG.—A labourer, aged 42, had noticed two weeks previous to admission a swelling in his leg "like a bit of stick," his attention having been called to it by the sensation of pain. He gave an indefinite history of injury to the part. In the peroneal region of the left leg was a hard mass about four inches long and the thickness of an ordinary cedar pencil. The skiagram revealed a shadow in the situation of the mass. An incision was made over it and the swelling excised. It was situated in the superficial fascia of the leg, and was not connected with the peroneal tendons as was first supposed. Microscopical examination after decalcification showed fibrous tissue only. (Male, iv. 857.)

AFFECTIONS OF THE NECK.

Hydatid Cyst of the Neck causing Dyspnœa.

A schoolboy, aged 12, noticed two years ago a small swelling in the right side of the neck. It never caused him any inconvenience until six months ago, when he first experienced difficulty in breathing. On admission to the Ward he was found to have a large elastic swelling in the region of the thyroid. His dyspnœa was extreme and his respiration even stopped. Operation for tracheotomy was commenced, but on making the incision a quantity of clear yellowish fluid was evacuated from the cyst, and after a short period of artificial respiration, normal breathing was re-established. A few days later the swelling began to refill, and the dyspnœa was again urgent. An operation was then undertaken to remove the cyst, which proved to be a hydatid cyst about the size of an orange. After the removal all the symptoms disappeared. The patient had an uneventful recovery. (Male, iv. 408.)

AFFECTIONS OF THE TRUNK.

Retro-peritoneal Fibro-Myoma.

A gardener, aged 44, was admitted complaining of abdominal pain and constipation. There was some resistance and some tenderness above the pubes, but nothing else abnormal found in the abdomen. Laparotomy was performed, and a large hard growth found in the posterior part of the abdomen. The operation was difficult, and before the tumour, which seemed to be connected with the retro-peritoneal tissue, could be removed, a loop of the small intestine had to be cut through and was afterwards united by means of a Murphy's button. The growth microscopically proved to be a pure leio-myoma. The patient died two days later from peritonitis. (Male, i. 189.)

A woman, aged 45, was admitted with a large swelling in the iliac region, for which she had worn a truss without relief. At the operation a small, reducible inguinal hernia was discovered, and growing from the sub-peritoneal tissue was a large tumour ten inches in diameter. Microscopically this proved to be a leio-myoma. The patient made a good recovery. (Female, i. 1534.)

Sacro-coccygeal Tumour.

A girl, aged 8½, was admitted with a swelling in the ano-coccygeal region which had existed since birth and had increased proportionately with the growth of the child. On admission this tumour was four inches by six inches in diameter. It lay at the back of the rectum, which was pressed forward under the pubic arch. The bladder was pushed up into the abdominal cavity. An extensive operation was undertaken for its removal. A transverse incision was made between the tubera ischii and the tumour was dissected out from the rectum in the front, part of the sacrum having been resected. In this way the whole tumour was successively removed, and though the wound suppurated for some time the patient was eventually discharged cured. (Female, v. 2189.)

INJURIES OF THE UPPER EXTREMITY.

Dislocation of Shoulder.

A boy, aged 15, was admitted with a sub-clavicular dislocation of the right shoulder which had occurred in 1899. There was much wasting of the deltoid and pectoralis major muscles. A skiagram revealed the fact that the head and shaft of the humerus were thinner than on the opposite side, and that the outline of the head was irregular. An incision was made through the deltoid muscle and the head of the humerus resected. The subsequent course of the case was not very satisfactory in spite of massage, passive movements, and frequent wrenchings. When the patient left the hospital there was very little movement of the arm independent of the scapulæ. (Male. v. 872.)

One other case was admitted, but patient refused operation. (Male, iv. 894.)

INJURIES OF THE LOWER EXTREMITY.

Dislocation of Hip.

Four cases, all males, were admitted.

A carman, aged 40, was knocked down by a horse, which fell on him. Patient fell on his back with his leg flexed on his abdomen, the weight of the horse coming on the flexed leg. On admission the head of the left femur was found dislocated on to the dorsum ilii. The dislocation was easily reduced under an anæsthetic. (Male, iii. 461.)

A boy, aged 15, while getting out of a van, fell, striking the ground on his left foot, with the thigh abducted. Dislocation of the dorsum ilii occurred. The dislocation was easily reduced under an anæsthetic. (Male, i. 575.)

A schoolboy, aged 9, was run over by a cart, the wheel passing over his thigh. On examination no fracture was discovered, but a dislocation into the obturator foramen. The head was successfully replaced, by manipulation, under an anæsthetic. (Male, ii. 49.)

A boy, aged 10, slipped on a piece of banana peel and fell with his leg doubled under him. In this case a pubic dislocation had occurred, and was easily reducible. (Male, iii. 2585A.)

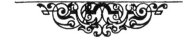

SUB-TABLE, SHOWING THE NUMBER OF CASES OF ERYSIPELAS, PYÆMIA, &c., IN THE SURGICAL WARDS.

DISEASES.	Under 5 M	Under 5 F	5—10 M	5—10 F	10—20 M	10—20 F	20—30 M	20—30 F	30—40 M	30—40 F	40—50 M	40—50 F	50—60 M	50—60 F	60—70 M	60—70 F	70—80 M	70—80 F	TOTAL M	TOTAL F	Deaths M	Deaths F
CUTANEOUS ERYSIPELAS—																						
Admissions	...	4	1	3	2	4	4	7	1	...	4	1	1	...	1	...	...	...	14	19	1	...
Occurring in Hospital	...	...	...	...	...	...	...	...	...	...	1	...	...	...	...	...	...	...	1	...	1	...
Occurring after operation	...	...	1	...	...	...	1	...	1	...	...	...	1	...	...	...	...	...	4	...	...	...
CELLULITIS—																						
Admissions	4	2	4	...	8	6	17	7	13	2	9	4	5	1	2	7	...	...	62	29	2	1
PYÆMIA AND SEPTICÆMIA—																						
Admissions	2	1	1	...	1	2	...	...	...	...	...	...	...	...	1	...	...	...	5	4	5	3
Occurring in Hospital	...	...	...	...	...	...	...	...	...	...	...	...	...	...	...	...	...	...	...	...	1	...
Occurring after operation	1	...	...	...	...	...	...	...	1	...	...	...	...	...	...	...	...	...	1	...	...	...
DELIRIUM TREMENS—																						
Admissions	...	...	...	...	...	...	...	...	...	...	...	...	...	...	...	...	...	...	...	...	...	...
Occurring in Hospital	...	...	...	...	...	...	...	...	...	...	...	...	...	...	1	...	...	...	1	...	...	...
Occurring after operation	...	...	...	...	...	...	...	...	...	...	...	...	...	...	...	...	...	...	...	...	...	...

APPENDIX TO SUB-TABLE OF ERYSIPELAS, PYÆMIA, &c.

ERYSIPELAS.—Cutaneous.

Two patients admitted with this disease died. One was a man, aged 65, who was admitted with erysipelas of the face and signs of septicæmia. He died three days after admission, and no post-mortem was performed (Male, i. 3016).

PYÆMIA AND SEPTICÆMIA.

Five men and four women were admitted with symptoms of this condition, or the symptoms developed shortly after admission. All died except one child (Female, iv. 2275*).

Of the other cases three were associated with suppurative otitis media (Male, ii. 1702, iv. 3408 ; Female, ii. 2397).

One with cellulitis of the leg (Male, iii. 829), one with necrosis of the jaw (Female, iv. 1728), one with periostitis of the femur (Female, iv. 2763), one with multiple septic arthritis (Male, v. 3337), and one with erysipelas of the face.

Occurring after Operation.

One small boy, aged 15 months, died with cellulitis of the scrotum and septicæmia after a circumcision which had been performed three weeks previously in the Surgery. (Male, iii. 2054.)

General Statistics of Cases of Appendicitis and their Complications during a period of ten years. Years 1894—1903 (inclusive).

Year.	Total No. of cases.	Total No. of operations.	Total No. of deaths after operation.	Total No. of deaths without operation.	Operative mortality.	General peritonitis.	Subphrenic abscess.	Empyema.	Pyæmia and multiple abscesses.	Fæcal fistula.	Thrombosis of veins.	Liver abscess.	Bronchitis and pneumonia.	Strangulation of intestine.
1894	41	10	7	0	70 %	5	...	...	...	...	...	...	...	...
1895	38	12	8	2	25 %	2	...	...	...	3	...	...	1	...
1896	81	45	14	2	31·1 %	12	...	...	...	2	1	...	1	1
1897	85	40	10	3	25 %	7	1	...	...	2	...	...	...	...
1898	97	60	9	1	15 %	8	1	...	2	3	...	...	...	...
1899	122	80	16	2	20 %	10	2	...	...	2	...	...	...	...
1900	120	89	12	0	13·4 %	13	...	...	...	4	...	...	...	1
1901	166	123	25	0	20·03 %	20	1	2	...	4	1	1	2	...
1902	205	171	19	1	11·1 %	19	2	...	3	4	...	...	1	...
1903	215	165	21	1	16·3 %	19	1	1	1	6	2	...	...	1

Complications occurring in Cases of Appendicitis recovering after Operation (in the same period of ten years).

Year	Total No. of operations	Total No. of recoveries	General peritonitis	Subphrenic abscess	Empyema	Localised peritonitis or residual abscess	Faecal fistula	Thrombos-s of veins	Sinus on discharge from hospital	Ventral hernia	Bronchitis and pneumonia	Parotitis
1894	10	3	...	...	...	...	...	...	...	...	...	...
1895	12	9	...	...	...	...	2	...	...	...	...	...
1896	45	31	1	...	...	...	1	1	1	...	1	...
1897	40	30	1	...	...	...	1	...	...	...	...	...
1898	60	51	1	...	...	1	2	...	4	1	...	...
1899	80	64	...	...	...	...	2	...	1	1	1	...
1900	89	77	1	1	1	1	2	...	1	...	1	...
1901	123	98	2	...	...	...	2	1	5	...	2	1
1902	171	152	2	...	...	4	4	1	6	5	1	...
1903	165	144	1	...	1	...	5	2	2	...	...	...

INDEX

to Register of Post-mortem Examinations.

SURGICAL, 1904.

BY THE SURGICAL REGISTRAR.

⸺ ⸺ ⸺

NUMBER OF SURGICAL POST-MORTEM EXAMINATIONS MADE
DURING THE YEAR—205.

(The figures refer to the pages of the Surgical Post-mortem Register kept in the Library.)

ABSCESS—
    Breast—203.
    Cerebrum—163.
    Cerebellar—48, 117.
    Lung—132.
    Psoas—151.
    Perimetric—166.
    Retro-pharyngeal—124.
    Subdiaphragmatic—1, 45, 64, 196.

ACTINOMYCOSIS—115.

AMPUTATIONS, Thigh—168.

AMYLOID DISEASE—124, 193.

ANEURYSM—
    Abdominal Aorta—94.
    Thoracic Aorta—112, 129.

ANTHRAX—134.

AORTA, Aneurysm—94, 112, 129.

APPENDICITIS—*See* Vermiform Appendix.

ARTERY, Aorta, Atheroma—90, 105.
    Laceration—49, 142.

ARTHRITIS, Suppurative—51, 199, 203.

ASCITES—30, 100, 114, 149, 197.

BLADDER—
    Carcinoma—172.
    Inflammation—9, 60, 63, 96, 172, 95.
    Papilloma—211.

BRAIN—
    Absoess—48, 117, 163.
    Hæmorrhage—32.
    Laceration—71, 97, 142, 156.
    Softening—213.

BREAST, Carcinoma—100, 149.

BRONCHI, Bronchitis—14, 57.

BURNS AND SCALDS—43.

CALCULI—
    Biliary—23, 76, 201.
    Renal—42.

CARCINOMA—
    Bladder—172.
    Breast—100, 149.
    Colon—26, 82, 84, 127, 138.
    Gall Bladder—123.
    Kidney—19, 198.
    Larynx—83.
    Liver—27, 35, 122, 198, 213.
    Lung—27, 198.
    Lymphatic Glands—17, 19.
    Œsophagus—5, 27, 40, 56, 129, 132, 182, 189, 198.
    Ovary—16, 58, 114, 139, 213.
    Peritoneum—31, 114.
    Pleura—114.
    Pylorus—10, 159, 175, 180.
    Rectum—35, 36, 137.
    Rib—122, 149.
    Sigmoid Flexure—92, 185.
    Spleen—198.
    Stomach—31, 59, 121, 126, 129.
    Testis—122.
    Tongue—17, 19, 116, 154.
    Urethra—215.

CELLULITIS—
    Arm—57, 187.
    Hand—72, 194.
    Leg—62.
    Scrotum—135, 215.

CIRRHOSIS, Liver—149.

COLON, Carcinoma—26, 82, 84, 127, 138.

CRANIOTABES—13.

CYSTITIS—See Bladder.

DUODENUM—
    Rupture—169.
    Stricture—41.
    Ulcer (Perforated)—4, 125, 131, 177, 208.

EAR, Inflammation of Middle—47, 48, 52, 111, 117, 143, 157, 191, 192, 200.

EMPHYSEMA—See Lung.

EMPYEMA, Pleura—45, 72, 74, 89, 111.

ENDOCARDITIS—192, 206.

EXTRAVASATION OF URINE—9, 63, 211.

FALLOPIAN TUBES—*See* Uterine Appendages.

FEMUR—
    Fracture—11, 73.
    Periostitis—206.

FIBULA, Fracture—136, 167.

FISTULA—
    Intestinal—37.
    Tracheo-œsophageal—5, 179.

FRACTURE—
    Femur—11, 73.
    Fibula—136, 167.
    Humerus—136.
    Jaw—73, 141.
    Patella—156.
    Pelvis—8, 49, 61, 68, 167.
    Radius and Ulna—7, 73.
    Rib—7, 14, 44, 70, 71, 136, 167, 179.
    Skull (Base)—97, 136, 141, 142, 145, 156, 167, 204.
       „ (Vault)—71, 142, 145.
    Spine—71.
    Sternum—179.
    Tibia and Fibula—136, 167.

GALL BLADDER—
    Carcinoma—123.
    Cholecystitis—41.
    Sarcoma—79.

GALL-STONES—*See* Calculi.

GANGRENE, Foot—23.

GASTRIC ULCER—38, 45, 54, 171, 212.
    Perforated—1, 77, 80, 99, 155.

HÆMOPHILIA—2.

HÆMORRHAGE—
    Into Brain—32.
    Into Peritoneal Cavity—7, 21, 44, 98, 120, 165, 207.
    Intracranial—97, 145, 204.

HÆMO-THORAX—*See* Pleura.

HARE LIP—22.

HEART—
    Dilatation—90, 103, 197.
    Endocarditis—192, 206.
    Morbus Cordis—11, 40, 57.

HERNIA—
    Strangulated—6, 18, 103, 205.
    Umbilical—173.

HIP, Tuberculous Disease—3, 193.

HUMERUS, Fracture—136.

HYDROCEPHALUS—78.

HYDRO-NEPHROSIS—*See* Kidney.

HYDRO-SALPINX—*See* Uterine Appendages.

ILEUM—*See* Intestine.
INTESTINE—
    Laceration—8, 50, 68, 120, 169.
    Obstruction—16, 26, 106, 118, 127, 137, 138, 144, 181, 183, 214.
    Sarcoma—75.
    Tubercle—3.
    Ulcer (Perforating, Typhoid)—12, 91, 209.
    Ulceration—158.
INTUSSUSCEPTION—34, 55, 88, 161.

JAW—
    Fracture—73, 141.
    Necrosis—160.

KIDNEY—
    Calculi—*See* Calculi.
    Carcinoma—19, 198.
    Nephritis, Acute—110.
        Chronic Interstitial—11, 14, 23, 70, 105, 201.
    Pyelo-nephritis—42, 60, 66, 170, 172, 195.
    Pyo-nephrosis—66, 96.
    Rupture—44, 70, 96.

LARYNX, Carcinoma—83.
LATERAL SINUS, Thrombosis—47, 52.
LIVER—
    Abscess—107 165.
    Carcinoma—27, 35, 198, 213.
    Cirrhosis—149, 173.
    Hydatid Cyst—74, 153.
    Pylephlebitis—15.
    Rupture—21. 44, 70, 98, 120, 207.
    Sarcoma—147.
LUNG—
    Abscess—132.
    Bronchitis—14, 57.
    Carcinoma—27, 198.
    Congestion—5, 18.
    Emphysema—11, 100, 195.
    Infarcts—66, 111. 117, 199, 206.
    Laceration—44, 167.
    Œdema—54, 103.
    Pneumonia—61, 83, 89, 142, 143, 154, 179, 182, 189, 195, 196.
    Sarcoma—176.
    Tubercle—3, 35.
LYMPHATIC GLANDS—
    Carcinoma—17, 19.
    Sarcoma—86, 147.

MARASMUS—22.
MEDIASTINUM, Suppuration—179.
MENINGITIS—
    Cerebral—13.
    Purulent—24, 52, 78, 95, 157, 191.
    Tuberculous—133, 163.

NECROSIS—160.

NEPHRITIS—*See* Kidney.

ŒDEMA, Glottis—134.

ŒSOPHAGUS, Carcinoma—5, 27, 40, 56, 129, 132, 182, 189, 198.

OTITIS MEDIA—*See* Ear.

OVARY, Carcinoma—46, 58, 114, 139, 213.

PALATE, Cleft—22.

PANCREAS—
    Suppuration—108.
    Chronic Pancreatitis—201.

PARALYSIS—210.

PATELLA, Fracture—156.

PELVIS—
    Fracture—8, 49, 61, 68, 167.
    Sarcoma—147.

PERICARDIUM—
    Adherent—53.
    Inflammation—89, 110, 174, 206.

PERIOSTITIS—174, 206.

PERITONEUM—
    Carcinoma—31, 100, 114, 139.
    Hæmorrhage into—7, 21, 44, 120.
    Inflammation—4, 6, 12, 15, 20, 29, 33, 34, 35, 39, 45, 50, 55, 59, 65, 69, 77, 80, 81,
        82, 91, 99, 102, 104, 106, 107, 113, 119, 125, 127, 128, 131, 140, 152, 155, 158,
        162, 164, 169, 170, 177, 178, 184, 185, 186, 190, 202, 205, 208, 209, 214.
    Tuberculous—37, 53, 101.

PHTHISIS—*See* Lung.

PLEURA—
    Carcinoma—114.
    Effusion—27, 61, 62, 114.
    Empyema—45, 72, 74, 89, 111.
    Hæmo-thorax—70, 112, 136.
    Sarcoma—176.

PLEURISY—*See* Pleura.

PNEUMONIA—*See* Lung.

PROSTATE—
    Enlarged—195.
    Sarcoma—60.

PYÆMIA AND SEPTICÆMIA—25, 51, 62, 72, 134, 135, 146, 160, 192, 194, 199, 200, 203,
    206.

PYELO-NEPHRITIS—*See* Kidney.

PYLEPHLEBITIS—15.

PYLORUS—
    Stenosis—54, 114.
    Carcinoma—10, 159, 175, 180.

PYO-NEPHROSIS—*See* Kidney.

PYO-SALPINX—*See* Uterine Appendages.

RADIUS, Fracture—7, 73.

RECTUM, Carcinoma—35, 36, 137.

RIB—
 Carcinoma—149, 189.
 Fracture—7, 14, 44, 70, 71, 136, 167, 179.

RICKETS—53.

SARCOMA—
 Gall Bladder—79.
 Intestine—75.
 Liver—147.
 Lung—176.
 Pelvis—147.
 Pleura—176.
 Prostate—60.
 Thyroid Gland—176.

SCALDS—See Burns.

SEPTICÆMIA—See Pyæmia.

SIGMOID FLEXURE, Carcinoma—92, 185.

SKULL, Fracture—71, 97, 136, 141, 142, 145, 156, 167, 204.

SPINA BIFIDA—13, 24, 78, 95.

SPINE—
 Fracture—71.
 Caries of—124, 151, 210.

SPLEEN—
 Carcinoma—198.
 Laceration—7, 44, 70.

STERNUM, Fracture—179.

STOMACH—
 Adhesions—33, 38, 105.
 Carcinoma—31, 59, 121, 126, 129.
 Dilatation—10, 90, 114, 159.

TESTIS—
 Sarcoma—86.
 Carcinoma—122.

THROMBOSIS OF VEINS—23, 166.

THYROID—176.

TIBIA, Fracture—186, 167.

TONGUE, Carcinoma—17, 19, 116, 154.

TUBERCLE—
 Glands—3.
 Hip—3, 193.
 Intestine—3.
 Kidney—96.
 Lungs—3, 35.
 Peritonitis—37, 53, 101.
 Spine—124, 151, 210.
 Meningitis—153, 163.

ULCER, Typhoid—12, 91, 209.

ULNA, Fracture—7, 73.

URETHRA—
    Carcinoma—215.
    Stricture—9, 63.
    Laceration—61.

URINE, Extravasation—9, 63, 211.

UTERINE APPENDAGES, Pyo-salpinx—39, 144, 152, 170.

UTERUS, Fibroid—69.

VERMIFORM APPENDIX—
    Gangrene—104, 119, 162, 184.
    Inflammation—16, 64, 65, 81, 102, 118, 128, 183, 186, 190, 196, 202.

WOUNDS—
    Neck—93.
    Throat—85.

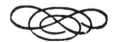

Lightning Source UK Ltd.
Milton Keynes UK
UKHW020623120219
337137UK00005B/551/P